Life & Health

Targeting Wellness

Acknowledgments

We gratefully acknowledge the expert advice and assistance of the following people, who by their careful reading and suggestions have helped to guide work on this book at various stages during its development:

Dale Anderson	California State University—Long Beach
Barbara Beier	University of New Mexico
John Bonaguro	University of Ohio—Athens
Jerry Braza	Stress Management Resources
William Chen	University of Florida
Jacqueline Corn	Johns Hopkins University
Peter Cortese	California State University—Long Beach
Darrell Crase	Memphis State University
John Curtis	University of Wisconsin—La Crosse
Richard Detert	University of Wisconsin—La Crosse
Steve Dorman	University of Florida
Mal Goldsmith	Southern Illinois University—Edwardsville
Frederick Goldstein	Drug Interaction Services Corporation
Renee Guitierrez	Mayo Clinic
Marsha Hoagland	Modesto Junior College
Herbert Jones	Ball State University
David Lowing	Slippery Rock University
David Macrina	University of Alabama at Birmingham
Katherine Martin	North Carolina Baptist Hospital
Warren McNab	University of Nevada at Las Vegas
Jill Moore	University of North Carolina—Chapel Hill
Leslie Oganowski	University of Wisconsin—La Crosse
Woody Powell	Essex Community College
Martha Prince	Springfield College
Ruth Reese	Arizona State University
Donna Richards	Mountain View College
Judie Stepner	DeAnza College
Victor Strecher	University of North Carolina
Lucy Stroble	University of Maine—Presque Isle
Laurette Taylor	University of Oklahoma
Bill Wallace	University of Tennessee—Knoxville
David Weissman	Medical College of Wisconsin
Lawrence Wilson	L. D. Wilson Consultants, Inc.
Richard Wilson	Western Kentucky University
Mike Young	University of Arkansas—Fayetteville

Life & Health

Targeting Wellness

Marvin R. Levy
Temple University

Mark Dignan
Bowman Gray School of Medicine, Wake Forest University

Janet H. Shirreffs
Arizona State University, West Campus

McGraw-Hill, Inc.

*New York   St. Louis   San Francisco   Auckland   Bogotá
Caracas   Lisbon   London   Madrid   Mexico   Milan
Montreal   New Delhi   Paris   San Juan   Singapore
Sydney   Tokyo   Toronto*

LIFE & HEALTH: Targeting Wellness

5 6 7 8 9 0   VNH   VNH   9 0 9 8 7 6

ISBN 0-07-037494-5

This book was set in Palatino by York Graphic Services, Inc. The publisher was Barry Ross Fetterolf, the editors were Charles C. Roebuck and Bob Waterhouse, and the development staff included Carol Ciaston, Cheryl Morrison, Carol Klitzner, Mike Buchman, Lorraine Steefel, Cindy Mooney, Isabelle Tourneau, and Elaine Silverstein. The production supervisor was Anita Crandall. Drawings were done by Vantage Art, Inc., anatomical art by Paul Gioni, and photo research by Cindy Cappa. Text design was by Howard Petlack, cover design by Max Crandall. Von Hoffman Press, Inc., was printer and binder.

Developed and produced by Visual Education Corporation, Princeton, New Jersey.

Library of Congress Catalog Card Number: 91-60807.

Photo Credits

Cover Photo

David Madison

Chapter Opening Photos

2 F. Stuart Westmorland/Tom Stack & Associates; **28** Charles Harbutt/Archive; **54** Timothy Eagan/Woodfin Camp & Associates, Inc.; **84** Chris Brown/Stock, Boston; **110** Leonard Speier; **138** Mark Bolster/International Stock; **168** Matthew Naythons/Stock, Boston; **196** Ellis Herwig/ The Picture Cube; **224** George Malave/Stock, Boston; **256** James J. Broderick/International Stock; **286** Bill Pierce/Rainbow; **312** Martin M. Rotker/Taurus Photos; **336** Tom Dunham; **370** Tom Dunham; **388** Tom Dunham; **406** Grapes-Michaud/Photo Researchers, Inc.; **434** Burk Uzzle/Woodfin Camp & Associates, Inc.; **458** Ben Michalski/Taurus Photos; **482** Leonard Speier; **508** Frank Siteman/The Picture Cube

Table of Contents Photos

v Bill Aron/PhotoEdit; **vi, top** Eunice Harris/Photo Researchers, Inc.; **vi, bottom** Birgit Pohl; **vii, top** Tom Dunham; **vii, bottom** Tom Dunham; **viii, top** Richard Hutchings/ InfoEdit; **viii, bottom** Alexander Tsiaras/Science Source/Photo Researchers, Inc.; **ix, top** Joseph Nettis/Photo Researchers, Inc.; **ix, bottom** Tony Freeman/PhotoEdit; **x, top** Doug Plummer/Photo Researchers, Inc.; **x, bottom** Arthur Sirdofsky/The Stock Shop; **xi, top** Robert Brenner/ PhotoEdit); **xi, bottom** Courtesy American Cancer Society; **xii, top** Tony Freeman/PhotoEdit; **xii, bottom** Tony Freeman/PhotoEdit; **xiii, top** Owen Franken/Sygma; **xiii, bottom** Tom Dunham; **xiv, top** Porterfield-Chickering/Photo Researchers, Inc.

Contents

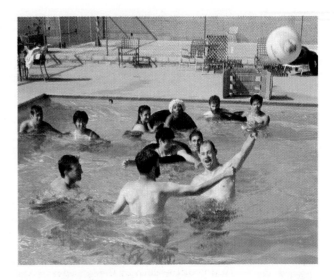

4. Activity, Exercise, and Physical Fitness 84

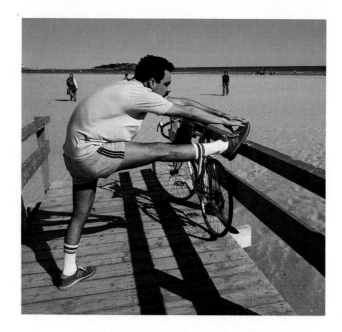

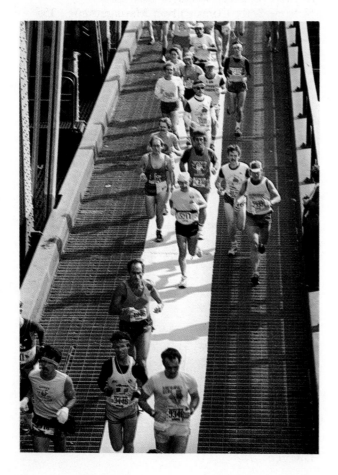

5. Diet and Nutrition 110

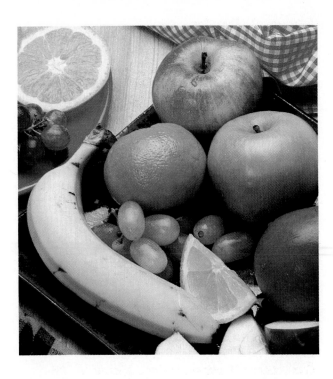

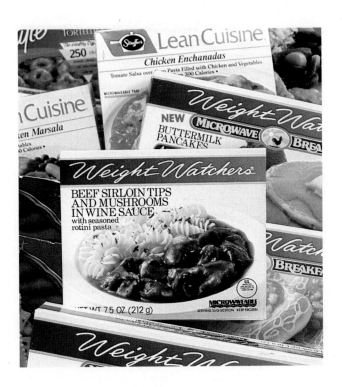

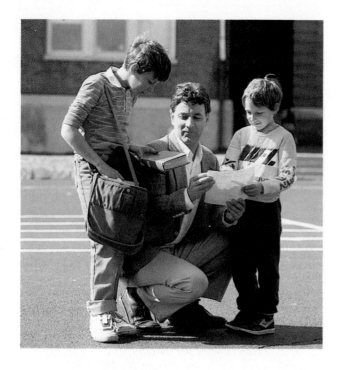

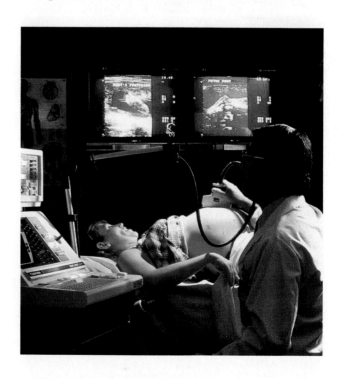

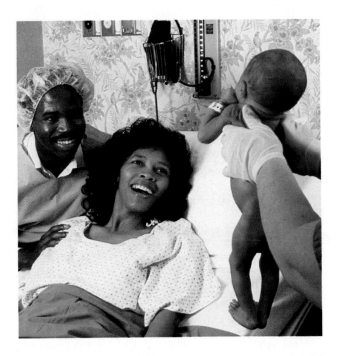

Part Four. Meeting Challenges: Health and Illness   255

10. Communicable Diseases   256

11. Cardiovascular Health and Disease   286

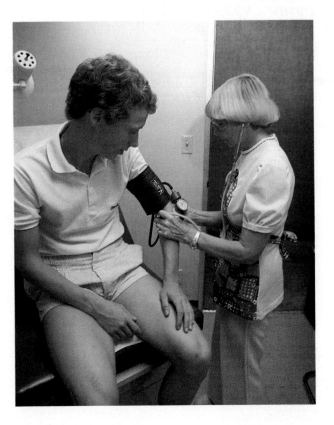

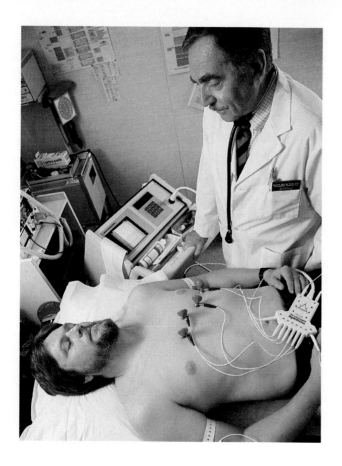

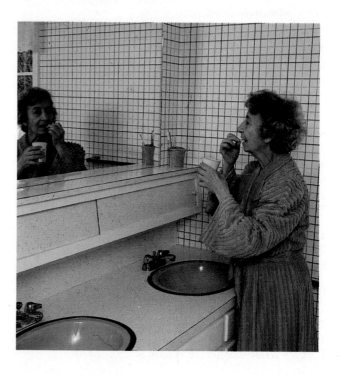

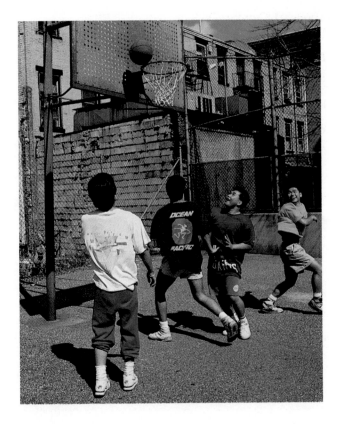

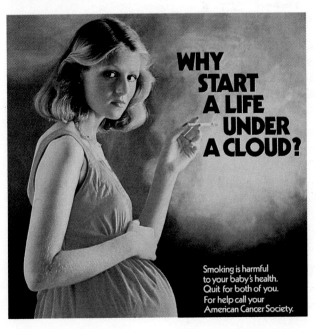

WHY START A LIFE UNDER A CLOUD?

Smoking is harmful
to your baby's health.
Quit for both of you.
For help call your
American Cancer Society.

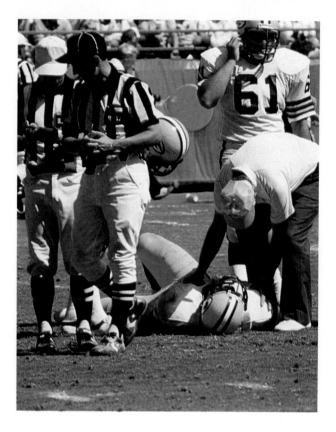

*Part Six. Caring for Others:
Health, Life Span, and
Society* 433

17. Lifestyle and Growing Older 434

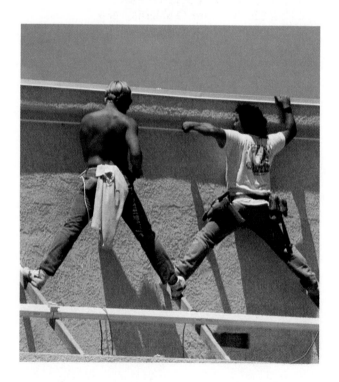

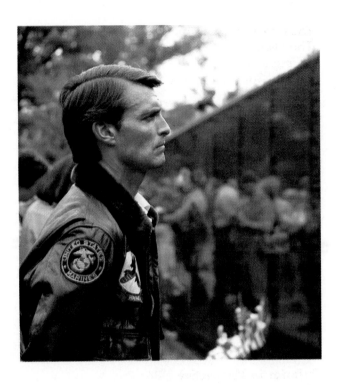

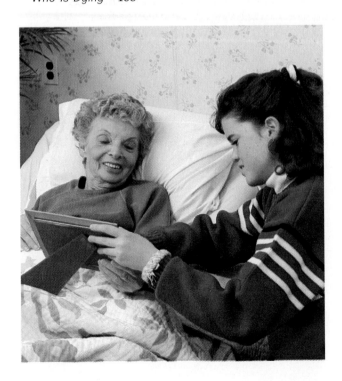

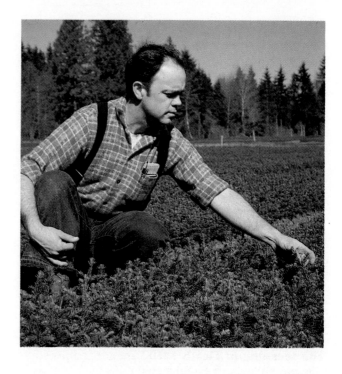

To The Student

Among all the subjects that you will study in college, health can be one of the most relevant to your life, one of the most interesting, and one of the most challenging.

Its relevance is hardly open to question: everyone can benefit from a basic knowledge of how the human body and mind work and how to lead a healthy lifestyle. Such knowledge can help us to function at our highest level from day to day. It can help us to maximize our potential for the future; to minimize our risks of disease and injury; and to develop our physical, emotional, intellectual, social, and spiritual resources for a longer, more productive, and more satisfying life.

Studying human health is also fascinating. The human body and human behavior are remarkable creations: though everyone has a personal and subjective understanding of them just through being alive, viewing them through the more objective eyes of science can bring home to one just how remarkable they are. Of all the subjects that can inspire awe and amazement—literature, art, music, geology, and astronomy are only a few examples—the study of the human body and mind are the nearest to us, and also in many ways the most amazing of all. Human beings are the most complex of all living things; understanding this complexity can deepen our appreciation of some of the mysteries of life.

Life and Health: Targeting Wellness is a new textbook published by McGraw-Hill, presenting current information for a person wishing to optimize his or her potential for wellness. It is based in part on two earlier texts we developed for Random House: *Life and Health*, fifth edition, and *Essentials of Life and Health*, but the materials have been thoroughly reworked based on the latest research. Equally important, it is designed to convey an understanding of the subtlety and complexity of human life, to increase awareness of the challenges of health, and to help develop self-efficacy: a confidence that can inspire each individual to rise to those challenges and make progress toward a healthier lifestyle.

One challenge of health arises from the fact that health is a dynamic concept. The information that has been discovered about human health during the past 300 years—and especially during the last 25 years—is staggering. But the process of discovery has not stopped; if anything, it is accelerating. New insights are continually being generated by researchers, studied and checked by their colleagues, and published in scholarly journals and in the popular press. Thus, learning about the current state of health knowledge, as you will do in this course, is important not only because it gives you the best chance of making sound health decisions now, but also because it provides you with a basis for understanding new health discoveries and evaluating their implications for your health care in the future.

The second challenge of health lies in the fact that every person is unique and continues to change throughout life, both in terms of personal needs and of personal goals. For this reason, there is no single prescription for good health that will apply to everybody: the road to wellness involves a continuing process of self-discovery, of learning some general principles about life and health and then applying these principles to one's own particular changing situation.

This textbook has been designed to help you meet both of these challenges; key elements are specifically directed at one or the other of them:

- *Conclusions drawn from classic and recent studies* are presented not as rules, rather as recommendations which can be examined on the basis of evidence given.
- *End notes after each chapter* familiarize you with scholarly and popular sources of up-to-the-minute health information, and allow you to evaluate specific topics from the text in more depth.
- *Straightforward language and illustrations* clarify significant ideas and important complexities of human health as it is understood by health experts today.

- *Technical terms of the health field*, are highlighted with bold-face type and defined where they first appear, in marginal notes, and in a glossary. This will help you to interpret and apply accounts of new discoveries in health that you may read about, and also to communicate with health professionals about these and other matters.
- *Additional marginal notes* provide useful supplementary information to the concepts presented in the text.

Life and Health: Targeting Wellness also includes many boxed features designed to help you to personalize the information presented in the book. There are six types of features:

- *"Thinking Critically"* features look at a significant health issue from two possible viewpoints. You are not expected necessarily to agree with either of them, but instead to ponder the issues being explored and to adopt a position that is consistent with the full range of your own understandings, values, and beliefs.
- *"My Story"* features present a personal account of someone's experience with a particular aspect of wellness or illness. These accounts are usually anonymous; in some cases useful readings are cited that can provide further perspectives on the situation described.
- *"A Broader View"* features look at the wider implications of a particular health topic, presenting international implications, for example, and illustrating how research and actions designed to benefit individuals may have far-reaching global implications.
- *"Comfort Level"* features explore a concept described earlier in this preface: the importance of applying health knowledge to your own life in a way that is in harmony with your goals and values. In this way you can feel confident and comfortable with the actions and behaviors you adopt.
- *"Self-Assessment"* features are brief self-tests designed to help you evaluate your present behaviors and beliefs and relate them to the health topic being discussed. Often based on diagnostic instruments prepared for health professionals, these questionnaires will give you important insights into your own needs and behaviors.
- Finally, *"Communicating About"* features are designed to guide you through some of the many pitfalls in communication associated with various health topics, and to encourage you to discuss some of these topics in a meaningful way.

As the authors of this book, we urge you to get involved in the topics presented. Strive to understand the major concepts and to incorporate them into your own lives as thoughtfully as possible. As you will read in the first chapter and throughout this book, personal health is an area in which each of us can really "make a difference," both for ourselves and for those around us.

MARVIN R. LEVY
MARK DIGNAN
JANET H. SHIRREFFS

Life & Health
Targeting Wellness

PART 1

Enhancing Your Life: Health and Lifestyle

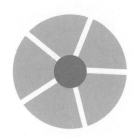

Although this book is titled *Life and Health*, it could well be called *Health and Lifestyle*. Your future health, as well as your present health, depends to a large extent on how you live.

Chapter 1 examines the concepts of health and lifestyle, urging the importance of a balanced approach to health. It then explores setting goals for life and health, examining lifestyle, and making lifestyle changes.

Chapter 2 explains the physiological and mental effects of stress in your life and lifestyle, in both the short term and the long term. It suggests how you can sometimes benefit from the positive impact of these effects, and how you can lessen their negative impact at other times.

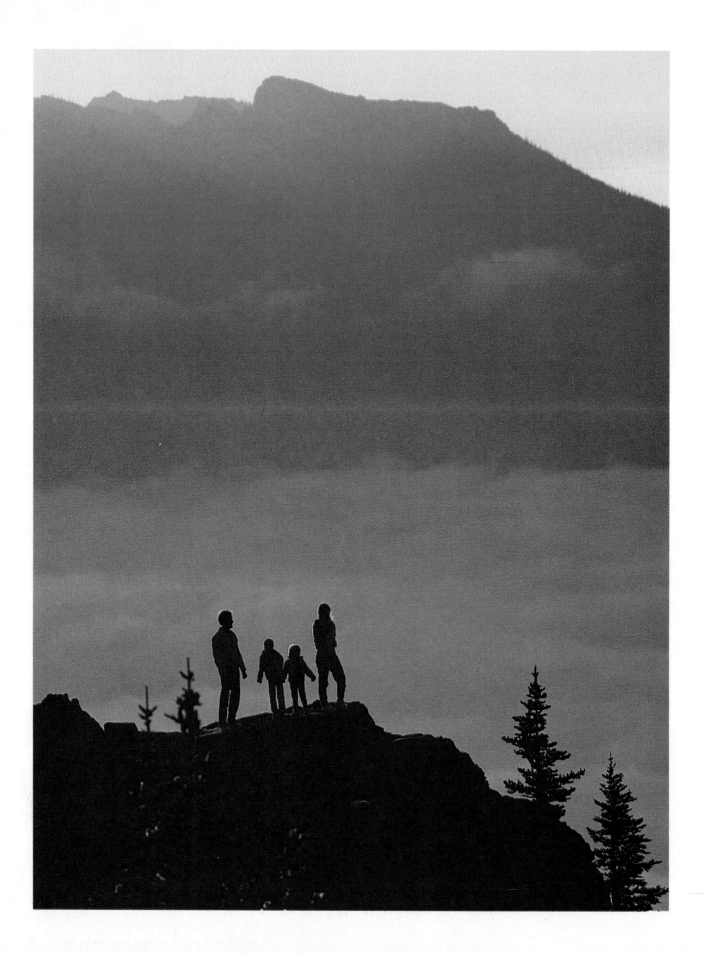

Chapter 1

The Concept of Health

To Guide Your Reading

When you have studied this chapter, you should be able to:

- Define health in terms of a balance between five distinct but interrelated dimensions.

- Analyze the importance to health of the components of lifestyle, as elements that can largely be controlled by individuals for the benefit of their health and feelings of self-efficacy.

- Explain how health goals can be refined by relating them to needs and wants, personal goals both short-term and long-term, and the priorities and trade-offs that make an individual feel most comfortable.

- Describe a process of setting health goals through realistic self-assessment.

- Distinguish between the immediate effects of active involvement in health-enhancing behaviors and the long-term benefits that can be gained by changing health-related aspects of one's lifestyle.

Good health—what does it mean to you? Many people take health for granted, assuming that they are as healthy as they can be and will probably remain so. They accept their general level of health as a given; and though they may on occasion feel sick, or miserable, they expect to recover and be back to their normal selves soon. They do not think of their health as a matter of choices.

Yet many aspects of our health are affected by what we choose to do. With the right information, we can choose sensibly and improve both our health and our lives—for the healthier one is, the more vigor and enthusiasm one has to focus on, and achieve, important goals. By contrast, lack of knowledge can lead to significant limitations, caused by health problems that we may or may not recognize.

Almost everyone has parts of their lives which seem quite healthy, and other parts which might be improved. Darlene, for example, is an attractive 21-year-old and a star on the college swimming team. To stay in good physical condition and strengthen her athletic skills, she follows a regular exercise routine and spends several hours every day in the pool. Darlene also wants to earn good grades because she would like to enter medical school, and so she spends a lot of time doing schoolwork. Her studies and swimming leave Darlene almost no time for socializing, however. She sometimes wishes she had more friends, but she is very shy and takes a long time to feel comfortable with new people. She rarely dates.

Barry, who is 41 years old, is a very gregarious person with many close friends and acquaintances. He is involved in many activities, including playing trumpet in a jazz band, and often goes drinking with his fellow players. Barry earns a living as a taxi driver and appreciates the flexible work schedule, though he finds the job stressful and tiring. His doctor tells him he should stop drinking and get more sleep, but Barry does not feel strongly motivated

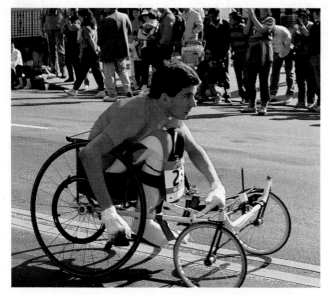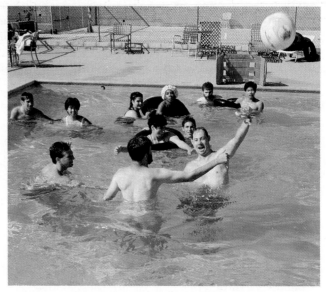

Good health does not require one to be in perfect physical shape—it is a state that each individual can reach for and enjoy. (Vicki Silbert/PhotoEdit; Bill Aron/PhotoEdit)

to do so. He enjoys smoking, too—he depends on cigarettes to keep him alert on the job.

A bright and energetic person, Melissa, in her middle thirties, has worked hard as a receptionist to support her children since the death of her husband. She has a reputation among her friends and coworkers as a stable and trustworthy individual. Although as a teenager Melissa smoked and experimented with illegal drugs, she has found other outlets as she has grown older. At work she relaxes through the occasional use of meditation techniques, and at home she reads and sometimes writes poetry. Recently she enrolled part-time in a community college computer science program in order to earn a degree and find a better career. However, these activities have made it hard for Melissa to get regular exercise—she is 15 pounds overweight. Because of the history of heart disease in her family, she is trying with her usual determination to control her weight through diet but is finding it difficult.

Despite his arthritis, Luis, who is 68 years old, always seems to be in high spirits. He attributes much of his positive attitude to his religious faith, which he says has helped him through difficult times. His wife, children, and grandchildren are also a source of support and joy. Because of his personality, people of all ages seem to come to Luis for advice; they know he is willing to listen to their problems. Luis goes to the doctor for a checkup every few months. So far he has had no major problems other than arthritis, although his blood pressure and total serum cholesterol are higher than they should be. He has managed to lower them somewhat by changing his diet and exercising a little more.

Health and sickness are not necessarily opposites. Even healthy people get sick. The difference is a matter of how sick they get, how often they get sick, and how quickly they recover.

Darlene, Barry, Melissa, and Luis are typical Americans, the kind of people you might see in a restaurant or meet in class. None of them could be considered completely healthy or completely unhealthy; certain parts of their lives seem healthier than others. The question is: What is it about each of their lives that can be recognized as being healthy?

Health and Well-Being

Traditionally, different people have defined health in different ways. An athletic director might have said that health entails exercising regularly and eating carefully to maintain normal weight and good physical conditioning. A physician might have considered health to be the absence of disease. A psychologist might have argued that health includes the ability to cope with emotional problems and traumas. Today, however, most health professionals regard these and many other common definitions of health as incomplete. According to these professionals, the prevention and treatment of health problems requires a broader definition of the concept of health.

What Is Health?

The modern view is that health has several dimensions—emotional, intellectual, physical, social, and perhaps spiritual—each of which contributes to a person's well-being. To maintain good health, a person must examine each of these dimensions and make choices that enable him or her not only to live a long time but also to enjoy life to the fullest.

The word *health* originally meant "whole-th," or "wholeness."[1] When health professionals speak of health, they are acknowledging the original meaning. The World Health Organization stated in 1947 that health is "complete physical, mental, and social well-being and not merely the absence of disease or infirmity."[2] Health is seen as involving the whole person within the total environment.

Health is a process in which all the parts of a person's life work together in an integrated way. No aspect of life functions by itself. Body, mind, spirit, family, community, country, job, education, and beliefs are all interrelated. The way in which these aspects jointly contribute to the richness of a person's life helps determine that individual's uniqueness as well as health.[3]

Perhaps the most important objective of this textbook is to help you discover these aspects of your life: to realize your uniqueness and identify the ways in which you can sustain good health now and throughout your life.

The Dimensions of Health

Health includes more than a smoothly functioning body. It also involves the mind—emotions and intellect, social relationships, and spiritual values. To better understand health, then, it is necessary to examine more closely each of these dimensions, which together constitute overall health and well-being. The dimensions will only be introduced here (Figure 1.1); they will be dealt with in more detail throughout this book.

Emotional Health   To a large extent the quality of a person's health reflects that person's emotions, the feelings he or she has toward self, situations, and other people. Essentially, emotional health includes understanding one's emotions and knowing how to cope with everyday problems and stress as well as being able to work, study, or pursue activities productively and with enjoyment (Chapter 3).

While they are important in themselves, emotions can also influence physical health. Occasionally a startling incident calls attention to the relationship between the mind and the body: a person dies from what appears to be sheer terror, for example,[4] or is made well through the use of a *placebo* (a medication that contains no active ingredients but that the patient believes is effective).[5] However, physicians frequently see less dramatic demonstrations of the mind-body connection. For example, people with good emotional health have a low rate of stress-related diseases such as ulcers, migraine headaches, and asthma.[6] When stress or emotional turmoil continues for a long time, however, the immune system can shut down,[7] increasing the risk of developing these and other diseases.

In recent years some researchers have argued that a personality trait called hardiness may help strengthen the immune system against the damaging effects of stress.[8] **Hardiness** is defined as the possession of an optimistic and committed approach to life, viewing problems, including disease, as challenges that can be handled (Chapter 2).

*The term **health professional** includes anyone who has received specialized training in the care and treatment of people's health concerns. Physicians, dentists, registered nurses, health educators, and dietitians are health professionals.*

hardiness—*a personality trait which gives a person an optimistic and committed approach to life, so that he or she is able to weather life's ups and downs.*

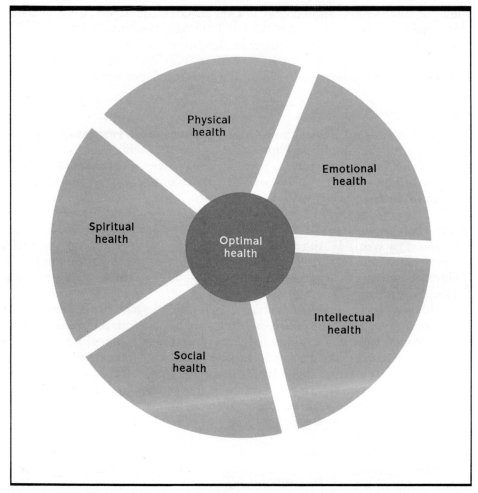

Figure 1.1 Health is an inclusive concept comprised of several components. One person may choose to emphasize one component, whereas someone else may focus on a different one; but none of the components should be neglected. All are interrelated and can help to provide an overall balance in a person's life.

Intellectual Health Intellect—the part of the mind which contributes to sound decision making—can play a crucial role in a person's overall health and well-being. Although intellectual capacity varies among individuals, all people are capable of learning how to acquire and evaluate information, choose between alternatives, and make decisions about health issues as well as other important questions. Critical thinking and decision making are important aspects of intellectual health.

Intellectual health is sometimes included with emotional health as a part of mental health. However, though closely interwoven with emotions, intellectual thought is obviously distinct from them. Emotions can impair a person's ability to think and confused thinking can make emotional problems harder to deal with, but this relationship does not mean they are the same. The ability to think effectively is an important and distinct sign of human health.

Physical Health Physical health refers to the condition of the body and its responses to damage and disease. To stay in good physical health, it is important to behave in ways that enhance one's physical well-being. For example, avoiding cigarettes, drinking alcohol only in moderation, and eating breakfast daily are habits that promote good physical health. Adequate exercise, balanced rest and work, maintenance of normal weight, and intelligent choice of foods also help to keep the body healthy.[9]

Comfort Level

Thinking about Health Priorities

When it comes to being healthy, it sometimes seems there are too many guidelines. A woman who is 5 feet, 4 inches tall should maintain a weight range of 108 to 138 pounds, according to the National Academy of Sciences, but the desirable weight given by the Metropolitan Life Insurance Company's chart ranges from 114 to 151 pounds, depending on age and body type. To promote physical fitness, the American College of Sports Medicine recommends 20 to 60 minutes of exercise at least three times a week. Other experts suggest that as little as 12 minutes of exercise per day can be beneficial.

Choosing among different guidelines can be confusing, especially when each one comes from a prestigious organization or individual. The guidelines differ because they are for different purposes and make different assumptions, but they can all serve as useful starting points for a decision so long as you are willing to accept them.

Health guidelines, as the term suggests, are not meant to set a rigid course but to guide people so that they can find their own pathways to health. Within each set of guidelines, an individual needs to identify a comfort level—a point at which it is possible to optimize the particular dimension of health involved without sacrificing other important dimensions.

Finding one's comfort levels in health entails asking a few key questions. First, what are your overall life goals? Do you want to excel in work that is physically demanding, or is the career you have chosen less strenuous and more intellectual? The health choices that face an athlete are quite different from those which challenge a computer scientist. Each can live a long and fulfilled life by pursuing different health practices.

Second, what values underlie your goals? A person who values achievement may be willing to increase his or her exercise schedule at the expense of social life but be unhappy if it affects his or her career plans. Someone who places a high value on friendships will feel differently about this choice, as may somebody with a deeply religious background. If a health decision is going to work counter to your values, you will rarely feel comfortable with it, and it will be that much harder to achieve.

Third, are you able to accept the full consequences of the change you have planned? Making one change in your lifestyle will almost certainly involve other changes too. Are all of them acceptable, or does one change undercut another? Suppose a dieter has set an ambitious weight-loss target and finds it impossible to achieve even after much deprivation. Rather than giving up or settling in for a life of misery, it may be much better to try to find a compromise comfort level. The weight goal should still be within a recommended range for good health, but compromises to avoid the discomfort and guilt of failure are certainly more healthful than is suffering endlessly for an unattainable goal.

Fourth, is your view of health a truly balanced one? It is necessary to guard against emphasizing one aspect of health at the expense of all the others. Comfort levels arise from a balanced attitude and nearly always lie between the extremes of becoming fanatical about an aspect of health and completely ignoring it. The ancients very aptly advised that "virtue stands in the middle." For each person the "middle" falls in a different place, and finding your individual comfort levels will help you discover that middle and achieve wellness, success, and satisfaction.

Based on ideas in George Will, "Grandmother Was Right," *Newsweek* (January 16, 1967): 68.

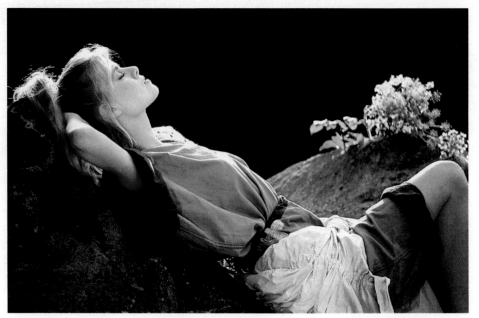

When thinking about physical health, do not forget the importance of rest as well as exercise. (Gunther/Photo Researchers, Inc.)

Good physical health requires that a person pay attention to the messages the body sends about what it needs—more sleep or different foods, for example—and respond to those messages accordingly. Basic self-care skills can help people cope with small health problems on their own.[10] However, it is also important to know how to deal knowledgeably with health care providers such as doctors and hospitals if more serious medical problems develop. Taking responsibility for receiving regular checkups may help prevent major medical problems or allow them to be detected early enough for effective treatment (Chapter 19).

Social Health Social health refers to the ability to perform one's role in life as a son or daughter, parent, spouse, friend, neighbor, perhaps lover or citizen effectively, comfortably, and with pleasure, without harming other people. Each of these roles entails different responsibilities and risks. All require the give-and-take of effective communication—healthy relationships are never one-way. The fulfillment of human needs for love, intimacy, and companionship is an important factor in social health. People who are deprived of these needs may develop behaviors that threaten their overall health and well-being.[11]

Spiritual Health The final dimension of health is spiritual health, a feeling that one's behavior and basic values are in harmony. Not everybody believes in the spiritual dimension, and those who do may describe it in several different ways,[12] but many health professionals hold that spiritual forces affect and are affected by overall health. Spiritual health may include a sense of awe at nature's beauty and majesty, a deeply held religious faith, or a sense of inner peace in regard to one's life. It grows from the struggle to develop a meaningful relationship with the universe and with life itself.

Some people relate spiritual health to energy. They believe that positive conditions such as joy and peace promote the flow of energy through the body and nurture bodily functioning. Negative feelings, by contrast, can block the flow of energy and promote disease.

A number of recent studies have indicated an association between religious affiliation and low rates of chronic disease and mortality. For example, Mormons and Seventh-Day Adventists have lower rates of certain kinds of cancer than does the general population.[13] Some people attribute these effects to religious rules, stating that religion can discourage behaviors that can lead to serious health problems, such as sexual promiscuity, use of tobacco, and excessive alcohol consumption. However, others have asserted that religious affiliation may contribute directly to health and general well-being.[14]

The Integration of Health

Each person assigns a different degree of importance to the five dimensions of health. Some people are more interested in emotional or intellectual health than in physical health; they care less about whether they can run long distances than about their ability to solve problems or grasp new ideas. Others may derive more satisfaction from their relationships with others or their involvement in working for religious ideals.

However, the dimensions of health are all integrated—each has an effect on the others. Suppose you have a job you feel is beneficial to humanity and to the world; in other words, your work is in harmony with your basic values. This harmony may contribute to your spiritual health. Sound spiritual health in turn can have a profound effect on your emotional health, on how you feel about yourself, your life, and other people. Sound emotional health can enhance your social relationships, and sound spiritual, emotional, and social health may enable your body to cope better with physical disease.

All the different dimensions of health—emotional, intellectual, physical, social, and spiritual—work together to determine how well you function and how much you enjoy life. The cultivation of any one dimension may also enhance the others. Similarly, the neglect of any single dimension may have serious consequences for one's overall health and well-being. To maintain your health, then, pay attention to each dimension, recognize the links among them, and attempt to keep them in balance so that they work best for you.

Health and Balance

Such balance is important because it affects the body's balance at a basic physiological level. The human body is a remarkably resilient organism. During our lives, we must respond to a variety of threats, including disease, physical injury, and stress. The body is capable of combating or adapting to many of these threats on its own, healing itself, and returning to a normal state.

To achieve this, the body continually seeks to maintain a balance between factors such as temperature, heart rate, blood pressure, water content, and blood sugar level. This natural equilibrium, or **homeostasis,** is achieved through the functioning of automatic mechanisms within the body. For example, human beings tend to maintain a normal temperature of 98.6 degrees F (37 degrees C). In hot weather the body perspires to cool itself and prevent damage from overheating; in cold weather it shivers to increase muscle activity, thus burning nutrients and producing warmth.

Returning to a normal balanced state is also a key factor in healing or combating disease. The human body can automatically **regenerate,** or replace, most damaged cells on a regular basis: when your skin is cut, new skin cells are created to replace those damaged by the injury, and new blood cells are regenerated to replace those lost during bleeding. Having healed the wound and replaced the materials used in the healing process, the body is thus able to return to a homeostatic condition. Similarly, defenses against disease also work to take care of threats to health and restore the body to a state of balance (Chapter 10).

Two other important aspects of good health are **managing stress** *and* **being safety-conscious.** *Stress is discussed in Chapter 2; preventing injuries is covered in Chapter 16.*

homeostasis—*the body's natural equilibrium, achieved through automatic mechanisms that control temperature, heart rate, blood pressure, and so on.*

regenerate—*to replace damaged cells on a regular basis.*

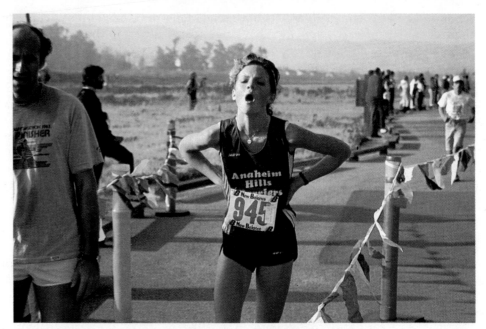

The deep breaths of a runner after a race illustrate homeostasis—the body's automatic effort to return its systems to balance. (Tony Freeman/PhotoEdit)

Such defenses are not only a function of the body, however. As indicated earlier in this section, emotional states can have physiological effects, and can thus play an important part both in destroying and in restoring our physiological equilibrium. As a part of emotions, the brain produces various chemicals that enter the bloodstream and affect the body's homeostatic processes. Because emotions arise in response to all areas of life, intellectual and spiritual as well as social, a balance in all the dimensions of health is important for the proper functioning of the body.

Health and Lifestyle

The dimensions of health can be influenced by several factors and determinants. One obvious factor is the availability of competent medical care and sound health education, both of which can benefit an individual not only physically but mentally and socially as well. Other, more general environmental factors are also important: the safety of homes and neighborhoods, the public services that are available, and negative factors such as the amount of toxic waste in the soil, air, and water. Several of these factors can be controlled to some extent by a person's choice of where to live, and others can be influenced through political action; however, for most people they are features of life that are given and can be changed only with difficulty.

Even harder to control are hereditary factors: aspects of life which are driven by genes. **Genes** are inherited "code" chemicals found in every cell of the human body; they control many aspects of an individual's development and functioning, from gender to tendencies toward certain diseases. They do not affect only physical health; emotions, intellect, and even social life have been found to be strongly influenced by genetics. These are basic aspects of a person's life and health; they cannot be controlled by the individual, though they often can be compensated for.

While all these factors are important in health, the most important influence in the developed world is lifestyle—and lifestyle is a factor one *can* control.[15] This is another important message in this textbook and in every health course: to a large extent you own your own health. While heredity and envi-

genes—inherited "code" chemicals found in every cell of the human body. They control many aspects of an individual's development and functioning.

Conditions that tend to be hereditary include Tay-Sachs disease, sickle-cell anemia, diabetes, Parkinson's disease, and allergies. Several mental tendencies also seem hereditary.

Is Your Lifestyle Good for Your Health?

As this chapter demonstrates, your lifestyle includes many components: the ways you work, relax, communicate, and perform other activities. The following assessment is designed to help you explore your lifestyle choices and determine whether they are affecting you positively or negatively. Your responses will help you understand the impact of your lifestyle on your health.

Directions: Respond to each of the statements with one of the following designations: 5—definitely true; 4—mostly true; 3—not sure; 2—mostly false; 1—definitely false.

Write the number that corresponds to your answer in the blank at the left.

_____ I am doing well in school.

_____ I am enjoying myself, not feeling bored or angry.

_____ I have satisfying relationships with other people.

_____ I express my emotions when I want to.

_____ I use my leisure time well and enjoy it.

_____ I am satisfied with my sexual relationships.

_____ I am satisfied with what I accomplish during the day.

_____ I am having fun.

_____ I am making use of the talents I have.

_____ I feel physically well and full of vitality.

_____ I am developing my skills and abilities.

_____ I am contributing to society.

_____ I am helpful to other people.

_____ I have a sense of freedom and adventure in my life.

_____ I feel joy or pleasure on most days.

_____ I feel that my body is fit enough to meet the demands made upon it.

_____ I feel rested and full of energy.

_____ I am able to relax most of the day.

_____ I enjoy a good night's sleep most nights.

_____ I usually go to bed feeling happy and satisfied about the day.

Scoring: Add up the numbers in your answers.

If your score was 90 to 100, you are making lifestyle choices that promote good health. Your lifestyle is making a very positive contribution to your health.

If your score was 80 to 89, you are doing well in many areas. Many of your lifestyle choices are healthful ones. Look at the statements that you marked with a 1, 2, or 3 for areas that need improvement.

If your score was 61 to 79, there are a number of aspects of your lifestyle that could use improvement. Statements to which you responded 1, 2, or 3 indicate areas where you could do better. Your lifestyle choices may be negatively affecting your physical, emotional, intellectual, social, or spiritual health.

If your score was 60 or below, your lifestyle puts your health at high risk. Carefully review your responses, focusing on statements that you marked with a 1 or 2, and decide what you can do now to make better lifestyle choices. Altering your lifestyle will help you preserve your health.

Statements adapted from the Quality of Life Test in Robert Allen and Shirley Linde, *Lifegain* (Burlington, VT: Human Resources Institute, Inc., 1981): 25–26. Used with permission.

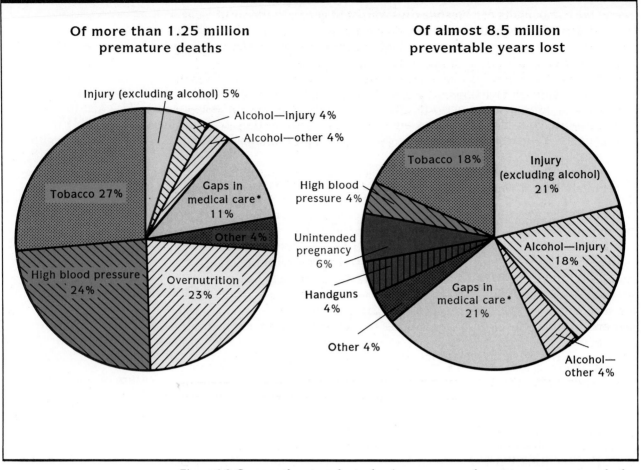

Of more than 1.25 million premature deaths

Injury (excluding alcohol) 5%
Alcohol—injury 4%
Alcohol—other 4%
Tobacco 27%
Gaps in medical care* 11%
Other 4%
High blood pressure 24%
Overnutrition 23%

Of almost 8.5 million preventable years lost

Tobacco 18%
High blood pressure 4%
Unintended pregnancy 6%
Handguns 4%
Other 4%
Injury (excluding alcohol) 21%
Alcohol—injury 18%
Gaps in medical care* 21%
Alcohol—other 4%

Figure 1.2 Compare these two charts showing precursors of premature, unnecessary deaths in the United States (estimated in a recent study to include more than three-fifths of all deaths). While more moderate use of alcohol could have prevented 8 percent of premature deaths, it might have saved 22 percent of the years lost because injuries due to alcohol kill a relatively large proportion of young people.

*Gaps in medical care include inadequate access to care, mistaken diagnosis, and failed primary care.

Source: Adapted from Robert Amler and Donald Eddins, "Cross-Sectional Analysis: Precursors of Premature Death in the United States," in *Closing the Gap,* Robert Amler and H. Bruce Dull (eds.) (New York: Oxford University Press, 1987): 181–187. With permission.

ronment play a large role in your health status, the choices you make about your lifestyle affect your health even more (Figure 1.2).

Lifestyle refers to an overall way of living—the attitudes, habits, and behaviors of a person in daily life. According to the Centers for Disease Control (CDC), lifestyle contributes greatly to 7 of the 10 leading causes of death in the United States.[16] People who smoke cigarettes, for example, are far more likely than are nonsmokers to develop a wide range of diseases affecting the heart, lungs, stomach, kidneys, bladder, mouth, and blood vessels.

Though not all components of lifestyle are under an individual's control—poverty, for example, limits opportunities for many—all people encounter many lifestyle choices that directly affect their health and well-being. A third goal of this book is to help you identify alternatives when you are making decisions or setting goals that will have an impact on your short-term and long-term health.

The Components of Lifestyle

Lifestyle includes a number of different components that include the ways in which people carry out major parts of their lives: how they work, play, eat, cope, and so forth. The word *style* implies a pattern rather than an isolated

lifestyle—*a person's overall way of living—the attitudes, habits, and behaviors of a person in daily life.*

Chronic diseases have surpassed acute infectious diseases as the main cause of illness and death for Americans. Today the major causes of death and disability are heart disease, cancer, accidents, stroke, and chronic lung disease such as emphysema. All are strongly associated with lifestyle.

event; the components of a lifestyle thus consist of general patterns of behavior. For example, going out with friends frequently, as you saw Barry do at the start of this chapter, indicates a highly social lifestyle, at least during recreational time; attending only one party a year does not.

Each individual develops a lifestyle largely through trial and error. People try different courses of action and generally adopt as habits those behaviors which are most successful and satisfying. These behaviors can be grouped into a number of overlapping patterns that make up the components of a lifestyle (Figure 1.3). Each component can have an effect on several dimensions of a person's health.

Working Style The ways in which people produce, create, and study constitute their working styles. Some people are perfectionists who strive to make every aspect of their work perfect. Others may be more concerned with the quantity of work they produce than with the quality.

Traditional physical work has been linked with healthy longevity: a very high proportion of the longest-lived Russians reside in rural agricultural communities.[17] Other types of work stimulate the mind and help maintain intellectual health. Some people, however, choose to spend so much time working that they have little time for social relationships or other types of activity. Darlene has this type of problem, and her social health and emotional health have suffered as a result.

Recreational Style How people spend their leisure time—their recreational style—also affects many dimensions of their health and well-being. People can engage in recreational activities that provide exercise, stimulate the mind, and nurture relationships with other people. Some recreational styles, however, can be harmful.

For example, too much emphasis on competition and aggression—whether in playing basketball, poker, or Scrabble—can harm one's social relationships

Figure 1.3 Lifestyle is such a complex concept that it is helpful to consider it as being made up of several components. Although these components will overlap differently for different people, they can help one think about many of one's general patterns of behavior and how these fit together.

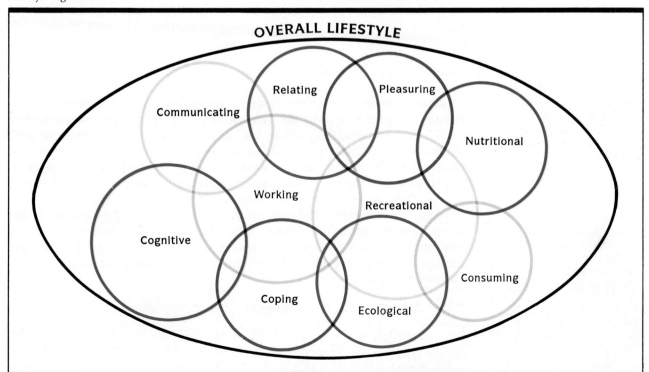

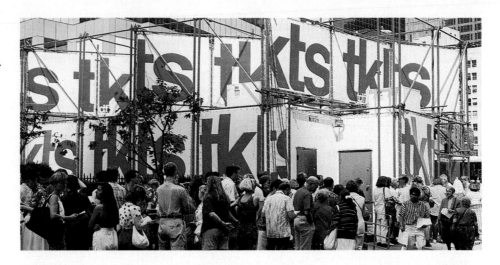

or contribute to stress. People like Barry, whose recreational style focuses on the use of alcohol or other drugs, may be courting serious physical and social health problems.

Pleasuring Style How does a person give pleasure to the important people in his or her life? By making them laugh? By cooking foods they like or giving them expensive presents? How does that person receive pleasure from others? The things people do to make themselves and others feel good and the ways in which they receive pleasure from others define their pleasuring style.

People like Luis are very unselfish in giving to others, while other people may be motivated more by self-interest. An individual who receives something from another person may be gracious and thankful or perhaps suspicious and ungrateful. The ways in which people give and receive pleasure can influence their social, emotional, physical, and spiritual health.[18]

Coping Style Stress is an unavoidable part of life. Financial setbacks; disagreements with relatives, friends, or employers; unexpected difficulties in carrying out tasks; accidents, illnesses, and deaths—these and other stressful events occur in everyone's life.

The way in which people cope with such occurrences is highly individual. One person may handle a family conflict by lashing out angrily, whereas a person like Melissa may try to mediate the dispute calmly and find a solution that is satisfactory to everyone; someone else may prefer to avoid involvement completely.

Cognitive Style Cognitive style refers to the ways in which people think, seek knowledge, and make decisions. Some people are very methodical in their approach to problem solving; they consider all the alternatives and carefully base their decisions on as much information as possible. Other people rely much more on intuition and tend to make quick decisions based on feelings or some other factor, or they may be fearful of making decisions at all and rely on others to tell them what to do.

Cognitive style may be related to the conditions of a person's social and spiritual health; it also reflects one's intellectual health. For example, a person who frequently makes important decisions with little consideration for the consequences may need to strengthen his or her intellectual abilities.

Certain facial expressions (laughter, anger, fear) seem to be universal, suggesting a genetic basis for this type of communication.

Communication Style The ways in which people let others know what they need, want, feel, or think and the ways in which they respond to the thoughts and feelings of others are all part of their communication style. Some people use words to express their feelings, while others may be uncomfortable talking about their emotions. However, there are a variety of ways of communicating besides speaking.

Health and Illness: Whose Responsibility?

Skyrocketing prices for health insurance have resulted from the cost of new medical procedures and from rising fees at hospitals and doctors' offices. One reason for those rising fees is malpractice suits: doctors are blamed for people's ill health, and so they have to buy insurance against lawsuits. But is it all their fault? The first speaker says that doctors are generously paid to keep people well, and when they do not, they should take the blame. The second speaker assigns the blame more broadly and includes other people, even the patients themselves.

Doctors Should Take Responsibility for People's Ill Health If I get sick, I rely on a doctor's help to get me better. Doctors are very well paid. Visiting the doctor is expensive—and gets more so as employers and insurance companies cut back on health coverage. As a result, patients have to lay out more themselves. With the kind of money doctors make, I think they *should* take responsibility.

So I'm alarmed by the recent trend toward doctors involving patients in health care decisions. Auto mechanics get paid less than doctors and study less, but they make decisions on their own. They locate the problem and fix it. Doctors should do the same.

Have you read how the American system of medical care is based on cures for disease rather than prevention? The situation may be getting better, but doctors still learn more about sickness and its treatment than they do about basic health, and standard insurance policies still don't cover physicals and other prevention services.

Of course, patients have some responsibility. If we don't follow the doctor's orders, then *we* are to blame. But doctors only advise us when we're sick—they rarely see us when we're well. So we have to figure out how to stay well from the media: TV, books, and newspapers. And the advice is conflicting— one diet says we must eat more protein; another recommends less protein. We need guidance even when we're well.

Uncertainty about how to act on an important topic causes stress—and what could be more important than health? But stress has been found to be a reason why people suffer from disease. So by not giving us basic health advice when we are well and by trying to make us take part in health decisions, I think doctors fail their responsibility. And I mean it: *their* responsibility.

Health Decisions Are Shared Decisions in Which Patients Are Also Involved You can't pin the blame for ill health on one person. Health is too complex and too important to lay on one pair of shoulders. As hospital admission forms state, "Medicine is not an exact science." It requires judgment, sensitivity, and cooperation.

Think about it. People are born different: different strengths, different weaknesses. The weaknesses are obvious in some people, but in others they become apparent only in response to specific diseases. How can we blame a doctor for that? There's no one to blame—it's just life. However, if we're lucky, for most health problems, doctors *can* help.

But doctors aren't gods. If they regularly advised healthy patients as well as those who are sick, doctors would be incredibly busy and we'd pay far more for health care. And they still couldn't give us all the answers, because the answers just aren't known. Anyway, how many people *want* to see the doctor when they're well?

And remember, it's your own life and health that are on the line, not the doctor's. When you go to a doctor, you don't change that or change your feelings about what *you* want. There are some decisions no one else can make for you. Are you willing to undergo major surgery? Doctors can advise you about what would be best on the basis of known probabilities, but they cannot be 100 percent certain that your condition is critical or that the surgery will work. They can't force you; balancing your feelings about the probabilities *has* to be your own decision.

What is your opinion? Do you agree that doctors should be blamed because people are unhealthy? Should people blame themselves? What is the most reasonable position to take?

Ideas drawn from Dan Brock and Steven A. Wartman, "Sounding Board," *New England Journal of Medicine* 322 (May 31, 1990): 1595– 1599.

People probably sense Luis's approachability from his facial expressions, gestures, and body language, for example. A person who is withdrawn and shy may have difficulty developing social relationships. Someone who does not express emotions may suffer social and emotional tensions, which could lead to physical problems as well.

Relating Style   Communication is only part of the way in which people relate to each other; an individual's relating style involves other types of interaction as well. Within a group, for example, some task-oriented people may tend to assume a leadership role while others are more comfortable letting someone else take the lead. Other aspects of relating style include the ways people approach others they would like to know better and the types of relationships people have with their families and friends.

Some relationships may be based on trust, mutual respect, or equality; others, on fear, awe, or subordination. Social health and emotional health depend in part on one's ability to deal with interpersonal relationships in ways that satisfy one's personal needs and desires.

Nutritional Style   A person's attitude toward and approach to food and eating constitute that person's nutritional style. For some people, food is a major source of pleasure; for others, it is merely a fuel required by the body. A meal can consist of various courses shared with other people over a couple of hours or a slice of pizza eaten quickly while one is going from one appointment to another.

A person's physical health depends to a large extent on what he or she eats. Food can also have an impact on one's intellectual health, and the way in which food is eaten—whether on the run or in a relaxed manner, alone or with other people—can affect one's social and emotional well-being. How do you imagine Darlene eats most of her meals?

Consuming Style   Another component of lifestyle consists of the ways in which people select and use products and services—their consuming style. A person shopping for a home may be more concerned with either comfort or appearance. How pleasant a home is to live in may affect one's physical well-being, while the image the home presents may have an impact on one's social relationships and emotional satisfaction.

People also use products and services in different ways. Some individuals use them carefully in order to preserve them as long as possible; others are more careless and discard things hastily when they become worn or outdated.

Ecological Style   The decisions a consumer makes also affect ecological style—the way in which a person interacts with the physical environment. One's ecological style reflects the level of one's concern for preserving a healthy environment. It involves decisions about nearly everything people do: whether they run errands by car, on foot, by bus, or by bicycle; how much heat or air-conditioning they use; how actively involved they are in recycling; and so forth.

Virtually every human action affects the environment. The way in which people treat the environment influences their own physical health as well as the physical health of others. The use of toxic chemicals, for example, can ultimately threaten the health of everyone on the planet. Some people view interactions with the environment as an important part of spiritual health; for them, concern for nature and the environment reflects a feeling of connectedness among humans, all living things, the planet Earth, the universe, and perhaps a higher power.

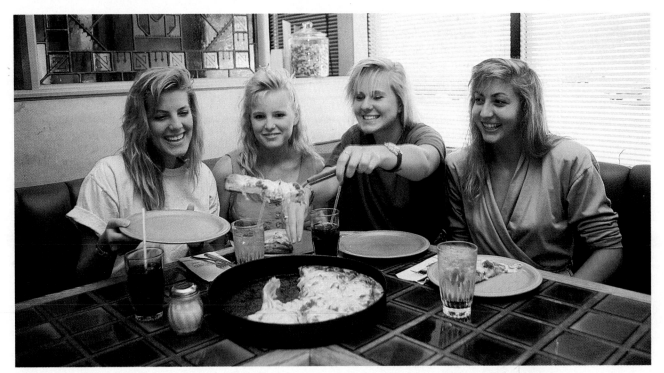

The components of lifestyle are not always separate from each other: the role of consumer often contributes to people's pleasure and social life as well as nutrition. (Felicia Martinez/PhotoEdit)

Lifestyle, Health, and Self-Efficacy

The multiple behaviors which make up a person's lifestyle indicate that lifestyle is a very complex entity affected by many variables and suggest that it is hard to control and change. However, in the United States people enjoy a high degree of individual freedom over the various components of their lifestyles. This may give Americans greater "ownership" of their health than is enjoyed by the citizens of other nations. People can make decisions about the work they do, where they live, how they spend their leisure time, and how they treat other people. They can decide what to eat, what to think, how to communicate with others, and how to treat the environment.

This freedom gives Americans the potential to develop a high level of self-efficacy, which is another important contributor to health. **Self-efficacy** means confidence in one's ability to plan and control one's own behaviors, one's lifestyle components.[19] No one can control every aspect of health, of course; a person cannot do anything to change his or her heredity or age, and no individual has much control over the quality of air or water. However, people do have options about the medical care they receive and are free to make many important decisions about their lifestyles that can have positive effects on health and well-being.

Suppose a person has inherited a tendency to have high levels of cholesterol; perhaps high cholesterol contributed to the early deaths of several relatives. Although that person shares this predisposition with other family members, he or she will not necessarily have the same fate; it is possible to learn how to keep cholesterol at a safe level. Of course, one must accept the fact that doing so will require a greater effort than it would for a person without this problem; that is something that cannot be changed. But people can set health goals and then make changes in their diet, exercise routine, or use of nicotine and other drugs. Such changes can greatly improve one's chances of having a longer, more comfortable life.

People equate lifestyle and behavior patterns with "habits," both good and bad. Habits are often hard to break, but achieving healthy behaviors often entails breaking old habits.

self-efficacy—confidence in one's ability to plan and control one's behavior and lifestyle components.

Self-efficacy does not merely help someone plan sound health behaviors—of itself it contributes to health as much as self-esteem does.

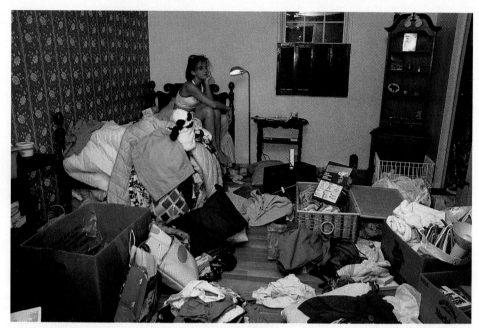

Having control over one's life does not always mean that everything is in order, but you need to feel ready to take care of important things such as your health. (Paul A. Hein/ Unicorn Stock Photos)

Health Goals

To be effective, the health goals people set for themselves should be based on a sound understanding of health information and issues. Another purpose of this book is to provide such information. What are the usual outcomes of different types of behavior patterns? What techniques are most effective in changing these outcomes? Such information is invaluable for anyone who seeks to develop self-efficacy.

However, health goals cannot be based on health information alone; they must also be compatible with the broader goals that every individual has. One person may want to gain or lose weight in order to look more attractive. Another may need to lose weight to help control high blood pressure or diabetes. Yet another may decide that despite having weight problems, other issues are more vital to his or her life; combating anxiety or developing a network of friends may be more important health goals. Objective information about weight control can be important in setting health goals, but people also need to examine goals in the context of their personal needs and wants.

Needs and Wants

Although most people have the same basic needs—food, shelter, safety, contact with other people, a sense of satisfaction in work and other activities—within these categories there is a wide range of possibilities that constitute people's wants. For example, although everyone needs to eat, the amount and types of foods people want vary a great deal. Similarly, while everyone needs human contact, people want it to different degrees and in differing circumstances, depending on their personalities, experiences, and values. Neglecting universal human needs makes it difficult for a person to enjoy good health and a satisfying life, but neglecting particular wants and interpretations of those needs may also have serious consequences.

Health professionals frequently cite the model of human needs formulated by psychologist Abraham Maslow.[20] According to Maslow, individuals progress through a *hierarchy of needs,* all of which must be met for a person to lead a satisfying and fulfilling life. The lower levels of Maslow's hierarchy consist of basic physiological and psychological needs such as water, food, shelter, sleep, human contact, safety and security, and love and acceptance. All these needs are "basic" in the sense that they are vital to positive human functioning (Figure 1.4).

Moving up Maslow's hierarchy, one finds growth needs, such as self-esteem, truth, goodness, justice, order, individuality, and self-sufficiency; self-actualization needs, which are basically drives to behave responsibly and morally toward oneself and others; and "transpersonal, transhuman, and transcendent" needs, which are experiences that allow people to transform their lives. As one moves higher in Maslow's model, interpretation of the needs becomes more personal: individual wants play a greater part in achieving satisfaction and fulfillment. However, these higher-level needs and wants are also important aspects of overall human health.

Defining Personal Goals

Defining personal goals is an important step in achieving the satisfaction and fulfillment described by Maslow. If needs and wants are not translated into specific goals, they may remain ideas only, awakening feelings of frustration rather than concrete plans for change.

Without goals, there is no way to measure progress or gauge success in meeting one's needs or satisfying one's wants. Goals are also important so that individuals can experience the satisfaction and sense of accomplishment that come with achieving them.

Effective goals, of course, must be realistic. Suppose two people have set themselves the goal of entering a marathon next year and finishing the race in under 5 hours. One is in good physical condition, has no serious handicaps,

Figure 1.4 Maslow's model of human needs has five levels. Lower-level needs such as exercise and a safe environment are the foundation of health, but a person cannot feel vibrant and whole without getting satisfaction from social life, achievement, and personal fulfillment.

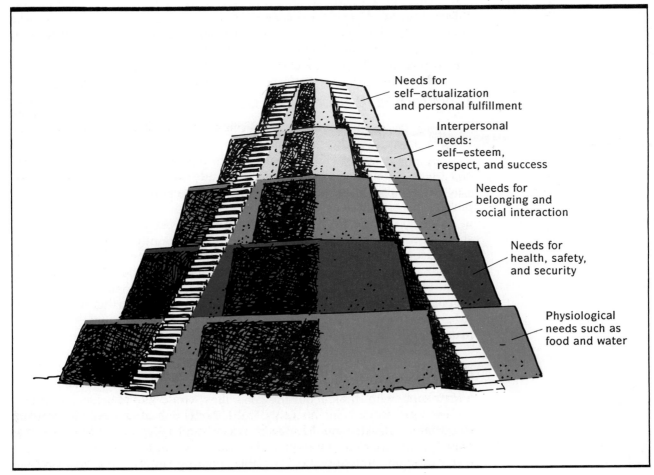

Needs for self–actualization and personal fulfillment

Interpersonal needs: self–esteem, respect, and success

Needs for belonging and social interaction

Needs for health, safety, and security

Physiological needs such as food and water

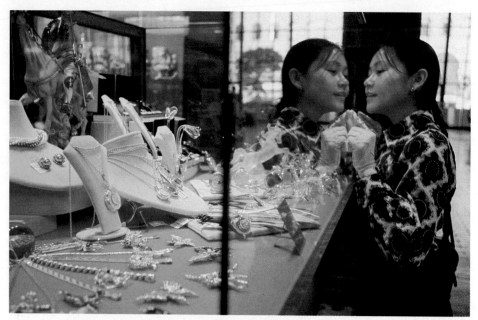

Window-shopping is merely the beginning of goal setting; it is like dreaming of becoming a sports star. Wants and dreams become goals as you decide they are realistic and develop plans to achieve them. (Alan Oddie/PhotoEdit)

and can reasonably be expected to achieve that goal with the proper exercise and training. The other is in poor physical condition and has little time for training; for that person, the marathon is obviously an unrealistic goal. A heart condition or another medical problem would make this goal not only unrealistic but dangerous.

Defining realistic goals that are appropriate to a person's needs, wants, and abilities provides opportunities for experiencing success and satisfaction, which help build self-esteem. Unrealistic goals may lead to failures that can undermine self-esteem and may even endanger one's physical health.

Long-Term and Short-Term Goals

The goals people set for themselves can be either long-term or short-term. Long-term goals, such as obtaining a graduate degree, may require years to achieve and are often closely connected to one's deepest needs and wants. Short-term goals, such as earning a good grade on a test, can be accomplished quickly and then forgotten. Short-term goals can, however, often be stepping-stones toward achieving long-term goals. For example, a long-term goal of losing 50 pounds over the next year can be broken down into a series of short-term goals of losing about 4 pounds each month.

Since long-term goals may seem overwhelming even when they are realistic, it is easy to become pessimistic about the likelihood of accomplishing them. Short-term goals, by contrast, seem much more manageable to most people. Approaching a long-term goal as a series of short-term goals provides a way to experience a more immediate sense of achievement and helps make long-term goals easier to accomplish.

Priorities, Trade-Offs, and Comfort Levels

Most people who think about the goals they would like to achieve find that the list goes on and on. As goals are defined, one also needs to establish **priorities** by deciding which needs, wants, and goals are most important. Many people try to do more than they can reasonably expect to accomplish given the time and resources available. Finding time for the goal of daily

priority—*a need, want, or goal that is more important than another.*

exercise was hard for Melissa at the start of this chapter, and Darlene's social life also suffered because of a heavy schedule. Similarly, it can be difficult to balance the need for personal independence with family responsibilities or the demands of a career. Establishing priorities can help a person resolve such difficulties so that the most important needs and goals are taken care of first.

Equally important when there are many competing needs and goals are **trade-offs**—decisions that certain needs or wants have to be sacrificed or met in other ways. Some trade-offs are fairly obvious. For example, alcohol may seem an important part of someone's pleasuring style, perhaps because it seems to ease stress and enhance one's relationships with others. Alcohol consumption, however, is not without major physical and emotional health risks. A full understanding of these risks may encourage people to give up or limit alcohol consumption for the sake of their overall physical and emotional health. It also may prompt them to develop alternative ways of relating to people or coping with stress that are less dependent on the use of alcohol.

Other trade-offs may be less obvious. For example, a person who wants to reduce the amount of stress in his or her life may be unsure about how to do this. A better understanding of stress and its causes may suggest some strategies. Depending on the source of stress, a person may try to alter his or her relating style so that relationships with other people are less stressful. That person may learn how to cope better with stressful events such as the death of a loved one or a major illness. He or she may also develop new ways to express feelings in order to reduce emotional stress.

Making trade-offs involves determining individual **comfort levels**—the levels of compromise a person feels comfortable making among different goals in order to maximize overall benefits (see the feature on comfort level in this chapter). Young people and older people as well sometimes worry that they are slower, more intellectual, or less active sexually than their peers. Extreme differences *may* signal real problems, but there is a wide range of "normal" behaviors and conditions. If people could become more comfortable and accept their actual levels of behavior, they might find that they have fewer things to worry about and thus can devote more time and energy to goals that are of greater importance to them. Establishing genuine comfort levels is a significant aspect of all health-related decisions.

Taking Stock of Your Health

The process of setting health goals that are realistic and appropriate starts with a thorough assessment of one's current health and capabilities. This self-assessment is a continuous process rather than a one-time task. It may be necessary to reconsider priorities, trade-offs, and comfort levels from time to time to accommodate changes in your body, wants or needs, and general circumstances. As some goals are reached, you may need to set new ones. Also, if a goal proves unattainable, it may have to be replaced with another, more realistic one with which you still feel comfortable.

Self-assessment includes several important steps (Figure 1.5).

1. **Clarify your health needs and wants.** The first step in self-assessment is to focus on your current health status and on tentative areas in which to consider change—tentative because it may be necessary to modify them as the assessment proceeds. Are there particular health goals that you already have or problems you wish to solve? Usually the two go together. If you want to improve your physique, it is because you feel inadequate in some way; if you feel that your energy level is low, you already have the general goal of becoming more active. Start by clarifying your areas of concern: for example, are you really overweight by objective standards? If so, what kind of action appeals to you? Do you favor a diet, or an exercise program, or both?

trade-off—*a need, want, or goal that has to be delayed, postponed, or given up in order for a priority to be accomplished.*

comfort level—*the level of compromise a person feels comfortable making among different goals in order to maximize overall benefits.*

In some areas of life, comfort levels can be chosen at will. It is all right to settle for a C in a course, but you must be sure you can live with the consequences. In terms of health, although there is a range of acceptable behaviors, it is possible to go too far: drinking while driving is never acceptable.

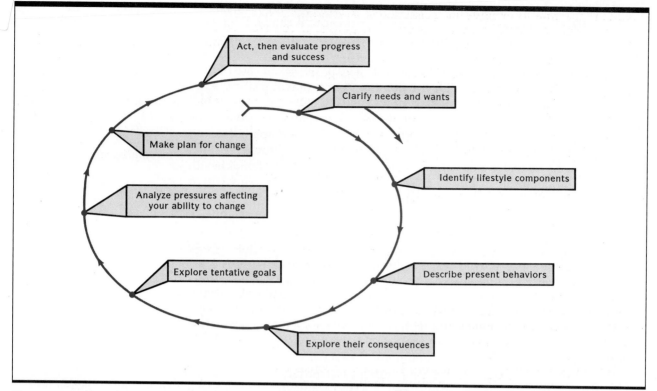

Figure 1.5 Making changes in one's behavior patterns may be desirable, but do not expect it to be easy. There are often hidden pressures not to change—if you do not anticipate and deal with them, you will find that they block your progress. To be sure that the attempted behavior change really meets your needs, the change process should be spiral—as you evaluate your success, you should be thinking again about your needs: Is further action necessary?

Two types of consequences may "block" changes in behavior: positive results from existing habits ("Smoking is relaxing"), and negative (or feared) results from proposed changes ("If I give up cigarettes, I'll be uptight all the time"). The struggle often involves circumventing these blocks.

2. **Identify the lifestyle components involved.** Clarify to yourself which parts of your lifestyle are most closely related to each area of concern. Is it your nutritional style, your recreational style, or both that are important in regard to your physique? Perhaps your sedentary working style is a factor. With some concerns it may be relatively easy to make this decision. Others—for example, the problem of having low energy—may be harder to analyze. Coping style may be involved; so may nutritional style; so may relating style or pleasuring style.

3. **Describe your present behaviors in regard to these components.** What are your typical relating behaviors? Are you generally relaxed or tense with other people? Do you get upset when others do not do what you want? How do you cope with these feelings? Is this what makes you withdraw into inactivity? Or do you feel socially at ease but still lacking in energy? Perhaps you are not eating right. What is your typical meal, and how often do you eat? These types of questions will help you explore the problem you are trying to deal with.

4. **Explore the consequences of these behaviors.** While a person's actions do not always have the same results, they can be typically successful or unsuccessful. Even if you suspect that irregular eating is the reason for your lack of energy, this eating pattern may have other consequences. Perhaps it allows you to stay involved in projects of interest to you or makes it easier to fit in spontaneously with your friends' activities; perhaps it gives you the satisfaction of annoying people who want to make you join them at mealtimes. All behaviors have many consequences, some of which seem good and some bad. A few may make you wish to give up the behavior, but others probably encourage you to continue. You should try to understand your feelings about all these consequences, because they contribute both to your willingness to keep your behavior patterns and to your annoyance with them.

5. **Explore your tentative goals and other possible solutions.** So far you have considered the behavior patterns in your lifestyle that appear to be causing you problems, the ones you want to change. You probably also have ideas about the changes you would like to make—perhaps you want to reevaluate the dreams or goals which led you to consider changing in the first place. Do you want to improve your physique?

Now is the time to explore the possibilities. A changed behavior pattern will have both good points and bad points. If you sign up at a health club, you have an excellent chance of improving your physique, but it will take time and you may experience embarrassment in the early months of your membership. In fact, it is possible that the bad points of this solution outweigh the good so that you will give up your effort. Think about other ways you might improve your physique and also about whether a better physique is really the answer to your problem. Maybe your problem is really shyness and there are easier ways for you to impress people than by building your muscles. Explore these possibilities too, both their good points and their bad points, and make a decision about which would be the best solution to try first.

6. **Analyze the forces and pressures that influence behavior.** After identifying the changes you want to make, think about why you have not made them already. This may give you ideas for strategies for changing behavior that are likely to work.

Various factors keep people from changing their lifestyle habits. Even when they know they should make changes, they often cling to old patterns of behavior. Sometimes, as suggested above, people do this because the existing behavior pattern is convenient or brings them pleasure. But maybe they do not know what to do instead or lack the self-confidence to try something new. Also, behaviors sometimes seem unavoidable, as when people knowingly expose themselves to hazards in order to earn a living.

It is possible, however, to lessen the effect of forces that block healthy change and strengthen those which promote it. If the benefits derived from an old behavior have kept you from changing it, think of other ways to obtain similar benefits. Have you resisted changing your diet because certain foods bring you pleasure? Be adventurous, and you may find healthful alternatives that you enjoy eating just as much or even more. Or try getting more pleasure from other things, such as activities, hobbies, and friendships. Also, find out what others have done to change similar behaviors and, if possible, get their support.

When you are trying to change a habit, it is important to reinforce the new behavior. In addition to being rewarded by reaching your ultimate goal, you can give yourself special rewards for successes along the way—for reaching short-term goals. These more immediate rewards can help provide the incentive needed for you to continue. Select as treats things that are meaningful to you, that you enjoy and are willing to work toward.

There are often many ways to solve problems and reach goals. The more open-minded you are, the more likely you are to come up with a solution which meets your needs. (Anne W. Krause/Take Stock)

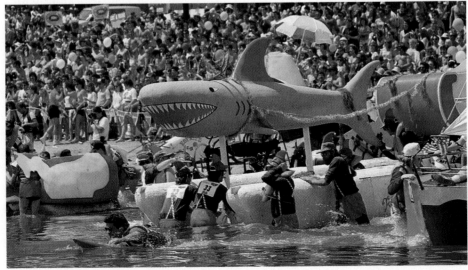

7. **Make specific plans for change, including resources and a schedule.** Identifying a specific goal to aim for and useful strategies for change is only the first step in effecting real change in your life and health. You also need a detailed plan and a reasonable timetable you are likely to follow.

   In their initial enthusiasm, people may set an unrealistic schedule for achieving their goals; this should be avoided. Spending 2 hours at a gym every day of the week may be difficult for someone with a family who works 10 hours a day. Failing to keep that schedule may result in feelings of failure and disappointment that can destroy your confidence in making a change. Scheduling three 1-hour workouts a week would be more realistic and would still provide a significant amount of exercise. Following the less demanding schedule successfully will help build your self-esteem and support the overall effort to improve your health.

   It is equally important to line up resources. There are usually many resources available that can help a person make and sustain a desired change in behavior. Arrange for the different types of resources you need and utilize them whenever possible. If your goal is to increase the amount you exercise, sign up at the gym or join the swimming club. Purchase a bicycle or even just a good pair of walking shoes.

   Do not forget to consider human resources as well. The support, encouragement, and even participation of family members and friends can help you change your behavior. Try to enlist their help. Tell them about your goals and let them know you would appreciate their help. Group support networks such as Weight Watchers and Alcoholics Anonymous are important resources for people who are trying to change certain behaviors.

Remember that monitoring personal behaviors in order to maintain and improve health is a lifelong process.

8. **Evaluate your progress and success.** Once you have started your program for change, it is important to evaluate the progress being made from time to time. Satisfactory progress encourages a person to continue. Decide in advance how to measure or evaluate your level of success. Written records of efforts and actions may be helpful. For example, if your goal is to run 2 or more miles three times a week, keep a log showing your days and distances. Visible evidence of success may encourage you to continue running or to run even more.

   If there seems to be no progress, an evaluation can often help determine what is blocking success, and plans can then be adjusted accordingly. If the written records show that your goals are not being met, try to identify the reasons why. Think about how your goals could be adjusted to make them more attainable. Perhaps you would be more likely to run early in the morning than late in the afternoon. Or maybe running in the morning would be easier if you went to bed earlier at night.

   Continue to keep records as you adjust the plan. This not only will help show you what works and what does not but also will help you find other ways of reinforcing your efforts.

Health and Your Future

Americans have begun to take a more active role in the pursuit of health and well-being. Half the participants in a study of health practices conducted by the National Center for Health Statistics reported that they are doing a good job taking care of their health; 15 percent said they are doing an excellent job.[21] According to a recent Harris survey, Americans are practicing more health and safety measures, including stress management, than ever before. Seventy percent of those polled reported that they take specific steps to manage stress, and 81 percent said they take steps to prevent accidental injury.[22] The 1989 Gallup Leisure Audit showed an increase in "back to nature" sports such as bicycle touring and racing, camping, hiking, and boating and a slight decline in "body image" activities such as weight lifting.[23]

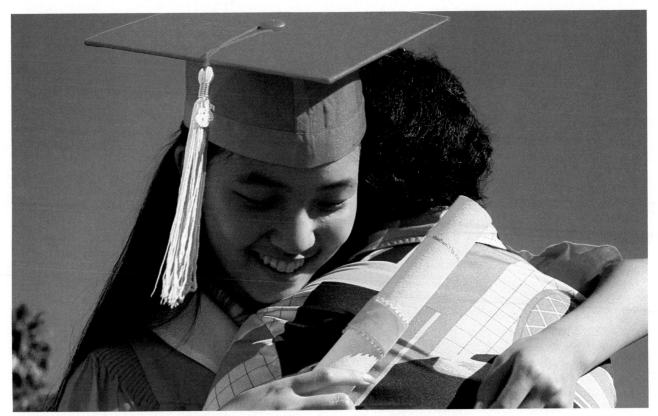

Many human endeavors provide great short-term satisfactions, but the real benefits are felt throughout one's life. Health is no different: what you do today and tomorrow will affect your whole future. (Alan Oddie/PhotoEdit)

Although many Americans are taking a more active role in their health, most people tend to focus on the immediate advantages and disadvantages of health-related behaviors rather than on long-term results. Most people, for example, concentrate on losing 5 pounds in 3 weeks rather than on developing a lifelong plan for maintaining ideal weight. Solving a current problem usually takes precedence over working to prevent problems that may occur later. People are more motivated to seek immediate benefits than to work toward goals that may be years or even decades ahead.

Many aspects of human behavior, however, affect long-range health even more than immediate, short-term health and conditions. The things you do today may not affect your health noticeably for years to come; even the immediate effects may be barely noticeable. A good example is cigarette smoking. In the beginning the negative health effects of smoking may seem slight or nonexistent. While some people may feel a little light-headed or nauseated, they do not feel the toxins building up in their lungs or the mucus clogging their breathing passages. Such damage is cumulative; it may take several years to develop smoker's cough or chronic shortness of breath, and lung cancer is most likely to strike people who have been smoking for decades.

The positive effects of behavior on health can also be cumulative and subtle. Early environment and behavior—whether your mother avoided alcohol and other drugs while pregnant, what you ate as a child, whether you got enough sleep, how you learned to express or cope with feelings—have a lot to do with your health today. They play an important role in determining your physical characteristics, emotional and intellectual state, and relationships with other people. Similarly, your environment and behaviors now are helping to determine the condition of your health during later life. The earlier you incorporate positive attitudes and behaviors into your life, the more apt you are to remain vigorous and energetic as you age.

Chapter Summary

- Health is a complex concept with several aspects, including physical, mental (emotional and intellectual), social, and perhaps spiritual dimensions.
- Health involves more than the absence of disease; it is a process that contributes to enjoyment and well-being.
- Emotional health refers to the ability to express and cope with one's emotions in a productive way.
- Intellectual health includes the ability to evaluate information and make sound decisions.
- Physical health has many components and involves behaviors that enhance health, the ability to deal with minor health difficulties, and, in the case of major health problems, one's understanding of health care systems.
- Social health is the ability to handle, enjoy, contribute to, and benefit from relationships with other people.
- Spiritual health refers to a sense of consistency, harmony, and tranquillity that appears to promote energy and nurture overall health.
- Although different people may focus on different dimensions of health, all these dimensions are interrelated. Positive effects in one dimension are likely to enhance other dimensions too, and negative influences in one dimension will probably cause problems in the other four.
- A balance between the dimensions of health is important. Balance is a key health concept—to maintain and restore itself, the body seeks homeostasis.
- All the dimensions of health are affected by many factors, which can be grouped into health-care-system factors, general environmental factors, genetic factors, and lifestyle factors.
- Lifestyle factors are in many ways the most influential on overall health; they are also the factors that are most under the individual's control.
- Lifestyle can be viewed as a conglomeration of different components—sets of behavior patterns that affect different areas of one's life. These components include working style, recreational style, pleasuring style, coping style, cognitive style, communication style, relating style, nutritional style, consuming style, and ecological style.
- Although lifestyle is complex, it is under personal control and "ownership," dictated by the ability to make wise choices that can benefit one's life and health.
- Making choices for health involves more than objective information: it also requires an understanding of the individual's overall goals in life.
- Human goals are in general based on human needs, most of which all people share, and wants, which are much more personal and may involve individual interpretations of those needs.
- Defining realistic goals enables people to make specific efforts toward attainable objectives.
- Short-term goals can make it easier to reach long-term goals.
- When many goals are competing for one's attention, it is useful to consider priorities, trade-offs, and comfort levels.
- Goal setting can be handled on a rational basis through self-assessment. This is a continuous process of examining one's many needs and wants, exploring behavior patterns in one's lifestyle that facilitate or hinder those needs and wants, and then planning appropriate changes in behavior.
- Just as many health-threatening behaviors, such as smoking, are more damaging in the long term than they are in the near future, the development of health-enhancing behaviors has not only short-term benefits but long-term benefits.

Key Terms

Hardiness (page 5)
Homeostasis (page 9)
Regenerate (page 9)

Genes (page 10)
Lifestyle (page 12)

Self-efficacy (page 17)
Priority (page 20)

Trade-off (page 21)
Comfort level (page 21)

References

1. M. L. Dolfman, "The Concept of Health: An Historic and Analytic Examination," *Journal of School Health* 48, no. 8 (1973): 491.

2. Constitution of the World Health Organization, *Chronicle of the WHO* 1 (1947): 1.

3. Carl A. Hammerschlag, *The Dancing Healers: A Doctor's Journey of Healing with Native Americans* (San Francisco: Harper & Row, 1988).

4. S. J. Lachman, "A Psychophysiological Interpretation of Voodoo Illness and Voodoo Death," *Omega* 13 (1982–1983): 354–360.

5. W. H. Greene and B. G. Simons-Morton, *Introduction to Health Education* (New York: Macmillan, 1984): 91.

6. Emrika Padus, *The Complete Guide to Your Emotions and Your Health* (Emmaus, Pa.: Rodale Press, 1986); Larry A. Tucker et al., "Stress and Serum Cholesterol: A Study of 7,000 Adult Males," *Health Values* 11 (1987): 34–39.

7. Robert Ornstein and David Sobel, *The Healing Brain: A New Perspective on the Brain and Health* (New York: Simon & Schuster, 1987); Sally Squires, "The Power of Positive Imagery: Visions to Boost Immunity," *American Health* (July 1987).

8. Suzanne C. Kobasa, "Stressful Life Events, Personality, and Health: An Inquiry into Hardiness," *Journal of Personality and Social Psychology* 37, no. 1 (January 1979): 1–11.

9. N. B. Belloc and L. Breslow, "Relationship of Physical Health Status and Health Practices," *Preventive Medicine* 1 (August 1972): 409–421.

10. Lowell S. Levin, "The Layperson as the Primary Care Practioner," *Public Health Reports* 91(May–June 1976): 206–210.

11. G. M. Moss, *Illness, Immunity and Social Interaction* (New York: John Wiley, 1973); S. Gore, "The Effect of Social Support in Moderating Health," *Journal of Health and Social Behavior* 19 (1978): 157–165.

12. Greene and Simons-Morton, op. cit., p. 9.

13. L. J. Lyon et al., "Cancer Incidence in Mormons and Non-Mormons in Utah during 1967–1975," *Journal of the National Cancer Institute* 65 (1980): 1055–1061; F. R. Lemon, R. T. Walden, and R. W. Woods, "Cancer of the Lung and Mouth in Seventh-Day Adventists: Preliminary Report on a Population Study," *Cancer* 4 (1964): 486–497.

14. Gordon W. Alport, *The Individual and His Religion* (New York: Macmillan, 1950); William James, *The Varieties of Religious Experience* (New York: New American Library, 1958).

15. M. Lelonde, *A New Perspective on the Health of Canadians: A Working Document* (Ottowa: Government of Canada, 1974); U.S. Department of Health, Education and Welfare, *Healthy People: The Surgeon General's Report on Health Promotion and Disease Control,* USPHS, DHEW (DHS) Pub. No. 79-55071 (1979); Mary Weisensee, "Evaluation of Health Promotion," *Occupational Health Nursing* (January 1985): 9–14.

16. DHEW, op. cit., pp. 2–3.

17. Bill Thomson, "In Search of Longevity," *East/West* (December 1989): 94–95.

18. Robert Ornstein and David Sobel, *Healthy Pleasures* (Menlo Park, Calif.: Addison-Wesley, 1989).

19. Albert Bandura, "Self-Efficacy: Toward a Unifying Theory of Behavioral Change," *Psychological Review* 84, no. 2 (1977): 191–215.

20. Gary F. Render and David Lemire, "A Consciousness/Spirituality Domain Based on an Elaboration of Maslow's Hierarchy," *Holistic Education Review* (Summer 1989): 29–33.

21. National Center for Health Statistics, "Basic Data from the National Survey of Personal Health Practices and Consequences," in *Vital and Health Statistics* 15 no. 2, DHHS Pub. No. (PHS) 81-1163, Public Health Service, Washington, D.C., USGPO (August 1981).

22. Louis Harris, Louis Harris Poll, "Prevention Index" (1989).

23. George Gallup and Frank Newport, "1989 Gallup Leisure Audit," *Gallup Poll Monthly*, no. 295 (April 1990).

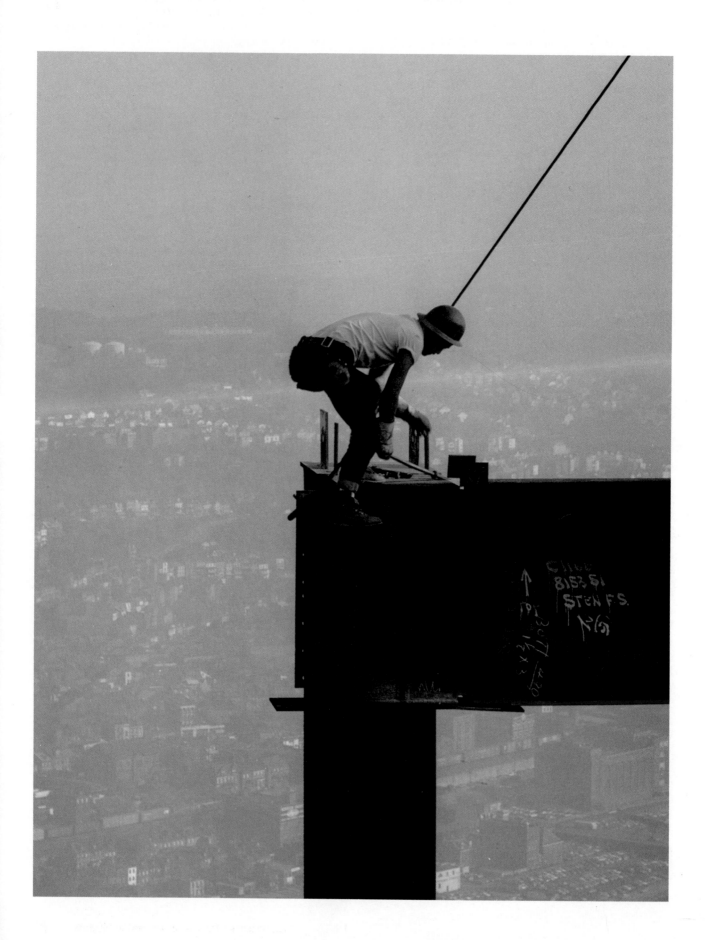

Chapter 2

Stress and Its Management

To Guide Your Reading

When you have studied this chapter, you should be able to:

- Define stress as the body's response to perceived challenges or stressors, some of which may give rise to considerable achievements, others to withdrawal and even ill health.

- Explain how the nervous system and chemicals in the bloodstream cause specific stress-related effects in the body that may lead to long-term damage if the stress is allowed to continue without relief.

- List some of the effects that stress can have on an individual's life, ranging from self-destructive behaviors such as excessive drinking to long-term damage to vital body systems.

- Describe different strategies that can be used to manage stress: ways to relax in the face of stress or to change one's perception of stressors; and approaches that give the body and mind greater resistance against stress in general.

Do you remember how you felt when you were about to speak before a group of people for the first time? No doubt your heart was racing and pounding, your breathing was rapid, and you felt nauseated or had an ache in your stomach. As you began to make your opening remarks, you found that your mouth was dry, your palms were sweating, and your hands were shaking. Anyone who has experienced sensations like these in response to a situation perceived as demanding or threatening has experienced stress.

Among the many influences that life and lifestyle exert on our health, stress is one of the most pervasive. People encounter a variety of stress-producing situations throughout their lives. For very young children, it may be the first time their parents leave them alone with a baby-sitter. For students, it may be the thought of impending exams or trying to combine studies with a job or other responsibilities. For employees, it may be the burden of a demanding, high-pressure job. For parents, it may be the demands of combining career and family or concerns about the welfare of their children. For older people, it may be the approach of retirement or moving to a new home.

Stress is a normal and necessary part of life from which people cannot escape. It can cause temporary discomfort and can also have long-term consequences. Yet while too much stress can threaten an individual's health and well-being, a certain amount of stress is needed to survive. Stress may result in a reduction of normal functioning or illness, but it can also help a person in danger and contribute to heightened achievement. Although some people feel burned out by stress, others respond to it positively. Studies of young animals have shown that some stress in infancy is necessary in the development of the processes of learning, sensing, and perception that equip the young animal with normal adaptive behavior patterns. Humans may need a moderate degree of stress for the same reason—both as children and as adults.[1]

The Nature of Stress

To some experts, stress is an event that produces tension or worry. Others regard stress as an individual's perception of an event—how a person interprets it in his or her mind. Most experts, however, define **stress** as the psychological and physiological response to any stimuli that an individual perceives as threatening, regardless of whether they are actually a threat.[2] Such threatening events or stimuli are called **stressors.**

People perceive situations very differently. One person may dread flying in an airplane (a stressor) because he or she perceives it as threatening. Another person, however, may look forward to flying because he or she enjoys it and is not afraid. A person's perception of a stimulus or event is often linked with thoughts and feelings that have been learned, often in childhood. For example, a student rejected by a graduate school may feel devastated because of subconscious associations with unhappy experiences of rejection during childhood. A student with less unpleasant experiences of rejection as a child may view the rejection as a challenge instead of as a failure. Although the stressor (rejection by the graduate school) is the same for both students, their perceptions and ultimately their responses to it are quite different.

The Sources of Stress

Burnout is the result of a high level of stress over a period of time. It is a state of physical and emotional exhaustion caused by stress from a person's job or other responsibilities.

Stress can be brought on by a wide variety of situations or events, ranging from the death of a spouse, parent, or child to a change in sleeping or eating habits. The amount of stress brought on by these stressors may vary a great deal, depending not only on an individual's perception but also on factors such as the type of stressor and its intensity and duration.

Types of Stressors Three general categories of stressors have been described. *Cataclysmic stressors* are sudden calamitous events, such as the earthquake centered near San Francisco, California, in October 1989. Such events often disrupt a person's life and may initially evoke a dazed response. Since cataclysmic events usually affect many people at the same time, large support networks tend to form to help people deal with stress. *Personal stressors* are events such as the death of a parent or the breakup of a marriage. Powerful enough to challenge a person's ability to adapt, these stressors affect individuals rather than groups. As a result, there are fewer and smaller support networks, if any, to help individuals deal with the stress. *Background stressors* are persistent, repetitive, almost routine events that are part of everyday lifestyle. Although less potent than cataclysmic or personal stressors, these daily hassles may pose an equally serious threat. For example, the cumulative pressures of dormitory living, a high-pressure job, or caring for young children or an aged parent may overtax a person's adaptive abilities.[3]

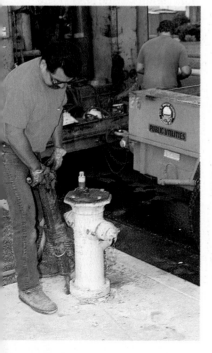

Job-related stress is as often generated by physical factors such as noise as it is by emotional ones. (Tony Freeman/ PhotoEdit)

Situational Stressors Cataclysmic stressors generally arise *outside* a person's normal life. Personal and background stressors, however, can arise from a variety of situations *within* a person's everyday life, including the physical environment, emotional conflicts, intellectual challenges, relationships with other people, and ethical or moral dilemmas.

Stressors that make people physically uncomfortable and force their bodies to adapt are called *physical stressors.* Loud noise, glaring lights, sickness, chronic headaches, and extremes of temperature and humidity are a few common examples. These and other physical stressors—such as jet lag, sunburn, and a lack of sleep—can hamper a person's performance and productivity as well as that person's health and well-being.

Disturbing or upsetting feelings and emotions are another source of stress. Such *emotional stressors,* including arguments with parents or loved ones, the beginning or ending of an intense love affair, and worry over a friend's ill-

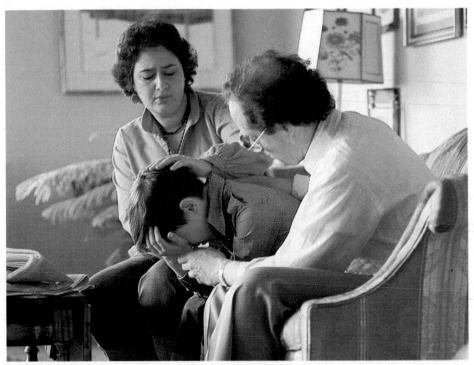

The trauma of a child's illness can cause as much emotional stress for parents as do problems in their own health. (Richard Hutchings/InfoEdit)

ness, can cause a great deal of emotional upset. Emotional stressors may even affect people's physical well-being by causing them to eat improperly, neglect their physical health, or behave in ways that can lead to injury.

Stressors that challenge the intellect or affect one's ability to think and reason are referred to as *intellectual stressors*. Studying for exams, taking difficult courses, calculating income tax, and making quick decisions in dangerous situations can all induce stress. Feelings of being overwhelmed by intellectual stressors often result when a person worries more about being unable to solve a problem than about how to solve it.

Demands placed on an individual by family members, friends, or other people are called *social stressors*. For example, a teacher or boss who will not or cannot communicate effectively with students or subordinates is a major source of stress for many people. It is very frustrating when the person in charge does not effectively explain to others what is expected of them. Social situations and family expectations can also be sources of stress.

Spiritual stressors are conflicts in personal, ethical, and moral beliefs. A person whose religious beliefs are challenged by new ideas may feel stress because of a conflict between what he or she has been taught to believe and the new ideas. For example, a person may have been raised to believe that premarital sex is wrong but later is persuaded to engage in it nonetheless. Philosophical issues that challenge individual beliefs, such as animal protection, euthanasia, abortion, apartheid, capital punishment, nuclear war, and pollution are significant spiritual stressors.

Threats to a person's basic beliefs are powerful stressors that can cause a great deal of inner conflict and uncertainty. The stress brought on by such stressors can be aggravated if a person feels pressured to hold on to old beliefs despite an inclination to consider change.

Pressures from parents and other adults to excel in school or sports can produce severe stress in children and young adults. So can excessive discipline and overpermissiveness.

Acute and Chronic Stressors

Several factors affect the impact that stressors have on an individual. One factor is the intensity of the stressor—whether it is mild or severe. Another is the stressor's duration—whether it occurs for a short or long period of time. Intense stimuli of relatively short duration are called *acute stressors*. Examples are the shock of a loud explosion and a fall off a ladder. Stimuli that tend to persist over an extended period are called *chronic stressors*; these stressors are often milder than acute stressors, but their effects may be quite severe.

The type of prolonged stress brought on by chronic stressors can be particularly injurious. Chronic stress often erodes an individual's ability to adapt and may lead to serious health problems. Although chronic stress may be difficult to manage, its effects can be reduced somewhat if a person has a strong social support network of people to rely on. Several studies have shown that these networks can help ameliorate unhealthy mental states such as depression and conditions associated with increased risk of illness such as elevated blood pressure and a high cholesterol level.[4]

Bad Stress versus Good Stress

Essentially, stress challenges a person's ability to adapt. Some people are able to adapt rather well; a stressor may encourage them to achieve more and can make their lives more interesting. Many people, for example, study and learn better under the stress of an impending exam. Getting married or leaving a job, although stressful, may lead to rewarding relationships and greater happiness.

Other people do not adapt well to stress, and this may result not only in poor performance and low productivity but also in illness. Employees who are continually overloaded with work or have too much responsibility not only may perform inadequately but may become ill or incapacitated. A person who is unable to deal with the death of a spouse may sink into depression, neglect work or other responsibilities, and do things that endanger his or her health.

The anticipation and excitement of the most joyful times in life can be major stressors. (Alan Oddie/PhotoEdit)

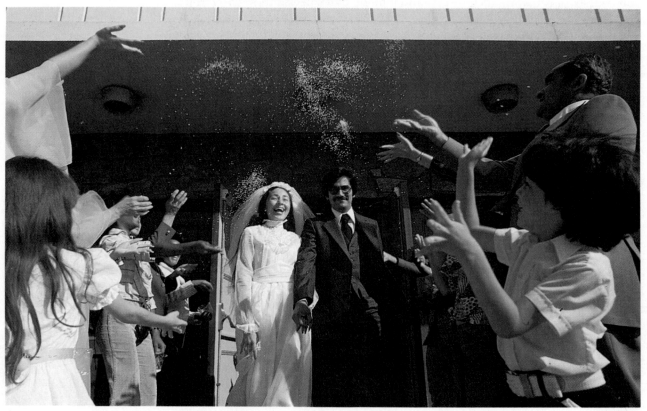

Stress can thus have either a positive or a negative effect and can act as either a helper or an inhibitor. Stress that has a positive effect—**eustress**—can help a person meet challenges more effectively. Stress that has a negative effect—**distress**—can take a heavy toll on the mind and body.

eustress—*stress that has a positive effect.*

distress—*stress that has a negative effect.*

Evaluating Stressors

Certain stressors have been shown to play a significant role in illness. In the early 1970s Thomas H. Holmes at the University of Washington in Seattle and Richard H. Rahe at the San Diego Naval Health Research Center attempted to quantify stressful major life events. The scale they developed—the Social Readjustment Rating Scale, or Holmes-Rahe scale—gives a numerical value to events in a person's life that have occurred within a given period of time. (See Self-Assessment feature for a version of this scale adapted to college-age people.) To determine his or her stress level for that period of time, a person could add up the number of life change units (LCUs) that correspond to the events listed on the scale. According to Holmes and Rahe, a high stress score—the result of several life changes within a relatively short time—indicates an increased susceptibility to illness.[5]

Until recently the Holmes-Rahe scale was widely used to assess the effects of stress on health. Recent research, however, has suggested that everyday stressors, or hassles, are more significant than are major life events.[6] Was it the stress of a final exam which made a student susceptible to the flu, or was it the cumulative everyday hassles of the working student's lifestyle in balancing job, family, and college responsibilities?

Studies contrasting life events and hassles have generally revealed that *hassles*—the persistent, repetitive, and almost routine events of everyday life—are better predictors of health outcomes than are major life events.[7] High on the "Hassle Scale" are such things as concern about weight, concern over the health of a family member, concern about rising prices, and having too much to do. These small daily worries seem to erode emotional and physical health more than major life events do. When such hassles are chronic and long-term, their effects on health are even more pronounced.[8]

The General Adaptation Syndrome

While the nature of stressors and a person's perception of them are important factors in stress, stress is also defined as a physiological response to a stressor. Pioneering stress researcher Hans Selye observed certain similarities in human physiological responses to stress. He determined that the body reacts to any stressor with the same series of responses: pale skin, rapid breathing, quickened heart rate, elevated blood pressure, and often extreme mental alertness, muscle tension, nausea, vomiting, and diarrhea. This is the body's way of mobilizing itself to do battle with stressors. Selye and other researchers identified a three-stage process the human body goes through in adapting to stress: the **general adaptation syndrome (GAS).**

The GAS begins with the *alarm stage,* in which physiological adjustments take place as the body reacts to a stressor. Next comes the *resistance stage,* in which the mind and body struggle to combat the stressor—to learn to live with it. Finally, if the stressor is not removed or if the individual is unable to overcome it, the body reaches the *stage of exhaustion:* the body's adaptation energy is used up, and the person or animal may actually die.[9]

general adaptation syndrome (GAS)—*a three-stage process the body goes through in adapting to stress. The three stages are alarm, resistance, and exhaustion.*

The importance of the GAS lies in its depiction of how stress can lead to physiological damage.[10] The body's ability to deal with stress is limited, and if it is not able to return to a state of balance, or homeostasis, the damaging effects of stress may accumulate, leading to uncomfortable symptoms (such as stomachaches) or disease (such as stomach ulcers).

How Stressed Are You?

Unless stressors are cataclysmic (for example, earthquakes and other major disasters), they come in two forms: basic hassles and major life changes. This stress quiz will help you look at both types of stressors in your life, identify areas where stress affects you the most, and decide whether you need to take steps to reduce your level of stress.

First, what is your HS (Hassle Score)? Though hassles are usually small, you may not have time to recover from one before the next one hits, and so your body stays revved up for action. How frequent and how severe on average are the following types of hassles in your life? Indicate low frequencies and low severities with a 1 in the appropriate column, and high frequencies and severities with a 5. Write 2, 3, or 4 to indicate gradations—3 would mean medium. (Use your own judgment to decide what is frequent and what is severe.)

	Frequency	+	Severity	=	HS
Schoolwork hassles (too much schoolwork, doing worse than expected, problems with a professor)	____	+	____	=	____
Job hassles (job is boring, boss or coworker problems, cannot find a job, work too demanding)	____	+	____	=	____
Money hassles (not enough money to stay in school, not enough money to have fun, not enough money for family/clothes/car, worry about debts)	____	+	____	=	____
Housing hassles (not enough room to live, noisy neighbors, place poorly kept up, bad neighborhood)	____	+	____	=	____
Family hassles (trouble with one or more close family members, difficulties between other members of family, family member has emotional or health problems)	____	+	____	=	____
Love life hassles (arguments with spouse or boyfriend/girlfriend, arguments with in-laws or loved one's family, cannot find right partner)	____	+	____	=	____
Other social hassles (no friends, difficulty with roommates, too many obligations, background of acquaintances too unlike that of own family)	____	+	____	=	____
Other chronic problems (continuous pain from injury or long-term illness, close friend or family member suffering from same, general fears about future)	____	+	____	=	____
Total:					____

Before Selye's research, stress was considered an emotional response only. Selye described a physiological component of stress.

When Selye proposed the GAS, he thought that the physiological reactions to stress are the same in all stressful situations. The body, in other words, does not differentiate between different kinds of stress. Instead, it responds with the GAS regardless of whether a stressor is "good" or "bad." Critics of Selye, however, contend that he failed to recognize that an individual's interpretation of an event may have much to do with whether that event is perceived as a threat. As pointed out earlier, some people may interpret the loss of a job as rejection and failure while others may view it as an opportunity to do something more challenging. Richard Lazarus and other researchers dispute Selye's contention that the stress response is automatic in a potentially stressful situation. Lazarus suggested that unless the person consciously views a situation as threatening, he or she will not experience stress.[11]

Now add up the frequency and severity scores for each type of hassle in the HS column and total these figures. This indicates the stress baseline of your overall lifestyle today.

Next, major life changes. Although these changes have generally been the focus of more research, they have recently been given less weight in overall accounts of chronic stress. On the following list of stressful life changes, circle the numbers beside any that have happened to you in the past 3 months; then sum the figures you have circled for your life change total.

(100) Death of spouse	(48) Lost financial support for college
(92) Female partner, unwed pregnancy	(47) Failed important course
(80) Death of parent	(45) Sexual difficulties
(77) Male partner, unwed pregnancy	(40) Serious problem with loved one
(73) Divorce	(39) Placed on academic probation
(70) Death of close family member	(37) Changed major
(65) Death of close friend	(36) New love interest
(63) Divorce of parents	(31) Increased work load at college
(61) Jail term	(29) Outstanding personal achievement
(60) Major personal illness or injury	(28) First months of freshman year
(58) Flunked out of college	(27) Serious conflict with instructor
(55) Marriage	(25) Lower grades than expected
(50) Fired from job	(24) Transferred to new college
___ (Subtotal)	___ (Subtotal)
	Total: ___

Interpreting Your Scores

If your hassles total is higher than 50, you should see whether you can lighten your basic level of stress, especially for the types of hassles for which your HS exceeded 6. If your life changes total is above 150, your stress level is excessive and could make you more vulnerable to illness unless you can find ways to adjust to stress. People with excessive scores on both halves of this quiz should definitely try some of the remedies for stress suggested in this chapter.

Based on ideas in T. H. Holmes and R. H. Rahe, "The Social Readjustment Rating Scale," *Journal of Psychometric Research* 2 (1967): 213–218; Nancy Burks and Barclay Martin, "Everyday Problems and Life Change Events: Ongoing versus Acute Sources of Stress," *Journal of Human Stress* (Spring 1985): 27–35. Reprinted with permission of Heldref Publications, Washington, DC.

The Stress Response

When a person reacts to a stressor, whether good or bad, an intricate physiological stress mechanism is set in motion that upsets the body's homeostatic balance. One of the earliest descriptions of this mechanism characterized stress as the body's reaction to a perceived threat and called it the fight-or-flight response.[12] This response can be visualized operating in the early days of the human race, when a typical stressor was the sight of an enemy or a menacing animal. Stress gears the body to defend itself by either fighting or fleeing the stressor. It may instead cause the body to freeze and be unable to move in any direction—even this would have been a successful outcome if the predator thought the individual was dead and left the person alone.

How the Stress Mechanism Works

When confronted by a stressor, a person must decide how to cope with it. In effect, the stressor represents a problem that must be solved. Some scientists believe that stress generates an increased blood flow to the parts of the brain that are crucial to problem-solving, or "coping," activities. The brain's arousal level increases, putting the rest of the body on red alert. Meanwhile, it also activates two interrelated physiological systems: the autonomic nervous system (ANS) and the endocrine system (Figure 2.1).

The Autonomic Nervous System The ANS is primarily concerned with controlling the inner workings of the body. It has two divisions: the sympathetic nervous system and the parasympathetic nervous system. In general, the sympathetic system arouses or mobilizes the body for action and the parasympathetic system reduces the level of output and conserves resources.

In highly emotional or stressful situations, the sympathetic system is activated and causes the following reactions: blood pressure rises, and the pulse quickens; blood races toward the brain and skeletal muscles for fast action; digestion slows so that energy can be devoted to combating the stressor; and the pupils enlarge to take in more information. These reactions help the individual cope with short-term stress, such as running to catch a plane and reacting to an immediate danger. Once the crisis has passed, the parasympathetic system—responsible for nonemergency functions such as digestion and respiration—takes over and helps return the body to homeostasis.

The Endocrine System A mechanism involving the endocrine system is also activated by stress, especially long-term stress. This system includes a collection of structures known as **endocrine glands,** which release a variety of chemical substances called **hormones** directly into the bloodstream. Hormones act as messengers within the body and help regulate the body's responses. They play an important role in many bodily functions in addition to the stress alert. The hormones that are secreted during stress tend to decrease urine output and raise the levels of certain chemical substances in the blood, including glucose, which helps produce energy. The two main types of stress-activated hormones are adrenal hormones and pituitary hormones.

One of the key glands in the stress-alert reaction is the *adrenal medulla*, the inner portion of the paired adrenal glands just above the kidneys. In response to a stress signal from the brain, the adrenal medulla secretes the hormones epinephrine (adrenaline) and norepinephrine (noradrenaline) into the bloodstream. These hormones are known as catecholamines. Norepinephrine increases the heart rate, constricts blood vessels, inhibits gastrointestinal activity, and speeds up a number of other bodily functions. Epinephrine produces similar effects, although it is more effective in stimulating the heart and less effective in constricting blood vessels.

At the same time the brain sends signals to the adrenal glands, it sends signals to the pituitary gland, a tiny "master control gland" at the base of the brain. In response, the pituitary gland secretes hormones that travel through the bloodstream to the adrenal, thyroid, and other glands. One of the most important pituitary hormones is adrenocorticotropic hormone (ACTH), which stimulates the outer portion (cortex) of the adrenal glands, causing the production of hormones called corticosteroids. Corticosteroids are very different from catecholamines, although they also appear to be involved in stress responses. There are two basic forms of corticosteroids: the glucosteroids, which help regulate glucose levels in the blood, and the mineralocorticoids, which affect the utilization of mineral substances and regulate electrolytes in the blood. Studies have found high corticosteroid levels in men who were starting underwater demolition training or jumping out of helicopters into the ocean and in people who were going through periods of anguish and anger over personal disappointments and changes in their work.[13]

endocrine glands— *structures that produce and secrete hormones directly into the bloodstream (ductless glands).*

hormones—*chemical substances that act as messengers within the body to help regulate many bodily functions.*

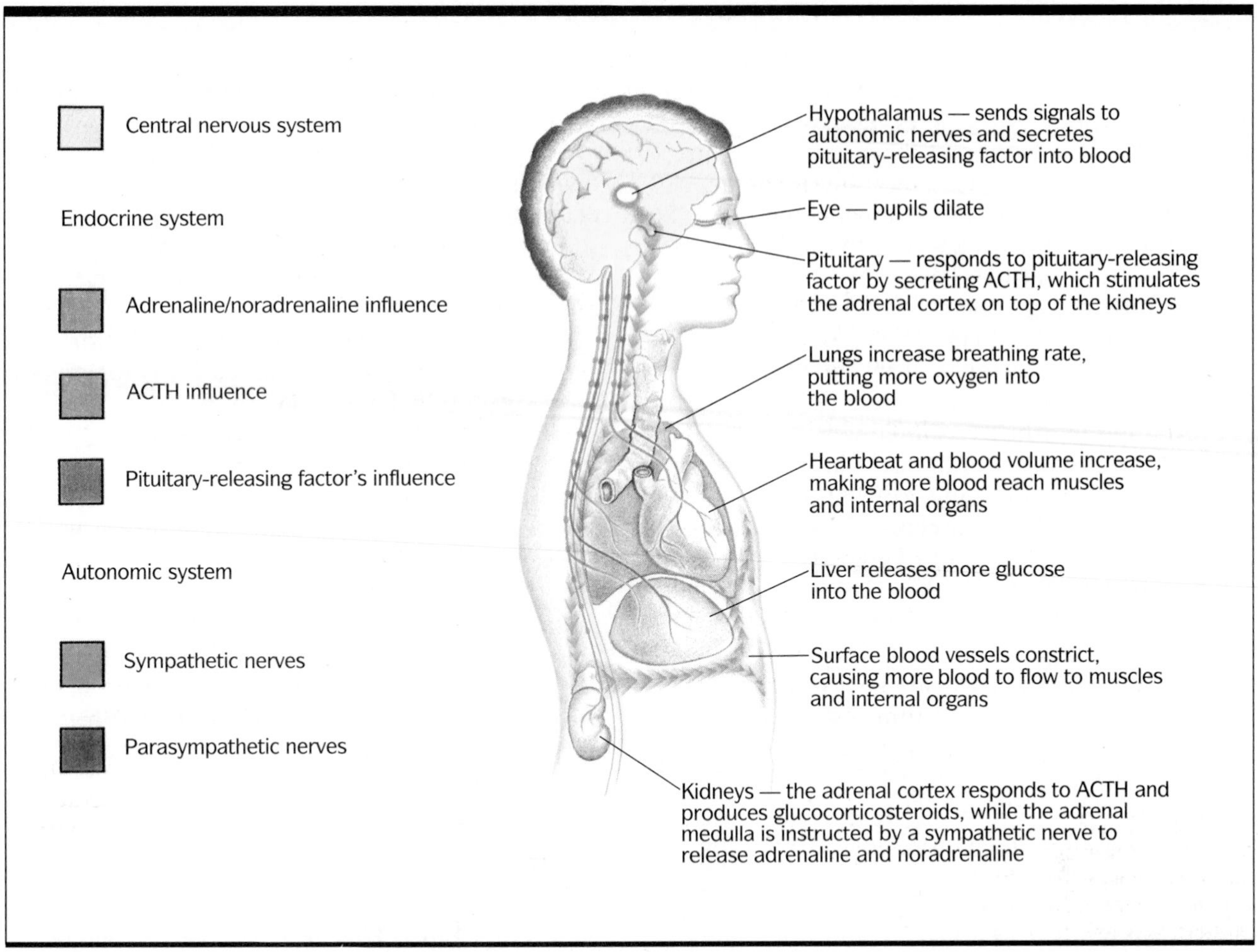

Central nervous system
Endocrine system
Adrenaline/noradrenaline influence
ACTH influence
Pituitary-releasing factor's influence
Autonomic system
Sympathetic nerves
Parasympathetic nerves
Hypothalamus — sends signals to autonomic nerves and secretes pituitary-releasing factor into blood
Eye — pupils dilate
Pituitary — responds to pituitary-releasing factor by secreting ACTH, which stimulates the adrenal cortex on top of the kidneys
Lungs increase breathing rate, putting more oxygen into the blood
Heartbeat and blood volume increase, making more blood reach muscles and internal organs
Liver releases more glucose into the blood
Surface blood vessels constrict, causing more blood to flow to muscles and internal organs
Kidneys — the adrenal cortex responds to ACTH and produces glucocorticosteroids, while the adrenal medulla is instructed by a sympathetic nerve to release adrenaline and noradrenaline

Figure 2.1 Stress activates the endocrine system to increase its output of both adrenal and pituitary hormones. It also works directly through the autonomic nervous system. Both processes prepare the body for emergency action.

The Stress Mechanism's Effects on the Body

The fight-or-flight response is useful if a physical reaction such as dodging a speeding car is called for or if a person has to meet a short-term psychological challenge such as giving a speech or taking an exam. The body is equipped to handle such stress without damage *if* it is able to relax after its physical resources have been mobilized to take short-term action. After the stressful situation has passed, the body must have a chance to regain its original homeostasis, returning to a normal blood pressure and normal hormone levels.

Trouble arises when one arousal reaction is piled on top of another and the body does not get a chance to return to normal. Today people are continually bombarded with a host of different stressors, from physical disease to emotional distress to value conflicts. As a result, the body is often unable to return to normal. Thus, stress tends to build up and disrupt the body's functioning, particularly through the action of hormones released under stress. Epinephrine, for example, may keep the muscles tense and the blood pressure and heart rate high for several days or even longer. It also may interfere with the immune system, lowering a person's resistance to disease. As a result, a person may develop one or more of many different, sometimes subtle symptoms without being aware of the degree of stress he or she is under.

The Role of Personality

Personality is often a mediating factor in the way people respond to stress and therefore affects the impact of stress on the body. Some people seem to invite disproportionate amounts of stress into their lives. Everyone has seen people like this, impatiently blowing their car horns, glancing nervously at their

Coping with Type A Behavior

Whenever I was angry at my job, people down the hall could hear me voicing displeasure. Anger, aggravation, and impatience could have been my middle names. Before anyone could finish a sentence, I completed it for them. Then I would continue with a defense of my unshakable opinion. I talked, walked, ate, and did everything in a hurry, sometimes simultaneously. I was the classic Type A personality: hard-driving, constantly on the go, extremely time-conscious, uptight when my environment got out of control.

Somewhere in the back of my mind I knew that I should lighten up. My father had died of a heart attack when I was very young. Already I had angina pains in my chest. But I was a go-getter who got things done. It was easy to deny that anything could go wrong when I had so much going for me. Then I suffered a heart attack.

It took a life-threatening illness to jolt me into recognizing an important reality: I really am mortal. Like so many others, I began to evaluate my life. My body would no longer support my frantic lifestyle and the resulting stress. I had to make changes and choices. As I recovered from the heart attack, I asked myself some important questions: What are my values? What do I really want from life?

I knew that my work was important to me. It gives me a great deal of satisfaction. For me, cutting back too much would be more stressful than working. Being in my own work environment, doing what I love, makes me feel good. I was a workaholic, wondering whether I could change—and not wanting to change too much.

But I did make some major alterations in my life. I quit smoking, learned to make healthier diet choices, and started exercising regularly. I cut back my work hours, too, although this wasn't easy because people still expected me to work every minute. However, I managed to hold my ground. When people tried to push me around, I told them to back off. So while I kept the same job, I did improve my lifestyle and lessen my level of stress.

Once I started playing a major role in my own health, it made me feel more in control of my life. It was easier to say no to stressful situations and yes to healthier lifestyle decisions. I knew I was making a difference in my own health.

I talked these choices out with my doctor, and he understands how difficult it is for me to modify my behavior. As he said, "If you take the honest-to-God Type A and try to turn him into anything else, you'll have a very unhappy person." Even my doctor realizes that there are limits to how much you can get people to change.

For example, I tried very hard to stay calm in stressful situations in the months after the heart attack. Then one morning, there I was caught in traffic, banging on the steering wheel—which I swore I'd never do. So despite many changes, I'm still the same person.

But I've made progress. I realized this clearly recently when a teenager crunched along the passenger side of my car. The damage was awful—rear light destroyed, side bent and scraped bare of paint, and a hole in the door. Can you imagine how I would have reacted before my operation? I felt like exploding in just the same way. But I thought, "What's a hole in the door compared to heart surgery?" Even though I still get mad easily, I've got a whole new perspective. I don't sound off like I usually would.

Another good sign is that people who have always been important in my life have begun to take on new meaning. I started to realize the importance of caring and being cared about. Others in my position describe their change of heart as taking time to smell the roses. It's true, I did begin to appreciate things and people more. And I also gained a better realization of me, what I'm like and how I operate.

From *Mr. King, You're Having a Heart Attack* by Larry King and B. D. Colen. Copyright © 1989 by Larry King. Used by permission of Dell Books, a division of Bantam Doubleday Dell Publishing Group, Inc.

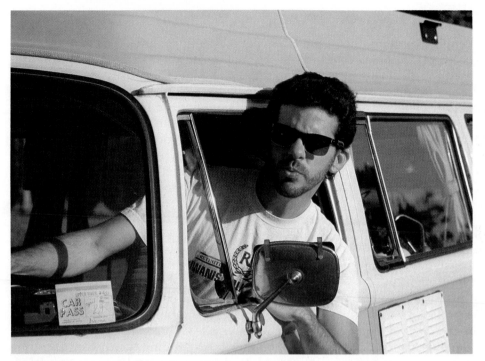

The Type A personality frequently appears to be aggressive and impatient at seemingly minor delays but often chooses occupations and schedules in which such delays are routine. (Tony Freeman/PhotoEdit)

watches all the time, consistently working 18 hours a day, or aggressively competing in everything they do. People who behave this way are exhibiting Type A behavior, a pattern of behavior characterized by impatience, competitiveness, and a work-against-the-clock style. Such people seek to control their environment through verbal aggression; when their control is threatened, they often overreact to a situation.[14] In contrast, a person who exhibits Type B behavior is generally low-key, contemplative, and relaxed.

In many ways Type A behavior resembles the traditional goal-directed orientation so common in American society. If kept within limits, such behavior may be viewed as adaptive; many success-oriented middle-class college students are competitive and show other Type A behavior patterns.[15] In excess, however, Type A behavior has been linked to high levels of stress and thus may lead to health-related problems. In one study of women those with Type A behavior were found to be four times more likely to have heart disease than were their Type B counterparts.[16] In another study it was found that people exhibiting Type A behavior are more likely to suffer from minor illnesses and have more severe symptoms than are those who are more relaxed.[17]

Not all stress experts agree that Type A and Type B behavior patterns by themselves can be linked with the presence or absence of health-related problems. These experts identify another personality disposition, called hardiness, which may act as a mitigating factor.[18] Hardy individuals show three basic personality dispositions: they tend to become deeply involved in what they are doing, usually act in the belief that their work will make a difference, and view the majority of life changes as normal and beneficial for personal growth.[19]

Because of their greater feeling of self-efficacy, people with hardy personalities seem able to withstand the impact of stress.[20] Some researchers also contend that hardiness acts as a buffer against illness. Personality hardiness appears to be related to lower blood pressure, lower levels of serum triglycerides (fatty acids) in the blood, less psychological distress, increased happiness, and even happier marriages.[21]

A person with Type A behavior may

- *Be very competitive*
- *Always seem in a hurry*
- *Demand perfection*
- *Be ambitious*
- *Try to do many things at once*
- *Be impatient*
- *Be hard-driving*
- *Overreact*
- *Never be late*
- *Have few interests outside work*
- *Be aggressive*

A person with Type B behavior may

- *Seem relaxed*
- *Be noncompetitive*
- *Be easygoing*
- *Enjoy leisure time*
- *Take things one at a time*
- *Have many interests*
- *Be low-key*
- *Be contemplative*

Many people, of course, display both types of behavior. They have been called "AB personalities."

The Impact of Stress

People may think they are adapting successfully to stress, but in resisting or becoming acclimated to a stressor, they are often unaware of the compromises and adjustments they are actually making. They may not consciously recognize the stress generated by situations such as being late for an important meeting, doing heavy physical labor in extreme heat, and carrying on a frustrating romantic relationship. They may think that they have become accustomed to poor eyesight, insufficient light, loud noise, or continuing family conflict.

In the short term stress can have a detrimental effect on a person's behavior, resulting in an inability to function normally or act in ways that promote good health. In the long term stress may have a serious effect on a person's vulnerability to illness and disease. In either case the impact of stress can be felt not only by the individual but by society as a whole.

Stress and Behavior

Drug abuse can be either a cause or an effect of stress.

Alcohol abuse, drug abuse, smoking, overeating, and lack of exercise—behaviors that raise health care costs— are linked to stress.

Stress can have an impact on a person's behavior in a variety of ways. As was mentioned earlier, stress can affect the way a person deals with disease and responds to discomfort. Stress may also make a person irritable, withdrawn, cautious, energetic, outgoing, or optimistic, depending on whether the stress is perceived as positive or negative. While eustress can have a beneficial effect, distress can be detrimental if it leads to maladaptive behaviors such as drug abuse and under- or overeating or to behaviors that can lead to injury. These and similar behaviors represent negative ways of coping with stress.

Many people turn to drugs, including tobacco, alcohol, and illegal substances, to relieve stress. For example, adolescents who are under a great deal of pressure and cannot cope with it effectively have been shown to abuse drugs. One study linked cigarette smoking to adolescents who experience stress as a result of a stressful major life event. The same study also found a relationship between heavy alcohol use among adolescents and subjective stress—an event or stressor that people perceive as stressful.[22]

Stress does not necessarily lead to abuse, however. It used to be argued that there is a link between stress and the onset of or an increase in drinking

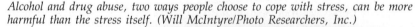

Alcohol and drug abuse, two ways people choose to cope with stress, can be more harmful than the stress itself. (Will McIntyre/Photo Researchers, Inc.)

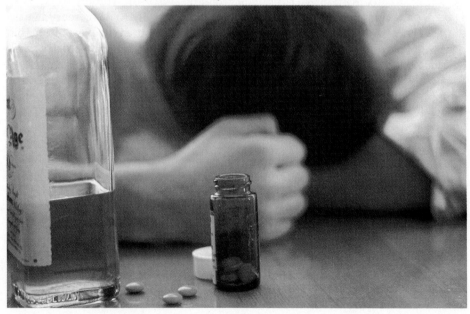

among the elderly. Drinking was considered a reaction to or a means of coping with stressful major life events typical of that age group, such as retirement or the death of a spouse. Recent research, however, has suggested that elderly persons who are generally successful at coping do not resort to such escapist strategies for dealing with stress[23] (Chapters 13, 14, and 15).

Stress may also affect a person's eating behaviors. Some people tend to eat less when they feel stressed, while others eat more. In the short term this may not be a problem, but chronic stress can contribute to weight problems and problems associated with poor diet and nutrition (Chapter 5). Research has shown that some foods trigger the production of natural painkillers (called *endorphins*) in the brain that ease stress and discomfort. Researchers have noted that the more stress a person is under, the higher the endorphin level in the blood. While the nature of these connections is unclear, it is interesting to examine the possible links between endorphins, a craving for certain foods, and eating disorders.[24]

Stress may also affect behavior in ways that can increase the risk of suffering an injury. For example, if stress leads to depression, lack of concentration, disregard for personal safety, or feelings of a lack of control, a person may behave in ways that can lead to injury. A person's driving ability may be impaired if that person is under severe stress. Similarly, a lack of concentration may be dangerous if it causes a person to disregard risk factors (unsafe conditions, potentially dangerous situations, and so on) within his or her environment.

Suicidal behavior may also be linked to stress. Researchers at the New York Psychiatric Institute have concluded that most suicides in young people are precipitated by stressful events such as getting into trouble with the law, breaking up with a girlfriend or boyfriend, and problems at home or school.[25]

Stress and Disease

If an individual already has a disease such as heart disease or diabetes, the increased muscle tension and elevated blood sugar caused by the stress response can aggravate the condition. Research has shown that prolonged stress may also be linked to the onset of illness and disease.[26] The degree to which stress contributes to the development of disease and the specific diseases it can contribute to are still unclear; researchers continue to study these questions.[27]

While research has demonstrated a strong correlation between stress and certain physical and psychological responses, it has not yet proved a direct cause-and-effect relationship. Thus, it cannot be concluded that stress in itself actually causes any specific disease. There is growing evidence, however, that stress can depress the ability of the immune system to fight diseases such as viral infections, autoimmune diseases (disorders in which the immune system seems to go out of control and attack body tissues), and some forms of cancer.[28] Furthermore, it is known that stress may affect the way in which people deal with disease, such as making them slower or faster in recognizing that something is wrong or altering the way they react to discomfort. With these cautions in mind, consider some of the connections between stress and diseases that have been suggested.

Hypertension Since an individual's blood pressure rises temporarily in reaction to a stressor, researchers have come to suspect a possible connection between stress and hypertension. Chronic hypertension—a condition of sustained abnormally high blood pressure that can be a forerunner of cardiovascular disease—is believed to be stress-related. A number of studies have revealed that people who work under great psychological pressure (such as airplane pilots) and those who are subjected to sustained environmental stress (such as people who work in places with high noise levels) are more

Emotional reactions to stress:

- *Nervousness*
- *Anger*
- *Anxiety*
- *Excitement*
- *Lack of concentration*
- *Fear*
- *Irritability*
- *Mild depression*
- *Withdrawal*
- *Alcohol or drug abuse*
- *Overeating*
- *Loss of appetite*
- *Hurrying*
- *Crying*
- *Sexual dysfunctions and disorders*

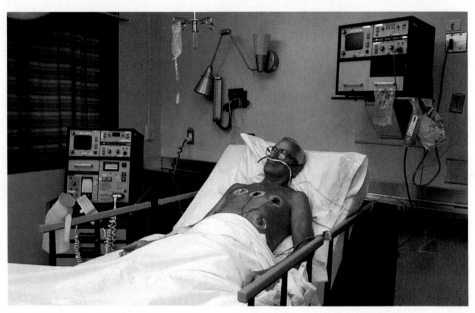

Chronic stress is a hidden factor which can cause major illness later in life. (Stan Levy/Photo Researchers, Inc.)

likely to develop high blood pressure than are people who live and work in a less tension-filled atmosphere.[29]

Once again it should be remembered that perception plays an important role in stress. One study of a group of people with hypertension found that they subjectively rated their stress levels as high during the period preceding illness. The researchers concluded that a person's subjective rating of overall stress may be more meaningful than an objective measure of actual events.[30]

Heart Disease Many researchers consider stress to be a contributing factor in heart disease. A Duke University study found links between heart disease and certain Type A behaviors that already were associated with high levels of stress. According to the study, a coronary-prone personality is one who mistrusts the motives of others, feels anger frequently, and aggressively expresses hostility toward others with no regard for their feelings.[31]

Other researchers, however, are not convinced that there is a link between Type A behavior and heart disease. One study suggests that the risk factors for heart disease seem to relate not to Type A behavior and aggression but to emotional problems such as an inability to perceive and verbalize negative emotions (expressing anger, for example) and to cope effectively.[32] At this point the consensus seems to be that although stress may be a secondary factor in the incidence of heart disease, it should not be considered a primary factor.

Cancer The role of stress in the development of cancer is much debated. Nevertheless, there are indications that tensions may play a role in the onset of cancer in certain individuals who, because of genetic, constitutional, and environmental factors, may be predisposed to contract the disease. Although the National Cancer Institute (NCI) states that there is as yet "no convincing evidence that certain emotions or personality traits might increase a person's risk for cancer," it adds that the possibility of such a relationship is still under study.[33] In contrast, researchers at the Memorial Sloan-Kettering Cancer Center in New York City have concluded that psychological states and traits can affect the transformation of normal cells into cancer cells. They have identified three types of psychosocial risk factors: stress, personality traits (or coping styles), and personal habits (for example, smoking).[34]

Physical conditions linked to stress:

- *Fatigue*
- *Frequent colds*
- *Sleep disturbances*
- *Shortness of breath*
- *Tension headaches*
- *Migraine headaches*
- *Cold hands or feet*
- *Aching neck and shoulder muscles*
- *Indigestion*
- *Menstrual problems*
- *Nausea or vomiting*
- *Diarrhea*
- *Ulcers*
- *Heart palpitations*
- *Constipation*
- *Lower back pain*
- *Allergy or asthma attacks*
- *Alcoholism or drug addiction*
- *Colitis*
- *Hypertension*
- *Diabetes*
- *Cancer*

It is somewhat more widely accepted that once an individual is diagnosed as having cancer, his or her emotional state will be one of the factors that determine the success of treatment. The medical annals are full of reports of patients who believed they would get well again or discovered something to live for and went into *remission* (a state in which the disease's symptoms disappear) or recovered completely. Conversely, severe emotional traumas have been associated with the reappearance of cancer in certain patients who had been in remission.[35]

Infectious Disease and the Immune System By altering the body's hormonal and nervous systems, persistent stress somehow creates a fertile climate for disease—researchers do not know exactly how. Stress can have direct effect on the immune system—the group of mechanisms in the body that work together to fight infection—by reducing its ability to function effectively.[36] Stress can also act indirectly on the body's resistance to infection if it causes a person to eat poorly, neglect exercise, lose sleep, smoke or drink too much, or behave in other ways that may be injurious to health.

Many people who experience long-term psychological distress as a result of stressful life events (such as those on the Holmes-Rahe scale) appear to have adverse immunologic changes that can lead to infections as well as malignant disease. Indeed, several human and animal studies have suggested a relationship between exposure to stress and an impaired immunologic system.[37] Whether someone actually does become ill, however, also depends on the harmful agents to which he or she has been exposed and the health of the person prior to the stressful life event.[38]

The NCI recognizes certain links between emotions and the endocrine and immune systems. At present, the NCI believes that stress activates the endocrine system, which in turn can cause changes in the body's immune response.[39] Reaction to stress has been associated with an increase in the secretion of cortisol (like the corticosteroids, a hormone produced in the adrenal cortex). Cortisol increases the sugar content of the blood in order to meet the energy demands of the fight-or-flight response, but it also decreases the number of T lymphocytes, which are key white blood cells that help fight invading microorganisms. The result is a compromised immune system[40] (Chapter 10).

Diabetes and Peptic Ulcers Both diabetes and peptic ulcers have been linked more directly with stress.[41] In the case of diabetes, when stress increases the secretion of cortisol, causing the glucose (sugar) level of the blood to increase, cells in the pancreas called beta cells react by producing insulin, a hormone that helps regulate blood sugar levels. Chronic stress can exhaust these cells, which cannot be replaced, seriously diminishing the ability of the pancreas to make the insulin needed to control the blood sugar level. The result is a higher risk for the onset of diabetes, especially among individuals who have a genetic predisposition for the disease.

A peptic ulcer is a sore in the lining of the stomach that is thought to be caused by excessive secretion of gastric acid (a digestive aid). A peptic ulcer often produces severe stomach pain and can cause internal bleeding if it perforates the stomach wall. Although the cause of peptic ulcers is not known, it is generally accepted that stress can aggravate the condition.[42]

Asthma and Allergies Since stress affects the body's immunologic response, it has been linked to asthma and other allergies, such as hay fever. These conditions often result from the reaction of the body's immune system to an invader. The invading organism causes a chain of events in which the body produces substances called antibodies. The antibodies in turn stimulate the release of chemicals that cause physiological changes, many of which may be more irritating and harmful than the original invader.

For example, the chemical histamine will cause the mucous membranes of the bronchial tubes to swell; this constricts those air passages and impedes the flow of air to the lungs, making it difficult to breathe. On occasion, this condition has resulted in death.[43]

Skin Disorders Stress is believed to aggravate several skin conditions, the most severe of which is eczema, an inflammatory condition characterized by redness, itching, and oozing lesions that become scaly, crusted, or hardened. Eczema tends to recur and persist for months or even years. Many physicians have found that when stress is reduced in a person's life, eczema and other skin disorders often improve.[44]

Mental Disorders Stress causes emotional upset, which can aggravate an existing emotional disturbance. It is difficult to ascertain, however, the role stress plays in causing emotional and mental disorders (Chapter 3).

Mental health practitioners have developed a number of theories about the possible relationship between stress and mental dysfunction, and studies have noted a high incidence of stressful major life events shortly before the onset of schizophrenia, depression, and nonpsychotic disorders. According to one theory, some individuals are born with a predisposition to mental disorders, which may surface under unusual stress.[45]

The Economic and Social Costs of Stress

In addition to its potential effects on the health and well-being of individuals, stress has economic and societal impacts. Stress can lower job performance and productivity and thus affect the economic well-being of businesses and, ultimately, the economy as a whole. It may also contribute to societal tensions that manifest themselves in frustrations toward leaders and other authorities as well as impatience toward and intolerance of others.

Economic Cost Occupational, or job-related, stress is an increasingly common complaint in the United States. Its causes include having little input in decision making, doing too much or too little work, unclear work objectives, and facing conflicting demands.[46]

The top causes of workplace stress: work overload, lack of recognition, unpleasant work environment, insufficient pay, unclear communication, and limited growth opportunities.

It has been estimated that job-related stress costs American industry about $150 billion a year. On any given workday, an average of a million workers are absent from their jobs because of such stress-related disorders as backaches, headaches, ulcers, insomnia, anxiety, depression, heart problems, hypertension, and gastrointestinal complaints. Surveys by the U.S. Department of Health and Human Services have suggested that stress accounts for 11 percent of occupational disease claims, 85 percent of industrial accidents, and 75 to 90 percent of visits to primary-care physicians.[47] Courts throughout the United States are struggling with worker's compensation claims that invoke injury as a result of stress; such claims have proliferated during the past 15 years.[48]

Particularly troublesome in today's workplace is *job burnout,* a syndrome characterized by physiological and emotional exhaustion and often caused by chronic frustration with a job coupled with having too much work to do. The symptoms include increased use of drugs and alcohol; depression, low self-esteem, pessimism, and loneliness; increased lateness and absenteeism; fatigue, irritability, muscle tension, and stomach complaints; and a loss of one's sense of humor and an increase in feelings of guilt.[49]

Job-related stress is not necessarily bad. If the tension and stress associated with a job are used constructively, the businesses and individuals involved can benefit. Some job-related stress can stimulate creative thinking, enhance performance, and increase productivity. Few companies, however, attempt to harness job-related stress in this way.[50]

Social Cost Stress may have not only an economic cost but a social cost as well. American society contains a diversity of individuals and groups of people whose needs and wants, attitudes, beliefs, and ways of living differ and sometimes compete. The society's stability depends in part on maintaining an acceptable equilibrium among these groups. Stress, however, may upset this balance. People under stress sometimes take out their frustrations on others, and their impatience and anger may contribute to greater intolerance of the ideas, attitudes, and behaviors of people different from themselves. Stress may also make them less willing to consider the needs and wants of others if those needs and wants compete with their own. If stress becomes chronic, these effects may harm the delicate fabric of society, leading to greater disharmony among people and increased frustration at the nation's authorities and institutions.

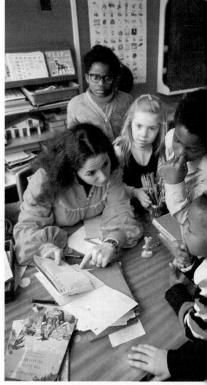

Many different occupations can lead to job burnout. The stress caused by a class of primary school students can be as great as the stress from making million-dollar business decisions. (John Moss/The Stock Shop)

Managing Stress

Stress is an inevitable part of people's lives. In the short term it can make life unpleasant and difficult; in the long term it can lead to a variety of stress-related illnesses. Rather than blaming stress itself for such problems, however, it is more accurate to say that the fault lies with a person's inability to cope with and manage stress. Learning to manage stress effectively is therefore the best defense against the discomfort or harm it can cause.

Some of the ways in which people attempt to manage stress—using alcohol and drugs, for example—not only are potentially dangerous but usually offer only a temporary escape from stress and often take away a person's sense of control. There are other, more healthful ways of relieving stress that are longer-lasting and reinforce an individual's sense of self-efficacy.

Keep in mind that the objective is not to eliminate all stress from your life. Stress, after all, not only is inevitable but also may be beneficial in some instances. Rather, you should try to evaluate the nature of stress in your life, determine your personal comfort level where stress is concerned, use eustressors to enhance the quality of your life, and attempt to reduce the negative effects of the distressors you experience.

A number of stress management techniques may prove beneficial in your attempts to cope with stress. They range from various relaxation techniques to psychological approaches to changes in attitude and behavior.

Stress can and should be managed, but it is incorrect to believe it can always be avoided. Avoiding stressful events can cause one to miss many opportunities to challenge and enrich one's life.

Relaxation Techniques

Relaxation involves more than just reducing tension. It is a positive and satisfying feeling of peace of mind and simply of being.[51] Studies have shown that relaxation results in reductions in anxiety, improved adjustment, and lower levels of psychophysiological arousal.[52] A person can achieve a state of relaxation through the use of various techniques, including progressive relaxation, meditation, autogenic training, and biofeedback.

Progressive Relaxation More than 50 years ago, long before the scientific study of stress, Edmond Jacobson, a physiologist, developed a technique he called **progressive relaxation** for relieving muscle tension. This technique requires that the individual deliberately tense and then relax his or her muscles in order to learn the sensations of tensing and letting go. It is "progressive" because it moves through the various muscle groups in the body—from the hands and arms to the head, eyes, mouth, neck, shoulders, back, chest, abdomen, buttocks, thighs, calves, and feet. Jacobson extended his system to exercises for mental relaxation as well: the individual alternately imagines sensory experiences—sights, sounds, smells, shapes, and tactile sensations—and then lets go of the images.[53]

progressive relaxation—*a technique for relieving muscle tension in which the individual tenses and relaxes various muscle groups in turn.*

Coping with Stress

Stress is a part of everyone's life, yet there are many different ways to view stressors and their effect on a healthy lifestyle. Health experts agree that a person's attitude toward stressful events has an effect on how that person will react. Two ways of coping with stress are discussed below. The first point of view suggests making lifestyle changes to avoid some stressors and lessen the effect of others. The second point of view recommends viewing stress as a source of energy that can be channeled to enhance a person's life and help a person accomplish individual goals.

Find Ways to Avoid or Reduce the Effects of Stress High levels of stress have been correlated with health problems. Stress has been suspected as a contributing factor in such illnesses as high blood pressure, heart disease, and ulcers. Too much stress may also compromise the immune system and make a person more susceptible to infection.

Coping with stress successfully means avoiding the damaging effects of stressors in one's life. One way to do this is to discover how certain stressors can be avoided. Suppose a student knows that sitting in traffic on his route to school makes him tense and irritable. Perhaps he can avoid this daily

traffic problem by finding an alternative route to school that utilizes less congested highways. Maybe he can wake up a half hour earlier and avoid the rush hour altogether. An elementary school teacher may feel that large class sizes and lack of preparation time at her school are causing stress. Discussing these pressures with her colleagues and principal may help her. She may want to consider another teaching position that better meets her needs and goals.

If stressors cannot be avoided, it is possible to lessen their negative effects by making other changes in one's life. Plenty of sleep and regular exercise are important. Eating a balanced diet and cutting down on alcohol and caffeine may also help. Many people find that meditative and relaxation techniques help counteract the effects of stress. A network of positive relationships can also provide support and encouragement.

Overall, there are many ways to alleviate the stresses of modern life. Individuals must identify the causes of stress and find ways to avoid or reduce it.

Make Stress Work for You Certain self-defense techniques are based on using an

---

Meditation Meditation is not a single, easily defined technique; rather, it encompasses a variety of diverse methods. The aim of the different meditative techniques, however, is the same: to focus attention on an image or thought with the goal of clearing one's mind and producing inner peace. Effective meditation produces a state of deep physiological and mental repose by reducing blood pressure, muscle tension, the pulse rate, and the level of stress hormones in the blood.

One well-known meditation method, developed by Dr. Herbert Benson of Harvard University, is called the **relaxation response.** Practicing this method for at least 20 minutes daily is said to increase the alpha brain waves associated with relaxation and well-being. The relaxation response can also help lower blood pressure in people with hypertension and discourage body tissues from responding to stress hormones as strongly as they would otherwise.[54] This method involves the following steps:

relaxation response—*a method of stress management similar to meditation; involves muscular relaxation and conscious breathing.*

- Sit quietly in a comfortable position and close your eyes.
- Deeply relax all your muscles, beginning at the feet and progressing up to the face. Keep them relaxed.
- Breathe easily and naturally through your nose. Become aware of your breathing. As you breathe out, say the word *one* silently to yourself.
- Continue for 10 to 20 minutes. You may open your eyes to check the time, but do not use an alarm. When you finish, sit quietly for several minutes,

attacker's own energy against him or her. The force designed to throw a victim to the ground can also be used to throw the attacker off balance. This can be a valuable image for coping with sources of stress. Most people think of stress as a negative, damaging thing: high levels make people unhappy and tense and may even cause illness. Yet there is another way of looking at stress—as a form of energy.

Looked at in this way, stress is a challenge to be managed and used to enhance one's life. Dr. Robert Ritvo, dean of the University of New Hampshire's School of Health and Human Services, points out that stress can drive people to reach their goals. Dr. Peter G. Hanson notes that "students maximize their learning curves with the stress of an upcoming exam. Athletes set world records only with the stress of stiff competition."

In other words, stress can make people perform better. The key lies in a person's attitude toward stressful events. Is a demanding professor only a source of extra work in a busy semester? Or can the professor's teaching style provide an opportunity to gain knowledge and improve one's skills? Is the end of a romantic relationship merely a loss? Or is it an opportunity to examine one's values and renew relationships that may have been neglected?

Stress can have its most devastating consequences when a person feels a sense of helplessness. Instead of identifying sources of stress as problems, individuals should strive to see them as challenges to be met. Finding ways to use stress to one's advantage gives a person more control over stressful situations, and this success boosts self-esteem and helps the individual face life's events with courage and confidence.

Which method do you think is better for handling stressful situations? List some current sources of stress in your life and decide how you might resolve them. Would you try to reduce or avoid the stressor, or could you use the stress to your advantage? Do you think that one of the strategies discussed above might work more successfully than the other for certain individuals or under different conditions? Why?

Based on ideas in Paul Martin, "The Power of Positive Stress," *Better Homes and Gardens,* March 1990 and in Peter G. Hanson, *Stress for Success* (New York: Doubleday, 1989).

at first with your eyes closed and later with your eyes open. Wait several minutes before standing up.

- Do not worry about whether you are successful in achieving a deep level of relaxation. Maintain a passive attitude and permit relaxation to occur at its own pace. When distracting thoughts occur, try to ignore them by not dwelling on them, and return to repeating *one*. With practice, the response should come with little effort.
- It is recommended that this be done twice a day, but not within 2 hours after any meal (an active digestive system interferes with meditation).

Autogenic Training **Autogenic training** is based on the premise that the mind can compel the body to relax and return to a homeostatic balance by consciously focusing on sensations such as heaviness and warmth. A key principle of autogenic training is that the body will naturally balance itself when it is directed into a relaxed state. With practice, a person can learn to induce this relaxed state when necessary. Autogenic training has been shown to be effective in medical case studies of people with peptic ulcers, high blood pressure, migraine headaches, asthma, sleep disturbances, and other conditions.[55] The typical instructions for performing autogenic imagery are as follows:[56]

autogenic training—*a method of self-induced relaxation in which the person imagines certain relaxing sensations.*

- Begin the exercise in a comfortable and relaxed sitting or reclining position with your eyes closed. Distractions should be kept to a minimum.

Table 2.1   Other Stress Management Techniques

There are a number of other things people can do to manage and alleviate stress.

Do not overload your schedule with too many things to do; students, for example, should avoid overloading their schedules with too many courses.

Take time to meet new people and develop new friendships and try out new activities.

Spend a little time regularly in self-talk or self-evaluation of your concerns and stressors.

Get help from a relative, friend, counselor, or other sympathetic person if you feel that stress is becoming unmanageable.

Get involved in a regular exercise program, even if it involves only walking briskly for 30 minutes every other day.

Pursue a hobby or do some light, enjoyable reading a few hours each week.

Set realistic goals based on your interests, strengths, and weaknesses.

- Imagine that you have just completed a long walk and are feeling very tired; your legs are especially tired. Try to feel the heaviness in your legs. Let them weigh themselves down.
- Now imagine that your legs feel very warm and then try to feel that warmth. Keep your legs relaxed and feel how heavy and warm they are.
- Enjoy the feeling of heaviness and warmth in your legs and try to retain it as long as possible.
- As you end the exercise, imagine that you are refreshed and alert. Take a deep breath and stretch.

Biofeedback   In progressive relaxation, meditation, and autogenic training, a state of relaxation is verified by the individual's subjective evaluation. A more objective measure can be attained through biofeedback.

biofeedback—*a technique for developing conscious control over involuntary body processes such as blood pressure and heartbeat.*

Biofeedback is a technique for developing conscious control over involuntary body processes such as blood pressure and heartbeat. This technique has helped some people cope with various problems, including hypertension, headaches, menstrual cramps, and gastrointestinal disorders.[57]

In most biofeedback training sessions a person listens to tape-recorded relaxation instructions while receiving auditory or visual feedback about what is happening to various physiological functions, such as heart rate, skin temperature, and muscle tension. Gradually the person becomes aware of the state of mind, attitudes, or thoughts associated with these functions and can summon them at will without the biofeedback machine.[58]

Many of the skills of biofeedback are difficult to master alone, and biofeedback devices are not always available to the public. People who are interested in the technique should seek the help of a professional. Certified biofeedback therapists and clinics are sometimes affiliated with a university medical center.

Psychological Approaches to Stress Management

Some methods of coping effectively with stress are primarily psychological. These methods focus on helping people learn healthier ways of looking at things. As you learned earlier, the amount of stress a situation evokes relates to the way in which a person perceives that situation. For example, if a boss walks by without even a nod of acknowledgment, a subordinate may worry that he or she has done something wrong. One psychological technique for learning different ways of perceiving such a situation is called **cognitive appraisal.**

cognitive appraisal—*a psychological and intellectual technique for analyzing stressors and learning different ways of responding to stress.*

Cognitive appraisal teaches people to consider less threatening explanations for any situation that is construed as harmful, threatening, or challenging. Perhaps the boss was distracted or not feeling well at the time. This explanation is less stressful to the individual who was ignored. The cognitive appraisal approach is consistent with the time-honored advice "Don't take it personally."

Such an approach to stress management can be tried independently; it can also be undertaken with professional guidance. Such psychotherapy has been well worth the cost to the many people it has helped. A psychologist, psychiatrist, or social worker can help a person develop healthier ways of perceiving and dealing with anxiety-provoking situations as well as gain insight into his or her responses to particular situations.

Changing Behavior to Avoid or Reduce Stress

It is generally agreed that the night owl, the couch potato, and the junk-food addict are examples of people with poor health habits. Researchers studying the relationship between poor health habits, stress, and illness have found that people may become ill after experiencing a stressor partially because they do not maintain good health behaviors.[59]

Changing poor health habits therefore may make a difference between stress and illness and relaxation and good health. Four areas in which a person can readily make changes to avoid or reduce stress and increase health are exercise, nutrition, time management, and mental outlook.

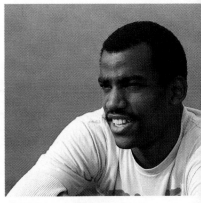

A positive outlook is a key factor in reducing stress. (David Young-Wolff/PhotoEdit)

Exercise Runners have frequently reported a sense of well-being related to their exercise. Not only does running strengthen their bodies, it also may raise their endorphin levels. Current studies strongly suggest that individuals who exercise regularly are less susceptible to stress-induced deteriorations in health than are those who exercise less frequently.[60] Researchers are also finding that even brief periods of low-level exercise have a positive effect on a person's mood.[61] The real benefit of exercise is that it enables the body to rid itself of the by-products of stress, such as adrenaline and noradrenaline; also, because it helps reduce fatigue, exercise increases the body's capacity to cope with stress.

Exercise is a good way to manage stress. It raises the body's level of endorphins; this helps reduce anxiety and keep a person mentally fit (Chapter 4).

Nutrition Although diet is obviously a factor that affects health, the specific role of nutrition in stress management is controversial. High levels of vitamin C and certain B-complex vitamins are purported to be necessary during times of stress to keep the body's nervous and endocrine systems functioning properly, but there is no consensus on this (Chapter 5). It is generally accepted, however, that a person who exercises regularly, is physically fit, and eats well-balanced meals is in a good frame of mind and body to handle stress.[62]

Time Management For many people, the fast pace of modern life and the numerous demands placed upon their time lead to highly stressed lives. Reducing that stress and becoming more productive in the time available require that a person learn to manage time better.

Successful time management requires that you plan everything you do carefully and really get tough with yourself about putting aside nonessential tasks and doing essential things *now.* It also requires that you set aside the idea that you have to do everything at the same time. Some things can wait. It is also important to realize that you are not indispensable and that it is not possible to be the center of all activities.

A good start in learning how to manage time is to assess your goals and values, decide which ones really matter, and proceed from there. An organized checklist of priorities will help you work toward achieving one thing at a time with a minimum of stress. Without such priorities, it is easy to spend time on nonessential tasks or waste time. When that happens, you worry about how to fit more and more things into less and less time. Anxiety develops, frustration sets in, and you move faster but still do not accomplish what you set out to do.[63]

You should, of course, bear in mind that priorities are flexible and subject to revision if emergencies or conflicts arise. It would be self-defeating to use time-management techniques to lock yourself into a pattern that imposes more stress. The idea is to learn to manage time, not to let time manage you.

Developing a Healthy Mental Outlook Personal attitude is an important element in coping with stressful events and a stressful lifestyle. People who develop a positive, healthy outlook toward life and its problems can minimize the effects of stress on their health and well-being. The story of writer and editor Norman Cousins demonstrates how a positive attitude can affect health. In his book *Anatomy of an Illness* Cousins discussed how attitude helped him beat the odds of recovering from a serious arthritic-type disease. Despite the stress of his illness, Cousins found humor and hope in his life. He watched old funny movies and laughed a lot, took megadoses of vitamins, and tried other ways of taking charge of his feelings and health. Unwilling to give up in the face of adversity, Cousins faced it with a positive, healthy outlook. In doing so, he improved his health and his life.[64]

Learning to manage stress in your life can bring great health benefits. Try to be open to change; view it as a challenge rather than a defeat. Develop a sense of involvement in your life by controlling and influencing life events. Draw on sources of strength such as friendships, physical fitness, and positive, flexible attitudes. The sense of self-efficacy and confidence these sources bring will help you make desired changes in your life and lifestyle, changes that can affect your overall health, well-being, and longevity. Attitudinal and emotional strength is an important foundation of overall health and well-being.

Chapter Summary

- Stress is the psychological and physiological response to a stimulus (or stressor) an individual *perceives* as threatening.
- The three general categories of stressors are cataclysmic stressors, personal stressors, and background stressors.
- There are five general sources of stress within a person's life: physical, emotional, intellectual, social, and spiritual stressors.
- Stress that has a negative effect on a person is called distress; stress that has a positive effect is called eustress.
- The Holmes-Rahe scale, a measure of major life events, has been used to assess the effects of stress on health.
- Major life events are powerful personal stressors, for example, the death of a spouse or a major illness; hassles are persistent, repetitive, and almost routine events that cause stress.
- The general adaptation syndrome (GAS) is a three-stage process the body goes through in adapting to stress; it includes the alarm stage, the resistance stage, and the stage of exhaustion. The GAS helps explain how stress can cause physiological damage.
- When it is under stress, the body reacts with a specific physiological response that represents its attempt to cope with a stressor. This re-

sponse is regulated by the autonomic nervous system and the endocrine system.
- Normally, the body is able to return to a state of balance after reacting to stress. Chronic stress, however, can interfere with the body's ability to return to normal; this can have a damaging effect on the body.
- Certain types of behaviors seem to be linked to high levels of stress and stress-related problems; hardy personalities seem to experience less stress.
- Stress can affect a person's behavior as well as physical well-being; it may lead to maladaptive behaviors such as drug abuse, overeating, and depression or may lead to increased drive and energy as one strives to meet challenges.
- Research shows a correlation between stress and certain diseases, such as hypertension, heart disease, cancer, and infectious diseases. While a causal relationship has not been demonstrated scientifically, stress may aggravate these diseases.
- Stress has a direct effect on the immune system, reducing its ability to function effectively.
- Job-related stress can reduce a person's performance and productivity, causing problems for the worker and the business where he or she is employed.

- Stress costs American industry millions of dollars each year in lost productivity, absenteeism, and accidents; it may also lead to disharmony within American society.
- Some people attempt to manage stress in ways that may be harmful, such as drugs.
- A positive strategy for managing stress is to use one of a variety of relaxation techniques, including progressive relaxation, meditation, autogenic training, and biofeedback.

- Cognitive appraisal techniques, which usually require the assistance of a health professional, help teach people to perceive events in less threatening ways so that they are less stressful.
- Changes in behavior, such as better nutrition, exercise, and time management, can help a person manage stress better.
- A positive, healthy outlook on life and problems can help minimize the effects of stress on an individual's health and well-being.

Key Terms

Stress (page 30)

Stressor (page 30)

Eustress (page 33)

Distress (page 33)

General adaptation syndrome (GAS) (page 33)

Endocrine glands (page 36)

Hormones (page 36)

Progressive relaxation (page 45)

Relaxation response (page 46)

Autogenic training (page 47)

Biofeedback (page 48)

Cognitive appraisal (page 48)

References

1. Seymour Levine, "Stress and Behavior," *Scientific American* 224, no. 1 (January 1971): 26–31.

2. D. S. Jewell, "The Psychology of Stress: Run Silent, Run Deep," *Advances in Experimental Medicine and Biology* 245 (1988): 341–352.

3. Richard S. Lazarus and Joseph B. Cohen, "Environmental Stress," in *Human Behavior and the Environment: Current Theory and Research*, vol. 2, I. Attman and J. F. Wohlwill (eds.) (New York: Plenum, 1977).

4. S. Gore, "The Effects of Social Support in Moderating the Health Consequences of Unemployment," *Journal of Health and Social Behavior,* 19 (1978): 157–165; K. Nuckolls et al., "Psychosocial Assets, Life Crises, and the Prognosis of Pregnancy," *American Journal of Epidemiology* 95 (1972): 431–441.

5. Thomas H. Holmes and Richard H. Rahe, "The Social Readjustment Rating Scale," *Journal of Psychosomatic Research* 2 (1967): 213–218.

6. A. D. Kramer, J. C. Coyne, and R. S. Lazarus, "Comparison of Two Models of Stress Management: Daily Hassles and Uplifts versus Major Life Events," *Journal of Behavioral Medicine* 4, no. 1 (1981): 1–39.

7. R. S. Lazarus, "Puzzles in the Study of Daily Hassles," *Journal of Behavioral Medicine* 7, no. 4 (1984): 375–389; J. J. Zarski, "Hassles and Health: A Replication," *Health Psychology* 3, no. 3 (1984): 243–251.

8. Carolyn M. Aldwin, Michael R. Levenson Spiro III, and Raymond Bosse, "Does Emotionality Predict Stress? Findings from the Normative Aging Study," *Journal of Personality and Social Psychology* 56, no. 4 (1989): 618–623.

9. Hans Selye, *The Stress of Life* (New York: McGraw-Hill, 1976): 36–38.

10. Becky deVillier, "Physiology of Stress: Cellular Healing," *Critical Care Quarterly* (March 1984): 15–20.

11. James W. Mason, "A Historical Review of the Stress Field," *Journal of Human Stress* 1 (1975): 22–36.

12. Walter B. Cannon, *The Wisdom of the Body* (New York: W W Norton, 1932).

13. Richard H. Rahe, Robert T. Rubin, and Ransom J. Arthur, "The Three Investigators Study: Serum Uric Acid Cholesterol, and Cortisol Variability during Stresses of Everyday Life," *Psychosomatic Medicine* 36, no. 3 (May–June 1974): 258–268.

14. David Murray et al., "Type A Behavior in Children: Demographic, Behavioral, and Physiological Correlates," *Health Psychology* 5, no. 2 (1986): 159–169.

15. Alfred B. Heilbrun, Jr., and Eric B. Friedberg, "Type A Personality, Self-Control, and Vulnerability to Stress," *Journal of Personality Assessment* 52, no. 3 (1988): 420–433.

16. J. Howard et al., "Personality (Hardiness) as a Moderator of Job Stress and Coronary Risk in Type A Individuals: A Longitudinal Study," *Journal of Behavioral Medicine* 9 (1986): 229–244; K. M. Nowak, "Type A Hardiness and Psychological Distress," *Journal of Behavioral Medicine* 9 (1986): 537–548; Kevin McNeil et al., "Measurement of Psychological Hardiness in Older Adults," *Canadian Journal on Aging* 5 (1986): 43–48; Julian Barling, "Interrole Conflict and Marital Functioning amongst Employed Fathers," *Journal of Occupational Behavior* 7 (1986): 1–8.

17. Jerry Suls and Christine A. Marco, "Relationships between JAS—and FTAS—Type A Behavior and Non-CHD Illness: A Prospective Study Controlling for Negative Affectivity," *Health Psychology* 9, no. 4 (1990): 479–492.

18. Deborah J. Weibe and Debra Moehle McCallum, "Health Practices and Hardiness as Mediators in the Stress-Illness Relationship," *Health Psychology* 5, no. 5 (1986): 425–438.

19. Nowak, op. cit.

20. Thomas Ashby Wills, "Stress and Coping in Early Adolescence: Relationships to Substance Use in Urban School Samples," *Health Psychology* 5, no. 6 (1986): 503–529.

21. Howard et al., op. cit.; K. M. Nowak, op. cit.; McNeil et al., op. cit.; Barling, op. cit.

22. Wills, op. cit.

23. Anthony J. LaGreca, Ronald L. Akers, and Jeffrey W. Dwyer, "Life Events and Alcohol Behavior among Older Adults," *The Gerontologist* 28, no. 4 (1988): 552–558.

24. Paul Raeburn, "Eater's High," *American Health* (December 1987): 42–43.

25. "Suicide," in *Injury Prevention: Meeting the Challenge*, National Committee for Injury Prevention and Control, *American Journal of Preventive Medicine* (1989): 252–260.

26. Richard H. Rahe, "Anxiety and Physical Illness," *Journal of Clinical Psychiatry* 49, no. 10 (suppl.) (October 1988): 26–29.

27. Roberta Gerry, "CME Update: Stress on the Rise," *Physicians' Travel and Meeting Guide* (October 1989): 26–27.

28. Ibid.

29. H. P. R. Smith, "Heart Rate of Pilots Flying Aircraft on Scheduled Airline Routes," *Aerospace Medicine* 38 (1967): 1117–1119; J. A. Roman, "Cardiorespiratory Functioning in Flight," *Aerospace Medicine* 34 (1963): 322–337; R. T. Rubin, "Biochemical and Endocrine Responses to Severe Psychological Stress," in *Life Stress and Illness*, E. K. E. Gunderson and R. H. Rahe (eds.) (Springfield, Ill.: Charles C Thomas, 1974).

30. A. Jalowiec and M. Powers, "Stress and Coping in Hypertensive and Emergency Room Patients," *Nursing Research* 30, no. 1 (1981): 10–15.

31. Gerry, op. cit.

32. Liisa Keltikangas-Jarvinen and Jaana Jokinen, "Type A Behavior, Coping Mechanisms and Emotions Related to Somatic Risk Factors of Coronary Heart Disease in Adolescents," *Journal of Psychosomatic Research* 33, no. 1 (1989): 17–27.

33. Gerry, op. cit.

34. Ibid.

35. Gotthard Booth, "Psychobiological Aspects of 'Spontaneous' Regressions of Cancer," *Journal of the American Academy of Psychoanalysis* 1 (1973): 303–307; Theodore R. Miller, "Psychophysiologic Aspects of Cancer," *Cancer* 39 (1977): 413–418.

36. George F. Solomon, Alfred A. Amkraut, and Phyllis Kasper, "Immunity, Emotions and Stress," *Psychotherapy and Psychosomatics* 23 (1974): 209–217.

37. Robert Ornstein and David Sobel, *The Healing Brain: A New Perspective on the Brain and Health* (New York: Simon & Schuster, 1987).

38. J. K. Kiecoltk-Glaser and Ronald Glaser, "Psychological Influences on Immunity: Making Sense of the Relationship between Stressful Life Events and Health," *Advances in Experimental Medicine and Biology*, 245 (1988): 237–247.

39. Gerry, op. cit.

40. Ornstein and Sobel, op. cit.

41. S. Cobb and R. M. Rose, "Hypertension, Peptic Ulcer, and Diabetes in Air Traffic Controllers," *Journal of the American Medical Association* 244 (1973): 1357–1358.

42. Alexander L. Strasser, "Outside Stress Factors May Underlie Variations in Workplace Productivity," *Occupational Health & Safety* 58, no. 3 (March 1989): 20.

43. National Center for Health Statistics, "Advance Report of Final Mortality Statistics, 1987," *Monthly Vital Statistics Report* 38, no. 6 (suppl.) (1989).

44. Dennis G. Brown, "Stress as a Precipitant Factor of Eczema," *Journal of Psychosomatic Research* 16 (1972): 321–327.

45. G. W. Brown et al., "Life Events and Psychiatric Disorders," parts 1 and 2, *Psychological Medicine* 3 (1973): 74–87, 159–176; B. Cooper and J. Sylph, "Life Events and the Onset of Neurotic Illness: An Investigation in General Practice," *Psychological Medicine* 3 (1973): 421–435; Arthur Schless et al., "The Role of Stress as a Precipitating Factor of Psychiatric Illness," *British Journal of Psychiatry* 130 (1977): 19–22.

46. Christopher T. Cory, "The Stress-Ridden Inspection Suite and Other Jittery Jobs," *Psychology Today* (January 1979): 13–14.

47. "Briefing," *Benefits Management* (Blue Bell, Pa.: National Health Resources, 1989).

48. John A. Davis, "Workers' Compensation Claims for Stress-Related Disorders," *Journal of Occupational Medicine* 27, no. 11 (November 1985): 821–824.

49. John W. Jones, "A Measure of Staff Burnout among Health Professionals," presented at American Psychological Association meeting, Montreal (September 1980).

50. Penelope Want, Karen Seringer, Tom Schmitz, and Mary Bruno, "A Cure for Stress?" *Newsweek* (October 12, 1987): 64–65.

51. Herbert Benson, *The Relaxation Response* (New York: William Morrow, 1976).

52. Robin Ludwick-Rosenthal and Richard W. J. Neufeld, "Stress Management during Noxious Medical Procedures: An Evaluative Review of Outcome Studies," *Psychological Bulletin* 104, no. 3 (1988): 326–342.

53. Edmond Jacobson, *Progressive Relaxation*, 2d ed. (Chicago: University of Chicago Press, 1938).

54. Herbert Benson, with Miriam Z. Klipper, *The Relaxation Response* (New York: William Morrow, 1975).

55. Vera Fryling, "Autogenic Training," in *The New Holistic Health Handbook: Living Well in a New Age*, Shepherd Bliss (ed.) (Lexington, Mass.: Stephen Green Press, 1985).

56. Jerrold S. Greenberg, *Student-Centered Health Instruction* (Reading, Mass.: Addison-Wesley, 1978).

57. D. G. Danskin and M. A. Crow, *Biofeedback: An Introduction and Guide* (Palo Alto, Calif.: Mayfield, 1981); M. D. Litt, "Mediating Factors in Non-Medical Treatment for Migraine Headache: Toward an Interactional Model," *Journal of Psychosomatic Research* 30 (1986): 505–519.

58. Ruth Rosenbaum, "The Body's Inner Voices," *New Times* (June 26, 1978): 48.

59. Wiebe and McCallum, op. cit.

60. Jonathon D. Brown and Judith M. Siegel, "Exercise as a Buffer of Life Stress: A Prospective Study of Adolescent Health," *Health Psychology* 7, no. 4 (1988): 341–353.

61. Andrew Steptoe and Sarah Cox, "Acute Effects of Aerobic Exercise on Mood," *Health Psychology* 7, no. 4 (1988): 329–340.

62. Jewell, op. cit.

63. Danskin and Crow, op. cit., p. 196.

64. Norman Cousins, *Anatomy of an Illness* (New York: W W Norton, 1979).

PART 2

Feeling Well: Health in Mind and Body

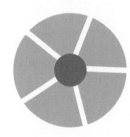

The second part of this text explores strategies for promoting basic fitness in mind and body. Beginning with the mental dimensions of health, the part continues by exploring changes you can make in your lifestyle to improve your physical condition.

Chapter 3 considers the human mind, both its emotional and its intellectual functioning, and indicates how to identify problems and effective ways to deal with them.

Chapter 4 explores the physical benefits of exercise, recommending how to develop a well-structured exercise program if your lifestyle does not include overall physical exertion on a regular basis.

Chapter 5 discusses the importance of eating right: selecting appropriate foods to provide optimal nutrition for your body. It provides a theoretical framework for understanding the body's nutritional needs and practical advice for meeting them.

Chapter 6 emphasizes the importance of body composition, describes some of the dangers of ignoring it, and explains how it can usually be managed through a combination of exercise and diet.

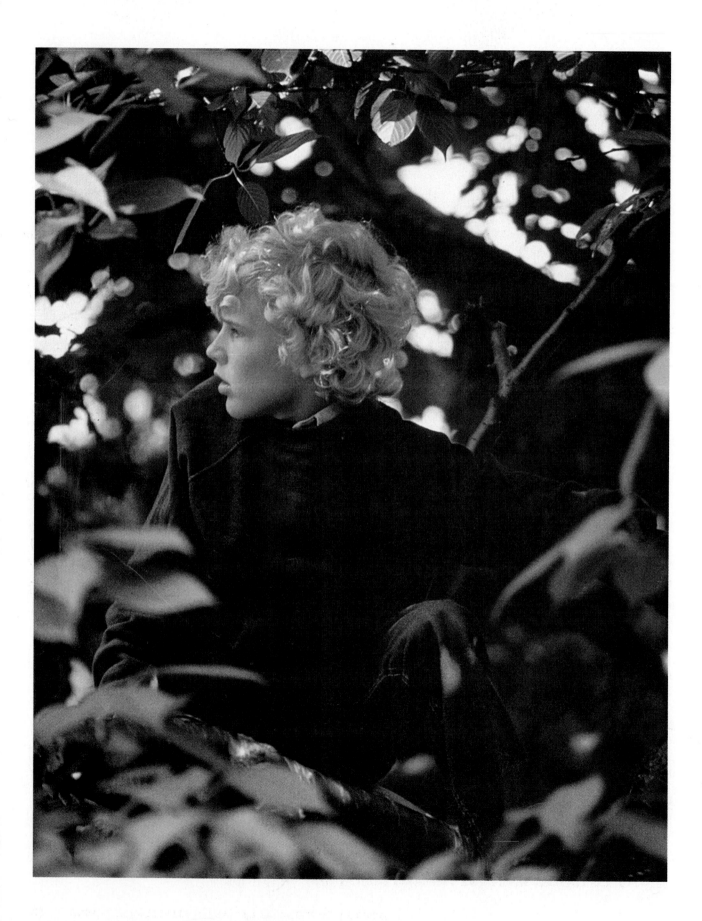

Chapter 3

Emotional Health and Intellectual Well-Being

To Guide Your Reading

When you have studied this chapter, you should be able to:

- Identify two basic dimensions of the human mind and explain how they have an impact on each other and on health.

- Describe six physiological responses that are linked to the emotions.

- Explain how emotional responses are learned and how people can deal with their negative emotional states to achieve emotional health.

- Name and describe several types of nonpsychotic disorders and psychotic disorders.

- Distinguish between the two main components of intellect and describe the activities for which they serve as a foundation.

- Explain how self-concept, different types of therapy, and individual attention can help people develop a healthy self-image and work on mental health problems.

As you read in Chapter 1, health has several different dimensions that can be viewed separately but are intricately interrelated. Even though health is most commonly considered a physical attribute, it can also be thought of in mental, social, and spiritual terms; of these, the mental—emotional and intellectual—aspects can be viewed as a key to all the rest. In the end, the satisfactions that people gain from their health and their lives are perceived as thoughts and feelings. The pleasure of enjoying good music, the pleasure of feeling at ease with friends, the pleasure of a strenuous game of racquetball and of relaxing after it—all these are feelings that are experienced in the mind.

It is also in the mind that people decide about the trade-offs involving health comfort levels that they make. Are you willing to put up with being above your ideal weight because you prefer to devote more time to reading or painting than to physical exercise? Do you deserve the pleasure of a festive meal with your family or friends, and are you content with the long-term risks such behavior may entail if you overdo it? Should you be planning for the future and devoting more time to improving your mind, or can you take time off to read a romantic novel? Perhaps you could put off dealing with your social problems and watch television or play a video game. All these decisions are made in the mind—even the last two.

Even at the unconscious level, the mind is a key to health. The brain coordinates the rest of the body. In Chapter 2 you read how body chemistry mediates the fight-or-flight reaction, and how this process is initiated and guided by the brain and the autonomic nervous system. Physical health and social and spiritual health do affect mental functioning, but it is the mind and brain that can control, and benefit from, decisions people make about all aspects of health.

The human mind has two basic dimensions: affective (emotional) and cognitive (intellectual). The affective dimension allows people to experience a

Mental health means far more than not being mentally ill. It includes how people see themselves, how they view and get along with other people, and how they meet the demands of life.

wide range of feelings—love, hate, anger, sadness, despair, hope, and so on. People react emotionally to things they see, hear, touch, smell, and taste. The cognitive dimension lets people store and recall an enormous amount of information. It also enables people to think abstractly, ponder the meaning of an idea, and develop new systems of thought and belief.

There is a constant interaction between these two dimensions of consciousness. Recalling an event or a person can make a person feel sad, happy, or angry. Pondering an idea can elicit feelings of frustration, joy, or despair. Fear can motivate people to think through and solve a problem, but it can also block rational decision making, especially when the emotional response is intense.

Emotion and intellect both have a significant impact on health, as does the interaction between them. On occasion the intellect can get in the way of experiencing one's emotions and feelings; by thinking about them too much, one becomes less spontaneous. But when emotional conflict leads to problems and unhappiness, the human intellect can be used to help understand these emotions. In regard to other dimensions of health, too, the ability to learn, remember information, solve problems, and make decisions is crucial in developing a healthy lifestyle.

Emotions

Emotions such as love, hate, anger, joy, and fear are powerful forces within people's lives. They represent the feeling, nonrational side of the mind and provide the emotional ups and downs that everyone experiences. Emotions are also related to physical health—feeling bad emotionally may cause a person to feel bad physically as well. A person facing a difficult problem may get a tension headache; a child fearful of going to the dentist may complain of an upset stomach; someone whose lifestyle includes habitual stress may develop a **psychosomatic disease** (a physical problem caused by the mind), such as a stomach ulcer or colitis.

psychosomatic disease—*a disease in which mental or psychological factors play an important role in the pathological process.*

Conversely, feeling well emotionally can help a person feel better physically. Surgeons routinely evaluate their patients' emotional state before operating on them because it has been learned that these emotional states can have an important effect on a patient's chances for recovery. For example, as related at the end of Chapter 2, the late writer and editor Norman Cousins used laughter and a positive attitude—good emotional states—to aid his recovery from a degenerative spinal disease that physicians were unable to treat.[1] Improving one's emotional health can thus be a powerful tool in the treatment of physical disease.

The Physiology of Emotion

Although most people think of an emotion as something which takes place solely in the mind, there are actually physical components to the emotions (Figure 3.1). When a person experiences an emotion, the body reacts with certain physical changes. The person perceives and interprets these changes as feelings of happiness, sadness, depression, fear, and so on. An emotion is a complex combination of mental perceptions and physiological changes.

How does the intricate relationship between emotions and physiological changes work? The answer lies in the organization of the nervous system. The nervous system has two levels: the **central nervous system (CNS),** which includes the brain and spinal cord, and the **peripheral nervous system (PNS),** which includes all the other nerves in the body.

central nervous system (CNS)—*the brain and spinal cord, which together regulate all bodily functions.*

peripheral nervous system (PNS)—*all the nerves in the body other than those in the central nervous system; divided into the somatic nervous system and the autonomic nervous system.*

The CNS is the command post of the body; it regulates and integrates all bodily functions, receiving and processing information and directing body movements. The spinal cord—a mass of nerve tissue organized into segments

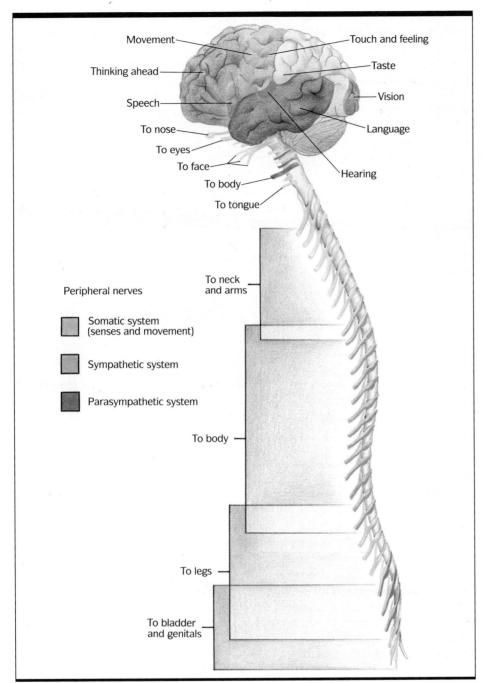

Figure 3.1 Although much remains to be discovered, scientists have made considerable progress in determining the functions of different areas of the central nervous system. The part of the brain involved with emotions (the limbic system) is in the center of the underside of the brain. It includes the hypothalamus and is connected with the autonomic (sympathetic and parasympathetic) nervous system.

that are associated with particular muscles, organs, and functions—is responsible for receiving and transmitting tactile and motor information.

The PNS is divided into two distinct systems: the **somatic nervous system (SNS),** which is connected to the voluntary muscles and consists of nerves that run between the sensory and motor organs, and the **autonomic nervous system (ANS),** which is linked to the involuntary muscles, for example, the heart, arteries, and glands.

The ANS is the part of the nervous system involved most directly with the emotions. (Its connection with the stress response was described in Chapter 2.) It is through the ANS that the physical expression of emotion is controlled: increased secretion by the sweat glands and tightening of the abdominal muscles, among other reactions. When you stand in front of a class to give a report and your eyes survey the sea of faces waiting to hear the first word, the ANS causes your hands to turn clammy and your stomach to churn.

somatic nervous system (SNS)—*the part of the peripheral nervous system that controls the voluntary muscles; it consists of nerves that run between the sensory and motor organs.*

autonomic nervous system (ANS)—*the part of the peripheral nervous system that coordinates involuntary muscles such as the heart.*

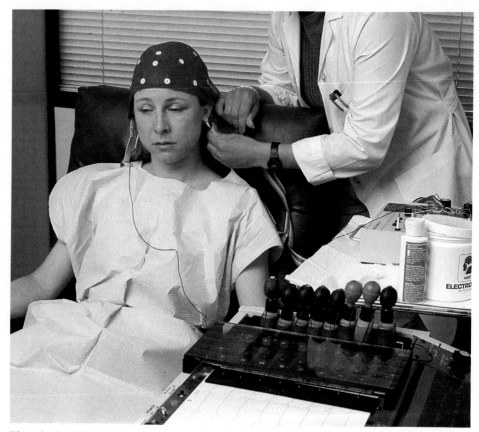

Though the EEG was developed more than 60 years ago, it is still used for diagnosis of many brain abnormalities. It only charts large-scale brain activity near the surface, however; more modern techniques are available for probing other irregularities. (Melanie Brown/ PhotoEdit)

Scientists commonly look at six physiological responses linked to the emotions: heart rate, blood volume, blood pressure, electrodermal responses, muscle potential, and brain wave patterns (electroencephalograms). All are controlled by the nervous system.

Heart Rate This is the physiological response people think of first in connection with emotional situations, because it is easy to recognize a thumping heart. Heart rate can fluctuate a great deal depending on a person's emotional state and other factors.

Blood Volume Blood vessels constrict and dilate (expand), altering the rate at which blood flows through them. When someone grows pale with fear, the flow of blood to the face has been restricted. In a person whose face is red with embarrassment, the same blood vessels have dilated, moving a greater volume of blood to the face.

Blood Pressure This term refers to the force exerted by the heart as it contracts to push blood out of the arteries and then relaxes. During highly charged emotional states, blood pressure can change drastically: anger can produce physical effects similar to those experienced during a highly strenuous activity.

Electrodermal Responses The skin, like the rest of the body, can conduct electricity. People sweat during strongly emotional states, and the added moisture makes the skin better able to conduct electricity than it is at other times. The degree of conduction can be measured by placing metal electrodes on the skin, frequently on the palms.

Muscle Potential Muscles often give visible signs of emotion: the tightening of the jaw during anger, the activation of the facial muscles that form a smile. To measure what is happening to a muscle during a frown or smile, scientists have devised a way to study the muscles' electrical potential. Each use of a muscle generates a burst of electricity; a small needle inserted in a muscle can help record the amount of electrical energy flowing through it, which indicates the degree of emotional activity.

Electroencephalogram The brain emits electric waves that can be measured by placing electrodes on the skull. The resulting pattern of waves is called an **electroencephalogram (EEG).** There are four types of brain waves, but only two are measured frequently in adults: alpha waves, which are the rhythms of the awake and relaxed adult, and beta waves, which indicate an alert or excited state, that is, a state of strong emotion.[2]

electroencephalogram (EEG)— *the pattern of electrical waves that can be measured by placing electrodes on the skull.*

The Psychology of Emotion

The responses just described are physiological changes connected with all emotions. They are related to psychological feelings in a complex way. The process begins with an environmental stimulus such as the sudden noise of a balloon popping. This is relayed to the brain, causing an immediate reaction in the autonomic nervous system, leading to symptoms such as increased heart rate and blood pressure.

The person experiencing such physical reactions interprets them as an emotion, but what determines whether a person interprets particular physical reactions as fear, amusement, annoyance, or another emotion? It depends greatly on what the person has experienced in the past. People learn over their lifetimes how to interpret their experiences and emotional sensations. They learn emotional responses in two basic ways: by association and by observing the experiences of others.

Learning by Association The process that underlies learning by association is classical conditioning, which is mentioned later in this chapter. Most psychologists agree that emotional responses are particularly susceptible to classical conditioning.[3] One student who experiences fear and discomfort

Some common positive emotions are love, joy, happiness, confidence, peace, humor, passion, affection, and excitement.

The environment can have a calming effect on the emotions, an observation well known to children as well as adults. (Gilles Peress/Magnum)

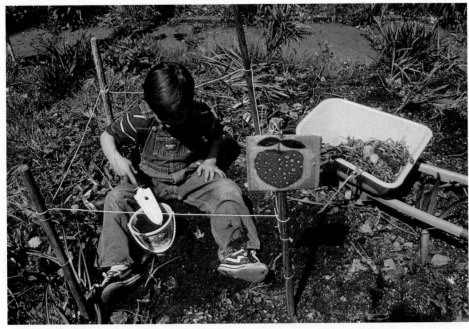

during an exam for which he or she is ill prepared may experience the same feelings as soon as another exam is mentioned; another student may even feel uncomfortable every time he or she goes to school. These students have learned to associate the painful emotions of a particular experience with a whole category of objects and events—a process known as **generalization.** In fact, emotional responses can generalize even more broadly: the same student may begin to feel uncomfortable in any school setting.

generalization—the association of the emotions involved in a particular experience with a whole category of objects and events.

Learning by Observation   People also learn emotional responses by observing the experiences of others. Consider the first experiences of a small child at the circus. Circus clowns move wildly, make very loud noises, and wear aggressively colored clothes. They often run through the audience. When a little child is first confronted with a clown, the first reaction may be to cry or even feel terror. However, thanks to the laughter of others, the child realizes that the clown is harmless and is able to convert the feelings of fear into joyous amusement.

Negative Emotions and Emotional Conflict

Happiness, affection, excitement—these and other pleasant emotions make life seem wonderful. Everyone wants his or her life to be filled with such good feelings and strives to achieve this. But obviously, people's lives are not filled with pleasant, positive emotions all the time. Many events in life are stressful and produce unpleasant, negative feelings. Such emotions can be triggered by a wide variety of conditions or events, including job dissatisfaction, conflict, lack of intimacy, noise, boredom, and even the anticipation of one of these or other situations.[4] The negative feelings that result can disrupt a person's emotional well-being.

An important part of emotional health involves learning to cope with negative emotions. Coping represents an attempt to remove or resolve a stressful situation or insulate oneself from the negative emotions that it can cause.

Negative feelings may result directly from unhappy situations such as fear of harm and sadness at loss. Everyone's life includes situations which give rise to such emotions, and they must generally be accepted and lived through. If a person is able to cope with a situation successfully, he or she will return to a normal state of emotional well-being.

Other negative feelings may arise from conflicts between different emotions, and in these cases it can be helpful to understand what is happening. Anger, for example, can be a positive force for doing good, but open displays of anger are disapproved of in most societies. This makes people feel conflicted about being angry. Other negative feelings, such as anxiety and depression, also often result from feelings that people do not wish to acknowledge.

Some common negative emotions are anger, frustration, resentment, guilt, fear, sadness, anxiety, depression, annoyance, and boredom.

Anger   Anger is a natural human response. Some people, however, feel angry and frustrated much of the time. Perhaps they are more vulnerable to external stressors and need to desensitize themselves or learn to filter out more of the hurts and hostilities the world throws in their direction. They may also need to look behind their anger to find out what other feelings—rejection, sadness, loneliness—it may be covering up and try to deal with those feelings.

If you feel that you are reacting with anger too often, try some of these techniques to cope with your angry feelings.

- Practice stress management techniques (Chapter 2) and work to develop feelings of security and self-esteem.

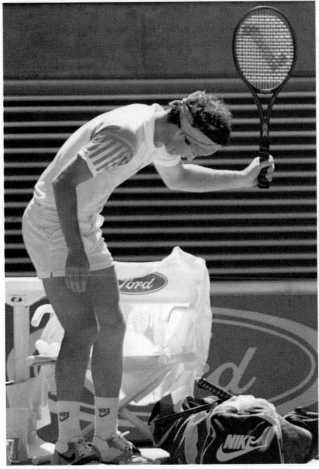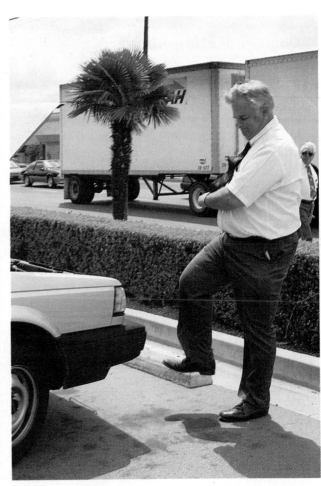

Anger is a natural human reaction to unpleasant moments and frustrating circumstances. Sometimes expressing the emotion can spur one to higher achievement; at other times it merely releases the tension. (left: Reuters/Bettman; right: Ron Grishaber/PhotoEdit)

- Try to reduce competitive feelings so that you are not constantly going forth to do battle with work, play, or other people. This will help you ignore what might otherwise seem painful challenges in your environment.
- Figure out why you are reacting so strongly to a particular situation. Is it because you are overly sensitive to criticism? Are there certain types of people who annoy you? Avoid situations and people who make you angry or see if you can change the way you perceive the situation. For example, your sensitivity to criticism may stem from the fact that you are already blaming yourself for some shortcoming. Try to stop beating yourself up and see if you can be more relaxed about receiving criticism from others.
- Sometimes anger is caused by frustration. Take a look at the situation and see if you can figure out what is frustrating you—and then do something about it.
- Anger can get even worse if you ventilate it. This is particularly true if you feel helpless to cause change. In such cases, yelling at an adversary escalates the hostility and anxiety rather than clearing the air. Talking to a sympathetic third party may confirm your anger but still fail to solve the problem. It is better in some situations to assert yourself and deal with the underlying difficulties or let the matter drop and simply walk away from the situation.[5]

Anxiety Anxiety usually occurs when a person feels fear that is related to an expected loss or hurt, though occasionally people feel "free-floating" anxiety, in which they cannot identify the reason for their apprehensiveness. It does

Communicating about Anger

Problems involving anger occur for two almost opposite reasons. Some people seem to be perpetually angry. For them, the problem is a matter of trying to identify cases where that anger is appropriate and, when it is not, finding other ways of dealing with it. Many of the strategies suggested in this chapter may be helpful for such people.

Other people err in the opposite direction by trying to avoid expressing their anger to other people altogether. They may suppress angry feelings by deliberately ignoring something that bothers them or even by unconsciously blocking their angry feelings so that they are not even aware of them.

Everyone has reason to feel angry from time to time. It is impossible to have a relationship with anyone—friends, parents, spouses, coworkers—without occasional conflict. Anger is a natural human response to conflict and to unmet expectations. However, anger that is not handled properly can cause problems.

The most primitive expression of anger is largely physical: the angered person physically attacks the object of his or her rage or shouts and threatens to attack unless specific demands are met. Although this may get results in some situations, it is very destructive to social relationships. Friendships rarely survive many of these bouts of anger.

Rather than using anger to try to enforce one's demands, it is often more productive to communicate about the anger itself. This can help a person vent the feelings without creating further problems. For example, instead of angrily telling your roommate to be sure to stick to the dishwashing schedule next time, say that having to do the dishes again has made you very angry and upset.

By focusing on your own feelings rather than making demands, you have a better chance of resolving the conflict. Angry demands often provoke refusal, but if you let your anger indicate how annoyed the situation has made you, your roommate is more likely to understand your behavior and respond to the issue in a rational manner.

In addition to emphasizing feelings rather than demands, try to focus on the specific situation or problem. Do not let your angry remarks become destructive generalizations or threats. Say "I'm annoyed about the mess in our apartment today" instead of "I'm angry at you because you're a slob and always leave things strewn about." Say "We need to work together to keep our place organized. When you're not doing your part, I get upset because I think you don't care." Remember, you usually like this person; you just do not like the situation that has developed.

Also, even in a loud and angry quarrel, try to avoid side issues, old quarrels, and vulnerabilities. If a wife is angry about the fact that her husband bought something without consulting her, neither of them should bring up her mother's spending habits, his low salary, or last year's battle about buying a new car. Comments about such issues are likely to hurt the other person's feelings while contributing nothing to resolving the issue at hand.

Expressing your anger effectively is only one part of arguing productively. You must also try to understand the other person's point of view fairly. Listen to what the person is saying and even make a point of restating the main arguments to be sure you understand them correctly. Finally, try to find common ground. Look for possible solutions and compromises. If you are friends, you want to resolve this conflict in a way that is comfortable for both of you.

Based on material in James McCary, *Freedom and Growth in Marriage* (Santa Barbara, Calif.: Hamilton Publishing, 1975). See also George Bach and Peter Wyden, *The Intimate Enemy* (New York: Avon Books, 1976).

not matter whether the expectation is real or imagined; the fear is very real. In most cases the fear is over some loss or hurt that may occur in the future, such as offending an elderly parent or starting a new job. People often feel helpless at such times; they feel that things are out of their control, and thus the anxiety is heightened.

The most effective way to deal with anxiety is to work toward regaining a feeling of *self-efficacy*—the feeling that you can control the events in your life or at least your reactions to them. Start by admitting to yourself that you are afraid of being hurt or losing someone or something important to you. Sometimes simply admitting that you are vulnerable to a loss or hurt can help relieve the anxiety. Accepting your vulnerability may help you see that you can survive even if your worst fears come to pass.

Once the sources of anxiety are brought out into the open, they can be examined objectively. Imaginary fears can be seen for what they are, and real threats to your well-being or self-esteem can be better understood. You may think of a way to act that will solve the problem.

Minor Depression   Minor depression is sometimes referred to as the common cold of emotional disorders. Most people feel depressed at times. *Depression* is a "down" feeling that is usually associated with loss of self-esteem: depressed people often feel worthless. It also may be due to anger that is directed inward: depressed people often fight to hold anger back and in some cases lose sight of the original reason for being angry.

To get over depression, start by directing energy away from yourself. Exercise, gardening, reading, and other distracting activities can often help break a depressed mood. Make a daily schedule so that you can structure your activities toward a productive end. Also, try to identify any sources of anger and allow your trapped feelings to escape.

While it is common to feel depressed, some people are more likely to become depressed and stay depressed longer than others are. For example, in one study it was found that persistent depression among teenagers primarily affects those of minority race, low socioeconomic status, low school grades, and poor progress in school.[6] There is also evidence that children who experience severe depression are likely to continue experiencing depression into

Minor depressions are not uncommon and can bring a person down physically as well as emotionally. (Michael P. Gadomski/Photo Researchers, Inc.)

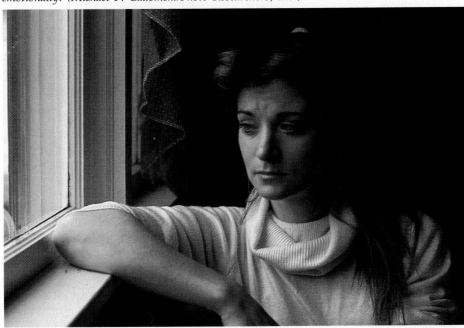

their adult years.[7] If a depression is unusually severe or persists more than a few weeks, the condition may be serious enough to require treatment.

The Use of Defense Mechanisms　Finding ways to cope with painful emotions is one of the most critical ongoing efforts of people's lives. Change is an inevitable part of the human condition: a family breaks up, a child leaves home, a mother or wife returns to work, a person finds a new job or goes to a new school. People are forced to adapt to all these changes. Luckily, the mind and body are adaptable. One of the ways people work through such adaptations is by using **defense mechanisms**—mental strategies for preserving one's sense of self by protecting oneself from the anxiety associated with painful emotions.[8]

Although defense mechanisms can lead to problems if they become a person's predominant or only way of dealing with painful emotions, they can also be used to help an individual adjust temporarily to stressful situations. People use several common defense mechanisms.

- **Repression** is considered the most basic defense mechanism. A person who is repressing denies any awareness of thoughts, feelings, memories, or wishes that are threatening. He or she refuses to acknowledge through speech, emotion, or behavior a response that would ordinarily be expected in specific circumstances. For example, a child who displays no anger or distress during his or her parents' divorce may be repressing fears and anxieties.
- **Rationalization** is a defense mechanism in which people assure themselves and others that they acted from better motives than was probably the case. A student who claims that she did not get work done on time because she was too busy helping others may be rationalizing negligence of responsibility for schoolwork.
- Repressed people cover up truths about themselves and their inner lives. **Denial,** by contrast, is a defense mechanism in which a person covers up truths about the outer world, ignoring those which threaten self-esteem or create anxiety. Thus, a person may not hear an insulting remark even though it is spoken clearly and within hearing distance. Similarly, a person may deny that certain physical symptoms require medical attention because of fear that the symptoms may be a sign of serious illness.
- **Projection** is an attempt to attribute one's undesirable feelings, wishes, and motives to other people or even inanimate objects. A man who is about to be married, for instance, may claim that his roommate is interested in every good-looking woman who walks down the street. He may be projecting onto his roommate the unacceptable feelings he has about other women.
- **Psychic contactlessness** refers to an inability to communicate with or become intimate with others. A person who is deeply afraid of being hurt by intimacy, perhaps because he or she has been hurt in the past, is suffering from psychic contactlessness. Such persons never get to know others well, nor do others get to know them. They keep their self-esteem intact: nobody can hurt them because nobody is allowed to get close enough to do so.
- A person who does not acknowledge that other people are fully human, with human feelings and emotions, is using a defense mechanism called **depersonalization.** Racial prejudice often contains strong elements of depersonalization: "That person doesn't experience the same needs or desires that I do, so it doesn't matter if he or she suffers socially or economically." Depersonalization has been used to justify slavery, pogroms, and other acts of violence against entire groups of people. On another level, depersonalization occurs when a person views others only in terms of their social roles, for example, as workers, husbands, or students.
- **Sublimation** refers to the substitution of socially acceptable behavior for unacceptable impulses such as hostility and aggression. Some people, for example, may become workaholics who work compulsively long hours each day rather than face the angry feelings they have about their home lives.

---

defense mechanism—*one of a number of mental strategies for preserving one's sense of self.*

repression—*a defense mechanism in which an individual has no conscious awareness of threatening thoughts, feelings, memories, or wishes.*

rationalization—*a defense mechanism in which an individual does not admit that his or her motives are anything but the highest.*

denial—*a defense mechanism in which an individual covers up truths about the outer world, ignoring the things that threaten his or her self-esteem and create anxiety.*

projection—*a defense mechanism in which an individual attributes his or her undesirable motives and feelings to other people or even to inanimate objects.*

psychic contactlessness—*a defense mechanism in which an individual is unable to communicate with or become intimate with others.*

depersonalization—*a defense mechanism in which an individual refuses to recognize that other people are fully human, with human feelings and emotions.*

sublimation—*a defense mechanism in which an individual substitutes socially acceptable behavior for unacceptable impulses, for example, conformity for hostility.*

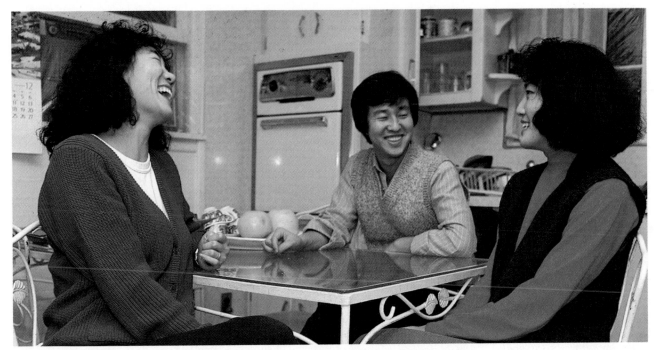

Many emotions bring people in a society together. If the emotions were unexpressed, people would feel more isolated from each other. (Robert Brenner/PhotoEdit)

The use of these various defense mechanisms is normal; everyone resorts to them to one degree or another. Nor are they necessarily negative; they can serve as a moderating force in people's lives when change is too stressful, giving people time to marshal their resources and gain the strength to face new challenges.[9] Many defense mechanisms thus serve important positive purposes. In one study, university students who used defense mechanisms were found to have reduced their tension and anxiety significantly.[10]

Basically, no defense mechanism is bad in itself; it depends on the degree to which a person uses it. A mentally healthy person uses a variety of defense mechanisms when necessary in order to adjust successfully to stress and problems. However, overuse of defense mechanisms has been found to be part of the chain of events that can lead to both violence and suicide.[11]

The terms sane and insane are basically legal terms that are rarely used by mental health professionals.

What Is Emotional Health?

What are the basic qualities associated with emotionally healthy people in American society? What is considered emotionally healthy depends to some extent on the culture. What Americans consider to be a normal way of dealing with emotional conflict may not be considered appropriate or healthy by the Japanese, who prefer not to confront others openly with their displeasure.

Most authorities agree that emotionally healthy people exhibit the following characteristics.

- They are able to understand reality and deal with it constructively.
- They can adapt to reasonable demands for change.
- They have a reasonable degree of self-efficacy.
- They can cope with stress.
- They are concerned about other people.
- They have the ability to love.
- They are able to work productively.
- They act in ways that meet their basic needs.

Emotional health is a complex quality. It is not a static condition but a dynamic process, and it does not imply total control over one's emotions. A person's emotional state varies day by day. All people have days when they feel good about themselves and the world around them and days when most things seem to go wrong and they feel bad about themselves. Emotional health implies a balance among the emotions.

A person who is emotionally healthy is not a person who has no problems but a person who has learned to adjust and cope successfully with the problems he or she encounters. Such a person feels capable of living with emotional ups and downs; the ups and downs do not get in the way and make it hard to lead an everyday existence.

From time to time, however, people are unable to cope effectively with their emotions. The result may be a temporary state of painful emotions or a long-term disruption of emotional health.

Emotional Disorders

Western psychology can be traced back to ancient Greece. Plato and Aristotle were concerned with the rational and irrational aspects of the mind and also with the nature of the soul.

Human behavior is far too complex to be easily categorized. It is sometimes very difficult to distinguish between a disorder and a behavior that is just "different" or between two distinct types of disorders. Most health practitioners and researchers have come to accept—if with occasional misgivings—the categories suggested by the American Psychiatric Association in its *Diagnostic and Statistical Manual of Mental Disorders* (DSM).[12]

The third edition of this manual, DSM-III, which was published in 1980, raised a storm of controversy because it eliminated or revised many standard classifications. The term *neurosis,* for example, was replaced by terms such as *anxiety* and *personality disorder.* DSM-IIIR, a revised edition of the manual published in 1987, further refined some of the classifications.

The categories discussed in this chapter all come from DSM-IIIR, although only a few of the main disorders are covered. It should be noted that although such a categorization is useful, one should not assume that each disorder is a separate, sharply defined condition. Sometimes an individual may suffer from more than one disorder.

Nonpsychotic Disorders

nonpsychotic disorder—a mental disorder in which the individual's functioning is seriously inhibited but in which his or her thought processes are not so grossly distorted that the individual loses contact with reality.

Health professionals view emotional and mental problems on a continuum, with many fine shadings between the "optimum health" end of the continuum and the end that represents serious mental illness. Between the negative emotions and feelings discussed previously and serious mental illnesses (psychoses), there are a variety of **nonpsychotic disorders.** While these disorders inhibit a person's full functioning, they do not distort thoughts and emotions so much that the person loses contact with reality. A person suffering from a nonpsychotic disorder recognizes and is disturbed by the symptoms. Moreover, that person is aware of how distressing and maladaptive his or her behavior is. In a sense, people with nonpsychotic disorders have a double anxiety: the anxiety associated with the disorder itself and the anxiety of knowing that something is wrong. Their behavior—morbid fears, panic attacks, unrealistic anxieties—does not actually violate social norms, but it may isolate them from others and cause them to feel chronically lonely, anxious, and sad.

Nonpsychotic disorders often respond to treatment; *getting help is therefore essential.* Without treatment, a disorder may become chronic, enduring for the rest of a person's life. It is important to recognize this fact, since so many people experience at least mild nonpsychotic symptoms at some point in their lives.

The causes of nonpsychotic disorders are not always clear. They appear to have no genetic basis. In response to an extremely stressful and painful life situation such as divorce or an accident, an individual sometimes develops an

Table 3.1   A Thesaurus of Phobias

Acrophobia	Heights	Claustrophobia	Closed spaces	Nyctophobia	Darkness
Aerophobia	Flying	Cynophobia	Dogs	Ochlophobia	Crowds
Agoraphobia	Open spaces	Dementophobia	Insanity	Ophidiophobia	Snakes
Ailurophobia	Cats	Gephyrophobia	Bridges	Ornithophobia	Birds
Amaxophobia	Cars, driving	Herpetophobia	Reptiles	Phonophobia	Speaking aloud
Aquaphobia	Water	Mikrophobia	Germs	Pyrophobia	Fire
Arachnophobia	Spiders	Murophobia	Mice	Thanatophobia	Death
Brontophobia	Thunder	Numerophobia	Numbers	Xenophobia	Strangers

Hundreds of phobias have been identified and given names based on Greek or Latin words. Here are 24 of the more common ones.

adjustment disorder—a response "in excess of a normal and expected reaction to the stressor." Other nonpsychotic disorders may be caused in part by faulty emotional development. However, in some cases no precipitating factors can be identified.

Anxiety Disorders   Anxiety can become incapacitating for some people. Unlike the type of anxiety most people experience, true **anxiety disorders** involve a severe and persistent level of fear or worry that can be almost as damaging to an individual's everyday functioning as a serious mental illness is. Two important types of anxiety disorders are phobias and panic disorders.

Phobias are characterized by a persistent and irrational fear of a specific stimulus—an object, activity, or situation—that leads to a compelling desire to avoid it. Many people experience unreasonable fear when confronted by a harmless stimulus such as a tiny spider. The fear is considered a phobia only if it becomes a significant source of distress or interferes with normal functioning. It is estimated that one in nine adult Americans suffers from some kind of phobia (Table 3.1).[13]

Panic disorders are often characterized by recurrent panic attacks that may occur unpredictably or as a result of a specific situation such as driving a car or

adjustment disorder—*a nonpsychotic disorder in which the individual's response to a painful event is more extreme than would ordinarily be expected or considered normal.*

anxiety disorder—*a nonpsychotic disorder involving a severe and persistent level of fear or worry that interferes with an individual's everyday functioning.*

phobia—*a type of anxiety disorder characterized by a persistent and irrational fear of a specific stimulus or activity, leading to a compelling desire to avoid it.*

panic disorder—*a disorder characterized by episodes of extreme anxiety that may occur unpredictably or result from a specific situation.*

Panic attacks can incapacitate people in situations that others find perfectly normal, for example, crossing a bridge. (Todd Jacobs/Custom Medical Stock Photo)

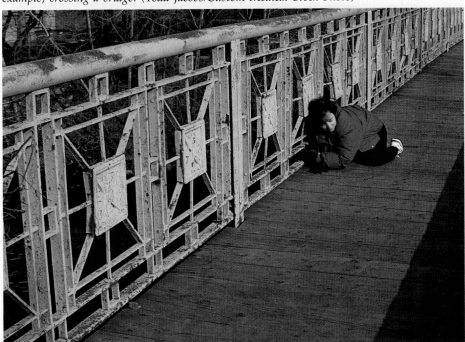

being in a crowded place. They are a common type of disorder, often starting in adolescence. The panic attacks may be confined to a period of several weeks or months or may become chronic. They involve sudden and intense fear that often is accompanied by physical symptoms such as palpitations, chest pain, dizziness, sweating, faintness, and trembling. Some people suffer few of these physical symptoms but feel more muscular tension and mental anxiety or apprehension instead.[14] The individual is often nervous between attacks, sometimes to the point of being unwilling to be alone or in public places away from home.

Personality Disorders   All people have distinct personality traits—characteristic patterns of perceiving, relating to, and thinking about their environment and themselves. In some cases these traits impair an individual's ability to function and cope with his or her environment. Such counterproductive styles of coping are termed **personality disorders.** People with these disorders may suffer from a continuing sense of failure, a feeling of resentment, or a sense of being exploited. Their usual emotional state is suppressed anger, and they have a rigid and repetitive style of interacting with others.[15]

There are a variety of different personality disorders. **Schizoid personality disorder** refers to a lack of desire to have social relationships; this can even include a total disinterest in sexual experiences with another person. **Narcissistic personality disorder** is typified by an exaggerated sense of self-worth, a constant need for praise and attention, and a tendency to exploit others. **Antisocial personality disorder** is marked by tantrums and behaviors which violate the rights of others, such as vandalism, aggressive actions, and theft. The treatment of personality disorders is difficult and time-consuming and may achieve only limited success.

Schizoid personality disorder, an impaired desire for social relationships, may cause people to withdraw from society completely, walking the streets in an aimless itinerary. (Will & Deni McIntyre/Photo Researchers, Inc.)

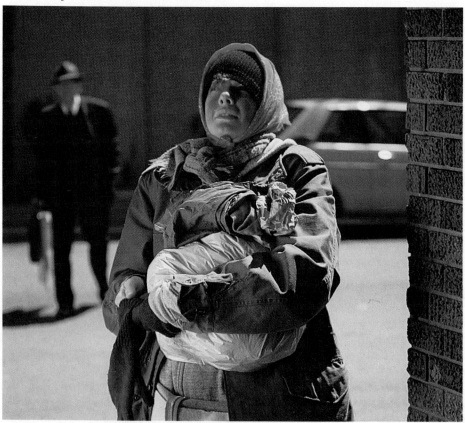

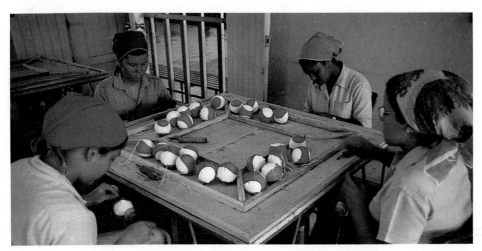

People suffering from major depression, schizophrenia, and other serious psychotic disorders require hospitalization; specialized psychiatric care may include occupational therapy. (Bill Aron/PhotoEdit)

Somatoform Disorders   The **somatoform disorders** are a group of mental disorders that are manifested as physiological symptoms. An individual may suffer from recurrent and long-term ailments that have no physical basis. The individual does not consciously invent these complaints; he or she actually feels ill but is unaware of the process by which the symptoms develop. One well-known somatoform disorder is **hypochondriasis,** in which a person imagines that every minor physical complaint—a headache, for example—is the first sign of a major illness. Many people with other mental disorders have somatic symptoms as well, but in such cases the condition is not considered a true somatoform disorder.[16]

Psychotic Disorders

Among the most serious mental problems are the **psychotic disorders.** Although it greatly oversimplifies this complex topic, psychotic disorders may be defined as those in which the individual has significantly lost contact with reality. Two of the most common psychotic disorders are affective disorders such as major depression and schizophrenia; the category also includes delusional, organic, and other disorders.

Affective Disorders   **Affective disorders** are serious disorders of mood or feeling. Minor depression is quite common; the National Center for Health Statistics reported over 6 million visits to therapists for treatment of minor depression over a 2-year period.[17] Some people, however, develop much more serious and incapacitating **major depression.** People who suffer from major depression experience a dysphoric mood—a profound unhappiness—and a loss of interest in all aspects of life, even their favorite activities. This persistent unhappy mood may be accompanied by appetite disturbance, change in weight, sleep disturbance, decreased energy, difficulty in concentrating, psychomotor agitation or retardation, feelings of worthlessness or guilt, and thoughts of death or suicide.

In **bipolar disorder,** a less common affective disorder, the person who is affected exhibits **mania,** a mood of extreme excitement, and depressive episodes are likely to occur as well. Mania usually impairs social and occupational functioning to a serious degree. When a person is manic, he or she is hyperactive, often planning and participating in several activities at once. The person becomes extremely sociable, optimistic, and reckless and is likely to show poor and hasty judgment. For example, he or she may spend a great amount of money on unnecessary things. The manic individual feels inflated

somatoform disorder—*a mental disorder that manifests itself in the form of physiological symptoms; hypochondriasis is a well-known example.*

hypochondriasis—*a somatoform disorder in which a person imagines that every physical complaint is the first sign of a major illness.*

psychotic disorder—*a mental disorder in which an individual has lost contact with reality.*

affective disorder—*a serious disorder of mood or feeling.*

major depression—*an affective disorder in which an individual experiences a dysphoric mood, loses interest in all aspects of life, and may suffer from other incapacitating symptoms.*

bipolar disorder—*an affective disorder in which an individual exhibits mania with or without depressive episodes.*

mania—*a mood of extreme excitement; an aspect of bipolar disorder.*

self-esteem, often accompanied by grandiose delusions. There is a decreased need for sleep. The mania may shift rapidly to depression, which can last for minutes, hours, or longer periods.

Bipolar disorder tends to manifest itself before age 30, and the frequency of the recurring episodes is variable. Research strongly indicates that bipolar disorder may be markedly influenced by genetic factors.

schizophrenia—*a psychotic disorder of the thinking processes in which the individual seems to be totally removed from reality.*

*A relatively rare psychotic disorder is **delusional (paranoid) disorder,** in which a person believes he or she is being followed, poisoned, infected, or deceived. The disorder may be brought on by severe stress. The person's life is usually disrupted, and full recovery is rare, although the person often appears to function adequately in most areas.*

Schizophrenia By contrast to these mood disorders, **schizophrenia** is primarily a disorder in a person's thinking processes. The term *schizophrenia* refers to a group of disorders that share certain essential features: duration of at least 6 months; failure to achieve an expected level of social development; a marked lack of initiative, interests, or energy; and disturbances in thought, perception, sense of self, relationship to the outside world, and psychomotor activity.[18] Schizophrenia appears to run in families, although nongenetic factors such as stress and socioeconomic status are also involved.

Schizophrenia is among the most serious psychotic disorders. Because those suffering from it seem to be totally removed from reality, it can be frightening both to the patients and to those around them. People with schizophrenia may hear voices, believe that electronic devices are monitoring their activities, and laugh and talk at inappropriate times. They may sit motionless, in silence; although they seem to feel nothing, they are actually suffering a great deal.

What is going on in these people's minds is just as disorienting as their behavior implies: their thoughts are connected in random order, with little or no meaning. When speaking, they may ramble, become increasingly vague, or repeat words or phrases without any awareness that they have lost the ability to connect ideas. Often, others have difficulty responding to people

These paintings done by schizophrenics reveal several patterns characteristic of the disorder. The solitary, partially faceless woman in a desolate setting suggests withdrawal and absence of emotion. The globe explosively splitting apart seems to represent the violence of a break with reality. The eyes in the trees convey a sense of sinister watchfulness. (Otto Billig, "Structures of Schizophrenic Forms of Expression," Psychiatric Quarterly 44 [April 1970]: 187–222)

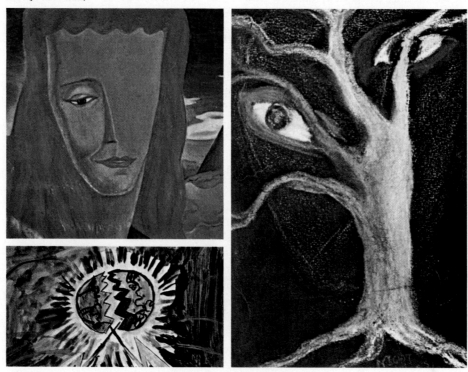

who suffer from schizophrenia with the sympathy and rationality that are needed. Instead, people with schizophrenia are met with fear and misunderstanding and become isolated.

Antipsychotic drugs have stabilized many people with schizophrenia to the extent where they can be released from the hospital permanently or for long periods. The relative calm that these drugs bring to the disordered life of many people with schizophrenia enables these people to benefit from family, group, or individual therapy as well as social and vocational rehabilitation.

Although schizophrenia is a grave disease, the outlook is not completely discouraging. Most patients do require hospitalization and drug treatment during the acute phases of the disorder, but the rest of the time they may live at home, interact socially, perhaps hold a job, and require only low maintenance doses of drugs for years at a time. About 55 percent of all people suffering from schizophrenia are chronically ill in this manner. In another 20 percent the illness is more devastating: these patients have only rare remissions despite treatment, but 25 to 30 percent recover fully after the first attack.[19]

*Involving symptoms such as delirium, dementia (mental deterioration), amnesia, and hallucinations, **organic mental disorders** are another class of mental illness, caused by physical damage to the brain. Such damage may occur as a result of disease, traumatic injury, or drug use.*

The Intellect

The other dimension of the human mind identified at the start of this chapter is **intellect**—the thinking, rational side of human consciousness. If emotions and emotional conflicts are often the cause of mental disorders, intellect can often be a part of the solution. Thinking through a problem either on one's own or with the help of a friend can enable a troubled person to explore and find possible solutions; it is also a part of many psychotherapies.

Intellect can be thought of as being composed of two main components: *memory*, which is the ability to learn and recall associated actions, ideas, and information, and *cognition*, a term that describes the several processes by which knowledge and action can be examined and improved upon. Together, they are the foundation on which people learn, create, solve problems, and make decisions—all of which are important in developing and maintaining a healthy lifestyle.

intellect—*the thinking, problem-solving, rational side of human consciousness.*

Learning and Memory

Learning is a complex and important subject. The ability to learn is essential for human survival and is also a sign of health—witness the importance of learning for the development of emotions. People who fail to learn by their mistakes are unlikely to survive very long, let alone be happy. Individuals, societies, and the human race as a whole depend on remembering what has been learned about health and satisfaction.

By studying animals, psychologists have discovered a great deal about the simpler aspects of learning. Much of what they have found can be applied to people as well. Out of their research have come various theories about how human beings learn. Two are briefly outlined below: both are very relevant to dealing with one's own health.

Conditioned Response Theories **Conditioned response theories** are very basic, mechanistic accounts of how animals learn to perceive simple stimuli and react with consistent responses. **Classical conditioning theory,** which was developed in Russia in the early 1900s by Ivan Pavlov, explores how sets of different objects or events (stimuli) become grouped, or associated in an animal's mind and are evidenced by its behavior. If two different stimuli are experienced together consistently, the animal soon reacts as though they were different aspects of the same thing. **Operant conditioning theory,** which was developed by American psychologists such as Edward Thorndike, John

conditioned response theory—*a basic, mechanistic account of how animals learn to perceive simple stimuli and react with consistent responses.*

classical conditioning theory—*a theory that explores how sets of different objects or events (stimuli) become grouped, or associated, in an animal's mind and are evidenced by its behavior.*

operant conditioning theory—*a theory that examines the conditions under which behaviors are learned.*

Watson, and B. F. Skinner, examines the conditions under which behaviors are learned. This theory explores the idea that an action is likely to be repeated if it is followed by a reward or pleasurable stimulus (positive reinforcement) and discouraged if it is followed by an unpleasant stimulus (punishment).[20] Although these are very simple ideas, conditioning theorists have been able to examine the phenomena in detail, finding, for example, that positive reinforcement is almost always more effective in encouraging desired behavior.

This is relevant not only to discipline in child rearing; it also helps people understand better ways to discipline themselves when they want to change their behavior. Blaming oneself for failure is not a very helpful course of action; it is far better to congratulate oneself on the positive things one manages to accomplish—or even to promise oneself a reward if one succeeds. A person is most likely to learn healthy eating behaviors if those behaviors are rewarded. Perhaps it will be enough to notice the loss of weight, increased energy, or enhanced self-image, because positive emotions such as joy, excitement, and triumph can be reinforcing in themselves. However, the learning may be more effective if the individual also celebrates by going out to a movie or devising another treat.

Social Learning Psychologist Albert Bandura has formulated a different learning model, based on the notion that children learn a great deal by imitating the adults around them. This model is called **social learning theory.**[21] It suggests that people acquire strategies, outlooks, and behaviors by listening to others and observing their actions. For Bandura, learning is a process which can take place independently of rewards or punishments.

Social learning theory is also a crucial model for understanding health-related behaviors. People's attitudes toward exercise, diet and nutrition, sexual behavior, and drug use are formed primarily as a result of social learning. People may have a poor eating pattern because that was all they knew as children. They may use drugs because their friends or family members use drugs. They may fear sexual intimacy because as children they learned from their parents that sex is bad.

social learning theory—*a learning model based on the notion that behavior is learned by observing the experiences and actions of others.*

Social learning theory argues that children tend to imitate bad as well as good behaviors from the adults they adopt as models. (Richard Hutchings/InfoEdit)

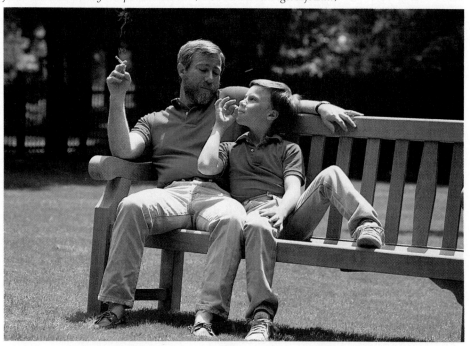

According to Bandura, reinforcement is more important in getting people to exhibit a newly learned behavior than in teaching that behavior in the first place. Thus, people may know how to exercise and understand that exercise is good, but that is often not enough. The reinforcement of being with friends may be needed to encourage a person to act on that knowledge.

Memory A healthy person can recall a vast number and variety of things—behaviors such as riding a bike or making a salad; a wide number of subjects, such as how to spell and do arithmetic; important events such as birthdays and anniversaries; and experiences such as meeting a loved one for the first time.

People's memory of information, events, and life experiences affects their current behaviors and reactions to situations. As such, memory is a factor in good health. It allows people to remember healthy behaviors and repeat them; it also allows them to review information that can have an important impact on their health, such as the nutritional value of food, the danger of using certain drugs, and techniques for relieving stress.

People often assess the mental health of the elderly by noting how sharp their memory is. In fact, memory is an important factor in all aspects of health; the decline of memory in some old people may be an important element in their overall declining health as they forget to eat the proper foods or take adequate precautions against disease and accidents. A serious disease that is associated with severe memory deterioration is Alzheimer's disease (Chapter 17).

Pioneer research on memory by Lloyd Peterson of Indiana University demonstrated that there are two types of memory: long-term and short-term. Information that is stored away for recall much later (several days) is considered long-term memory, while information to be recalled almost immediately (15 seconds) is considered to be in short-term storage.

Cognition, Problem Solving, and Decision Making

Learning and remembering are not the full story of intellect, of course; intellect also includes what one does with one's knowledge. *Cognition* is the creative part of mental activity; it involves thinking, judging, reasoning, imagining, synthesizing, making decisions, and solving problems. While these activities may seem quite disparate, they are all instances of creative thought and depend on the application of knowledge derived from learning and memory.

Everyone encounters numerous problems during his or her daily life and must make hundreds of decisions every day. The ability to solve such problems and make decisions is an important aspect of effective intellectual functioning and is essential to promoting and maintaining optimum health.[22] For example, unsolved problems are often at the root of stress and even of non-psychotic disorders. Successful coping may depend on a person's ability to understand and solve these types of problems. Decisions about health issues such as what to eat, whether to use drugs, and when to seek medical care can also have an impact on a person's health. Poor decisions in these areas may affect a person adversely by leading to weight gain, drug abuse, and health complications arising from lack of treatment.

The relationship between learning, memory, and cognition is not simple. Even to recognize an object, one must use one's cognition; people frequently remember best the facts they have deduced by themselves.

Understanding the Problem The first and perhaps most important stage in problem solving is understanding the problem. This involves interpreting the problem and viewing it in a way that makes it more easily understood. Suppose you are trying to deal with the anger that you feel at someone for the way that person treats you. If you see the problem as "How can I get them to change their behavior?" a solution may be difficult. However, if you see the problem in terms of your own behavior ("What is it that is making me so angry?" or even "Why am I staying in this situation and getting hurt?"), you may be much closer to establishing a solution that you can control. In other words, if you are having trouble solving a problem, go back and look at the problem in a different way.

Understanding a problem also involves identifying its causes. Depression, for example, may be due to anger, but it also may be caused by a low-grade

Assessing Your Self-Esteem

As this chapter stresses, self-esteem—how much you value yourself—is critical to psychological health. If you have a high level of self-esteem, you reward yourself continually because you generally approve of yourself. If you lack it, you punish yourself frequently with self-criticism, self-doubt, and often isolation from other people.

How much do you like yourself? This may seem a simple question, but a liking for yourself is reflected in many different aspects of your life: your feelings, your perceptions of the feelings of others, and your judgments of your own and others' behavior.

The following exercise will help you evaluate your level of self-esteem. Imagine that someone has made each of these statements to you; respond by deciding how similar to them you feel. If you identify readily with a statement, check "Like Me." If you rarely or never feel that way, check "Unlike Me."

	Like Me	Unlike Me
1. I often wish I were someone else.	_____	_____
2. I find it very hard to talk in front of a group.	_____	_____
3. There is much I would change about myself if I could.	_____	_____
4. I am generally quite decisive.	_____	_____
5. I am a lot of fun to be with.	_____	_____
6. I get upset easily at home.	_____	_____
7. It takes me a long time to get used to anything new.	_____	_____
8. I am popular with people my own age.	_____	_____
9. My family expects too much of me.	_____	_____
10. My family usually considers my feelings.	_____	_____

physical infection. Identifying the cause allows a person to deal with depression more effectively.

Selecting Suitable Strategies   When one is attempting to solve a problem, it is important to select a suitable strategy for reaching the solution. The best approach is to consider the options available and select the strategy most appropriate to the problem. For example, in dealing with depression caused by anger, a person might try to think a problem through, talk with friends or loved ones, or seek professional therapy. These strategies are not equally effective or advisable. Depending on the depth of depression, one strategy is usually more appropriate than the others.

As a person tries to solve a problem, it is often necessary to reevaluate potential solutions and perhaps try others if the first ones prove ineffective. When trying to lose weight, a person may find that a low-calorie diet without exercise is less effective than is a moderate-calorie diet coupled with a daily exercise program. Rather than give up when one solution does not work, a person should consider and try other possible solutions.

11. I do not give in very easily. _____ _____

12. It is pretty tough being me. _____ _____

13. Things are all mixed up in my life. _____ _____

14. Other people usually follow my ideas. _____ _____

15. I have a high opinion of myself. _____ _____

16. There are many times when I would like to leave home. _____ _____

17. I often feel upset at the work I do. _____ _____

18. I am not as nice-looking as most people. _____ _____

19. If I have something to say, I usually say it. _____ _____

20. My family understands me. _____ _____

21. Most people are more popular than I am. _____ _____

22. I usually feel my family is pushing me. _____ _____

23. I seldom get discouraged at what I am doing. _____ _____

24. Things usually do not bother me. _____ _____

25. I am pretty happy. _____ _____

Score your evaluation by giving yourself a point for each of these checks: "Like Me" for statements 4, 5, 8, 10, 11, 14, 15, 19, 20, 23, 24, and 25 and "Unlike Me" for statements 1, 2, 3, 6, 7, 9, 12, 13, 16, 17, 18, 21, and 22. A score from 20 to 25 indicates that you have a high level of self-esteem; a score from 15 to 19 shows that you have doubts about yourself; a score below 14 indicates low self-esteem, and you might consider counseling to improve your attitude toward yourself.

From *The Antecedents of Self-Esteem*, by Stanley Coopersmith. Copyright © 1967 by W. H. Freeman and Company. Reprinted with permission.

Making Decisions Considering possibilities and selecting an appropriate strategy are obviously useless unless decisive action is finally taken. However, the better able you are to understand a problem and evaluate different alternatives, estimating the advantages and disadvantages of possible outcomes, the better your ultimate decision will be and the more likely it will be to contribute to your health and well-being.

Toward a Healthy Personality

Emotional difficulties and disorders can make it hard to perceive or define problems and devise effective solutions. This chapter has already suggested strategies for controlling some negative feelings, but handling feelings is not easy: they can change very abruptly and can affect the way people look at things. What follows is a more general description of how one can "work on" mental health problems.

Concepts, Self-Concept, and Self-Esteem

In addition to initiating actions and making decisions, the intellect learns, examines, and explores ideas and concepts. A *concept* is a group of associated perceptions and thoughts about an object or something less tangible, such as an event, a movement, or even a theory. The human intellect, with its great ability to think and ponder, works with many ideas and concepts, creating and changing them and exploring the relationships between them. A person's self-concept is central to the whole structure of ideas that that person has. **Self-concept** refers to all the perceptions a person has about himself or herself—strengths and weaknesses, the potential for growth, and ways of acting. It is the result of thinking about oneself and evaluating what others think. The self-concept is not static; it evolves throughout life as people re-evaluate their beliefs, attitudes, and values.

Self-concept is important not only because it is central to the ideas that a person has but also because it is very basic to a person's overall mental health in that it has a powerful effect on the emotions. Self-concept is focused on knowing oneself. A well-developed realistic self-concept is vital to one's **self-esteem,** the feelings of worth and dignity which constitute an important part of overall health and well-being. In turn, a high level of self-esteem is vital to self-efficacy, the confidence that one can take care of important aspects of one's life and health. For example, a person who has high self-esteem is often better able to control the behaviors that contribute to being overweight than is someone whose self-esteem is low. Conversely, low self-esteem can be very damaging to health. There is much evidence that self-esteem and a sense of self-efficacy are lower in depressed people than they are in normal people.[23]

The relationship between self-concept and self-esteem is therefore vital. Self-esteem is an emotional matter that is affected by the events of the day and the opinions of others. Self-concept, however, can be a stabilizing influence; people can review their self-concepts and remind themselves of their strengths as well as the weaknesses which are causing emotional problems. They can also strengthen their view of themselves by acting on deliberate decisions: to organize their room or house, to master a topic they are studying, to try out a sport that looks like fun, or to make a new friend.

Getting Help

In the past people were often reluctant to seek help for emotional problems. Today, however, many people realize that it makes sense to get help dealing with problems they are having trouble coping with on their own. Research has shown that people with low self-esteem have a greater chance of developing mental disorders than do those with high self-esteem.[24] As a result, many methods for coping with emotional problems and mental disorders are aimed at helping people achieve greater self-esteem and increased self-efficacy. They are designed to help give people more control of their lives by removing or managing the symptoms that prevent them from functioning normally.

Individuals who realize they need help have a variety of options (Table 3.2). The choice is largely dependent on the individual's needs and the nature of his or her problem. The most common options are behavior therapy, psychotherapy, family and group therapy, and organic therapy.

Behavior Therapy **Behavior therapy** attempts to alter a person's symptomatic behavior without attempting to discover its root causes. It is based on the idea that a person learns, or acquires, behaviors under specific conditions and then transfers the feelings and attitudes associated with those conditions to other, inappropriate situations.

A behavior therapist tries to help a client get rid of troublesome behavior by creating learning situations in which the client can unlearn an unwanted response or learn an alternative response. For example, simple phobias have

Table 3.2 Know Your Therapist

Title	Qualifications	Main Function
Psychiatrist	M.D. (doctor of medicine) with a specialty in psychiatry	Provides psychotherapy, diagnoses physical illness, prescribes treatment, including medications
Psychoanalyst	Trained in the theories and techniques of Sigmund Freud and his followers; must have undergone similar treatment to that received by patient	Provides Freudian psychoanalysis, usually in private practice
Clinical psychologist	Usually a Ph.D. or Psy.D. in psychological research, assessment, and psychotherapy; must have undergone supervised internship.	Diagnoses mental disorders, gives psychological tests, provides psychotherapy
Counselor	Graduate degree in counseling psychology	Works in education or industry, provides counseling on personal problems, may refer some patients to clinical psychologists and psychiatrists
Psychiatric social worker	Master's degree, especially in social work, and practical training for 2 years	Provides individual, family, or group therapy
Psychiatric nurse	R.N. (registered nurse) with special training in psychiatric nursing	Under supervision of a psychiatrist, administers medication and provides informal therapy
Others	Teachers, physicians, clergy, and others without formal training in psychotherapeutic techniques	May provide useful counseling services, but usually less helpful for the severely troubled

been treated successfully with desensitization techniques in which patients are taught how to achieve deep muscle relaxation to reduce their anxiety and are then asked to imagine themselves in phobia-inducing situations for increasing lengths of time.

A behavior therapist may also try to teach new behavior by changing the environment so that the client is systematically rewarded for developing the desired responses. The behavior of some individuals with psychoses and other disorders has been changed considerably through positive reinforcement of desired behaviors. Some behaviorists practice cognitive behavior therapy, which seeks to alter patients' self-concepts and thought patterns by persuading them to look at themselves and their situations in new ways which can be linked to healthier behaviors. In treating depression, the therapist attempts to show the patient that his or her unhappiness is contributed to by negative thoughts that can be changed.

The purpose of therapies is to replace negative feelings with plans. Plans may take many forms, but they all add up to ways out of lost and hopeless feelings. In this sense, any objective person can provide real help to others. A good companion can be a good listener.

Psychotherapy Psychotherapy is based on the idea that people need to understand their problems. A psychotherapist meets regularly with a client to talk, listen carefully to that person's problems, and provide emotional support and acceptance. The therapist analyzes the patient's situation and suggests new ways of looking at problems. The goal of psychotherapy is to help the patient find insight into his or her problems and ways to function more comfortably and effectively.

*Freud believed there are three forces that interact to produce behavior. The **id** represents instinct and primitive, pleasurable desires; the **ego** is the conscious personality that controls the id's impulses; the **superego** represents conscience, moral and ethical codes, and social imperatives.*

Psychotherapy is changing in response to the changing needs of society.[25] For example, since many people do not have the time or money for long-term traditional psychotherapy, there has been an increase in the use of short-term therapy geared toward dealing with a specific set of symptoms. Specific forms of psychotherapy have also been developed to target the problems of specific groups within the population: the elderly, children, people with chronic pain, and so on.

Family and Group Therapies It is sometimes useful for a psychotherapist to work with a couple or an entire family as a unit so that the relationships that have contributed to a person's problems can be more easily untangled. Other people who are having problems with their lives can benefit from group therapy, which can give them the support and guidance of others who have similar problems. Group members learn to see themselves as others see them; they learn to understand other people's motivations and personality styles. Group cognitive therapy has been used recently as a treatment for depression, although some studies have indicated that it may not be as effective as individual cognitive therapy.[26]

Today there is also a tremendous variety of nontherapeutic groups: "12-step groups," assertiveness training groups, support groups, and marriage encounter groups, among others. Such groups focus on helping their members develop better skills in human relationships and thereby help them gain more satisfaction from life.

Self-help groups organized by laypeople who share common problems can be very effective in providing emotional support and reducing the emotional distress of their members. For example, there are self-help groups for single fathers, women in business, alcoholics (Alcoholics Anonymous), widows, parents who have lost children to crib death, and cancer patients.

organic therapy—a therapy that attempts to treat a person in a physical way rather than through learning or talking; the most common type of organic therapy involves the use of drugs.

Organic Therapies **Organic therapy** attempts to treat a person in a physical way rather than through learning or talking. The most common type of organic therapy involves the use of medications; drug or medication therapy is increasingly used to treat a variety of mental disorders.

Three basic categories of medications are used to treat mental disorders: antipsychotics, antidepressants, and anxiolytics. Each of these categories includes many different drugs, the use of which depends on an individual's emotional and physical condition.

The way in which antipsychotic drugs work is not clear. It has been found, however, that they are very powerful substances that can alter mental processes and thus benefit psychotic patients. These medications have potentially serious side effects, including drowsiness, irregular heartbeat, and persistent muscle twitching. Stelazine, Thorazine, and Haldol are three commonly used antipsychotic drugs.

Antidepressants such as Tofranil, Elavil, and Prozac relieve depression by mechanisms that are also not well understood. They are most effective for depression that is not brought on by an outside event, such as a death in the family. Potentially serious side effects from antidepressants include dangerously low blood pressure, disorientation, and confusion. Patients who cannot be treated with antidepressants because of medical problems occasionally can be helped by the use of stimulants such as Ritalin.[27]

electroconvulsive therapy (ECT)—an organic therapy, also known as shock treatment, in which an electric current is applied to the brain to induce convulsions.

psychosurgery—an organic therapy in which small amounts of brain tissue are irreversibly destroyed using laser surgery techniques.

The anxiolytics, sometimes known as minor tranquilizers, are the most commonly prescribed medications for mental disorders of all types. They reduce anxiety, induce sedation, and sometimes stimulate the appetite. They may also produce drowsiness, lack of muscular coordination, and confusion. Librium, Valium, and Xanax are perhaps the most commonly used anxiolytics.

Other organic therapy approaches include **electroconvulsive therapy (ECT;** shock treatment), and **psychosurgery.** In ECT, an electric current is applied to the patient's brain to induce a convulsion. The patient experiences very little

Comfort Level

Feeling Good about Yourself

Friends and family members are the people you feel comfortable with. You enjoy them because they have qualities you appreciate and admire and accept you for what you are without seeming to demand perfection. They feel at ease with you for the same reasons.

Think about your circle of family and friends. Perhaps you admire an uncle for his generosity and can accept the fact that he also has selfish motives from time to time. You love a close friend for her kindness and forgive her for an occasional thoughtless remark.

However, many people have difficulty accepting themselves in the same way. They may fail to give themselves credit for their positive characteristics and focus unduly on what they think are negative aspects of their appearance or personality.

For example, some people worry about the way they look even though others consider them attractive. Men may be concerned about being too short or losing their hair. Women may exaggerate perceived flaws in their appearance and think that their features are too large or their hips are too heavy. People often have an image of how they want to appear that is based on unrealistic standards.

However, being comfortable with the way one looks is an important part of accepting oneself. Mental health experts say that people who cannot accept imperfections in appearance and personality often develop a sense of shame that distorts their behavior and prevents them from enjoying life fully. This is a classic description of low self-esteem.

Such people often worry that their accomplishments do not measure up to the standards set by others when it is their own standards that are impossibly high. They may tend to be competitive, frequently feeling envious of those who accomplish more—and then they may feel guilty because they are envious.

Frequently, they are very concerned about what others think, even though they do not know those people very well or care very much about their opinions. They worry that others may be angry with them; if someone actually confronts them with criticism, they feel vulnerable. Fearing rejection by others, they may interpret a simple question as a criticism. They become elated over praise but at the same time have difficulty accepting compliments, suspecting that they are not sincere. Sometimes they may reject any praise by pointing out the minor mistakes they have made.

If you recognize any of these symptoms in yourself, your first response may be to view them as further evidence of inadequacy. Instead, you should consciously try to come up with a very different response. You should accept this recognition as a sign of growing self-awareness, which is a starting point for healthier behavior.

Also, think about how you accept imperfections in your family members and friends. Then try to see that some of your own "flaws"—maybe you have a hot temper— are not too harmful, after all. Perhaps you can live with the fact that you cannot carry a tune or your backhand may never improve. In fact, your friends may view these characteristics as part of what makes you uniquely you.

Everyone has weaknesses, but they should not color your whole view of yourself. Focusing instead on your strengths builds self-esteem, makes you better able to accept your limitations, and helps you develop a more realistic picture of yourself. Accepting oneself does not mean giving up on changing things you know can be improved, however. If you identify traits that you do in fact want to change, self-esteem can give you the confidence, motivation, and courage to do so.

Based on ideas in Joan Borysenko, "Ridden with Guilt," and Cheryl Sacra, "Mirror Images," *Health* (March 1990).

discomfort; before treatment he or she is given a sedative and injected with a muscle relaxant. In psychosurgery, small amounts of brain tissue are irreversibly destroyed using sophisticated laser surgery techniques. These forms of treatment are risky and controversial and are usually reserved for cases in which all other types of treatment have been unsuccessful.

Helping Others

Individuals can sometimes play an important part in helping others deal with emotional problems. When someone has a problem, it often helps him or her to talk about it with another person who will listen empathetically and uncritically. Verbalizing the problem in this way can be an important step in resolving it. The most helpful approach is to acknowledge the person's feelings with responses such as "I can tell you are very worried" and "I've been down and unhappy, too." It is best to then let the person work out a strategy for resolving the problem independently rather than rush in with advice or analysis. It is appropriate, however, to encourage and reassure the person.

If it becomes apparent that the person is not feeling better, it is time to seek outside help. It is better to get such help too early than too late. In many cases tragic outcomes might have been prevented if people who knew about the problems had sought outside help sooner (Table 3.3).

It is important to reinforce whatever inclination a troubled person has toward getting help. A good first contact might be a campus counseling service, a member of the clergy, a family physician, or another professional the person with the problem can trust. Most communities have mental health associations, clinics, and medical societies that can provide referrals and advice. If the person seems uninterested in seeking help, a friend or family member might investigate how to get help and perhaps arrange the first contact.

Crisis Intervention If an emotionally disturbed person poses a danger to himself or herself or to others, those nearby must get professional help even against the person's expressed wishes. One source of help is a hospital emergency room. If the person is too upset to be taken there without help, another source is the police, who in most communities are trained to intervene humanely and effectively.

Many communities have a crisis hot line for helping people deal with emergency situations. People can telephone at any time and receive immediate counseling, sympathy, and comfort. Hot lines have been set up for suicidal persons, alcoholics, rape victims, battered women, runaway children, gamblers, and people who just need a shoulder to cry on. Hot lines also provide information about other community services.

Recognizing a Potential Suicide Every year some 30,000 Americans are officially reported as having committed suicide. The true number of suicides, however, may be as high as 100,000 a year, and there may be 8 to 10 suicide attempts for every one that results in death. Suicide attempts among teenagers and young adults have increased dramatically in recent years; this has become a matter of great concern. The rate of death by suicide is second only to death by accidents among young adults.[28]

Many people who are contemplating suicide, particularly young people, are reluctant to seek professional help. Instead, they turn to peers when they are in distress or in need of emotional support.[29] To prevent tragedy, it is important to recognize the warning signs of a potential suicide.

- *Severe depression.* Suicidal people may be hopelessly depressed and so withdrawn or agitated that they cannot eat or sleep. Suicide is 500 times more likely among severely depressed people than it is among the general population.

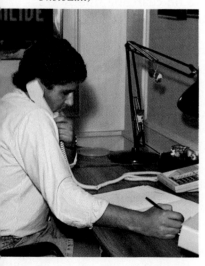

Only a phone call away, 24-hour suicide hot lines offer immediate support for people undergoing major emotional crises. (Mary Kate Denny/PhotoEdit)

Table 3.3 Sources for Help Coping with Emotional Problems

Campus counseling center	Most colleges and universities run counseling centers specifically to help students with problems they may face.
Campus health services	Psychiatric staff—psychiatrists, psychologists, and qualified nurses and social workers—are often available through student health services.
Campus ministry	Many students may prefer to go to the campus ministry office for counseling, also for referral services.
Academic departments	Help may be available through related academic departments, for example, clinical psychology, social psychology, sociology, social welfare.
Community mental health centers	Many communities provide comprehensive services, a major thrust of which involve preventive as well as intervention services.
Traditional therapists	In most areas of the country there are private facilities—psychiatric hospitals, mental health clinics, individual psychiatrists, psychologists, and psychiatric social workers.
Informal contacts: friend, relative, instructor, minister	Sometimes a person you trust can help you look at your problems and your feelings more objectively.
Other sources	Labor unions and company managements; social, religious, and civic organizations; philanthropic foundations; professional mental health associations; local and national governmental agencies concerned with mental health.

- *Extreme mood swings.* A person who is severely depressed one day, elated the next, and depressed again the day after may be struggling with the desire to live and the even stronger desire to die.
- *Giving away precious possessions.* The suicidal person may be indicating that he or she no longer has any reason to live.
- *A crisis that may precipitate a suicide attempt.* When suicidal individuals feel overwhelmed by external events—the loss of a job, the death of a parent, a pile of unpaid bills—they may feel that they cannot cope with life. With young people, the suicide of someone they know or one reported in the media may act as a precipitating event and increase the chance of suicide.[30]
- *Talk of death or suicide.* Suicidal people often talk about their death wish long before they try to kill themselves.

In addition to recognizing these warning signs, it is important to take every suicide attempt or threat seriously no matter how ineffective it may seem. People who quickly bounce back from a suicide attempt and act as if nothing happened may soon try to kill themselves again unless they receive help.

Helping others deal with their emotional problems can benefit both the person receiving help and the person giving it. A concern for others and an ability to help others in times of need are characteristic of an emotionally healthy person. The act of helping another person also contributes to one's self-esteem and self-efficacy.

Like all areas of health, mental health results from a careful balance of interrelated factors: helping and being helped, thinking and feeling, physical and psychological states, and positive and negative emotions. Mental health is also closely related to other components of health—helping to promote them but also benefiting from them. For example, not only do productive attitudes and a sound self-concept help a person who wants to improve his or her physical health, physical health can also contribute to one's mental stability and satisfaction. The next three chapters look at this aspect of health.

Chapter Summary

- The human mind has two basic dimensions: an affective (emotional) dimension and a cognitive (intellectual) one.
- Emotions do not occur only in the mind; they have an important physical component as well.
- These physiological responses, which include changes in heart rate, blood pressure, and brain waves, are controlled by the autonomic nervous system.
- People learn the meaning of their emotional responses in two basic ways: by association and by observing the experiences of others.
- Negative emotional states such as anger, anxiety, and minor depression are experienced by all people at times. Most people are able to deal with these feelings effectively.
- An important part of emotional health is learning how to cope with negative emotions. People employ a variety of defense mechanisms in their coping strategies.
- Sound emotional health allows a person to cope more effectively with the ups and downs of daily life.
- Some people experience nonpsychotic mental disorders, including anxiety, personality, and somatoform disorders. These disorders can seriously inhibit a person's ability to function and should be treated before they become chronic.
- Psychotic disorders such as major depression, bipolar disorder, schizophrenia, delusional disorders, and organic mental disorders are among the most serious mental problems. An individual with one of these disorders has significantly lost contact with reality; professional treatment is essential.
- Intellect is the thinking side of the mind. It has two components: memory and cognition.
- Conditioned response theory and social learning theory attempt to explain aspects of how people learn.
- Memory—the vast storehouse of information that one has learned—is an important factor in good health.
- Cognition is the process of knowing; it includes mental activities such as thinking, judging, reasoning, making decisions, and solving problems.
- The ability to solve problems and make decisions is an important element in effective intellectual functioning and is essential to promoting and maintaining good health.
- A healthy self-concept and sense of self-esteem and self-efficacy are vital parts of overall health and well-being.
- Many types of help are available for emotional problems, including behavior therapy, psychotherapy, group therapy, and organic therapies. The therapy that is chosen depends on the individual's needs and the nature of the problem.
- Individuals can help others deal with emotional problems by listening empathetically, encouraging them to seek outside help, and referring them to appropriate sources of help.
- Suicide is a significant problem in the United States, particularly among teenagers and young adults. Everyone should recognize the warning signs of a potential suicide and be available to help prevent it.

Key Terms

Psychosomatic disease (page 56)

Central nervous system (CNS) (page 56)

Peripheral nervous system (PNS) (page 56)

Somatic nervous system (SNS) (page 57)

Autonomic nervous system (ANS) (page 57)

Electroencephalogram (EEG) (page 59)

Generalization (page 60)

Defense mechanism (page 64)

Repression (page 64)

Rationalization (page 64)

Denial (page 64)

Projection (page 64)

Psychic contactlessness (page 64)

Depersonalization (page 64)

Sublimation (page 64)

Nonpsychotic disorder (page 66)

Adjustment disorder (page 67)

Anxiety disorder (page 67)

Phobia (page 67)

Panic disorder (page 67)

Personality disorder (page 68)

Schizoid personality disorder (page 68)

Narcissistic personality disorder (page 68)

Antisocial personality disorder (page 68)

Somatoform disorder (page 69)

Hypochondriasis (page 69)

Psychotic disorder (page 69)

Affective disorder (page 69)

Major depression (page 69)

Bipolar disorder (page 69)

Mania (page 69)

Schizophrenia (page 70)

Intellect (page 71)

Conditioned response theory (page 71)

Classical conditioning theory (page 71)

Operant conditioning theory (page 71)

Social learning theory (page 72)

Self-concept (page 76)

Self-esteem (page 76)

Behavior therapy (page 76)

Organic therapy (page 78)

Electroconvulsive therapy (ECT) (page 78)

Psychosurgery (page 78)

References

1. Norman Cousins, *Anatomy of an Illness* (New York: W W Norton, 1979).

2. William W. Grings and Michael E. Dawson, *Emotions and Bodily Responses* (New York: Academic Press, 1978): 6–19.

3. Camille Wortman and Elizabeth Loftus, *Psychology*, 3d ed. (New York: Knopf, 1988): 130.

4. A. Collins and M. Frankenhaeuser, "Stress Responses in Male and Female Engineering Students," *Journal of Human Stress* 4 (1978): 43–48; Gunnar Johansson, "Case Report on Female Catecholamine Excretion in Response to Examination Stress," in *Reports from the Department of Psychology* (Stockholm: University of Stockholm Press, 1977): 515; Jerome E. Singer et al., "Stress on the Train: A Study of Urban Commuting," in *Advances in Environmental Psychology*, vol. 1, A. Baum et al. (eds.) (Hillsdale, N.J.: Erlbaum, 1978); Marianne Frankenhaeuser, "Biochemical Events, Stress and Adjustment," *Reports from the Psychological Laboratories* (Stockholm: University of Stockholm Press, 1972): 368; Marianne Frankenhaeuser, "Quality of Life: Criteria for Behavioral Adjustment," *International Journal of Psychology* 12 (1977): 99–110; Marianne Frankenhaeuser, "Coping with Job Stress: A Psychological Approach," *Reports from the Department of Psychology* (Stockholm: University of Stockholm Press, 1978): 532.

5. Carol Tavris, *Anger: The Misunderstood Emotion* (New York: Simon & Schuster, 1983).

6. Carol Garrison et al., "Epidemiology of Depressive Symptoms in Young Adolescents," *Journal of the American Academy of Child and Adolescent Psychiatry* 28, no. 3 (1989): 343–351.

7. Harvey F. Clarizio, "Continuity in Childhood Depression," *Adolescence* XXIV, no. 94 (Summer 1989): 253–267.

8. The discussion of defense mechanisms is based on Sidney M. Jourard and Ted Landsman, *Healthy Personality*, 4th ed. (New York: Macmillan, 1980): 214.

9. G. E. Vaillant, "Introduction: A Brief History of Empirical Assessment of Defense Mechanisms," in *Empirical Studies of Ego Mechanisms of Defense* (Washington, D.C.: American Psychiatric Press, 1986).

10. Sidney M. Jourard and Ted Landsman, *Healthy Personality*, 4th ed. (New York: Macmillan, 1980): 211–245.

11. Alan Apter et al., "Defense Mechanisms in Risk of Suicide and Risk of Violence," *American Journal of Psychiatry* 146, no. 8 (August 1989): 1030.

12. American Psychiatric Association, *Diagnostic and Statistical Manual of Mental Disorders*, 3d ed. revised (Washington, D.C.: American Psychiatric Association, 1987).

13. A. T. Beck et al., *Anxiety Disorders and Phobias* (New York: Basic Books, 1985).

14. Rudolf Hoehn-Saric et al., "Symptoms and Treatment Responses of Generalized Anxiety Disorder Patients with High versus Low Levels of Cardiovascular Complaints," *American Journal of Psychiatry* 146, no. 7 (July 1989): 854–859.

15. F. Von Broembsen, "Role Identity in Personality Disorders: Validation, Valuation, and Agency in Identity Formation," *American Journal of Psychoanalysis* 49, no. 2 (1989): 115–125.

16. Wayne Katon and Joan Russo, "Somatic Symptoms and Depression," *Journal of Family Practice* 29, no. 1 (1989): 65–69.

17. National Center for Health Statistics, B. K. Cypress, "Patients' Reasons for Visiting Physicians, The National Ambulatory Medical Care Survey, United States, 1977–1978," in *Vital and Health Statistics*, Series 13, no. 56 (DHHS Pub. No. PhS82-1717), (Washington, D.C.: U.S. Government Printing Office, December 1981): 113.

18. Kenneth S. Kendler et al., "Psychotic Disorders in DSM-III-R," *American Journal of Psychiatry* 146, no. 8 (August 1989): 953–955.

19. Dr. Robert Cancro, cited in Maya Pines, "Darkness of Schizophrenia Begins to Lift, A Little," *New York Times* (May 26, 1982).

20. Wortman and Loftus, pp. 130–133.

21. Ibid., pp. 144–146.

22. The discussion of problem-solving steps is derived from Bootsin et al., *Psychology Today*, 6th ed. (New York: Random House, 1986): 259–265.

23. P. McC. Miller et al., "Self-Esteem, Life Stress and Psychiatric Disorder," *Journal of Affective Disorders* 17 (1989): 65–75.

24. Ibid.

25. T. Byram Karasu, "New Frontiers in Psychotherapy," *Journal of Clinical Psychiatry* 50, no. 2 (February 1989): 46–52.

26. Robert D. Zettle and Jeanetta C. Rains, "Group Cognitive and Contextual Therapies in Treatment of Depression," *Journal of Clinical Psychology* 45, no. 3 (May 1989): 436–445.

27. Sally L. Satel and J. Craig Nelson, "Stimulants in the Treatment of Depression: A Critical Overview," *Journal of Clinical Psychiatry* 50, no. 7 (July 1989): 241–249.

28. James C. Overholser et al., "Suicide Awareness Programs in the Schools: Effects of Gender and Personal Experience," *Journal of American Academy of Child and Adolescent Psychiatry* 28, no. 6 (1989): 925–930.

29. Ann Garland et al., "A National Survey of School-Based, Adolescent Suicide Prevention Programs," *Journal of American Academy of Child and Adolescent Psychiatry* 28, no. 6 (1989): 931–934.

30. David A. Brent et al., "An Outbreak of Suicide and Suicidal Behavior in a High School," *Journal of American Academy of Child and Adolescent Psychiatry* 28, no. 6 (1989): 918–924.

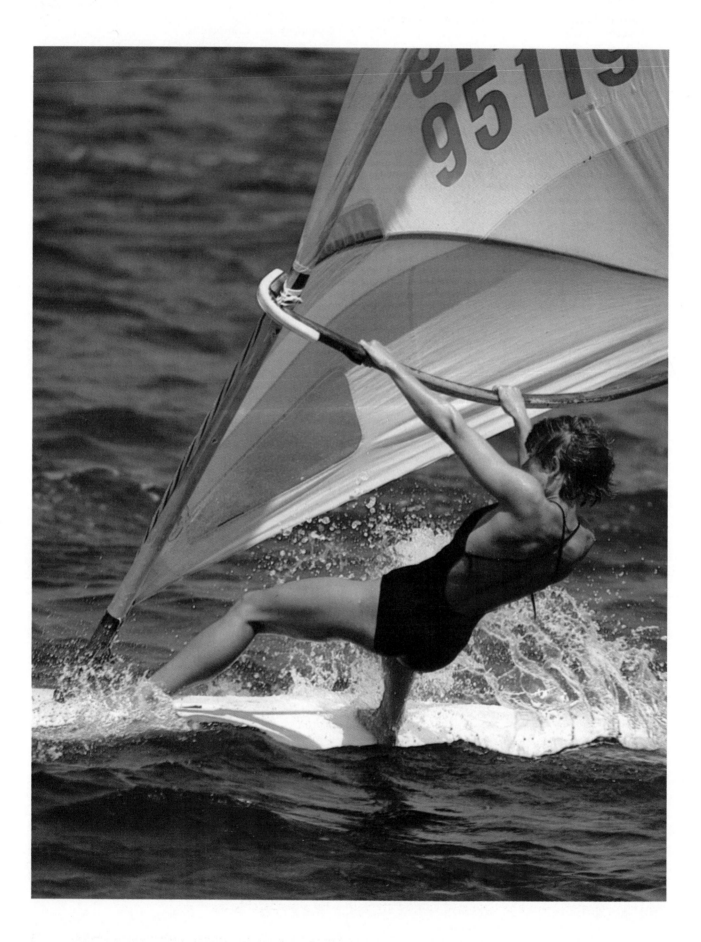

Chapter 4

Activity, Exercise, and Physical Fitness

To Guide Your Reading

When you have studied this chapter, you should be able to:

- Differentiate between activity and exercise and discuss the benefits and dangers of exercise.

- Define 11 different components of fitness, distinguishing between those which are skill-related and those which are health-related.

- Explore the benefits of flexibility, strength, endurance, and cardiovascular fitness, indicating which types of exercises promote each one.

- Name four general principles that should underlie every exercise program.

- Describe important stages in developing a sound exercise plan to meet personal goals.

- Explain why an exercise plan should become a permanent part of a person's weekly routine, adapted throughout the person's life span.

Fitness is fashionable; the evidence is everywhere. Models, entertainers, and other popular idols are not just thin anymore; they are lean and fit, with trim, toned bodies that radiate good health. In recent years the trend toward fitness has taken hold: health clubs have sprung up everywhere, exercise books and videos have become best-sellers, and warm-up suits have become standard clothing. More Americans than ever are exercising regularly—running, swimming, doing aerobics, and walking their way to physical fitness. Regular exercise not only helps them look and feel better physically, it also helps them feel more relaxed and energetic and increases their sense of inner power and self-esteem. Physical fitness enables individuals to lead more productive, creative, healthy, and emotionally balanced lives.

Despite the interest in fitness and exercise, a recent survey by the National Sporting Goods Association (NSGA) showed that only about 20 percent of Americans get a significant amount of regular exercise and that 45 percent of American adults do not participate in any fitness or athletic activity.[1] This indicates that despite the emphasis on fitness, many Americans are still not exercising regularly or at all. Of course, everyone knows that exercise promotes weight loss and lowers one's chances of developing heart disease and other illnesses. Somehow, though, many people have missed the message that exercise is for everyone, not just for the young and the athletic. In fact, a lifelong commitment to regular exercise may be one of the most important factors in promoting health and longevity. At every stage of life regular exercise is as important as regular meals.

In its objectives for the year 2000, the United States Public Health Service (PHS) has made the goal of getting more people to exercise one of its top priorities.[2] While PHS objectives used to stress vigorous physical exercise for at least 20 minutes a day, recent research has indicated that fitness is within the reach of many more people and can be attained with considerably less exercise than was thought previously. Some studies have shown that people can improve their fitness significantly with just 12 minutes of exercise three times a week.[3] The PHS's newest guidelines recommend that almost everyone exercise on a regular basis and indicate that this exercise need include only a moderately strenuous activity such as brisk walking in conjunction with warm-up, stretching, and cool-down activities.

When you consider the many benefits of exercise and the relatively small investment of time it requires, it is clear that a physical fitness program should be part of your health care plans. If you are already exercising regularly, this chapter can help you get the most out of a fitness program not just now but throughout your life. If you are not exercising now, you can learn what you need to know to start and continue a physical fitness program that is right for you.

Decisions about exercise are personal, based on what you want for yourself: a trimmer body, greater endurance or strength, cardiovascular fitness, and so on. You are free to decide what you want to get out of an exercise program and plan the program accordingly. Whatever you decide, be sure to block out time for exercise in your weekly schedule—and make it a lifelong habit. Exercise is vital for your health.[4]

Physical Fitness and Health

The human body was designed to be used—to be kept in fairly constant motion. Until recently, the daily tasks of life required physical work. Even 100 years ago, most people spent their days getting strenuous exercise: swinging a scythe in the fields, manipulating machinery in factories, or scrubbing floors and lugging tubs of wet laundry at home. Today, however, few people en-

Good news for those who prefer to exercise at a more leisurely pace: you burn the same number of calories whether you run a mile or walk a mile. The average person burns about 100 calories for each mile covered on foot.

Former Surgeon General C. Everett Koop suggested that even the busiest people can find ways to fit walking into their daily schedules. Among the examples he cited were the following:

- *Park your car or get off the bus or subway farther away from your destination than usual and walk the rest of the way.*
- *Take walks at lunchtime or during a daily break from work.*
- *Walk with family members or friends to make exercise a social occasion and help them get benefits as well.*

Table 4.1   *The Physical Benefits of Regular Exercise*

Major Benefit	Related Benefits
Improved cardiovascular fitness	Stronger heart muscle; lower heart rate; increased oxygen-carrying capacity of the blood; improved coronary circulation; possible improved peripheral circulation; reduced blood fat, including low-density lipoproteins (LDLs); increased protective high-density lipoproteins (HDLs); possible resistance to atherosclerosis; possible reduction in blood pressure; resistance to ''emotional storm''; less chance of a heart attack; greater chance of surviving a heart attack
Greater lean body mass and less body fat	Greater work efficiency; less susceptibility to disease; improved appearance; less incidence of self-concept problems related to obesity
Improved strength and muscular endurance	Greater work efficiency; less chance of muscle injury; decreased chance of low back problems; improved ability to meet emergencies; improved sports performance
Improved flexibility	Greater work efficiency; less chance of muscle injury; less chance of joint injury; decreased chance of low back problems; improved sports performance
Other benefits	Extended life; quicker recovery after hard work; decreased chance of adult-onset diabetes; less chance of osteoporosis; reduced risk of certain cancers

Source: Charles B. Corbin and Ruth Lindsey, *Concepts of Physical Fitness with Laboratories,* 7th ed. (Dubuque, Iowa: Brown, 1991). All rights reserved. Reprinted by permission.

gage in daily activities that require physical exertion. Most people's waking hours are spent sitting at a desk, behind the wheel of a car, or in front of a television set; even toothbrushes and pencil sharpeners are motorized. From the start, children do not get enough exercise. Many spend long hours watching TV or engaged in other passive activities. According to a recent government study, 50 percent of girls and 30 percent of boys under age 12 cannot run a mile in less than 10 minutes.[5]

Activity versus Exercise

Today, most people must make a special effort to get the amount of physical activity their bodies need for adequate health and fitness. Everyone engages in some **physical activity**—any bodily movement that results in an expenditure of energy. Physical activities include household tasks, work-related activities such as talking on the phone and typing, walking across a parking lot, and even studying. However, few people get enough physical activity to meet the body's needs. Even people who are sometimes quite physically active may have periods of inactivity. As a result, almost everyone needs some **physical exercise**—planned, structured, repetitive activities designed to improve or maintain one or more components of physical fitness.[6] It is not necessary to spend a lot of time and effort, but it is necessary to set aside time for regular physical exercise. The benefits in regard to overall physical fitness as well as physical and psychological health will be substantial.

physical activity—*any voluntary body movement that results in an expenditure of energy.*

physical exercise—*planned, structured, repetitive physical activities designed to improve or maintain one or more components of physical fitness.*

Physical Benefits of Exercise

Regular exercise is an important element in developing and maintaining overall physical health. There is mounting evidence that it reduces the risk of contracting many diseases, including heart disease.[7] In a landmark study of Harvard alumni whose health was followed for up to 40 years, the physically active men had much lower death rates. Men who burned as few as 500 calories a week through exercise and activity had death rates from all causes that were 15 to 20 percent lower than those of men who were more sedentary.[8] This finding was reinforced by a more recent study showing that death rates are inversely related to regular physical exertion, even in men at high risk for developing coronary heart disease. The decline in death rates was associated with a moderate increase in physical leisure-time activities such as gardening and home repairs.[9]

Exercise has also been shown to be related to the prevention and control of high blood pressure, osteoporosis (Chapter 17), and even cancer. One study even suggests that athletic women may cut their risk of developing breast and uterine cancer in half and the risk of developing the most common form of diabetes by two-thirds.[10] In addition, exercise can help prevent musculoskeletal problems such as back pain (Table 4.1).

The Centers for Disease Control now recommend promoting fitness activities that can ward off these and other chronic diseases. They further recommend that more research be done to determine the effect of regular physical activity on osteoarthritis, low back pain, and depressive episodes as well as on smoking and alcohol and drug abuse.[11]

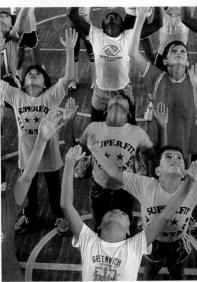

Regular exercise should begin in childhood and continue throughout one's life. (Charles Harbutt/Archive)

Exercise and Psychological Health

Exercise also promotes a feeling of mental and emotional well-being. People who walk, run, swim, or cycle regularly are familiar with the psychological and physical glow that often follows exercise. Exercise seems to discharge the tension that accumulates when the body is under stress. After a strenuous workout, the body naturally relaxes, and this has beneficial effects on the mind as well (Table 4.2).

Perseverance and Motivation

Many people who enjoy sports have no difficulty incorporating an exercise regime into their regular lifestyle. For many others, exercise turns out to be a short-term commitment if it becomes a commitment at all: they do not feel comfortable with the idea of regular exercise. They may work out when they have a goal to achieve—firmer muscles or weight loss—but either they reach their goal and then given up exercise or they just give up. These people miss out on the advantages of exercise which come only to those who persevere with regular physical workouts throughout their lives.

Exercise can indeed help you reach important goals, such as building strength or stamina, becoming more flexible, and losing weight. But perhaps more important, exercise can help you maintain those goals and contribute to a lower likelihood of developing heart disease and other chronic problems in later life.

Any exercise program you set up for yourself should be designed to help you achieve your short-term physical goals. This will help keep you motivated. However, the program should also be as much fun as possible; otherwise your willpower may fade early.

Fortunately, fitness experts, who once advised people to choose a single strenuous activity such as running or swimming as their main source of exercise, are now calling for exercise plans that include a variety of activities. You can run one day a week, do calisthenics or yoga on another day, and engage in a sport such as softball, basketball, or tennis on a third.

An exercise plan that includes a variety of activities has several advantages. It is more fun, and so you are less likely to abandon the exercise routine out of boredom. Sports such as softball and racquetball, which require short bursts of movement, complement sustained strenuous activities such as swimming and jogging. Different activities also tone up different muscle groups. Even those which use the same muscles use them in different ways.

The benefits gained from one kind of exercise may make it easier to pursue another. For example, cycling strengthens the leg muscles in a way that helps you run long distances, and running develops calf and hamstring muscles that are important in cycling.

Your exercise routine can alternate long, slow workouts with short, more intense activities. For example, if you run 3 miles in 18 minutes one day, your next workout might consist of a softball game or a long walk at a moderate pace. Remember to include days of rest in your exercise routine, too, especially if you tend to squeeze a lot of activities into the day. Exhaustion leaves you prone to illness and injury, which can interrupt your exercise routine—and the rest of your life—for much longer periods.

For those who still find that they cannot abide exercise, studies indicate that physical activity can provide many advantages even if it is not strenuous enough to make you sweat. For example, a recent study of mail carriers led researchers to conclude that regular mild physical work provides many of the benefits of exercise: a job which involves walking appears to raise the body's level of high-density lipoproteins, the "good" cholesterol.

There is no single fitness prescription that suits everybody, says a sports medicine specialist from New York. Instead, you should choose a mix of activities that can create an enjoyable "custom package" and be ready to change it periodically so that you stay challenged and interested.

Tailor your package to meet your goals and capabilities, but also be sure that you are comfortable with it and find it fun. That is the first step toward making exercise an integral part of your life.

Ideas based on Hal Higdon, "Base Fitness," *Walking* (February–March 1988): 38–43; "Mini Workouts Work," *East West* (August 1990); "Mix and Match" and "Smart Ways to Shape Up," *U.S. News and World Report* (July 18, 1988).

Table 4.2 The Psychological Health Benefits of Regular Exercise

Major Benefit	Related Benefits
Reduction in mental tension	Relief of depression; improved sleep habits; fewer stress symptoms; ability to enjoy leisure; possible work improvement
Opportunity for social interaction	Improved quality of life Increase in social support system
Resistance to fatigue	Ability to enjoy leisure; improved quality of life; improved ability to meet some stressors
Opportunity for successful experience	Improved self-concept; opportunity to recognize and accept personal limitations
Other benefits	Improved sense of well-being; improved self-concept; improved appearance

Physical exercise seems to reduce stress and help people manage it in at least two ways. First, exercise may use up the hormones and other by-products that stress produces in the body. Second, exercise seems to increase a person's tolerance for stressful situations.[12] In a sense, exercise seems to immunize the body against the harmful effects of stress.

To get the full benefits of stress reduction, however, it may be necessary to avoid activities that are highly competitive. Playing a competitive game of tennis or golf is not relaxing when a person's ego gets too involved. An individual activity such as walking, biking, or swimming may be more relaxing and enjoyable.

Researchers have found that regular exercise can help reduce anxiety and depression. For many people, exercise increases self-esteem as well. As a result, most people who begin a regular exercise program can expect to sleep better, work more efficiently, cope better with stress, have more energy, and feel more relaxed and self-confident.

Exercise and Physical Risks

Despite the pleasures and benefits it brings, exercise contains an element of risk. Doctors, clinics, and emergency rooms handle an estimated 3 million to 5 million sports-related injuries a year, and millions of other aches, pains, and pulled muscles go unreported. Some people have to stop exercising because of pulled muscles or minor joint injuries. Others struggle on despite pain or discomfort, believing in the maxim "no pain, no gain." Usually the cause of minor injuries or discomfort is exercising too hard and too long in the early stages of an exercise program. It is important to start slowly and build up the length and difficulty of the sessions gradually, particularly if a person has been inactive for some time. Do not try to make up for years of neglect in a day or a week.

Contrary to the saying, it is not necessary to feel real pain to improve fitness. Some soreness is to be expected when a person starts using muscles that have not been used recently. The soreness usually comes on gradually, and unless the exercise has been overdone, it is fairly mild. However, sudden or severe pain is always a signal to stop exercising. The body is warning you that something is wrong, and it is important to find out what it is. A person who experiences pain in the chest or repeated episodes of pain while exercising should stop and see a doctor.

While many people risk their health because they do not exercise enough, others become compulsive exercisers who may injure themselves by exercis-

Ankle injuries are particularly common among people who are starting out in racket sports, basketball, and volleyball—sports that require people to make sudden stops and turns. These people tend to try to do too much in one session, and the ankle is more likely to roll over during a sudden stop, when a person's legs are tired. For serious strains and sprains, experts recommend the RICE treatment: rest, ice, compression, and elevation.

ing too much. Sports medicine specialists suggest that excessive exercise is the primary cause of the increased number of sports injuries today.[13] Exercise addicts abuse exercise just as others abuse food, drugs, or alcohol. They risk injuries such as stress fractures, damaged cartilage, and *tendonitis* (an inflammation of the tendons), and they continue exercising even when injured. In women, the loss of body fat induced by too much exercise can lead to **amenorrhea** (loss of monthly menstrual periods) and a resulting loss of bone density that can result in fractures and other problems.[14] For everyone, moderation is the key to proper exercise.

Physical Fitness and Its Components

Physical fitness is made up of several separate components, which can be grouped into two broad categories: skill-related and health-related.

Skill-Related Components

The skill-related components of fitness are the ones that athletes in particular try to improve with exercise. These components include the following:

- **Agility**—the ability to change the position of the whole body quickly while controlling its movement.
- **Balance**—the ability to maintain or regain upright posture, or equilibrium, while moving or standing still.
- **Coordination**—the ability to use the senses of vision and touch together with kinesthetic, or muscle, sense to accomplish accurate, well-timed body movements.
- **Power**—the ability to do strength exercises quickly.
- **Reaction time**—the amount of time it takes to start moving once a person decides to do so.
- **Speed**—the ability to perform a movement or cover a distance in a short time.[15]

It is easy to see how each of these skill-related components is helpful to an athlete. To some extent, these skills are influenced by heredity; that is why people speak of the "natural athlete," a person who seems to have been born with superior physical abilities. Some, or perhaps all, of these components may not be important for your personal fitness goals. However, these qualities may be helpful to you if you include a skill-related sport such as tennis in your physical fitness program.

Anyone can improve these components of fitness through exercise. Many types of exercise are very useful for improving coordination, agility, speed, and so on. If you are an athlete, you probably do these kinds of exercises as part of your regular sports training. When you work on developing skill-related fitness, you will probably improve only to a certain level, because the body has limits for speed, agility, coordination, power, and so on. This knowledge will help prevent frustration if you cease to improve.

Health-Related Components

The health-related components of fitness are the ones that all people need and should work to develop and improve. These components include the following:

- **Flexibility**—the ability to use the joints fully and move them easily through their full range of motion.
- **Muscular strength** and **muscular endurance**—the amount of external force the skeletal muscles—those which are attached to the bones—can exert (strength) and the ability to use these muscles many times in succession without getting tired (endurance).
- **Cardiovascular fitness**—the ability to exercise the whole body for long periods and have the circulatory system supply the fuel—mostly oxygen—that keeps the body going.

amenorrhea—*suppression of monthly menstrual periods for reasons other than pregnancy or menopause.*

agility—*the ability to change the position of the whole body quickly while controlling its movement.*

balance—*the ability to maintain or regain upright posture, or equilibrium, while moving or standing still.*

coordination—*the ability to use the senses of vision and touch, together with kinesthetic (muscle) sense, to accomplish accurate, well-timed body movements.*

power—*the ability to do strength exercises quickly.*

reaction time—*the amount of time it takes to start moving once a person has decided to do so.*

speed—*the ability to perform a movement or cover a distance in a short time.*

flexibility—*the ability to use the joints fully and move them easily through the full range of possible motion.*

muscular strength—*the amount of external force the skeletal muscles can exert.*

muscular endurance—*the ability to use muscles continuously over a period of time.*

cardiovascular fitness—*the ability to exercise the whole body for long periods and have the circulatory system supply the fuel that the body needs to keep going.*

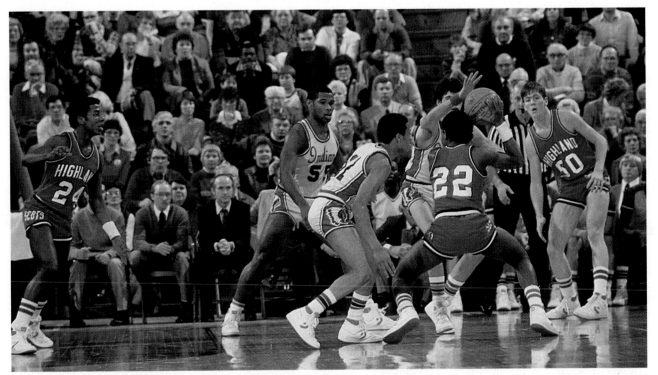

A fast-paced basketball game combines all the skill-related components of physical fitness: agility, balance, coordination, power, reaction time, and speed. (Joe McNally/Wheeler Pictures)

- **Body leanness**—the quality of having more than 75 to 80 percent of body composition as lean tissue (muscle and bone) and less than 20 to 25 percent as fat. A person who develops body leanness through exercise is likely to be healthier and have a longer life than is a person who is overly fat.[16]

body leanness—the quality of having more than 75 to 80 percent of body composition as lean tissue (muscle and bone).

All the health-related components are linked; a certain amount of strength is necessary, for example, to develop cardiovascular fitness. However, it is possible for the body to exhibit one or more of these qualities without exhibiting all five; a person may be strong but lack flexibility. Yet to be healthy, a person must be at least minimally fit in each of these areas.

Developing Health-Related Fitness

Since the health-related components of physical fitness are particularly vital for health and well-being, it is important to look at each one in greater detail. (Body leanness is covered extensively in Chapter 6.)

Flexibility

Flexibility involves the range of motion possible at the many joints in the body (Figure 4.1). It is largely dependent on the various muscles associated with the joints; when these muscles are developed and lengthened through appropriate exercise, they allow the joints to move through a wider range of motion. Different joints have different ranges of motion; for example, the knee joint has a more limited range of motion than the shoulder joint does. At each joint, the connective tissue—tendons, ligaments, and joint capsules—determines how far muscles can stretch and whether the joint can reach its full range of motion. Muscle tension can also affect a joint's range of motion. Relaxed muscles and elastic connective tissue allow one to achieve the greatest degree of flexibility.

Figure 4.1 The joints are highly complex systems. Powered by the muscles, they are surrounded by different connective tissues: tendons, which transfer movement from the muscles to the bones; ligaments, which hold the bones together; and cartilage, which cushions the bone ends. Warm-up and stretching increase the blood supply to the joint, making the muscles more efficient and making the other tissues softer, more flexible, and less likely to tighten or tear.

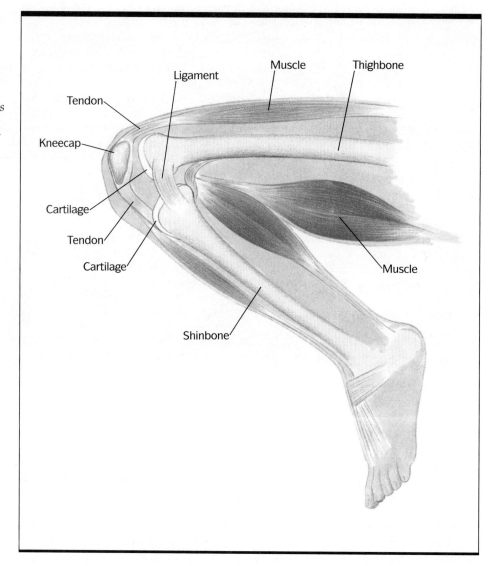

The sports most likely to result in back injury are football, weight lifting, and volleyball. The sports that are least likely to result in back injury include bicycling, hiking, and swimming.

In his book Stretching, Bob Anderson recommends stretching before and after physical activity but also at various times of the day. Among the examples he gives are the following:

- *In the morning, before the start of the day*
- *At work, to release nervous tension*
- *After sitting or standing for a long time*
- *When you feel stiff*
- *At odd times during the day: when watching TV or listening to music*

Benefits   Flexibility is necessary for many routine daily tasks, such as reaching for a plate on a high shelf and pulling a sweater over the head. Good flexibility also helps prevent musculoskeletal problems such as backaches. It is also vital in preventing injuries during exercise; a lack of flexibility impairs one's performance in many sports.[17] Many athletes, even those whose sports require minimal flexibility, recognize the importance of flexibility and incorporate appropriate exercises in their conditioning programs.[18]

Unfortunately, sedentary jobs, daily stress, and poor posture can cause muscle tightness and reduce flexibility. Chronic tension can also lead to shortening of the muscles and connective tissue, leading to muscle spasms and pain and then to more stress and tension.

Stretching Exercises   Static stretching exercises are the best and safest way to improve flexibility. Regularity and relaxation are the keys to a good stretching program. The objective should be to reduce muscular tension in order to promote freer movement.[19] Stretching also can be a stress management technique that can break the tension–muscle pain cycle and foster more relaxed muscles and a more relaxed state of mind. When engaging in a stretching program, you should follow these guidelines.

1. Do not start stretching without doing a preliminary warm-up first. When you increase the temperature of your muscles, they become more elastic so that stretching is safer and more effective. Walking is an

ideal warm-up activity because it is a nonjarring way to get the muscles moving and the blood circulating.

2. After you have warmed up, begin stretching gradually and then increase the intensity. Do not stretch too hard at first. In all stretching exercises, a good rule is to stretch until you feel mild to moderate discomfort. Do not stretch to the point of pain.

3. When stretching, get into position and reach until you feel a mild amount of stretch. Hold this position for 10 to 30 seconds, until you feel your muscles relax. If this does not happen, ease up and find a more comfortable position. Deep, slow breathing helps increase flexibility.[20] As you exhale, stretch a little farther and hold the position for 30 seconds more.

4. Stretch but do not strain. Do not bounce; the alternating tightening and stretching can pull your muscles too hard and too suddenly. Instead, relax into the stretch.

5. To improve flexibility in specific body areas, select stretching activities designed especially for those areas. Try to do several exercises for each area.

6. To achieve the best results, stretch four or five times a week. While stretching can be done on its own, it should also be included in the general warm-up for other, more vigorous exercises. Stretching is especially important to prevent the stiffness many older people experience after exercising. It is also very helpful for people whose jobs require them to sit long hours at a desk or computer terminal.

Muscular Strength and Endurance

Muscular strength is the maximum amount of force a muscle group can exert against resistance. It is often measured by how much weight a person can lift. Muscular endurance refers to the ability of a muscle to continue a prolonged or repetitive exertion without tiring. Many daily activities—washing windows, shoveling snow, using a handsaw, even vacuuming—may make use of both endurance and strength. (But using muscles and developing them are not the same.)

When muscles are used, they burn, or metabolize, two kinds of chemicals provided by the body: carbohydrates and fats. They usually need oxygen for this process. These chemicals reach the muscle by way of the bloodstream; this is why the heart is so important, though carbohydrates and fats also can be stored in small amounts within the muscle tissue itself.

To develop muscle, however, other chemicals are also needed, in particular proteins, from which the muscle fibers themselves are made. Proteins are also vital for the general repair of body tissue. In fact, muscle development is itself a special form of repair: heavy work causes a slight breakdown of the tissue, which is then rebuilt larger and stronger to compensate. Unfortunately, it will not stay larger; if the muscle tissue is not used for a while, it will **atrophy,** or grow smaller again.

atrophy—*to waste away or grow smaller, usually as a result of inactivity.*

Like the chemicals involved in muscle use, proteins are transported in the blood. You will read in Chapter 5 how proteins, along with carbohydrates and fats, are vital chemicals which first enter the body through the digestive system. (Oxygen, of course, comes through the lungs from the air one breathes.)

Benefits Building muscle strength and endurance, at least to a certain level, is an important element in fitness that helps prevent muscle damage and fatigue. Although slight tissue breakdown is good for the muscles and causes growth and development, excessive muscle overload may cause long-term damage, resulting in considerable pain and stress. People who fail to keep their muscles properly toned often suffer unexpected and painful sprains, such as the chronic backaches that can afflict older people with poor muscle tone.

Exercises for Muscular Strength and Endurance Strength and endurance can be improved through exercises that require the muscles to lift, push, or pull against resistance.[21] When one does these exercises, the work load on the muscles is systematically increased as they develop strength. Three kinds of programs are designed to develop muscular strength and endurance: isokinetic, isotonic, and isometric. They differ in the kinds of equipment used and the amount of resistance the muscles encounter at different points during a movement. Table 4.3 summarizes the advantages and disadvantages of each type of exercise.

isokinetic—*referring to the strength training of muscles through the use of special apparatus that provides resistance that is equal to the force the user applies.*

1. **Isokinetic** exercise relies on specialized apparatus, such as Nautilus and Cybex equipment, that provides equal tension at all angles over the full range of a joint's motion. When properly used, this equipment is effective in increasing both muscular strength and endurance. Unfortunately, since isokinetic training programs require special machinery that is usually available only at health clubs and gyms, not everyone has access to such equipment.

isotonic—*referring to the strength training of muscles through exercises that involve muscle contractions throughout a complete range of motion.*

2. **Isotonic** exercise involves lifting a constant weight through a full range of joint motion. Isotonic weight training, which involves the use of free weights such as barbells and dumbbells, can help increase muscular strength and endurance if it includes progressive resistance through a full range of motion. In other words, to execute a given exercise, you should warm up with a weight you can lift 10 times. For the next set, you should choose a weight you can lift only 8 times, and for the final set, you should select a weight you can lift only 6 times.

A major disadvantage of isotonic programs is that since the weight is constant, the heaviest weight that can be lifted through the full range of muscle motion is also the heaviest one that can be lifted at the weakest angle. Thus, a person who tries to lift too heavy a weight is likely to fail at the attempt or move the weight through less than the full range of motion.

Some experts believe that isotonic programs are superior to isokinetic exercises. When properly performed, they involve balancing a constant weight throughout the full range of movement, working many more muscles than isokinetic equipment does. Experts are still debating the relative safety and effectiveness of isokinetics and isotonics.

isometric—*referring to the strength training of muscles by pushing or pulling against a fixed or an immovable object through a relatively narrow range of motion.*

3. In **isometric** exercise, the individual pushes or pulls against a fixed resistance or an immovable object. Experts now consider this the least useful of these three methods. Because the range of motion is restricted, movement strengthens the muscle only at a particular angle.

Table 4.3   Rating Potential Advantages of the Different Types of Exercise

Advantage	Isometrics	Isotonics	Isokinetics
In small space	excellent	fair to good	fair to good
No equipment or low-cost equipment	excellent	fair to good	fair to good
Provides feedback for motivation	fair	excellent	fair
Can rehabilitate immobilized joint	excellent	poor	poor
Builds strength through full range of motion	poor	fair to good	excellent
Less apt to cause soreness	excellent	fair to good	excellent
Aids dynamic coordination	poor	excellent	good
Safe for hypertensive	poor	excellent	good to excellent
Amount of strength developed	fair	excellent	excellent
Dynamic exercises, controlled testing	poor	fair to good	excellent
Hypertrophy	poor	excellent	excellent
Power development	poor	good	excellent
Rapid improvement in strength	excellent	fair to good	fair to good
Can accelerate to resemble sport skill	poor	excellent	poor

Source: Charles Corbin and Ruth Lindsey, *Concepts of Physical Fitness with Laboratories,* 7th ed. (Dubuque, Iowa: Brown, 1991). Reprinted by permission.

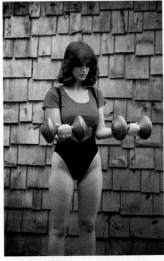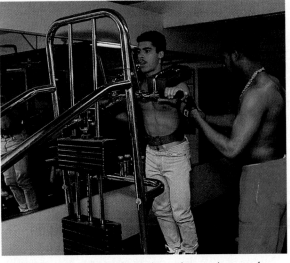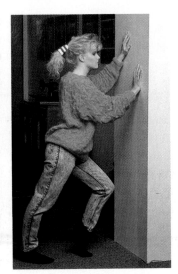

The three major approaches to developing muscular strength are isotonic exercises, such as weight lifting; isokinetic exercises, which require expensive equipment like that shown here; and isometric exercises, which involve pushing or pulling against a fixed resistance. Because they are designed to focus tension at all angles on a moving joint, isokinetic exercises require the use of specialized workout machines. (Burton McNeely; Robert Brenner/ PhotoEdit; David Weinstein/Custom Medical Stock Photo)

Building Strength and Endurance When properly designed and executed, such weight-training programs build muscular endurance as well as strength. If the emphasis is on developing strength, a relatively small number of repetitions should be performed with a heavy load. If the goal is to develop endurance, each exercise should include a relatively large number of repetitions using a low to moderate weight load.

Cardiovascular Fitness

Cardiovascular fitness is the quality that enables a person to mobilize energy and sustain movement over an extended period. It requires that the heart be strong, the lungs healthy, and the blood vessels unobstructed. Since life depends on the capacity of these organs to deliver nutrients and oxygen to the tissues and remove wastes, it is essential that they function efficiently. Cardiovascular fitness is thus the most important component of physical health.

How does exercise aimed at cardiovascular fitness improve physical health? First, it makes the heart and lungs work more vigorously and the blood vessels carry more blood. The body responds by adapting; that is, it becomes capable of accommodating future demands with less or no stress. In time, the muscles involved develop a more extensive network of blood vessels. This means that the blood has more routes for transporting the oxygen and nutrients it carries to all parts of the body. The body also develops more red blood cells (which carry oxygen) and a greater volume of blood (Figure 4.2).

In addition, there is typically an increase in the amount of air the lungs can take in and breathe out at one time **(vital capacity)** and in the amount of air the lungs can take in over a period of time **(maximum breathing capacity)**. The exchange of oxygen and carbon dioxide in the tiny chambers (alveoli) of the lungs becomes more efficient.

vital capacity—*the amount of air the lungs can take in and breathe out at one time.*

maximum breathing capacity—*the amount of air the lungs can take in over a period of time.*

Benefits With improved cardiovascular fitness, the heart becomes stronger and more efficient. Although the heart does not increase much in size, it pumps an increased amount of blood on each beat and is emptied more completely. Between beats, it can slow down and rest more. The normal adult resting pulse rate is around 70 beats a minute, and 80 to 90 beats is not unusual in sedentary individuals. In contrast, a physically fit adult usually has a resting pulse rate of only 55 to 60 beats a minute. (The pulse may be even lower. In trained athletes, such as runners, it is not unusual to see rates of 40 beats a minute.) Consequently, the heart makes thousands fewer beats per day, reducing wear and tear on heart valves and blood vessels.[22]

Cardiovascular fitness may also reduce some forms of hypertension (high blood pressure) because it tends to relax the tiny arteries (arterioles) that work much like nozzles in controlling blood pressure. Experts also believe that increased cardiovascular fitness may have a preventive effect on coronary heart disease: greater fitness levels increase the ratio of high-density lipoprotein (HDL) to total cholesterol, a condition associated with a lower risk of contracting heart disease.[23]

Aerobic Exercise Cardiovascular fitness is usually improved through **aerobic exercise,** sustained exercise of the whole body that increases the heart rate for a significant period of time. Examples of this kind of exercise include vigorous walking, running, jumping rope, bicycling (including stationary bicycles), swimming, cross-country skiing, and aerobic dancing (Table 4.4).

Every time the body performs an exercise, its oxygen needs increase. If the exercise is very strenuous, the heart and lungs cannot provide oxygen fast enough, and the effort thus cannot be sustained for long. Aerobic exercise is exercise done at a slightly lower level of intensity, allowing the body to keep going because it can meet its oxygen needs continuously.

Exercise of this type also uses the large muscles and puts the joints through a wide range of motion. Thus, cardiovascular fitness and muscle endurance can develop together: as cardiovascular fitness improves, the muscles get the oxygen they need to perform longer.

Ideally, an aerobic exercise session should begin with a warm-up and stretching period at least 10 minutes long, followed by a period of aerobic exercising that lasts 20 to 30 minutes and ending with a cool-down period of 5 minutes or more to let the heart rate return to normal. The cool-down is not a period of inactivity but rather a time of very light activity, such as slow walking or a less vigorous version of the exercise you have been doing. Do not neglect this cool-down period. If you stop moving abruptly, blood can collect in the blood vessels in your legs and you may feel light-headed or dizzy.[24]

aerobic exercise—*sustained exercise of the whole body that increases the heart rate, done at a level that allows the body to meet its oxygen needs.*

Think of your cooling-down session as a warm-up in reverse. Instead of doing exercises that gradually increase the heart rate, you are now doing the opposite: reducing your activities slowly to allow the heart rate to decrease slowly.

Cool-down activities are important after all strenuous activity. A runner's victory lap, a hurdler's work-out for tired muscles, a football player's jogging off the field and up to the locker room—all give the cardiovascular system a chance to stabilize. (Tony Freeman/ PhotoEdit)

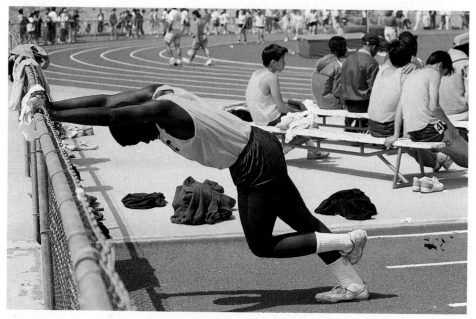

Table 4.4 Benefits of Regular Aerobic Exercise

Increased lung capacity	Increased muscle strength
Lower breathing rate	Increased flexibility
Lower resting heart rate	Increased skill
Lower heart rate during exercise	Increased muscle capacity
Increased blood volume per heartbeat	Increased insulin-receptor sensitivity
Lower blood pressure	Increased sense of physical well-being
Lower levels of low-density lipoproteins	Reduced depression and anxiety
Lower triglyceride levels	

Injuries to women who take part in aerobic dancing classes are quite common, and some physicians recommend restricting aerobic dance sessions to a maximum of three times a week. A research report from San Diego State University indicates that 76 percent of aerobic instructors and 43 percent of participants suffer injuries from time to time. The most common injuries reported were stress fractures.

Low-impact aerobic exercise can be just as effective in improving cardiovascular fitness as is more vigorous exercise, and it is less likely to result in injury. The jarring impact of many exercise routines can cause or aggravate joint and muscle problems. There are many kinds of low-impact aerobic exercises. Race walking, for example, is lower-impact than jogging but can be just as effective. There are low-impact aerobic dance and exercise routines, and swimming is by nature low-impact. Especially for older people but also for anyone with a history of back or knee problems, low-impact aerobic exercises are a good choice.

Anaerobic Exercise   Exercise that causes the body's demand for oxygen to exceed the supply—producing "oxygen debt"—is called **anaerobic exercise.** An example of anaerobic exercise is sprinting 100 meters. The runner exercises so intensely that he or she can replace only part of the oxygen the body uses during the sprint and has to make up for the oxygen debt afterward. For a well-conditioned athlete, both aerobic and anaerobic exercises can be helpful in building cardiovascular fitness. For those who are not well conditioned, however, anaerobic exercise is a poor choice because it may put excessive strain on an unfit heart and circulatory system.

anaerobic exercise—*exercise in which the body's demand for oxygen exceeds its supply, producing oxygen debt.*

Principles of Exercise

To get the maximum benefit from any kind of exercise, it is necessary to understand four basic principles: specificity, overload, progression, and regularity.

Specificity

Specificity means simply that to develop a certain component of fitness, one must work on that particular component. For example, exercises that increase flexibility may do little to develop strength or cardiovascular fitness. If your goal is to develop strength in your biceps, you will have to do arm curls with barbells or another biceps exercise. If you want to develop cardiovascular endurance, you must select an activity that offers continuous aerobic exercise, such as running or swimming.

specificity—*the principle that to develop a component of fitness, one must work on that particular component.*

Overload

As explained earlier in this chapter, for a muscle to become stronger, it must be **overloaded,** or worked against a greater load than usual. Systematic overloading can increase the strength, flexibility, and endurance of muscles. This does *not* mean starting out with an extremely strenuous routine, as this may cause a major injury. In the early stages of an exercise program, overloading a muscle can mean simply stretching it slightly, lifting a light weight, or moving

overload—*to work against a greater load than usual.*

How Fit Are You?

The President's Council on Physical Fitness and Sports has compiled a set of adult fitness standards to help people assess their physical fitness level.

The guidelines include four basic assessment tests: sit-ups for abdominal strength and endurance, push-ups for upper body strength and endurance, sit and reach for flexibility, and a 1.5-mile walk/run for cardiovascular endurance.

These tests can be self-administered. However, if you are over age 40, are a novice exerciser, or have a chronic medical problem such as diabetes, obesity, or coronary artery disease, check with your doctor before taking an exercise testing program.

Test 1   Sit-Ups (abdominal strength and endurance) Scoring standard: number completed in 1.5 minutes

Instructions: Lie flat on your back with the shoulders touching the floor, the knees bent, and the feet flat 8 to 12 inches from the buttocks. Curl upward, lifting the head, shoulders, and upper trunk off the ground. Slide the hands forward to the kneecap. Curl down and repeat. Continue until you are fatigued or for 1.5 minutes maximum. The test is completed at the point of any pause.

Fitness Rating for Sit-Ups (number completed)

	Under 30		30–39		40–49		50–59		60 and Over	
	F	M	F	M	F	M	F	M	F	M
Very high	45+	50+	45+	50+	40+	45+	35+	40+	35+	40+
High	35–44	40–49	35–44	40–49	30–39	34–44	25–34	39–40	25–34	28–39
Moderate	25–34	30–39	25–34	30–39	20–29	25–34	15–24	20–29	15–24	19–27
Low	15–24	20–29	15–24	20–29	14–19	19–24	10–14	15–19	8–14	14–18
Very low	0–15	0–20	0–15	0–20	0–14	0–19	0–10	0–15	0–8	0–14

Test 2   Push-Ups (upper body strength and endurance) Scoring standard: maximum number of push-ups you are able to do without pausing

Instructions: *Women:* Assume the bent-knee push-up position with the hands under the shoulders. Lower the body until the chest touches the floor. Return to the starting position with the arms extended. *Men:* Assume a straight-leg push-up position. Lower the body until the chest touches the floor. Return to the starting position with the arms extended. Continue the test to the maximum number of push-ups. No pauses are allowed.

Fitness Rating for Push-Ups (number completed)

	Under 30		30–39		40–49		50–59		60 and Over	
	F	M	F	M	F	M	F	M	F	M
Very high	49+	55+	40+	45+	35+	40+	30+	35+	20+	30+
High	34–48	45–54	25–39	35–44	20–34	30–39	15–29	25–34	5–19	20–29
Moderate	17–33	35–44	12–24	25–34	8–19	20–29	6–14	15–24	3–4	10–19
Low	6–16	20–34	4–11	15–24	3–7	12–19	2–5	8–14	1–2	5–9
Very low	0–5	0–19	0–3	0–14	0–2	0–11	0–1	0–7	0	0–4

Test 3 Sit and Reach (flexibility) Scoring standard: number of inches reached

Instructions: Warm up for this test with a few minutes of low-level movements such as arm circles or walking in place.

You will need a yardstick and tape for this test. Sit with the legs straight and the heels about 5 inches apart. Place the yardstick between your legs with the 15-inch mark aligned with your heels (you may want to tape the yardstick in place). While sitting in this position, slowly reach forward as far as possible and touch the yardstick. Your score is the number you reach on the yardstick. Repeat three times and record your best score.

Fitness Rating for Sit and Reach (inches)

	Under 30		30–39		40–49		50–59		60 and Over	
	F	M	F	M	F	M	F	M	F	M
Very high	24+	23+	24+	23+	23+	22+	23+	22+	23+	22+
High	20–23	19–22	20–23	19–22	19–22	18–21	19–22	18–21	19–22	18–21
Moderate	18–19	12–18	18–19	12–18	17–18	12–17	17–18	11–17	17–18	11–17
Low	14–17	9–11	14–17	9–11	12–16	8–11	11–16	8–11	10–16	8–9
Very low	0–13	0–8	0–13	0–8	0–11	0–7	0–10	0–7	0–9	0–7

Test 4 Walk/Run Test (cardiovascular endurance) Scoring standard: rating is based on the time it takes to walk/run 1.5 miles

Instructions: Warm up and stretch before doing this test. Walk or run 1.5 miles as quickly as possible but not until you become exhausted. Record your time. After the test, walk an additional 5 minutes and stretch to cool down. This test is recommended after about 6 weeks of training.

Fitness Rating for Walk/Run Test (minutes:seconds)

		Under 30	30–39	40–49	50–59	60 and Over
Very high	M	Up to 9:44	Up to 9:59	Up to 10:29	Up to 10:59	Up to 11:14
	F	Up to 12:29	Up to 12:59	Up to 13:44	Up to 14:29	Up to 16:29
High	M	10:45– 9:45	11:00–10:00	11:30–10:30	12:30–11:00	13:59–11:15
	F	13:30–12:30	14:30–13:00	15:55–13:45	16:30–14:30	17:30–16:30
Moderate	M	14:00–10:46	14:45–11:01	15:35–11:31	17:00–12:31	19:00–14:00
	F	18:30–13:31	19:00–14:31	19:30–15:56	20:00–16:31	20:30–17:31
Low	M	16:00–14:01	16:30–14:44	17:30–15:36	19:00–17:01	20:00–19:01
	F	19:00–18:31	19:30–19:01	20:00–19:31	20:30–20:01	21:00–20:31
Very low	M	16:01 or more	16:31 or more	17:31 or more	19:01 or more	20:01 or more
	F	19:01 or more	19:31 or more	20:01 or more	20:31 or more	21:01 or more

Adapted, with permission from The President's Council on Physical Fitness and Sports.

slowly in an aerobic exercise routine. It is important to go at your own pace; what is easy for one person constitutes overload for another and may send a third person to the emergency room.

Progression

progression—*the principle that once muscles adapt to an overload, the load should be increased slowly and gradually.*

Progression refers to the fact that once muscles adapt to an overload, the load should be increased slowly and gradually. You should stretch farther, lift greater weights, and move more quickly and for a longer period of time. If you progressively and gradually increase your exercise load, your fitness level will improve over time. As your fitness improves, continue to increase the exercise load until you reach an optimum amount of exercise. Do not exercise at too high or too low a level. Exercising at too high a level can be dangerous, perhaps resulting in injury; exercising at too low a level will not build fitness. Then you should maintain your exercise program at the optimum level to avoid atrophy and lessening of function.

Regularity

regularity—*the principle that exercise needs to be done frequently enough, with enough intensity, and for a sufficient period of time.*

For exercise to be effective in developing fitness, it must follow the principle of **regularity**; that is, it must be done frequently enough, with enough intensity, and for a sufficient period of time.

1. **Frequency.** Exercise must be performed regularly to be effective. Most fitness components require at least 3 days of exercise a week.
2. **Intensity.** Exercise must be hard enough to require more exertion than normal, as measured by heart rate (Figure 4.2), in order to produce an improvement in fitness. Too little will not improve fitness; too much may result in soreness or injury.
3. **Time.** An exercise period should be long enough to produce sustained, heightened activity in the muscles involved. For optimal fitness gains, 30 to 90 minutes is often recommended,[25] but several experts accept 20 minutes of vigorous exercise as a useful standard, and recent studies have suggested that exercise periods as short as 12 minutes can be beneficial.

One can benefit by deliberately exercising most of the muscles in one's body; however, one cannot directly exercise the heart, the muscle that ensures that oxygen and key nutrients reach all the other muscles. Prolonged repetitive exercise, especially vigorous exercise involving the long muscles of the legs and the other large muscles in the trunk and arms, ensures that the heart also gets a good workout.

Developing an Exercise Plan

When it comes to exercise, Americans often seem to do either too much or too little. They play football all Saturday afternoon and then get no exercise for the rest of the week. Regular exercise involving the whole body in a program that is tailored to the abilities and needs of the individual is essential for achieving lifelong fitness. Thus, a planned exercise program must take into account not only your present fitness level but also your fitness goals.

Evaluating General Fitness Goals

Exercise serves many purposes. A professional golfer may take up weight training to increase arm and upper body strength in order to put more force and speed into the golf swing. A senior citizen may undertake a series of exercises specially designed to improve back flexibility in order to relieve chronic low back pain. A fit, well-conditioned older college student may take up swimming because his schedule has become too busy to allow frequent games of tennis. A young woman who wants to improve her health and manage stress more effectively may begin a jogging program. Someone in a weight-loss program may use aerobic exercise to help speed weight loss. Some people simply need a minimal though scientifically based exercise plan—a "fitness-for-health" plan.

A fitness-for-health plan suits the individual who has no interest in becoming a marathon runner or world-class athlete. Such an individual wants the health benefits of basic fitness: flexibility, muscular strength and endurance, cardiovascular fitness, perhaps improved body composition (more muscle and less fat), relaxation, and improved emotional health.

Other people prefer a more ambitious plan—a fitness-for-its-own-sake or fitness-for-skill plan. A fitness-for-skill plan is geared to individuals who want to refine or improve skills, such as agility, speed, and coordination, which are needed in a specific sport or activity. Such a plan generally includes exercises that foster health-related benefits as well. A football player, for example, will follow a program of training with weights or other strength-training equipment; he will also engage in agility and cardiovascular exercises to improve his speed, strength, and endurance on the field. A long-distance runner will concentrate on aerobic exercise to increase cardiovascular fitness and will also include stretching and weight training to improve her flexibility and muscular endurance.

If you are interested in a fitness-for-skill program, you may want to receive guidance from a qualified trainer, coach, or exercise physiologist.

Assessing Fitness Needs

Once your general fitness goals have been set, an essential part of planning a fitness program is finding your current fitness level. This can be done with professional help, particularly if you sign up at a professional fitness facility. If you plan to exercise by yourself, you can take the National Fitness Test developed by the President's Council on Physical Fitness and Sports. This consists of four separate tests: sit-ups, push-ups, sit and reach, and a walk/run test. These tests are used to assess, respectively, abdominal strength and endurance, upper body strength and endurance, flexibility, and cardiovascular endurance. (See the Self-Assessment feature on pages 98–99 for additional information on these tests.) Such self-assessments will indicate the level at which you should begin your fitness program. Later, as your fitness improves, you can add to the pace or distance and increase the total time of workouts.

When choosing an exercise program, be conscious of any injuries you have suffered in the past. You may want to avoid activities that can aggravate that injury. For example, if you have a history of knee problems, it may be wise to leave jogging out of your plan—try swimming instead.

- *Evaluate your fitness goals*
- *Assess your fitness level*
- *Choose the exercises*
- *Get a medical checkup*
- *Decide when, where, and how often to exercise*
- *Chart your progress*

How Much Exercise Is Enough?

When you choose an exercise routine, which is the best goal to aim for? If your goal is health—to make yourself less susceptible to illnesses such as heart disease—moderate amounts of exercise may be enough. If you are also aiming for fitness— increased strength and endurance and a trim, more flexible body—you will have to work out longer and more strenuously. Here are two arguments— one for moderate exercise with health as the goal and one for strenuous exercise to achieve fitness.

Exercise Moderately for Health   People who exercise regularly face only half as much risk of developing heart attacks as do those who do not, according to the Centers for Disease Control. However, you need not spend hours jogging, swimming, or working out every week to maintain cardiovascular health.

A 30-minute workout three times a week leads to a heart rate that is one-third lower, saving 36,000 beats per day. It also lowers blood pressure, reduces stress, and strengthens the bones. Even 15 minutes of exercise three times a week can substantially improve your cardiovascular health.

A full-blown fitness effort takes a lot of time. To develop a perfect-looking body, you may have to spend an hour or two at a gym 5 days a week. But many people do not have that much time to spare.

Too much exercise can actually make you more susceptible to injury. Exercise fanatics also hurt themselves more often than do those who exercise moderately, and injuries cause some people to stop regular exercise altogether. Sports injuries are increasing, and excessive exercise seems to be the primary cause. Frequent long, hard workouts can also cause women to stop menstruating and can lower men's sperm counts. What's more, some people become exercise addicts, working out so compulsively that they neglect other aspects of their lives.

Exercise More Vigorously for Fitness as Well as Health   Frequent long, strenuous workouts—especially when combined with a careful diet—quickly produce results you can see, feel, and measure. You know your endurance has increased because you tire less quickly. You can measure the increased

strength by the greater amount of weight you can lift. People tell you how good you look. These rewards motivate you to continue.

When you exercise only moderately for health rather than fitness, you do not get these gratifying results. Your work may pay off by preventing heart disease later on, but you must take the results largely on faith. With nothing to show for your efforts, you may get discouraged and give up.

Furthermore, exercising vigorously for fitness may also increase the health benefits you get from workouts. One study which compared the calories people use up in exercise with death rates concluded that the more exercise people get, the less likely they are to die prematurely. Men whose regular exercise consumed 500 calories a week had death rates more than 15 percent lower than those of men who did not exercise. But among men who burned off 2,000 calories a week the death rates were 33 percent lower, and they were lower still for men who exercised even more. This trend continued up to about 3,500 calories a week.

One reason why some people exercise compulsively is simply that it makes them feel good. Long-distance runners, for example, talk about a runner's high. And what can be wrong with an addiction that makes you feel good, keeps your weight down, strengthens your body, and reduces your chance of contracting heart disease all at the same time? Furthermore, a focus on fitness may prevent people from becoming addicted to something more harmful, such as nicotine, alcohol, or other drugs.

What do you think? Is it better to adopt a moderate exercise program designed only to improve health? Or is it preferable to improve fitness as much as you can? Also, assuming that both courses of action have benefits, which would you choose for yourself?

Ideas based on Peter Aleshire, "Exercise: Do as I Write, Not as I Do," *Arizona Republic* (October 22, 1989); Hal Higdon, "Base Fitness," *Walking* (February–March 1988): 38–43; and "Smart Ways to Shape Up," *U.S. News and World Report* (July 18, 1988).

After evaluating your general fitness goals, assessing your present fitness level, and choosing the exercises you will use, you are almost ready to begin. Before starting, however, there are some things to decide: how often to exercise, what exercises to do, how hard to work, and how much time to spend in each exercise session, as well as when and where to exercise.

How Often Should You Exercise?   As was noted earlier in this chapter, researchers have found that exercising at least 3 days a week provides the greatest cardiovascular benefits; 2 days a week or less is not adequate. Furthermore, if more than 2 days pass between exercise sessions, "detraining" begins; that is, the beneficial effects of earlier sessions are lost. The guidelines of the American College of Sports Medicine (ACSM) recommend exercising three to five times a week. The ACSM sets five as the upper limit because studies have shown that exercising beyond that level increases the chances of injury.[26]

What Exercises Should You Do?   The mix of activities chosen for an exercise program depends on one's current fitness level, goals, and personal likes and dislikes. No single activity is best for all people. For optimal results, a fitness-for-health program should be planned around an aerobic exercise that you enjoy and that involves vigorous, continuous whole-body movement. In addition, it is recommended that two of your exercise sessions include strength exercises for the major muscle groups.[27]

Other considerations include the skill needed, the intensity of the exercise, and the length of time needed per session to produce a conditioning effect. Running, for example, is a more intense activity than cycling, and so exercising with a bicycle will require pedaling longer and faster to achieve the same level of conditioning. Therefore, the activity you choose may depend on how much time you want to spend in each exercise session. Above all, it is important to choose activities that feel good and that you enjoy. Generally, if you enjoy something and feel good doing it, you will do it.

How Hard Should You Exercise?   Recent studies have suggested that it is not necessary to exercise at high intensity to get benefits from a workout. Major health benefits can be obtained from exercise that is the equivalent of walking briskly for about 3 hours a week. Other research has shown that low-intensity exercise improves cardiovascular fitness nearly as much as high-intensity exercise does.[28] Not all experts agree on these findings, however. Some state that more strenuous workouts are necessary to produce a conditioning effect.

Of course, what is strenuous for one person may be easy for another person who is more physically fit. One way to measure the intensity of a workout is to take your pulse to determine your heart rate during exercise. During an exercise session, your pulse should not exceed your target heart rate. Traditionally, physical fitness experts have stated that a person's target heart rate during exercise should be 70 percent of the heart's maximum capacity for that person's age (Figure 4.2). Some recent findings have suggested that a target heart rate of only 50 percent of the heart's maximum capacity can still produce real benefits.[29] Perhaps the best approach is to try to work up gradually from a lower to a higher target heart rate as your fitness program progresses.

How Much Time Should You Spend Exercising?   The answer to this question depends partly on your comfort level about physical fitness. The ACSM recommends doing 20 to 60 minutes of continuous aerobic activity per exercise session.[30] Studies mentioned earlier in this chapter indicate that even 12 minutes of exercise per session can produce benefits, but many exercise physiologists recommend 20 to 30 minutes per session.[31] Remember that extra time must be allowed for warm-up and cool-down and for stretching. And

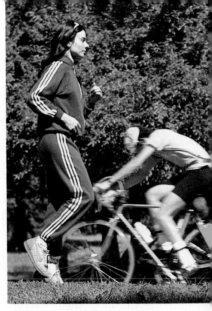

People can choose from a wide variety of exercise activities to match their interests, needs, and abilities. (Ken Karp)

Many fitness experts emphasize the importance of building rest days into an exercise program. Many people try to squeeze too many activities into their crowded lives and then "crash" with exhaustion. It is far better, say the experts, to schedule a day of rest— and enjoy it.

become, the lower the maximum heart rate and therefore the lower the recommended target heart rate for an exercise session. Doctors calculate maximum heart rates in relation to one's age and sex and calculate the target rate on the basis of maximum heart rate and general fitness.

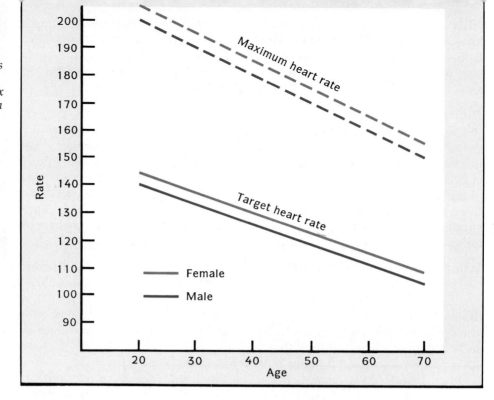

your additional exercises for developing strength and endurance will also require extra time in the same exercise session or a different one.

Playing It Safe: Getting Medical Approval

It is advisable to obtain medical clearance before beginning a fitness program, especially if you are inactive, over age 35, or under 35 and have documented or suspected coronary artery disease or significant risk factors. A number of medical conditions can be aggravated by physical exertion, and the possibility of your having such conditions should be ruled out by a medical examination and an exercise stress test before the exercise program begins. It is also a good idea to show the tentative plan for a fitness program to a doctor who is familiar with your physical condition and medical history.

Some colleges and universities have set up human performance laboratories that are equipped to conduct exercise tolerance tests on a treadmill. Find out whether your campus has such a facility, staffed by an exercise physiologist who can give you a graded treadmill test.

Deciding When and Where to Exercise

Once you have determined the type of exercise program you want to follow, you need to get down to the truly practical aspects: how can you fit the exercise into your weekly schedule, where do you plan to work out, and what alternatives do you have if the arrangements go wrong or you feel the need for a change? These are very important decisions: people are more likely to stick with a fitness program if they have carefully considered their options and alternatives.

Fitting Exercise into Your Schedule The time of day you choose to exercise depends on your schedule; no one particular time is best. Some people like to exercise early in the day; others find that jogging or biking after work or school provides a relaxing change of pace. (People who exercise outdoors after dark should wear reflective clothing.)

Weather can pose problems, and you may need to consider this in planning a schedule. Humidity may reduce the body's normal ability to dispel heat; on an extremely hot, humid day, body temperature may rise much more than normal, resulting in heatstroke. In hot, humid weather, you may be able to do your jogging or cycling by exercising very early in the morning, when it is coolest. Extremely cold weather can also pose problems. Such weather requires you to wear warmer clothing for protection, or you may have to switch to indoor activities.

Selecting Places to Exercise   Another point to be considered in planning an exercise program is deciding where to exercise. This decision may be affected by various factors, such as the type of exercise program chosen, the equipment or facilities required, and personal motivation. Many good forms of exercise, such as walking and bicycling, can be done almost anywhere. In fact, part of their appeal comes from the fact that different locations and routes can be planned to vary the experience. On vacations, one may find that enjoyment is added not only to the exercise but also to the visit: exercise can take one to places that one might otherwise never have visited. Once again, bad weather can require you to have alternative indoor plans.

Even exercise that requires special facilities, such as swimming, can often be done at several different locations. Do not consider only the school's facilities. There may also be a community recreation center that is less crowded or a YWCA or similar organization. In the summer, consider a local park, a private swim club, or even a local quarry or lake, but make sure lifeguards are present if you are not totally confident about your swimming ability. Perhaps you prefer to work out in one place only; even then, it is wise to have alternatives in case your regular exercise spot is closed.

For some people, exercise programs can be initiated quite easily at home. Even if equipment is required, many people are able to set up a home gym. Today's fitness equipment is often compact, and thus it is possible to use this equipment in the home. Before selecting equipment, though, it is important to consider personal fitness goals, the space available, and the cost.

There are exercise machines for two general categories of exercise programs: aerobic conditioning and strength training. For aerobic conditioning, there are a number of machines to choose from, including stationary bicycles, rowing machines, treadmills, and cross-country skiing machines. Strength-training equipment includes a range of products from barbells to weight stack machines like those found in health clubs.

Most home exercise machines take up about 15 square feet. Some can be folded up and stored when not in use. While some treadmills and weight stack machines take up a good deal of space and are not easily stored, a set of dumbbell weights is quite small and can be put away easily.

With the exception of dumbbell and barbell weights, most exercise equipment costs several hundred dollars or more. Before making such an investment in a piece of equipment, it is wise to check unbiased consumer ratings to be sure the equipment is safe, reliable, and effective. If possible, use the equipment at a gym first to make sure it is something you will use regularly.

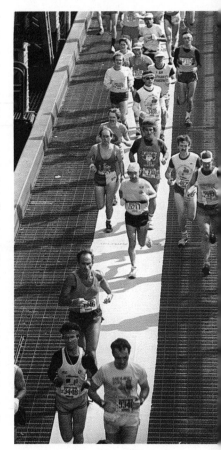

On occasion, exercise that is solitary can take place in very social and competitive settings. (Birgit Pohl)

The Health Club Option

People can usually design their own perfectly adequate fitness-for-health programs by following some simple guidelines, including those already discussed in this chapter. In fact, designing their own programs may help people stick to them longer because they have chosen activities they enjoy and have worked them into their own schedules. However, there may be valid reasons for a person to prefer working in a setting with other like-minded people under professional supervision. Some people therefore begin an exercise program by joining a health club.

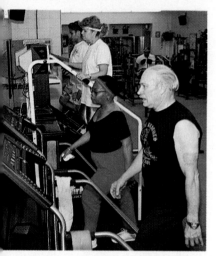

In addition to having more equipment available, health clubs offer the advantage of a social environment. This may encourage people not to slack off while exercising. (David M. Grossman/Photo Researchers, Inc.)

Reasons for Joining a Health Club   Many people feel that although they know about exercise and fitness programs, they cannot exercise properly on their own. They find that something always interferes with their plans to exercise at home. At a health facility, by contrast, the entire focus is on exercising and there are few distractions. Some people may feel that they need the help of the professionals at a health club to plan an exercise program. They should be sure, however, that the planned program is tailored to their likes, schedule, and needs. Otherwise they may need great determination to continue with the program.

Many people enjoy the social atmosphere of a health club, finding exercise more pleasant when it is done in a group. There is less temptation to skip part of an exercise routine when it is done with others. Motivation is a large part of exercise, and going to a health club may provide that motivation.

Choosing a Health Club   Unfortunately, many people drop out of or rarely go to their health clubs after spending hundreds of dollars on membership. Generally, health clubs expect 50 to 60 percent of their members to drop out.[32] People are clearly not finding what they wanted when they joined. Before joining a health club, therefore, it is important to shop around, visiting several clubs and comparing them. At each club, you should do the following:

- Visit during the time of day or evening you plan to use the facilities to see how many people are there. See whether there are long waits for the equipment and facilities you plan to use, such as the pool. Find out whether the club sets limits on enrollment to prevent overcrowding.
- Observe the facilities to see whether the atmosphere is comfortable or is too intense or social for your taste. Judge whether the equipment is well maintained and the club is clean and well ventilated. Ask people who belong to the club what their experience has been.
- Assess the convenience of the club. It is best to find a club close to home or work; a person is more likely to go to a club if it is convenient. People with children should check whether the club offers baby-sitting services.
- Determine the credentials of the instructors and find out what kind of instruction is offered. See whether the instructors are required to have a degree in exercise physiology or physical education and if they are certified by the ACSM as fitness professionals. Instructors should be certified in cardiopulmonary resuscitation (CPR). Be wary of a health club that requires only in-house training for its instructors.
- Find out what fitness-testing procedures the club uses. The club should take a health history and recommend that its members get medical approval before beginning an exercise program. Some clubs do fitness assessment testing to find a member's fitness level. After the initial assessments, the club should then set up a personalized exercise program to meet the individual's needs and goals.
- Find out the cost of membership and compare it to that at other clubs. Compare that cost to the amount you might spend on exercise classes, pool fees, and equipment if you did not join the club.

Staying with Your Plan and Modifying It

Many studies have shown that 60 to 70 percent of adults who start exercising drop out within the first month.[33] Once you have begun a fitness plan, how can you avoid being one of those who give up? Thinking ahead and anticipating pitfalls can help. Be sure to set realistic goals for improvement and know how much improvement to expect. Do not expect too much too soon; it may take a few months before the improvement is noticeable. If your goals are unrealistic, you may become discouraged and quit. Be aware of how quickly fitness can be lost and use that knowledge as an incentive to continue. Finally, be prepared to modify your exercise plan, change your activities, or revise your schedule if you have trouble sticking to the original plan.

Table 4.5 Amount of Exercise Needed to Maintain Conditioning after One Builds up to Optimal Fitness Level

Type of Exercise	Frequency (times per week)	Distance	Time (minutes)
Walking	3	4 miles	48–58
	5	3 miles	36–43
Running	3	2 miles	13–16
	5	1.5 miles	12–15
Cycling	3	8 miles	24–32
	5	6 miles	18–24
Swimming	3	1,000 yards	16–25
	4	800 yards	13–20

Source: Adapted from K. Cooper, *The New Aerobics* (New York: Bantam, 1983). Copyright by Kenneth H. Cooper. Used by permission of Bantam Books, a division of Bantam Doubleday, Dell Publishing Group.

How Fast and How Much Can Fitness Improve? During the first few weeks of exercise sessions you can expect a period of soreness and fatigue. This will abate as the program proceeds. After 2 or 3 months you will probably reach a plateau. Improvement beyond that point may be minimal if you stay at the same level of activity.[34] While this can be discouraging, you should keep your original fitness goals in mind. If you have been following a fitness-for-health plan, you will have improved your overall endurance and cardio-vascular fitness and probably will have lost some pounds or inches as well—a major achievement. To improve beyond this plateau, you will have to work harder. For example, although aerobic capacity can increase 20 percent in the first 2 or 3 months, improving another few percentage points will require exercising at a more intense level for another 3 months. The more fit you are, the harder it is to improve. Once you are really fit, however, maintaining that fitness is easier (Table 4.5).

How Quickly Can Fitness Deteriorate? Experts think that people get out of shape about as fast as they got into shape in the first place. So if it takes 3 months to attain a certain level of fitness, it will probably take 3 months to lose that fitness if you stop exercising. This is true even for people who have trained hard for a long time.

Modifying Your Plan It is important to evaluate your fitness program periodically and modify it as necessary. As was emphasized at the beginning of this chapter, exercise is not a temporary measure—it should be a part of your permanent routine throughout life. As you grow older, you may find that your overall fitness goals change: you have less time for athletic sports and want to move into a fitness-for-health program appropriate to your age, or you may wish to increase the intensity of your workouts to achieve optimum results. In addition, your interests may change; boredom may set in; and the availability of facilities, your personal schedule, and a change in season may all require modifications in your personal fitness plan. To be of maximum benefit throughout your life, your program should reflect your current schedule, needs, and interests. It should be flexible enough to change as your life changes; such flexibility will help ensure that exercise remains a part of your life rather than being dropped when it seems inconvenient.

Is Fitness Worth the Effort?

Physical fitness is definitely worth the effort. When you exercise regularly, you feel better and look better. At the same time, you probably will also feel more relaxed and energetic. Even when you are tired or unenthusiastic about things, exercise will help turn those feelings around and give you more en-

If you need an extra incentive to stay with an exercise program, consider getting a cholesterol test the day before you start and another after you have followed the program for about 10 weeks. Chances are that you will see a reduction in your cholesterol readings, especially if the exercise program is accompanied by a program of sensible eating.

ergy. Perhaps most important, the long-term benefits to your health from exercise are enormous. Exercise not only can improve your life expectancy, especially by reducing the risk of developing heart disease,[35] it also can retard the aging process and keep you fit and healthy longer. Few things in life are as beneficial to physical and mental well-being as a regular program of exercise and physical fitness.

Chapter Summary

- Interest in fitness is at an all-time high in the United States. However, only 20 percent of Americans get adequate exercise even though it can take less than an hour a week to gain some benefits.
- The vast majority of Americans today need more physical exercise than their jobs and lifestyles provide. They need planned and structured exercise.
- Exercise provides many health benefits, including a reduced risk of developing heart disease and protection against contracting osteoporosis.
- Exercise also provides psychological benefits, including stronger defenses against stress, anxiety, and depression.
- Because exercise carries a risk of injury, it is important to follow sound guidelines in creating and following an exercise program.
- Exercise contributes to many physical skills, some of which may be needed by relatively few people—athletes, for example. However, it also contributes to basic physical health, which is vital for everyone.
- Basic physical health includes flexibility, muscular strength and endurance, cardiovascular fitness, and body leanness.
- Flexibility refers to the range of motion in the joints. It is determined by the elasticity of connective tissue and the ability of muscle fibers to relax.
- A good exercise program begins with a basic warm-up routine that starts with simple muscle movement and ends with stretching exercises for flexibility.
- Strength and endurance are two qualities of muscles that are important in overall health. Besides the quality of the muscle tissue itself,

optimal muscle fitness requires a good supply of chemicals from the blood.
- There are three basic types of exercises for muscle strength and endurance: isokinetic (weight stack machine exercises), isotonic (barbell exercises), and isometric (stationary pressure exercises). Isometric exercises are considered the least effective type.
- Cardiovascular fitness refers to fitness of the circulatory system, including the lungs, heart, and blood vessels. The heart muscles are vital to cardiovascular fitness.
- Aerobic exercise is the type recommended for cardiovascular fitness. It lasts long enough to increase the heart rate significantly but does not starve the muscles of oxygen.
- To be effective, an exercise program should be designed for specific muscles and purposes and should slightly overload the muscles at which it is directed. The exercises should become progressively harder until the desired level of fitness is reached. Regular times should be set aside for exercise every week.
- To design a personal fitness program for oneself, one must consider one's fitness goals—general overall health versus preparation for specific activities, for example.
- One must also assess one's current fitness, select appropriate exercises at an appropriate level, get a medical checkup, plan a workable schedule, and decide where to exercise—at home or in a health club.
- Staying with a fitness program is also important. This will be easier if your expectations are realistic, you are ready to modify the program as you become fitter and as your life progresses, and you are aware of the real and continuing benefits of exercise to life both in the present and in the future.

Key Terms

Physical activity (page 87)

Physical exercise (page 87)

Amenorrhea (page 90)

Agility (page 90)

Balance (page 90)

Coordination (page 90)

Power (page 90)

Reaction time (page 90)

Speed (page 90)

Flexibility (page 90)

Muscular strength (page 90)

Muscular endurance (page 90)

Cardiovascular fitness (page 90)

Body leanness (page 91)

Atrophy (page 93)

Isokinetic (page 94)

Isotonic (page 94)

Isometric (page 94)

Vital capacity (page 95)

References

1. National Sporting Goods Association news release (October 1988).

2. United States Public Health Service, "Promoting Health/Preventing Diseases: Objectives for the Nation" (Washington, D.C.: U.S. Government Printing Office, 1980).

3. "12 Minutes Does It," *American Health* (June 1988): 41.

4. "Physical Exercise: An Important Factor for Health," position paper of the International Federation of Sports Medicine, *The Physician and Sports Medicine* 18, no. 3 (March 1990): 155–156.

5. Steven Findlag, "Smart Ways to Shape Up," *U.S. News and World Report* 105, no. 3 (July 18, 1988): 45–54.

6. Carl J. Casperson et al., "Physical Activity, Exercise, and Physical Fitness: Definitions and Distinctions for Health-Related Research," *Public Health Reports* 100, no. 2 (March–April 1985): 126–130.

7. Robert J. McCunney, "Fitness, Heart Disease and High Density Lipoproteins: A Look at the Relationships," *The Physician and Sports Medicine* 15, no. 2 (February 1987): 67–75, 78–79.

8. R. S. Paffenbarger et al., "Physical Activity, All-Cause Mortality and Longevity of College Alumni," *New England Journal of Medicine* 314 (March 7, 1986): 605–613.

9. Arthur Leon et al., "Leisure-Time Physical Activity Levels and Risk of Coronary Heart Disease and Death," *Journal of the American Medical Association* 258, no. 17 (November 6, 1987): 2388–2395.

10. R. Rish, American Association for the Advancement of Science, reported in *Time* 131, no. 9 (February 29, 1988): 68.

11. Kathryn Simmons, "The Federal Government: Keeping Tabs on the Nation's Fitness," *The Physician and Sports Medicine* 15, no. 1 (January 1987): 190–195.

12. D. Giordano et al., *Controlling Stress and Tension: A Holistic Approach* (Englewood Cliffs, N.J.: Prentice-Hall, 1990).

13. John Yacenda, "First Aid and Self-Care for Minor Sports Injuries," *Fitness Management* 4, no. 8 (October 1988): 56–57.

14. B. L. Drinkwater, "Amenorrheic Athletes: At Risk for Premature Osteoporosis?" Proceedings of the IOC World Congress on Sport Sciences (1989: Colorado Springs): 151–155.

15. Charles Corbin and Ruth Lindsey, *The Ultimate Fitness Book* (New York: Leisure Press, 1990).

16. Ibid.

17. Margareta Moller et al., "Duration of Stretching Effect on Range of Motion in Lower Extremities," *Archives of Physical Medicine and Rehabilitation* 66 (1985): 171–173.

18. Katy Williams, "Crucial to Performance and Injury Prevention, Warm-Up, Warm-Down Is Simple, Practical, and Adaptable to Every Sport," *Sportscare and Fitness* (1988): 35.

19. Bob Anderson, *Stretching* (Bolinas, Calif.: Shelter Publications, 1980).

20. Barbara Brehm, "The Importance of Mind and Muscle," *Fitness Management* (September/October 1987): 16–17.

21. Charles Corbin and Ruth Lindsey, *Concepts of Physical Fitness,* 5th ed. (Dubuque, Iowa: Brown, 1985).

22. R. S. Paffenbarger et al., "A Natural History of Athleticism and Cardiovascular Health," *Journal of the American Medical Association* 252 (1984): 496.

23. McCunney, op. cit.

24. Barbara Brehm, "Don't Forget to Cool Down," *Fitness Management* (September 1988): 15.

25. Corbin and Lindsey, *Concepts.*

26. Hal Higdon, "Base Fitness," *Walking Magazine* (February–March 1988): 38–43.

27. American College of Sports Medicine, "The Recommended Quantity and Quality of Exercise for Developing and Maintaining Cardiorespiratory and Muscular Fitness in Healthy Adults," pp. 265–274.

28. "New Rules of Exercise," *U.S. News and World Report* (August 11, 1986): 52–56.

29. Ibid.

30. American College of Sports Medicine, op. cit.

31. Higdon, op. cit.

32. *Consumers Digest* 26, no. 1 (January–February 1987): 60–65.

33. Kenneth E. Powell et al., "The Status of the 1996 Objectives for Physical Fitness and Exercise," *Public Health Reports* 101, no. 1 (January–February 1986): 15–20.

34. Higdon, op. cit.

35. "Physical Exercise: An Important Factor for Health," op. cit.

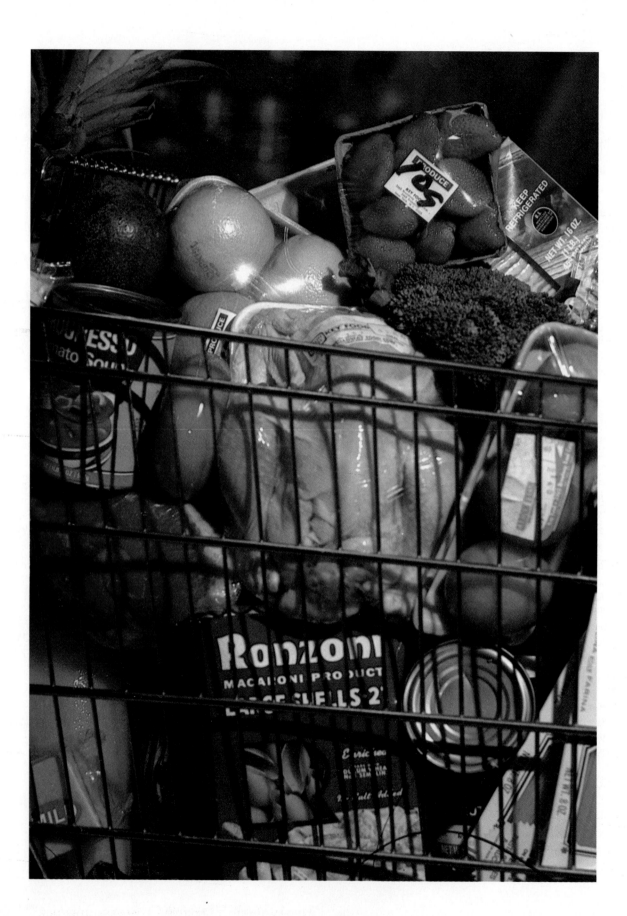

Chapter 5

Diet and Nutrition

To Guide Your Reading

When you have studied this chapter, you should be able to:

- Define nutrition and explain the importance of diet and proper nutrition to health.

- List seven different classes of components in food, including fiber and water, specifying foods which are good sources for each component.

- Explain some of the important functions of the major components and nutrients in food.

- Describe the two classic strategies for determining a proper diet and discuss the drawbacks of each one.

- Discuss the basic principles of a positive food strategy and analyze and plan a daily diet based on those principles.

- Explain some of the strategies for buying and preparing food that can help ensure that one eats a nutritious diet.

- Identify five universal principles that can provide guidance for anyone who wishes to eat healthily in today's world.

Americans are more interested in food and nutrition than ever before. Proper nutrition has come to be recognized as a major factor in achieving and maintaining a healthy lifestyle. As a result, people are much more concerned about making dietary choices that promote health and well-being. They realize that the choices they make can affect not just their physical health but all aspects of their lives. Not only does food provide the fuel for muscular activity and exercise, as described in Chapter 4, it also supplies energy for all the other functions of the body, including emotions and thoughts. Thus, nutrition affects every aspect of a person's life.

Americans have more food choices than any people in history, thanks to a high standard of living and advanced agricultural and transportation technologies. The quantity and variety of foods available are amazing. What were once mainly regional or seasonal foods can be found almost everywhere at any time, from Maine lobsters in Albuquerque to fresh Brazilian strawberries during a New England winter. With this increase in choices, however, have come increased expectations. People expect high-quality foods that taste good, look good, and are free of hazards. For the most part, such food is available, but the cornucopia of the American food market does not guarantee adequate nutrition. Alongside fresh fruits and vegetables in the market there are so-called junk foods—foods that contain high proportions of fat, sugar, or salt—and other foods of questionable value.

Thus, even with the great variety of American food products, a healthy and satisfying diet is not guaranteed. Only by learning about the nutritive substances in foods and using that knowledge to guide your choice of foods can you plan a diet that will promote and maintain a level of health and well-being with which you are comfortable.

What Is Nutrition?

Nutrition is the science of food—how the body uses it and its relationship to good health. Nutrition includes the study of the major food components: proteins, carbohydrates, fats, vitamins, minerals, water, and fiber. It is concerned with both how the body utilizes these nutrients and the effect of this process on health.

Food is vital to the good health of all people of all ages. When you eat, you are doing much more than filling an empty stomach. As indicated in Chapter 4, the body uses food for energy, growth, and the repair of damaged tissues. Food can also help strengthen the body against the effects of future stress and disease.

Before food can be used by the body, it must be broken down into substances the body can absorb. The process by which the nutrients in food are converted into body tissue and energy is called **metabolism;** it occurs as food moves through the digestive tract and as nutrients drawn from there into the bloodstream are chemically changed for use by the cells.

The conversion of food into body tissue is a very complex process (Figure 5.1). Nutrients are chemically changed before they are used; for example, the protein in steak is not used directly by the body but has to be metabolized into human protein. Another process of metabolism takes place as nutrients are converted into energy; that is, they are oxidized, or "burned," by oxygen carried in the bloodstream.

The energy potential of food is measured in units called **calories.** (A calorie is the amount of heat needed to raise 1 kilogram of water 1 degree Celsius.) Foods differ in the amount of calories they contain per unit weight and thus differ in their energy potential. An individual's caloric needs depend on age, weight, height, sex, and activity level.

Too little or too much food—or, worse, too much low-nutrient food—leads to poor health. There is evidence that poor dietary habits play a key role in 5 of the nation's top 10 causes of death—heart disease, cancer, stroke, diabetes mellitus, and atherosclerosis—according to a 1988 report from the surgeon general on nutrition and health.[1] Therefore, a knowledge of basic nutrition is necessary to enable a person to choose the proper balance of food nutrients that will safeguard health and improve the quality of life.

metabolism—*the process by which the nutrients in food are converted into body tissue and energy.*

calorie—*the amount of heat needed to raise 1 kilogram of water 1 degree Celsius; used to measure the energy potential of food.*

Eat most of your food before the evening. Calories consumed earlier are easier to burn off in the course of the day, when you are most active and your metabolism is most efficient.

The Basic Components of Food

All foods are composed of various chemical compounds, or nutrients. There are several basic groups of nutrients, which can be divided into two general classes: macronutrients and micronutrients. The **macronutrients**—nutrients the body needs in large amounts—consist of proteins, carbohydrates, and fats. The **micronutrients,** which are needed in smaller amounts, include minerals and vitamins. In addition to these nutrients, foods also contain two essential nonnutritives: fiber and water.

macronutrients—*nutrients the body needs in large amounts, such as proteins, carbohydrates, and fats.*

micronutrients—*nutrients consisting of minerals and vitamins that the body needs in small amounts for its essential functions.*

Proteins

Proteins are essential for the growth and repair of body tissues. The body uses proteins in muscle, hair, teeth, nails, bones, hemoglobin, and many other important components. Special proteins known as nucleic acids are found in the nuclei of all cells in the body. The job of these nucleic acids—which include ribonucleic acid (RNA) and deoxyribonucleic acid (DNA)—is to transmit hereditary characteristics. Another type of proteins—**enzymes**—play an important role in chemical reactions that build up and break down cellular material in the body. Each human cell contains several thousand kinds of enzymes.

protein—*a basic component of food that is essential for growth and the repair of body tissues.*

enzyme—*a type of protein that plays an important role in chemical reactions that break down cellular material in the body.*

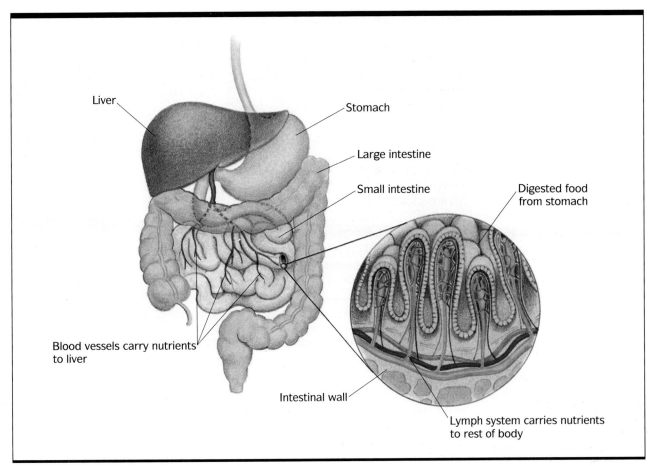

Figure 5.1 *Most people think of the stomach as the main organ in the digestive system. The stomach continues a process that begins in the mouth, physically and chemically breaking down the food into separate nutrients, but it ingests very little. Most nutrients are absorbed through the complex tissue of the intestinal wall, which carefully sorts them to travel to different parts of the body. There the nutrients are used to create human fluids and tissues. Much of this metabolism takes place in the liver.*

Proteins and Metabolism Proteins are made up of different amino acids, chemicals that are the building blocks of the body. Twenty-two amino acids are used to build human proteins. Of these, nine are called **essential amino acids** because the body cannot synthesize enough of them—they must be present in food. The body can manufacture the other 13 amino acids from other substances in one's diet.

The body assembles the forms of protein it needs by chemically linking amino acids in a specific order. For this to occur, however, all the amino acids must be available at the same time. Since amino acids cannot be stored in the body, you must keep supplying the nine essential amino acids through your food choices, including them in your diet at least twice a day.

One way to get protein is to eat foods of animal origin (meat, fish, poultry, eggs, dairy products). The proteins in these foods are known as **complete proteins** because they contain all nine essential amino acids.

You can also get protein from plant foods. However, proteins of plant origin (vegetables, seeds, grains, and nuts) almost invariably lack one or more of the nine essential amino acids—they are thus called **incomplete proteins.** As a result, vegetarians must combine plant proteins either with each other in specific combinations or with permissible animal proteins such as milk to get their full complement of amino acids. (Vegetarian diets are discussed later in this chapter.)

essential amino acids—*the nine amino acids that the body cannot manufacture in adequate amounts and that therefore must be present in the diet.*

complete protein—*a protein of animal origin (meat, fish, poultry, eggs, dairy products) that contains all nine essential amino acids.*

incomplete protein—*a protein of plant origin (vegetables, seeds, grains, and nuts) that lacks one or more of the nine essential amino acids.*

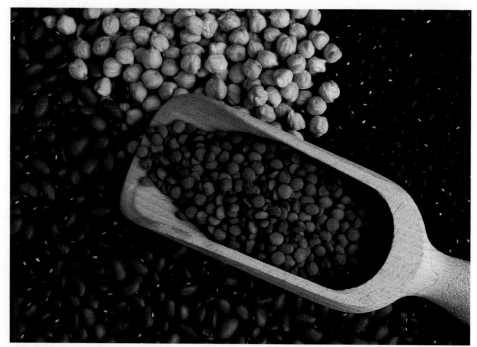

Beans and nuts are excellent sources of protein, but a strict vegetarian diet requires careful planning to supply the right kinds of protein for proper nutrition. (Felicia Martinez/ PhotoEdit)

Lean meat is less juicy than well-marbled meat, and so it can dry out easily when cooked. For lean meat to turn out moist and tender, it should be simmered in broth, marinated, or stir-fried quickly so that the juices do not have time to evaporate.

glucose—a type of sugar that is readily used by the body.

carbohydrate—a basic component of food that is found in bread, rice, potatoes, most fruits and vegetables, and certain other foods. Carbohydrates are the body's most immediate source of ready energy.

How Much Protein Do You Need? Clearly, it is vital to consume adequate amounts of protein every day. Getting too little protein can be dangerous. Low-protein fad diets (Chapter 6) can have undesirable results. The dieter can become seriously ill, though this is rare.

Even minor protein deficiencies will eventually cause fatigue and irritability and reduce the body's production of antibodies, resulting in greater susceptibility to infection and slower recovery from disease. Wounds and burns will heal more slowly as well. A continued protein deficiency may lead eventually to anemia and liver disorders.

However, it is desirable not to eat too much protein. If necessary, the body can convert protein to **glucose,** a fuel vital for energy, but excess proteins usually are converted to substances known as fatty acids, which are then stored in fat tissue.

Most Americans take in far more protein than is needed. The average daily consumption is about 100 grams, although most young men need about 56 grams, most young women need about 45 grams, and as people age they generally need less.[2] One quick way to get a rough estimate of your protein need is to divide your weight in pounds by three. Thus, if you weigh 150 pounds and divide this by three, your approximate daily protein need is 50 grams. That is roughly the amount of protein found in two 2- to 3-ounce servings of lean cooked meat, poultry, or fish. (These are considerably smaller portions than most people eat.)

Carbohydrates

Carbohydrates are found in abundance in all forms of plant life. They play an important role in metabolism as the body's chief source of energy. There are two basic types of carbohydrates: the simpler forms are sugars of various types, found in fruit and milk as well as in table sugar, and the more complex forms are starches and dietary fiber. (Fiber, however, cannot be converted into energy; its importance in the diet will be discussed later in this chapter.)

Carbohydrates and Metabolism While all the macronutrients can also be burned, or converted to energy, carbohydrates are the most economical energy source—the American Heart Association recommends that carbohydrates constitute 50 percent or more of total calories, with an emphasis on complex carbohydrates.[3]

Carbohydrates are metabolized in several stages by the digestive system and the liver and converted into a simple sugar called *glucose.* Sugars can thus enter the bloodstream rapidly, providing a quick burst of energy. Starches, by contrast, take longer to convert to usable energy; as a result, energy is released over a longer period of time. Some glucose remains stored in the liver and muscles as **glycogen,** ready for release into the bloodstream if blood glucose levels fall too low. The remainder of the glucose goes right into the bloodstream and is used directly by all the cells in the body for energy. Excess glucose—that which is neither stored as glycogen nor burned as energy—cannot be stored in large amounts; like excess protein, it is converted to fat.

Besides providing energy directly, carbohydrates play an important role in the metabolism of fat stores. To utilize fat stores efficiently, the body needs at least some dietary carbohydrate. If an individual consumes less than 125 milligrams of carbohydrate a day (about 1 percent of the minimum recommended daily allowance, or RDA), the body will not be able to burn its stored fats completely.

How Much Carbohydrate Do You Need? As with all food components, the ideal amount of carbohydrate in the diet depends on a person's size, activity level, and metabolic rate. The National Research Council recommends five or more daily servings of vegetables and fruits in addition to six or more daily servings of starches such as rice and potatoes and other complex carbohydrates, including pasta, whole-grain breads and cereals, and legumes. A single serving is one-half cup of vegetables, a medium-size piece of fruit, or a slice of bread.[4] Foods rich in carbohydrates include grains (rice, wheat, rye, millet, barley, and corn), tubers (potatoes, yams, and sweet potatoes), and a variety of processed foods (pasta, cereal, and whole-grain breads). Most fruits and vegetables also contain carbohydrates.

Fats

Fats are the only macronutrients that the body can store in large amounts. They thus serve as an important source of reserve energy. The energy they provide, however, is more limited than energy from carbohydrates; it is easily used in aerobic exercise but is much less useful for other types of activity. For example, fats cannot maintain brain function if carbohydrates are lacking.

In addition to storing and providing energy, fats play many other vital roles. They are an important ingredient in the walls of every cell, contribute to blood clotting and hormone synthesis, help store and carry important vitamins (A, D, E, and K), and insulate the body and surround vital organs, protecting them from injury.

Fats and Metabolism There are many kinds of fats in the human body. Also known as **lipids,** each type of fat fulfills a specific function. Most fats are combinations of fatty acids called **triglycerides,** but there are other types too, including the substance known as **cholesterol,** a fat which is thought to play a role in the development of heart disease.

The fats that people eat are easily converted into the forms of fat that the body needs. An important feature of fat metabolism, however, is the way in which fats are transported in the body. Because fat floats on water, fat in the bloodstream would always tend to push upward and would thus not be directed where the body needed it. Fat is carried in large molecules called **lipoproteins,** which are largely made of fats but have walls that are not repelled

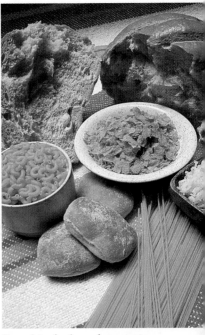

Found in foods such as pasta and rice, carbohydrates should provide more than 50 percent of the body's energy needs; they are metabolized more efficiently than are fats and proteins. (Tony Freeman/PhotoEdit)

glycogen—*a substance containing glucose that is stored in the liver and muscles and released into the bloodstream when blood sugar levels fall.*

lipids—*fats.*

triglycerides—*fatty acids into which excess glucose is converted and stored by the body's fat tissue.*

cholesterol—*a fatlike substance (many researchers would not technically define it as a fat) that is found in all foods from animal sources and is also manufactured by the human body.*

lipoproteins—*substances containing both fat and protein that transport fat molecules through the body.*

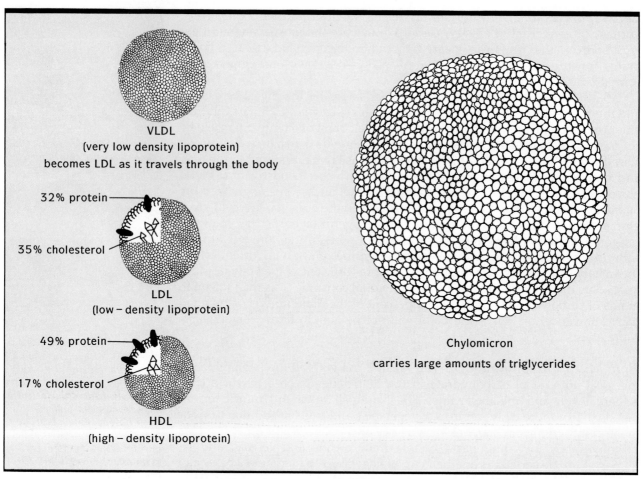

VLDL
(very low density lipoprotein)
becomes LDL as it travels through the body

32% protein
35% cholesterol
LDL
(low – density lipoprotein)

49% protein
17% cholesterol
HDL
(high – density lipoprotein)

Chylomicron
carries large amounts of triglycerides

Figure 5.2 Large particles called lipoproteins carry triglycerides and cholesterol and are coated with protein and phosphate so that they can travel in body fluids. Lipoproteins come in four different types, depending on their size and the proportion of different substances they contain. Note the high proportion of protein in HDLs (this accounts for their density) and the high proportion of cholesterol in LDLs. The huge chylomicrons are the main carriers of triglycerides from the intestine into the body.

by water (Figure 5.2). There are several kinds of lipoproteins, two of which play an important part in carrying cholesterol (Chapter 11).

How Much Fat Do You Need? Because fats are easily manufactured from the other macronutrients, they are not a vital part of most diets. There are, however, particular types of fat which, like the essential amino acids, must be included in what people eat, but these fats are needed only in very small amounts, and are present in many foods.

Most dietary fats (the fats in food) can be classified as either unsaturated or saturated (Table 5.1). **Unsaturated fats** include most vegetable oils; they are usually liquid at room temperature. They can be divided into two classes: polyunsaturated fats, such as corn, soya, sunflower, and cottonseed oil, and monounsaturated fats, such as olive oil. Polyunsaturated fats tend to lower blood cholesterol; monounsaturated fats do this to a lesser degree. The essential fats are unsaturated.

Saturated fats—found in meat, butter, coconut oil, palm oil, and whole milk—are usually solid at room temperature. They tend to raise blood cholesterol by serving as the starting material from which cholesterol is synthesized in the body. Thus, saturated fats are also associated with an increased risk of developing cardiovascular disease, and their consumption should be restricted.

When a label says "no cholesterol," it does not mean there is no fat. Products such as vegetable oils are cholesterol-free but still may contain saturated fats and be high in calories.

unsaturated fat—*a fat that is usually liquid at room temperature. Most vegetable oils are unsaturated fats.*

saturated fat—*a fat that is usually solid at room temperature; found in meat, butter, whole milk, and some oils.*

Table 5.1 Calories in Common Dietary Fats

Food	Measure (tablespoons)	Saturated Fat (calories)	Monounsaturated Fat (calories)	Polyunsaturated Fat (calories)
Butter	1	65	30	4
Corn oil	1	16	31	74
Lard	1	46	53	14
Margarine				
Hard	1	20	46	33
Soft	1	18	36	44
Olive oil	1	17	93	11
Peanut oil	1	22	59	41
Safflower oil	1	12	15	94
Soybean oil	1	19	54	48
Sunflower oil	1	13	24	83

Source: Eleanor Whitney and Eva Hamilton, *Understanding Human Nutrition*, 4th ed. (St. Paul, Minn.: West, 1987): H10–H12. All rights reserved. Reprinted by permission.

The American Heart Association recommends a diet in which total fat intake is less than 30 percent of total calories. At least one-third of this fat should be monounsaturated: saturated fat intake should be less than 10 percent of total calories, and polyunsaturated fat intake should not exceed 10 percent. In addition, cholesterol intake should not exceed 300 milligrams a day. This knowledge makes it possible to reduce the amounts of fats and cholesterol you take in by adjusting your choice of foods.

There is some controversy over whether these guidelines are applicable to children. Some experts maintain that children need more fat in their diets in order to meet the added nutritional needs of growth, especially during the adolescent growth spurt.

Unfortunately, many children get as much as 60 percent of their calories from fat, and this contributes to problems of obesity and can lead to high blood levels of cholesterol. Most experts agree that this amount is excessive. The Committee on Nutrition of the American Academy of Pediatrics recommends a diet of 30 to 40 percent fat for most children, except for those with highly elevated cholesterol levels. The American Heart Association recommends its figure of 30 percent or less for all persons over age 2.[5]

Minerals

Minerals are inorganic elements that the body needs daily to help form tissues and various chemical substances. They assist in nerve transmission and muscle contraction and help regulate fluid levels and the acid-base balance of the body. Since minerals are absorbed, used, and excreted by the body, they must be replaced continuously.

Minerals are needed in different amounts. The body requires fairly large quantities of the so-called macrominerals, or electrolytes, such as calcium, phosphorus, potassium, and magnesium. Iron, zinc, selenium, copper, cobalt, and manganese—the so-called trace minerals—are needed in only tiny amounts (a few micrograms) daily.

Minerals are contained in almost every food, and most people can obtain sufficient quantities of essential minerals by eating a variety of foods, particularly fruits and vegetables. Although there are many different minerals, this chapter will discuss only calcium, potassium, sodium, and iron in detail.

Calcium **Calcium** is the most abundant mineral in the body. It is essential for a wide range of vital bodily functions, including building bones and teeth and ensuring normal growth. A calcium deficiency during childhood will cause bone deformities such as bowed legs. Throughout adulthood, calcium is needed to maintain a strong, hard skeleton, because bones start losing

Margarine actually has the same number of calories per serving that butter does. It is recommended because it is made from vegetable oils and has no cholesterol.

About half the calories in nuts come from fat. Fortunately, most nuts are high in polyunsaturated fat and low in saturated fat. Raw unsalted nuts are the best choice.

The U.S. Food and Drug Administration is deciding the fate of fat substitutes, or "fake fats." These new products will take calories out of traditionally fat-filled foods but not affect their flavor or texture.

minerals—*inorganic elements that humans need in trace amounts daily to help form tissues and various chemical substances.*

calcium—*the most abundant mineral in the human body; essential for building bones and teeth and ensuring normal growth.*

Deciding about Food Additives and Irradiation

Food additives have been part of the food system for many years. Over the past several decades they have become a controversial topic as people have gained greater understanding about the effects of different substances in the body. The two speakers below discuss two sides of the issue.

Without Additives, Foods Would Be More Limited—and More Expensive

The bounty of America's harvests today is maximized and prices are minimized when as few foods as possible go to waste. This is ensured if items are purchased and consumed soon after they arrive at the market. Foods move faster from the store if people find they taste good, look good, and are good for them. Additives—flavors, food colorings, and nutrients—can contribute to all these qualities.

Waste is also minimized when foods are slow to spoil. Many traditional preservatives—for example, salt and sugar—are now recognized as carrying considerable health hazards; if modern chemical preservatives carry any risk, it is considerably less.

In fact, testing procedures ensure that additives are used with a considerable margin of safety—a margin larger than that for many substances that occur naturally in foods. Allergenic foods such as shellfish cause considerably more negative reactions than do additives, and many important nutrients—for example, vitamin A—can cause problems if too much is ingested.

The overall effect of food technology in the United States has been to improve the food supply. More people eat better now than was ever possible before the food industry began to use additives. And the technology is also continually improving: preservatives are beginning to be supplanted by food irradiation, which kills many insects and bacteria but leaves no residue. (Although radioactive materials are used, the food is not made radioactive.) Modern food technology provides a net gain, and an increasing gain, to our lives.

Additives Are Potentially Dangerous and Are Also Unnecessary

Even if food irradiation proves completely harmless to food, it leads to the risk of transporting and disposing of radioactive materials. But its effects on health—like the effects of food additives—take a long time to show up. While only a few additives, such as cyclamates and Red Dye No. 2, have actually been withdrawn after being approved, they certainly cast doubt on the others.

True, tests are required and performed, but no testing can be perfect, and tests for toxic risks to humans are particularly difficult. To start with, such tests cannot be performed on humans. In addition, the danger of additives in food may be long term, but the tests must be done in the short term, so they often use high concentrations. Third, tests cannot cover all the possible effects of an additive. Some hazards—for example, the effect of a substance on reactions to a particular medicinal drug—may not be discovered. Finally, the tests are usually done by the firms that produce the additives. These are all major imperfections in the testing procedure.

If the use of additives and similar procedures were the only way to ensure safe nutritious foods in the market, it would be one thing. But some additives are used for color and flavor, hardly vital qualities of food. Furthermore, nutritional additives are frequently used to replace nutrients destroyed by poor processing techniques or to overload foods with many more nutrients than would be needed in a balanced diet. Finally, in recent years the health food industry has shown that even today natural foods, produced and processed without chemical additives, can be successfully brought to the market at not too much added cost.

What is your opinion? Do you agree that food additives are largely safe and a beneficial part of our food production system? Or do you think that consumers should demand additive-free foods? How do the arguments above seem to apply to food irradiation?

Information drawn from Geri Harrington, *Real Food, Fake Food, and Everything in Between* (New York: Macmillan, 1987); "Food Irradiation: Is the Time Ripe?" *Nutrition Action Letter* (November 1986).

calcium during middle age. If calcium is not replaced by calcium-rich foods or calcium supplements, one's bones can become increasingly thin, brittle, and fragile, particularly with inactivity. Many older people are afflicted with osteoporosis, the painful and crippling bone disease described in Chapter 17. A diet rich in calcium can help prevent this condition. Since osteoporosis is eight times as common in women as it is in men, women should make sure they get enough calcium, especially after menopause or a hysterectomy.

Almost three-quarters of the calcium in the average American's diet comes from milk and milk products (cheese, yogurt, ice cream). The remaining one-fourth is supplied by foods such as leafy vegetables, salmon, and sardines with bones.

Potassium and Sodium A proper balance of **potassium** and **sodium** is essential for normal functioning of muscle tissue, proper conduction of nerve impulses, and maintenance of the body's acid-alkaline balance. Together, these two minerals are the primary **electrolytes**—substances that carry the electrical charges needed by cells to carry on their work.

Potassium is found in the highest quantities in beans, fruits (especially bananas), vegetables, whole grains, ocean fish, lean meat, and potatoes. It is more effective when consumed with vitamin B and moderate amounts of sodium. However, an excessive intake of sodium can decrease the body's supply of potassium, as can an excessive intake of sugar, aspirin, coffee, or alcohol.

Sodium is one of the most overconsumed nutrients. It is most commonly found in table salt (sodium chloride) but is a hidden ingredient in almost all processed foods and occurs naturally in many foods. In recent years there has been a great deal of concern about the relationship of sodium to high blood pressure, or hypertension. A high sodium intake is thought to be a contributing factor in this disorder. As a result, nutritionists and health authorities now recommend that all people limit their sodium intake somewhat.[6]

Iron Although it is only a trace mineral, **iron** is one of the most important nutrients, essential for the production of hemoglobin in red blood cells. However, it is also the most frequently deficient nutrient in the diet. Since about 80 percent of the iron in the body is found in the blood, iron losses are greatest whenever blood is lost. Iron-deficiency anemia is a fairly widespread health problem in the United States, particularly among women of childbearing age, who regularly lose considerable amounts of iron through the menstrual process. A woman's iron requirement is almost twice that of a man, and this is the one nutrient that frequently requires supplementation.

Everyone should try to include some iron-rich foods in the diet—meat and poultry, dried beans, dried fruits, dark-green leafy vegetables, and cereal that has been fortified with iron.

Vitamins

As you read earlier in this chapter, **vitamins,** along with minerals, are often referred to as micronutrients. Although they are needed only in small amounts, these substances are indispensable in triggering vital bodily functions. Vitamins do not form new compounds in the body as proteins, carbohydrates, and fats do. Rather, they help other chemical reactions take place and facilitate other bodily processes. For example, vitamin D helps calcium form strong bone structure. Vitamins play other important roles as well. Studies suggest that vitamin E may partially reverse the decline in immunity that occurs with aging,[7] and vitamin A strengthens the immune system and helps protect the body against the ill effects of radiation, drugs, and chemical pollutants.[8]

potassium—*one of the two primary electrolytes in the body; found in beans, fruits, vegetables, whole grains, fish, lean meat, and potatoes.*

sodium—*one of the two primary electrolytes in the body. It is found in table salt and in many processed foods and also occurs naturally in many foods.*

electrolytes—*substances that carry the electrical charges needed by cells to carry on their work. Potassium and sodium are the body's primary electrolytes.*

iron—*a trace mineral that is one of the most important nutrients; it is essential for the production of hemoglobin in red blood cells.*

vitamins—*substances found in food; they are needed in only very small amounts but are essential for triggering vital bodily functions.*

One stalk of broccoli, half a green pepper, and half a cantaloupe all contain 100 percent of the RDA of vitamin C.

Table 5.2   Vitamins and What They Do

Vitamin	A	B₁[a] (Thiamin)	B₂ (Riboflavin)	Niacin	B₆ (Pyridoxine)
Found in	Milk and other dairy products, green vegetables, carrots, animal liver	Whole-grain or enriched cereals, liver, yeast, nuts, legumes, wheat germ	Liver, green leafy vegetables, milk, cheese, eggs, fish, whole-grain or enriched cereals	Yeast, liver, wheat germ, organ meats, eggs, fish; can be synthesized from the essential amino acid tryptophan	Yeast, wheat bran and germ, liver, kidneys, meat, whole grains, fish, vegetables
Benefits	Helps maintain skin and tooth enamel, bone formation, and vision	Helps convert glucose to energy or fat; helps nervous system and appetite	Vital to all major nutrient metabolism; keeps skin in good condition	Hydrogen transport; maintenance of all body tissues; energy production	Essential to amino acid and carbohydrate metabolism
Recommended daily allowance (RDA)	Men: 1,000 RE[b] Women: 800 RE	Men: 1.4 mg Women: 1.1 mg	Men: 1.7 mg Women: 1.3 mg	Men: 16–19 mg Women: 13–14 mg	Men: 2.2 mg Women: 2.0 mg
Deficiency causes	Night blindness, decrease in growth, lack of tears	*Beriberi:* numbness in feet and toes, tingling legs, weak muscles, heart irregularities	*Ariboflavinosis:* sore skin, cracking of corners of mouth, bloodshot eyes, sensitivity to light	*Pellagra:* diarrhea, skin rash, mental disorders	Greasy scaliness around eyes, nose, mouth; mental depression
Excess causes	Swollen feet and ankles, weight loss, tiredness, eye bleeding	Excess of water-soluble vitamins is rare	Excess of water-soluble vitamins is rare	Excess of water-soluble vitamins is rare	Excess of water-soluble vitamins is rare

[a] The vitamins listed in the blue columns are water-soluble.
[b] RE = retinol equivalents, the standard measure for vitamin A.

Table 5.2 shows the specific functions of each vitamin, its food sources, RDAs, and the effects of deficiency and excess. Recently much attention has been paid to vitamins A and C.

Vitamin A and Beta-Carotene   The importance of vitamin A lies in its role in strengthening the body's protective mechanisms and contributes to bone formation. One of the richest sources of vitamin A is fish liver oil. In addition, a substance called beta-carotene, which occurs in many vegetables, is converted into vitamin A by the body. Beta-carotene is found in most yellow, orange, and dark-green leafy vegetables such as carrots, broccoli, and kale.

Vitamin A and beta-carotene improve the growth, reparability, elasticity, strength, and resistance of internal and external tissues. A deficiency of vitamin A or beta-carotene can harm the structure and function of these tissues and render them vulnerable to disease.[9]

Vitamin C and Bioflavonoids   Numerous studies have suggested that vitamin C both improves the immune system and effectively counteracts radiation and chemical toxins. It is now generally recognized that it plays a role in cancer prevention as well.

There is considerable controversy over the recommended doses of vitamin C. Nobel Prizewinner Dr. Linus Pauling, who stated that vitamin C can pre-

Folacin (Folic acid)	B$_{12}$ (Cyanocobalamin)	C (Ascorbic acid)	D	E	K
Liver, nuts, green vegetables, orange juice	Meat, liver, eggs, milk	Citrus fruits, tomatoes, cabbage, broccoli, potatoes, peppers	Fish oils, beef, butter, eggs, milk; produced in skin on exposure to ultraviolet rays in sunlight	Widely distributed in foods: yellow vegetables, vegetable oils, and wheat germ	Spinach, eggs, liver, cabbage, tomatoes; produced by intestinal bacteria
Necessary for production of RNA and DNA and red blood cells	Necessary for production of red blood cells and normal growth	Collagen formation and maintenance; protects against infection	Promotes absorption and utilization of calcium and phosphorus; essential for normal bone and tooth development	May relate to oxidation and longevity; may protect against red blood cell destruction	Shortens blood-clotting time
Men: 0.4 mg Women: 0.4 mg	Men: 0.003 mg Women: 0.003 mg	Men: 60 mg Women: 60 mg	Men: 0.005–0.0075 mg Women: 0.005–0.0075 mg	Men: 10 mg Women: 8 mg	Men: 0.07–0.14 mg Women: 0.07–0.14 mg
Anemia yielding immature red blood cells; smooth, red tongue; diarrhea	*Pernicious anemia:* drop in number of red blood cells; irritability; drowsiness; depression	*Scurvy:* rough, scaly, skin; anemia; gum eruptions; pain in extremities; retarded healing	*Rickets:* a softening of bones causing bow legs or other bone deformities	Increased red blood cell destruction	Poor blood-clotting (hemorrhage)
Excess of water-soluble vitamins is rare	Excess of water-soluble vitamins is rare	Excess of water-soluble vitamins is rare	Thirst, nausea, vomiting; loss of weight; calcium deposits in kidneys or heart		Jaundice in infants

vent and cure the common cold, recommended that the minimum daily intake for adults should be between 2,000 to 10,000 milligrams. The possible side effects of such massive doses are a matter of concern. Toxicity is rare because vitamin C is one of the **water-soluble vitamins**—this means that the body can excrete the amounts it cannot use. Nevertheless, regular daily megadoses of 5,000 to 10,000 milligrams may lead to a buildup that can result in diarrhea, kidney or bladder stones, skin rashes, and gout.

Bioflavonoids are water-soluble substances that often occur in fruits and vegetables as complements to vitamin C. When ingested together, vitamin C and bioflavonoids are more effective than vitamin C is when ingested alone. Because bioflavonoids appear to be completely nontoxic, they seem to be a highly desirable element in the diet. Foods high in vitamin C and bioflavonoids include cherries, rose hips, sweet and hot peppers, strawberries, spinach and other dark-green leafy vegetables, and citrus fruits.

Are Vitamin Supplements Necessary? Most people can get all the vitamins they need by eating a healthy, varied diet. Some, however, feel the need to take daily vitamin supplements to maintain health and ward off illness. One factor that complicates the issue of vitamin needs is a concept called **biochemical individuality**—the idea that some people need more of certain vitamins and minerals than others do.[10] Experts disagree about the need to

water-soluble vitamins—
vitamins that dissolve in water and that the body can excrete.

The skin of a baked potato has 75 percent of the potato's vitamin C. Use skim milk instead of butter or sour cream to keep the potato moist.

biochemical individuality—
the idea that some people need more of certain vitamins and minerals than others do.

supplement a varied diet with additional vitamins. Several factors suggest, however, that moderate supplementation may improve health and probably does not diminish overall well-being. Certainly, the American public has accepted supplementation, making vitamins a multibillion-dollar industry.

The current state of nutrition seems to favor supplementation to ensure that individuals receive sufficient vitamins and minerals. Vitamin needs increase in the presence of stressors such as illness, physical activity, and psychological pressures.[11] In addition, poor diets, including those aimed at quick weight loss (below 1,500 calories), call for multivitamin supplementation, as do chronic problems such as alcoholism and chronic diarrhea.[12]

Environmental pollution and chemical additives in food can also increase the body's need for vitamins. Finally, there is evidence that some medicines block or neutralize the effects of certain vitamins. Despite these factors suggesting supplementation, **most** individuals can get the vitamins they need by eating a varied and balanced diet rich in an assortment of vitamins and other micronutrients.

Potential Hazards of Vitamin Megadoses People who take vitamin supplements in megadoses—amounts far above the RDAs—may be adversely affecting their health. When consumed in large doses, vitamins are properly considered drugs; overdoses of vitamins A, D, E, and K—the **fat-soluble vitamins**—can cause illness or even death.[13] These vitamins cannot be excreted but are stored in the fatty tissues, where they may build to toxic levels.

fat-soluble vitamins— vitamins that are stored in the fatty tissues and cannot be excreted.

Fiber

Popcorn is a wholesome low-calorie, high-fiber munchie. Instead of loading it with salt and butter, try chili powder, garlic powder, or other seasonings to give it flavor.

Fiber is a nonnutritive carbohydrate that is composed of cellulose, the major structural carbohydrate of plants. Also known as roughage and bulk, fiber is found in fruits, vegetables, and grains. Bran and fruit skins are a common source.

Humans cannot digest the cellulose found in fiber; as a result, fiber is not technically a nutrient, providing neither energy nor materials for cell building. However, it plays an essential role in the digestive process. In the large intestine (colon), it binds other waste products with large amounts of water, forming an easily passed soft, large stool. Since fiber passes through the digestive system unchanged, it helps move food quickly through the intestines and out of the body. This in turn helps prevent constipation and diverticulitis, a physiological problem in which the wall of the large intestine weakens and balloons out.

There is some evidence that dietary fiber may also affect blood cholesterol levels.[14] It may help lower blood cholesterol levels by reducing the amount of time cholesterol-containing foods stay in the digestive tract.[15] Some researchers have suggested that fiber (found in foods such as oat bran, dried beans and peas, raw carrots, barley, and certain fruits) can directly reduce cholesterol levels.[16] The most recent evidence, however, suggests that this is not the case. One study compared people on both high-fiber and low-fiber diets and found that their cholesterol levels, while lower than normal, were virtually identical. (The low-fiber diets included large amounts of complex carbohydrates.) The researchers concluded that the drop in cholesterol levels resulted from a lower intake of saturated fats rather than from an increase in fiber.[17] Future studies may clarify the effects of fiber on blood cholesterol.

There are other documented benefits of dietary fiber. It provides a medium for the growth of certain bacteria that help the body synthesize nutrients such as vitamin K. A high-fiber diet has been associated with a reduced risk of developing diabetes, colon cancer, and obesity. In addition, since fiber can act as a dietary "filler" without adding calories, a high-fiber diet can be satisfying and help people manage their weight.

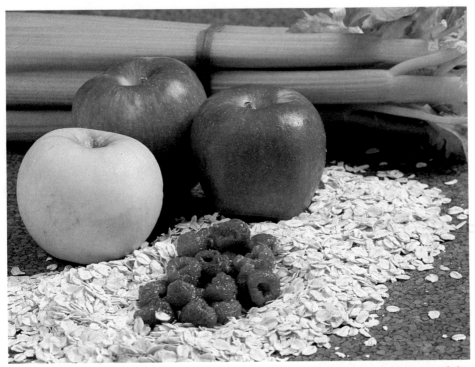

Fiber, an indigestible carbohydrate found in fruits and vegetables, is an essential part of the digestive process; people with little or no fiber in their diets run the risk of developing intestinal problems. (Tony Freeman/PhotoEdit)

Unfortunately, the diets of many Americans are lacking in adequate fiber. These diets consist predominantly of processed foods in which most of the fiber has been either milled out or peeled away. As a result, many traditional sources of fiber have disappeared from the diet. Moreover, Americans are not consuming enough fruits, vegetables, and whole-grain cereals, which are important sources of dietary fiber.

The National Cancer Institute recommends that people increase their dietary fiber intake to 20 to 30 grams daily, keeping it below 35 grams.[18] One's daily diet should include a variety of fruits and vegetables as well as whole-grain breads and cereals. Bran and other supplements are unnecessary unless a person has ongoing bowel problems, in which case a physician should be consulted.

Water

Like fiber, water has no nutritional value yet is a very important food component. It is the medium both for transporting nutrients to the cells and for removing cellular waste products. In addition, it acts as a medium for digestion, regulates body temperature, and, like fat, helps cushion the vital organs. An inadequate water intake will restrict the function of all body systems. Finally, water and some of the chemicals it carries are responsible for bodily structure. The cells in the body contain fluid, and there is fluid around the cells, too. As much as 80 percent of body weight may be water, although the average is closer to 60 percent.

While the body can survive for long periods without food, it can exist for only a few days without water. The actual amount of water the body requires per day depends on environment, physical activity, the season of the year, and the type of food eaten. Most people should drink six to eight glasses of water a day to maintain optimal health.

Toward a Balanced Diet

Knowing about food components is only the first step toward eating well. Virtually all foods contain nutrients, and most nutrients are so chemically complex that their effects on the body are not fully understood. In fact, most nutritionists would agree that it is not possible to create an "ideal" diet based on a balance of macronutrients and micronutrients. Knowledge about metabolic interactions is still incomplete, and individual dietary needs also vary greatly. Factors such as climate, body chemistry, and physical activity all affect the body's dietary needs.

How, then, can people choose the right foods to eat, attempt to achieve a balanced diet, and develop healthy dietary habits?

The Basic Four Food Groups

Pizza made with low-fat cheese and a whole-wheat crust is nutritionally preferable to hamburgers. Adding vegetables such as peppers, broccoli, and mushrooms increases the vitamin A and C content.

Probably the most widely known set of guidelines for determining proper diet is the basic four food groups system. This system, which was devised decades ago, groups food into four basic groups: meat, milk products, fruits and vegetables, and breads and cereals. The system was based on the RDAs established by the National Academy of Sciences–National Research Council.[19] The RDAs, which are reviewed for possible revision every 5 years, are estimates of the optimal quantity of each nutrient required—the most a person is likely to need (Table 5.3).

The four food groups plan specifies that a recommended number of servings be consumed daily from each group. However, despite much study, this system has recently been seen to have certain deficiencies. One problem is that the average energy content of a diet based on basic four food groups is 2,200 calories daily, which is high for people who are concerned about weight control. This means that a person whose calorie allowance is less than 2,200 finds few if any options for food choices in this plan.[20]

Another problem with the basic four food groups is that a person can follow the guidelines and still fail to meet the day's needs for certain nutrients, especially vitamin B_6, iron, magnesium, and zinc.

Finally, two of the four food groups consist of animal products: milk and meat. This gives many people the mistaken idea that half the amount of food consumed daily should consist of milk and meat, leading to a high fat consumption. In reality, the system recommends only two milk and two meat servings plus eight servings from the plant-food groups daily.

The Exchange System

Another method of determining diet is the exchange system. Unlike the basic four food groups system, which classifies foods by the nutrients they provide, the exchange system groups foods by the calorie content of their carbohydrate, fat, and protein components and by serving size.

Each food group in the exchange system identifies a typical food of that group and specifies a serving size. Each of these typical foods heads a group of other foods that may be exchanged for the "standard" food. Eaten in the specified serving size, each exchange food provides the same number of calories—in the form of protein, carbohydrate, and fat—as does the standard food in its group.

The exchange system is a complicated approach to developing a healthy diet. It takes time and interest to compute dietary intake according to its careful rules. Therefore, this system, like the basic four food groups system, is confusing for most people. Fortunately, there are guidelines to help people design a nutritional diet program.

Table 5.3 Recommended Daily Dietary Allowances for Adults

Total Intake in Energy (Kcal)	Men			Women[a]		
	19–22	23–50	51+	19–22	23–50	51+
	2,900	2,700	2,400	2,100	2,000	1,800
Major nutrients						
Protein (gm)	56	56	56	44	44	44
Carbohydrates	Carbohydrates and fats are not included in the RDAs because					
Fats	they are readily metabolized and are primarily energy foods.					
Vitamins						
A (RE)[b]	1,000	1,000	1,000	800	800	800
B (thiamine)[c]	1.5	1.4	1.2	1.1	1.1	1.0
B (riboflavin)	1.7	1.6	1.4	1.3	1.2	1.2
Niacin	19	18	16	14	13	13
B (pyridoxine)	2.2	2.2	2.2	2.0	2.0	2.0
Folacin	0.4	0.4	0.4	0.4	0.4	0.4
B (cyanocobalamin)	0.003	0.003	0.003	0.003	0.003	0.003
C	60	60	60	60	60	60
D	0.0075	0.005	0.005	0.0075	0.005	0.005
E	10	10	10	8	8	8
K	0.07–0.14	0.07–0.14	0.07–0.14	0.07–0.14	0.07–0.14	0.07–0.14
Biotin	0.07–0.14	0.07–0.14	0.07–0.14	0.1–0.2	0.07–0.14	0.07–0.14
Pantothenic acid	0.07–0.14	0.07–0.14	0.07–0.14	4–7	0.07–0.14	0.07–0.14
Minerals						
Calcium	800	800	800	800	800	800
Phosphorus	800	800	800	800	800	800
Magnesium	350	350	350	300	300	300
Zinc	15	15	15	15	15	15
Iron	10	10	10	18	18	18
Iodine	0.15	0.15	0.15	0.15	0.15	0.15
Potassium	1,875–5,625	1,875–5,625	1,875–5,625	1,875–5,625	1,875–5,625	1,875–5,625
Sodium	1,100–3,300	1,100–3,300	1,100–3,300	1,100–3,300	1,100–3,300	1,100–3,300
Manganese	2.5–5.0	2.5–5.0	2.5–5.0	2.5–5.0	2.5–5.0	2.5–5.0
Copper	2.0–3.0	2.0–3.0	2.0–3.0	2.0–3.0	2.0–3.0	2.0–3.0
Fluorine	1.5–4.0	1.5–4.0	1.5–4.0	1.5–4.0	1.5–4.0	1.5–4.0
Molybdenum	0.15–0.5	0.15–0.5	0.15–0.5	0.15–0.5	0.15–0.5	0.15–0.5
Chromium	0.05–0.2	0.05–0.2	0.05–0.2	0.05–0.2	0.05–0.2	0.05–0.2
Selenium	0.05–0.2	0.05–0.2	0.05–0.2	0.05–0.2	0.05–0.2	0.05–0.2

[a] Women who are pregnant or breastfeeding need special advice, as their requirements are considerably higher.

[b] RE = retinol equivalents, the standard measure for vitamin A.

[c] Except where specified, quantities are in milligrams. Note the extremely small requirements for some vitamins and minerals; they are, however, essential.

Source: Food and Nutrition Board, National Research Council, *Recommended Dietary Allowances,* 9th ed., and *Estimated Safe and Adequate Daily Dietary Intakes* (Washington, D.C.: National Academy of Sciences, 1979).

Finding the Right Diet for Yourself

Developing a personal diet is an excellent example of discovering and achieving a comfort level for yourself. There is no single ideal human diet—good diets differ from person to person. Nutritionists can set general guidelines and advise people to strive for overall proportions of the major nutrients and certain daily allowances of vitamins and minerals. However, the personal goals that can govern your diet are much more particular than those guidelines—and also more wide-ranging, covering not only your nutritional needs but your plans, tastes, principles, and lifestyle.

The differences between people's nutritional needs are not quite as simple as those reflected in daily allowance tables like Table 5.3, which makes different recommendations according to sex, weight, and age and mentions the effects of pregnancy and nursing. Everyone has his or her own particular metabolism, or biochemical individuality. Some people are thinner than average and never seem to get heavy no matter how much they eat or how little they exercise. Others eat very little but still have great difficulty losing weight. Between these extremes lies a great range of other types, some seemingly quite responsive to diet and exercise while others are less so. Add to this variety the many people who must watch their diets because they have food allergies or similar problems. People's nutritional needs can differ greatly.

However, people do not choose foods simply because of their nutritional needs. Many try to achieve certain specific goals through their eating. At the least, if they are satisfied with the way they are, they probably want to maintain their condition and maximize their chances of having a healthful old age. For these people, the general advice offered in this chapter is vital, but there are many other possible goals worth considering in connection with diet. Obviously, you can lose or gain weight, though this is easier for some people than it is for others. You can modify your choice of foods in a way that will help you prepare for a vigorous athletic event. You can help yourself through stressful times like final exams if you manage to eat

right, as described in this chapter. In the hospital or at home you may have a specific diet recommended by a physician to help you recover after an illness or operation.

Another obvious factor that influences people's diets is enjoyment. While most people dislike some foods, some have particular favorites that they like to eat again and again. For others, meals can be adventures in taste: they are always exploring new foods and combinations of foods. For still others, the main pleasure of a meal is the social occasion of being with friends; the food being eaten is incidental.

People's principles and lifestyles can be very important. Vegetarians usually choose to follow their diet because of their principles. Religious groups often have strict dietary rules. People dedicated to their work may not have time for a lot of thought about diet and may have a strong preference for packaged and fast foods. This chapter of the book focuses on nutrition because it is an important thing to consider in planning your life, but it is not the only thing.

Your health also depends on your success in reaching other goals. True, it is possible to succeed at more than one goal at a time; for example, you can eat out with friends at a fast-food restaurant and still eat positively by choosing the salad bar and drinking milk instead of a shake. However, such solutions are not always possible: compromises may have to be made. The human body is tolerant and can accept varied conditions.

There is no need to be a diet purist. The emotional stress this can cause may be worse than any physical stress brought on by occasional lapses from perfect eating. Sacrificing other parts of your lifestyle for the sake of perfect nutrition can create unnecessary problems. As with all things, find your own comfort level in matters of diet. Nutrition is important to your health, but do not let it ruin the rest of your life!

Material developed from Beatrice Hunter, "Food for Thought: Appreciating Individual Differences," *Consumer's Research* (December 1989): 8–9.

A Positive Food Strategy

Unlike these complicated approaches to diet, there is a simple strategy for choosing foods that provide maximum energy, vitality, and health. This strategy simply requires a basic understanding of foods that are preferred sources of nutrients and those which should be limited as well as guidelines for consuming the proper ratios of these foods. This food strategy, which could be called a positive food strategy, should not be followed for only a prescribed period of time; it should be the basis of a lifelong commitment to new and better eating habits.[21]

The positive food strategy includes four basic principles.

Many people think that starchy foods such as potatoes, bread, and pasta are fattening, but they are not. A lot of calories come from what they are served with—calorie-rich butter, margarine, sour cream, gravies, jams, and jellies.

1. Daily caloric intake should support normal growth in children and a desirable weight in adults. Eating just enough to maintain an ideal consistent weight is considered the key to increased longevity and an improved quality of life (Chapter 6).

2. The daily intake of food should include a relative ratio of five times as much complex carbohydrates as protein. The key here is that protein should never constitute more than one-fifth of a meal. This does not mean that it is all right to consume 12 ounces of meat and five times that amount of vegetables. Servings of protein should be limited to 3- or 4-ounce portions.

3. The basic goal of a positive food strategy is to increase the intake of complex carbohydrates, decrease the intake of protein, and limit the intake of fat.

The average American's diet contains far too much protein. It is much more healthy to prepare meals with large amounts of vegetables. (Richard Hutchings/InfoEdit)

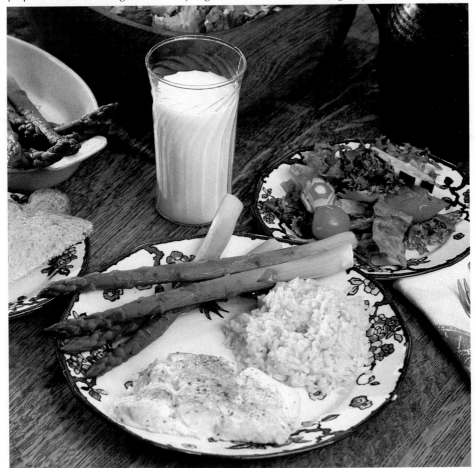

Table 5.4   Preferred Foods

Carbohydrates	
Preferred foods (complex carbohydrates)	Limited foods (simple carbohydrates)

Whole-grain products

Whole-wheat cereals, bread, rolls; tortillas, pasta, barley, brown rice, corn meal, popcorn, cracked wheat, bran, millet, old-fashioned oatmeal, rye

Cold cereal: puffed rice, corn flakes, shredded wheat, Grape-Nuts

Refined grain products

White flour, white bread and rolls, highly processed cereals, and cereals containing sugar

Vegetables

Legumes: richest source of vegetable protein; includes all dried peas and beans: lentils, black-eyed peas, chick-peas, kidney beans, soybeans, and foods made from soybeans

Tofu: soybean curd, an excellent source of vegetable protein

Fruits and dried fruits

Protein	
Preferred foods (protein foods low in fats)	Limited foods (protein foods with fat and cholesterol)

Fish

Poultry (no skin)

Meat (lean cuts, no choice or prime)

Processed meats: sausages, hot dogs, cold cuts

Dairy products

Low-fat: Non-fat milk, buttermilk, nonfat and low-fat yogurt, low-fat cheeses (cottage cheese and partially skimmed ricotta and mozzarella)

Dairy products

High-fat: Whole milk, half and half, cream, sour cream, ice cream, high-fat cheeses (cheddar, Swiss, blue, most cheese spreads)

Be aware of the high sodium content of some cheeses

Eggs: yolks are high in cholesterol

Other Protein

Other protein

Nuts and seeds: high in fat; buy raw nuts and seeds with exception of peanuts; buy dry-roasted, unsalted peanuts

Peanut butter: high in fat

4. Limit the intake of foods of poor nutritional quality and increase the intake of high-quality foods. Some foods are simply better than others because they contain more nutrients per ounce (Table 5.4).

Using this positive food strategy will help you become leaner and more energetic and will provide protection against diseases related to a poor diet. It will also enable you to enjoy all the foods you like—some in abundant quantities, others in moderation, and others in limited amounts. Although you have to limit the consumption of certain foods, you do not have to give them up entirely. Choosing foods based on their preferred or limited status (Table 5.4) will also help you plan meals and shop for food.

Table 5.4 Preferred Foods (continued)

Fats

Use of fats in the diet should always be limited

Butter is high in saturated fat and cholesterol
Margarine has no cholesterol but has the same number of calories as butter
Mayonnaise is high in fat and cholesterol
Commercial salad dressing may be high in one or both of these
For salads and cooking, use polyunsaturated oil such as corn or safflower oil; avoid margarines or anything that contains coconut or palm oil; these oils are highly saturated fats

Miscellaneous

Canned foods

Preferred foods (limited use of salt and sugar)	Limited foods (preserved with salt or sugar)
Vegetables: use when fresh are not available; canned tomato products make an excellent base for sauces	Canned vegetables with added salt, sugar, or preservatives
Fruits: should be packed in water or natural juices; no sugar added	
Fish: water-packed tuna, available with no or reduced salt	
Chicken or beef stock: contains less salt than bouillon	
Juices: fruit — unsweetened only; tomato and other vegetables: no salt added	

Frozen foods

Fruits and juices: unsweetened only	TV dinners: are usually high in salt and fats
Vegetables: unsalted only	Frozen french fries

Seasonings and Condiments

Herbs and spices, dried or fresh — are calorie-free	Salt and salt substitutes; artificial sweeteners — have chemical additives
Vinegars — can be used for salad dressings, sauces, and marinades	Catsup: high in salt and sugar
	Pickles and olives: high in sodium

Beverages

Water, herb teas	Coffee and nonherbal teas contain caffeine; even decaffeinated coffee has a small amount of caffeine
Skim and low-fat milk	Soft drinks: contain sugar and possibly caffeine
Vegetable juices: unsalted	Diet soft drinks: have artificial sweeteners and sometimes caffeine
Fruit juices: unsweetened only	Wine, liquor, beer: high in calories; little nutritional value

Adapted, with permission, from Jeanne Jones, *Jet Fuel: The New Food Strategy for the High Performance Person* (New York: Villard Books, 1984).

Meeting Special Needs

A diet based on the positive food strategy will meet the nutritional needs of most people. Some individuals and some situations, however, may require special attention and perhaps certain changes in food choices.

Food Choices for Vegetarians Vegetarianism has become more common among Americans. The vegetarian faces a special problem in diet planning— obtaining the needed nutrients from fewer food groups.

There are two major classes of vegetarians: ovolactovegetarians and vegans. Ovolactovegetarians eat eggs (*ovo-*) and dairy products (*lacto-*) as well as plant foods, while vegans eat plant foods only—no eggs, cheese, or milk.

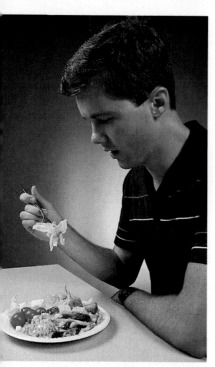

Although vegetarian diets are considered healthful by many nutrition experts, a completely meat-free diet can lead to serious vitamin and iron deficiencies; therefore, vegetarians must make informed choices to ensure good health. (Tony Freeman/ PhotoEdit)

Although either vegetarian diet can be adequate for health with the reservations expressed below, it is far easier to obtain the necessary nutrients from the ovolacto diet than from the vegan diet. Since proteins from eggs and dairy products are complete, ovolactovegetarians can meet their basic nutritional needs even after giving up meat. Proteins from plant sources, however, are usually incomplete; that is, they do not contain all the amino acids the body needs. Therefore, vegans must plan meals that combine incomplete proteins so as to form complete ones. Typically, this means a combination of grains and legumes, such as rice and beans, bread and peanut butter, or corn muffins and pea soup. By selecting appropriate food combinations and a wide variety of foods, a vegan can consume enough complete protein.

The real problem in the vegan diet is a lack of vitamin B_{12}, which is most often found in animal foods. Vegans must consume a source of B_{12} or suffer a deficiency. The nonmeat source may be a special form of yeast, soybean milk, or a B_{12} supplement. Besides vitamin B_{12}, iron may be a problem for vegans, since its best sources are animal foods. Vegans should make a special effort to eat plant foods high in iron (beans, spinach, prunes, tofu) and iron-enriched foods or take an iron supplement.

Food Choices for People under Stress   As was noted in Chapter 2, prolonged stress can damage the immune system, providing fertile ground for a wide range of ailments. Eating patterns are often disrupted during periods of stress, and as a result, the body begins to lose a number of important nutrients, including potassium, glucose, protein, fat, and calcium. This deprivation can be prevented if nutrients are stored in the body in much the same way money is saved for a rainy day.

Most people know the importance of eating a balanced and varied diet, but many are unaware that many nutrients literally go in one end and out the other if exercise is not used to make them "stick." Only muscles that are called on to work are able to grow and accumulate protein. The same is true of bones, which must be active to absorb additional calcium. Regular exercise— daily or every-other-day workouts—is the most effective means of retaining nourishment. This nutritional "money in the bank" can help one avoid becoming dangerously weak during periods of unavoidable stress.

Stress can have a significant effect on the appetite. Many people do not feel much like eating when they are under stress. This can be dangerous, because the more debilitated a person becomes, the harder it is to combat the stressor. Ideally, one should not let stress build to the point at which eating becomes impossible. It is important to eat whatever you can, eat small amounts, and drink fluids. Some experts also recommend that a vitamin-mineral supplement be taken every day to replenish important nutrients.

Other people may ravenously overeat in response to stress; for them, the best solution is, once again, exercise. Not only does exercise keep an individual away from the refrigerator, it fuels the body by building muscle and bone and prevents excess calories from being stored as fat.[22]

The consumption of some foods can add to stress by stimulating the body's stress response (Chapter 2). Certain substances found in these foods trigger this response. The most common of these substances is caffeine, which is found in coffee, tea, cola drinks, cocoa, and chocolate. It is advisable to limit the consumption of such foods.

Another connection between diet and stress is a phenomenon known as *vitamin depletion*. Excessive stress over prolonged periods can deplete the body of certain vitamins, such as vitamin C and the vitamin B complex. Such depletion can cause improper functioning of the endocrine and nervous systems. Sugar and sugar products have also been implicated as a factor in vitamin B complex depletion, and their consumption should be limited during periods of stress.

Sugar is the most widely used food additive. Sugar in food takes many forms— white, brown, raw, corn syrup, honey, and molasses.

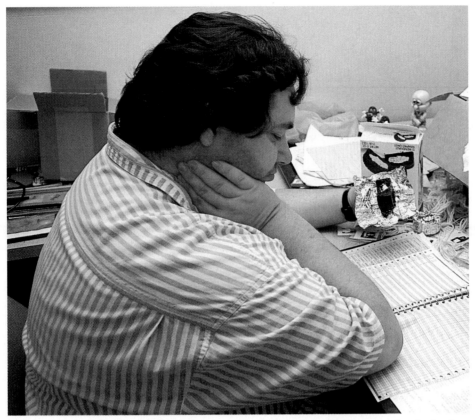

People who are in a hurry and under stress frequently snack on candy and other foods of low nutritional value. These foods lack nutrients that build up one's ability to cope with stress. (Tony Freeman/PhotoEdit)

Putting Nutritional Principles to Work

Once you know the nutritional value of foods and the best dietary strategies, it is necessary to develop the skills that will enable you to purchase and prepare the foods you need. These skills are essential if you want to make sure the nutritional principles you have learned will be put into practice wisely.

Buying Food

A key to shopping for food is to spend less time shopping in the center aisles of supermarkets and grocery stores. The majority of preferred foods identified in this chapter (Table 5.4) are found along the outer walls of most food stores. On these walls there are fresh fruits and vegetables; fresh fish, poultry, and meats; dairy products; and bread. The middle aisles, by contrast, are filled primarily with low-quality processed foods, although there are some exceptions, such as grains, pasta, cereals, and frozen and canned goods. As a general rule, therefore, it is wiser to shop from the outer walls to get the foods that will best meet your nutritional needs.

Of course, almost everyone buys processed or packaged foods from time to time. When you buy these foods, it is very important to be able to assess what you are buying and know the contents of the products. To some extent, this can be done by learning how to read the fine print on product packages.

Misleading Packaging In their zeal to sell products, companies often design product packages to appeal to health concerns. Thus, words associated

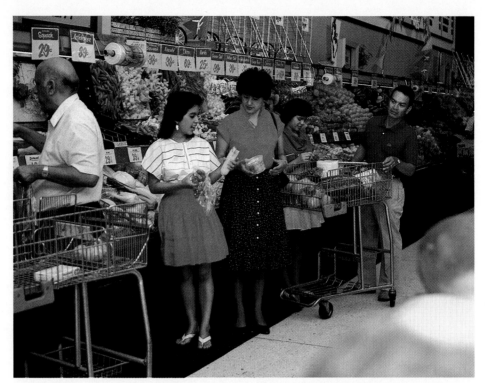

A wise supermarket shopper will avoid the junk food and processed food aisles in favor of the produce section, where nutritious fresh fruits and vegetables are found. (Stephen McBrady/PhotoEdit)

with good health—*organic, natural, bran, oat,* and *fruit,* for example—often appear in product names and claims. Such words conjure up images of fresh air, mountain streams, and healthy, active people. Claims about the healthfulness of foods can be deceiving, however. Some products that claim to be nutritious may actually contain many low-quality nutrients, including sugars, fats, and salt. For example, fruit drinks may contain mostly sugar with added color and flavor and only a small percentage of real fruit juice. Another example of misleading words is the term *natural,* which by law can be used to describe sugar, since sugar is a product of nature. The state and federal governments have not made consistent attempts to deal with this type of misleading language. It is possible, however, to determine the contents and nutritional value of most processed or packaged foods by reading their labels.

Fruit juice beverages, or fruit drinks, may contain as little as 5 percent real fruit juice. The remainder is mostly water and sugar.

Nutrition Labeling Except for a few standard products (for example, mayonnaise), the law requires that every processed food list its ingredients in the order of the quantity used, by weight. In addition, nutrition labeling is required for every food that has been enriched with additional nutrients or makes a specific nutritional claim. Such food labels must show the following:

1. Serving size
2. Number of servings per container
3. Per-serving amount of calories, protein, carbohydrates, and fat
4. Percentage of U.S. RDAs per serving for certain essential nutrients—protein, vitamins A and D, thiamin, riboflavin, niacin, calcium, and iron—calculated by weight

An ounce of the most highly sweetened breakfast cereals may have the equivalent of 3.5 teaspoons of table sugar. Shredded wheat, puffed wheat, and puffed rice are usually unsweetened, though they may contain the sugar maltose and certainly contain complex carbohydrates or starches.

Thanks to nutrition labeling, careful consumers are better able to avoid foods that have a significant amount of unhealthy ingredients and those which offer little nutritional benefit. For example, labeling can alert consumers to foods high in sugars (including ''pure cane sugar,'' corn syrup, molasses, and honey), fats, sodium, and potentially harmful additives such as sulfites, which are used to preserve food, and nitrites or nitrates.

Fats, Oils, and Shortening   Another area of labeling to be aware of concerns the fat, oil, and shortening in processed foods. Although cooking oils and shortenings provide an analysis of saturated fats on their labels, the ingredient lists on processed foods mention only the fats in question without specifying how much is saturated or unsaturated. Many labels are quite vague, stating only what the food ''may'' contain. Thus a consumer may read that the product contains corn oil, palm oil, and coconut oil but is not told how much is saturated or unsaturated. Worse, a vague term such as *vegetable oil* can refer to saturated fats such as palm kernel, palm, or coconut oil as well as polyunsaturated fats such as corn or safflower oil.

The habit of reading labels helps consumers get the right foods into their kitchens—and keep the wrong ones out. Despite misleading labels and the use of dubious ingredients, shopping need not be a grim exercise in extensive research and self-denial. You can tolerate some low-quality foods and some less-preferred ingredients so long as most of your shopping basket is filled with preferred foods.

Nutrition Information Per Serving	
Serving Size . . . . ½ Cup	
Servings Per Container Approx. 3	
Calories 100	
Protein. . . . . 2 Grams	
Carbohydrates . . . . 25 Grams	
Fat . . . . 1 Gram	
Sodium . . . . 300 Milligrams	
Percentage of U.S. Recommended Daily Allowances (U.S. RDA)	
Protein. 2	Riboflavin 2
Vitamin A 2	Niacin 4
Vitamin C 8	Calcium . . . . . *
Thiamine 2	Iron 2
*Contains Less Than 2% Of The U.S. RDA Of These Nutrients.	
Ingredients: Whole Kernel Golden Corn, Water, Sugar, Salt.	

The nutrition label from this can of kerneled corn reveals that the product contains a significant amount of sodium. This is a serious concern for people with hypertension. (Tom Dunham)

Avoiding Food Hazards

Americans in general have access to a great variety of safe high-quality food products. Even so, there are some potential hazards that consumers should recognize, understand, and guard against. The improper storage and handling of food may be hazardous to your health. For example, as many as one American in six may fall prey to food poisoning every year. Caused by bacteria, most of these cases are mild—perhaps consisting only of an upset stomach—but some require lengthy recuperation and may be life-threatening.

There are ways to protect yourself against this and other similar hazards.

- Never buy, keep, or use canned goods if the can is swollen or badly dented. Damaged cans may allow air to enter, contributing to bacterial growth.
- Keep all perishable food refrigerated or chilled at all times. Do not let foods sit out for extended periods. The growth of harmful bacteria is slowed by refrigeration.
- Wash your hands frequently while preparing food. Do not prepare food if you are ill or have a cut or infection.
- Scrub vegetables intended to be eaten raw to remove parasites or germs that have survived from the growing fields or retailer.
- Keep foods either hot (over 140 degrees F) or cold (below 45 degrees F).

Preparing Food

One of the keys to eating nutritiously is knowing the best ways to prepare and cook food. While a full discussion of cooking is beyond the scope of this chapter, here are some basic guidelines for preparing nutritious low-fat, low-salt, low-sugar meals.

1. Use water, defatted stock, juice, or wine instead of butter or oil to prevent food from sticking to the pan and burning while braising and sautéing it. Another technique is to use chopped onions and cook them slowly so that they release moisture, which will prevent sticking and burning.
2. Use vanilla extract, cinnamon, or concentrated fruit juice in place of sugar or artificial sweeteners. If you must use sugar, use one-half the amount called for in the recipe.

Food Selections, the Food Chain, and World Hunger

American consumers can choose from an enormous range of foods. The United States has the land resources and climatic conditions to produce a wide diversity of crops and livestock. In addition, the United States imports a large variety of foods grown or processed abroad: beef from Argentina, lamb from New Zealand, avocados from Mexico, tomatoes from Israel, tea from China and India, coffee from Colombia, and olives and olive oil from Spain and Italy, to name a few. The foods people select from this cornucopia affect not only their individual health but the health of the world's food supply as well.

Obviously, food choices can help ensure that the body is getting the nutrients it needs in the correct proportions and that as few toxins as possible are ingested. There is plenty of advice elsewhere in this chapter about selecting appropriate foods and avoiding those with the potential to cause harm. However, the concept of the food chain has not been discussed—and it is relevant both to personal health and to world hunger.

In the food chain foods are ranked according to their position on what might be called a predator scale. To simplify matters somewhat, plants are at the bottom of the chain because all their nutrients come from the soil, air, and water. Animals that eat plants (herbivores) are the next link up on the food chain; they may in turn be prey to carnivores and omnivores (creatures that eat all types of food), which are therefore even higher on the chain. Human beings are at the top of the food chain: people eat foods from all levels, including some carnivores. (Dog and snake are delicacies in some cultures, and shark and alligator can be found on the tables of some Americans.)

As a rule, food items lower on the food chain are less complex chemically; hence, plants do not contain the variety of amino acids that animals do. However, plants are also less likely to contain significant amounts of pesticides and other toxins, which tend to accumulate toward the top of the food chain. In other words, people may ingest some pesticides by eating plants but will ingest more if they eat animals whose diets are based on those plants. Note that foods lower on the food chain—grains, vegetables, and fruits—usually contain less saturated fats than do animal foods: this is another advantage of eating more vegetables and less meat.

There is also an argument, however, that where people eat on the food chain affects not only their own health but the amount of

---

3. Use herbs and spices to replace salt. They contain no calories and add greatly to the flavor and enjoyment of food. Use two to three times as many herbs and spices as you would normally use.

4. Whenever possible, steam or stir-fry vegetables. Broiling and baking are other health-conducive cooking techniques.

5. When preparing poultry, meat, and fish, remove all visible fat before cooking. Remove the skin of poultry either before cooking or before serving. Broil or bake meat products and avoid low-quality meat products that are high in fat.

6. Use oils sparingly and select those which are low in saturated fats. Monounsaturates such as olive oil may be best for frying, since heat can saturate polyunsaturated oils.[23]

Eating Right in Today's Fast-Paced World

Selecting, preparing, and eating nutritious food is a rewarding experience; not only is it enjoyable, it also promotes good health. Today's fast-paced lifestyle, however, sometimes causes people to neglect their nutritional needs. Some people spend their lives on the run, rushing to and from work

food available to people the world over. Some experts concerned with world hunger believe that this argument—and not individual health benefits—is the most compelling reason for selecting food from lower links on the food chain. They point out that livestock production is a highly inefficient way to produce protein. Beef cattle, for example, produce about 42 pounds of protein per acre. However, an acre planted with cereals can produce five times that amount of protein. Legumes (peas, beans, and lentils) can produce ten times more, and leafy vegetables fifteen times more.

If the Western countries decreased their demand for animal protein, therefore, they would not only improve the health of their own people, they would also encourage land-use decisions that would assure more food for everyone in the world. Land resources both at home and abroad are used to rear animals for Western tables and to grow animal feed. The same land could be used to provide vegetable foods for American tables *and* for the populations of the poorer countries. The excessive meat consumption of the Western world leads to the less than optimal use of agricultural land—which is a resource that could be used to help solve the pressing problem of world hunger.

Basing food choices on land-use efficiency does not entail eliminating meat from the Western diet altogether, of course. There are many high-grade sources of animal protein that do use resources efficiently. Large areas of land are more suitable for livestock grazing than for any other purpose. There are also many animals—for example, turkeys and chickens—that convert grain into animal protein more efficiently than do pigs, sheep, and cattle. However, the fact remains that by all standards of nutrition, affluent people eat far more meat than is good for them, not to mention how much food they need. Even a 10 percent reduction in the amount of meat we eat in America could mean enough grain to feed 60 million people—a population considerably larger than that of many nations.

Ideas based on Frances Moore Lappe, *Diet for a Small Planet* (New York: Ballantine, 1974); Frances Lappe and Joseph Collins, *Food First* (New York: Ballantine, 1978); Daniel Chiras, *Environmental Science: A Framework for Decision Making* (Redwood City, Calif.: Benjamin-Cummings, 1988).

and social engagements. As a result, nutritious meals are often replaced by readily available snacks or other fast foods.

Every year Americans spend billions of dollars eating out in regular restaurants and fast-food outlets. The tempting foods in these places sometimes present a health hazard. Finer restaurants frequently offer creamed sauces, rich meats, and other fat-laden foods that prudent eaters avoid, and fast foods are generally very high in fat, cholesterol, and salt.

How can you make good food choices in this eating environment? The simplest advice is to follow a few basic universal principles that can provide guidance for everyone in developing a healthy diet.[24]

1. **Eat moderately.** Eating too much at one meal or in one's total diet is stressful to the body. It may lead to poor digestion and can force the body to expend excess energy to digest large quantities of food, resulting in an energy deficit. A meal should leave you feeling light and energized, with a clear mind.
2. **Eat early in the day.** Eating too close to bedtime can lead to poor digestion and assimilation of food. Late-night snacks can easily turn to fat. Therefore, it is preferable to eat the majority of your dietary intake earlier in the day and taper off as evening approaches. Ideally, dinner should be the lightest, smallest meal of the day.

3. **Eat natural foods.** Foods in the natural state have their original nutrients; food processing, refining, preserving, aging, and cooking deplete these nutrients. Raw or lightly steamed fresh vegetables have more nutritional value than do those which have been overcooked; so do fresh, unprocessed fruits. While freezing some vegetables and fruits may capture vitamins that otherwise would be lost in shipping and storage, raw fruits and vegetables are best.

4. **Eat quality foods and avoid junk foods**—foods that have few nutritional benefits other than providing a source of quick energy. These include cookies, cakes, and highly refined foods, plus many heavily salted foods, such as potato chips. Eat foods that provide the best-quality fuel and nutrients instead. Such foods are packed with vitamins, minerals, and other essential nutrients (Table 5.4).

5. **Eat a wide variety of different types of foods.** This will help ensure that your nutritional needs are met. Dietary variety can also provide more novelty and be more satisfying, especially for people who are trying to change their eating habits.

Some additional strategies for life on the run include the following: (1) Do not skip meals; if you eat between meals, choose snacks that are healthy. (2) When eating out, select foods that are good for you; ask how foods are prepared and do not hesitate to make requests about the food you are served. For example, request broiled, baked, steamed, or poached meat, fish, or poultry or specify that sauces or salad dressings be served on the side.

Ideas about diet and nutrition are continually changing. New nutritional research will undoubtedly suggest additional strategies for healthy eating. This research and the strategies that will emerge are very important. While medical advances and public health policies have succeeded in eliminating many of the causes of disease and death, good nutrition and better eating habits can perhaps play an even more important role in the improvement of personal health.

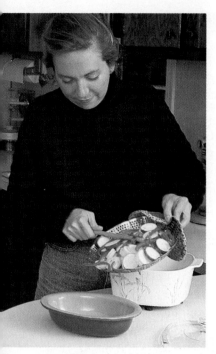

Most foods retain more nutrients when cooked in steam or baked. Boiling and frying tend to drain important nutrients. (Tom Dunham)

Chapter Summary

- Proper nutrition is now recognized as a major factor in developing and maintaining good health.
- Nutrition is the science of foods and how they are used in the body for energy, growth, and the repair of damaged tissues.
- There are several basic groups of nutrients in food—proteins, carbohydrates, fats, vitamins, and minerals. There are also two essential non-nutritive substances—fiber and water.
- Protein is composed of different amino acids, the building blocks of the body. Protein is essential for growth and the repair of body tissues. It is found in foods of animal origin (complete protein) and plant origin (incomplete protein).
- Carbohydrates are found in all forms of plant life and constitute the body's chief source of energy. Simple carbohydrates, or sugars, provide a quick burst of energy; complex carbohydrates, including starches, produce energy slowly.
- A certain amount of fat is essential; fat insulates the body, cushions the vital organs, and con-

tributes to other bodily functions. Saturated fats and cholesterol have been associated with cardiovascular disease, and their intake should be limited.
- Vitamins are essential for triggering vital bodily functions, such as helping chemical reactions take place; different types of vitamins play different roles. Some experts recommend that people take vitamin supplements to get adequate amounts.
- Minerals help in the formation of body tissue and various chemical substances needed for nerve transmission and regulation of the body's fluid levels. The body requires different amounts of the many different types of minerals found in a variety of foods.
- Though not a nutrient, fiber plays an essential role in the digestive process. A diet high in fiber has been associated with a reduced risk of developing diabetes, colon cancer, and obesity and may help reduce cholesterol levels.
- Humans cannot live without water; it acts as a medium for transporting nutrients to the cells

and removing waste products. It also aids in digestion, helps regulate body temperature, and cushions the vital organs.

- Classic strategies for choosing the proper foods to eat in the proper amounts include the basic four food groups and the exchange system but are now considered by many people to be inadequate or too complicated. What is needed is a basic understanding of which foods are preferred sources of nutrients and which should be limited, along with some simple guidelines for determining the quantities that should be consumed.
- People with special nutritional needs, for example, vegetarians and people under stress, must make sure to choose foods that will provide them with the nutrients they need.
- An important factor in proper nutrition is knowing how to buy the best-quality foods and prepare them in safe and nutritious ways.
- Nutrition labeling on food packages can be misleading, yet it is an important way to determine the quality of foods.
- Foods must be stored and handled properly to ensure safety; improperly stored or handled food may be dangerous.
- A few universal nutritional principles, such as eating high-quality, natural foods in moderate amounts, can provide guidance for everyone in developing a healthy diet.

Key Terms

Metabolism (page 112)

Calorie (page 112)

Macronutrient (page 112)

Micronutrient (page 112)

Protein (page 112)

Enzyme (page 112)

Essential amino acid (page 113)

Complete protein (page 113)

Incomplete protein (page 113)

Glucose (page 114)

Carbohydrates (page 114)

Glycogen (page 115)

Lipids (page 115)

Triglycerides (page 115)

Cholesterol (page 115)

Lipoproteins (page 115)

Unsaturated fat (page 116)

Saturated fat (page 116)

Minerals (page 117)

Calcium (page 117)

Potassium (page 119)

Sodium (page 119)

Electrolytes (page 119)

Iron (page 119)

Vitamins (page 119)

Water-soluble vitamins (page 121)

Biochemical individuality (page 121)

Fat-soluble vitamins (page 122)

References

1. *Surgeon General's Report on Nutrition and Health* (USDHHS [PHS] Pub. No. 88-50210, Washington, D.C.: U.S. Government Printing Office, 1988).

2. Food and Nutrition Board, National Research Council, *Recommended Dietary Allowances*, 9th ed. (Washington, D.C.: National Academy of Sciences, 1979).

3. Nutrition Committee, American Heart Association, "Dietary Guidelines for Healthy American Adults: A Statement for Physicians and Health Professionals," *Circulation* 77, no 3 (March 1988): 721A–724A.

4. From "Diet and Health: Implications for Reducing Chronic Disease Risk," in "The Latest Word on What to Eat," *Time* (March 13, 1984): 51.

5. Ellen Ruppel Shell, "Kids, Catfish, and Cholesterol," *American Health* (January–February 1988): 56.

6. N. A. Boon and J. K. Aronson, "Dietary Salt and Hypertension: Treatment and Prevention," *British Medical Journal* 290, no. 6473 (1985): 949–950.

7. Simin Meydam, "Vitamin E Might Help Elderly Battle Disease," presented at the American Chemical Society Meeting, Los Angeles, Calif., October 1, 1988. Reported in the *Arizona Republic* (October 2, 1988).

8. Eli Seifter, "Vitamin A and Beta-Carotene and Effects of Gamma Radiation," *Journal of National Cancer Institute* 73, no 5 (Nov. 1984): 1167–1177.

9. Ibid.

10. Roger Williams, *Nutrition against Disease* (New York: Titman, 1971).

11. D. Giordano et al., *Controlling Stress and Tension: A Holistic Approach* (Englewood Cliffs, N.J.: Prentice-Hall, 1990): 101.

12. Elaine Feldman, *Essentials of Clinical Nutrition* (Philadelphia: F A Davis, 1988): 334.

13. Ibid.

14. D. J. Fletcher and D. A. Rogers, "Diet and Coronary Heart Disease," *Postgraduate Medicine* 77, no. 5 (1985): 319–328.

15. Ibid.

16. Leslie Roberts, "Measuring Cholesterol Is as Tricky as Lowering It," *Science* 238, no. 4826 (October 1987): 482–483.

17. Jane E. Brody, "Small Study Challenges Role of Oat Bran in Reducing Cholesterol," *New York Times* (January 18, 1990): A24.

18. Elaine Lanza et al. "Dietary Fiber Intake in the U.S. Population," *American Journal of Clinical Nutrition* 46 (1987): 790–797.

19. Food and Nutrition Board, op. cit.

20. S. Chuck Clapp, "The Basic Four?" *Community Nutritionist* 2 (January–February 1983): 1–7.

21. Jeanne Jones, *Jet Fuel: The New Food Strategy for the High Performance Person* (New York: Villard Books, 1984).

22. Surgeon General's Report (1988).

23. Ibid.

24. Elson M. Haas, "Dieting with the Seasons," in *The New Holistic Health Handbook*, Shepherd Bliss (ed.), (Lexington, Mass.: Penguin Books, Stephen Green Press, 1985): 129–131.

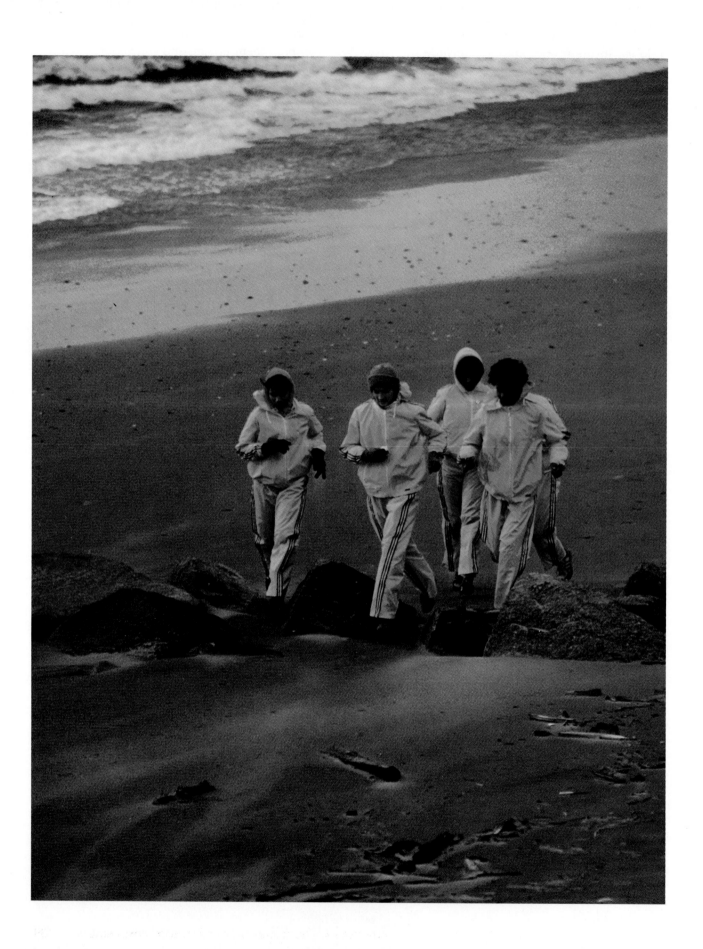

Chapter 6

Weight Management and Body Composition

To Guide Your Reading

When you have studied this chapter, you should be able to:

- Describe the relationship among weight, appearance, and body composition and list some of the problems associated with unhealthy body composition.

- Explain the different uses of fats in the human body, indicating which ones cause the most problems in regard to healthy body composition.

- Identify and comment on at least four different techniques Americans use to control and manage appearance and body composition.

- Characterize two approaches that underlie explanations of body composition problems and explain how to work on them.

- Explain how people can use natural management techniques for body composition.

- Name and describe three extreme conditions that occasionally affect body composition, indicating current ideas about their cause and treatment.

Weight. The topic is one of the most talked about and written about in the United States. Television shows, books, videotapes, spas, restaurants, and even manufacturers of frozen dinners all cater to Americans who wish to lose, or sometimes gain, pounds. Weight control has become a major industry; $74 billion is spent each year on low-calorie foods from crackers to nondairy creamers. Millions more are spent on diet books, diet aids, and equipment designed to help people shed pounds.[1]

For most people the scales may be the measuring tool, but the mirror is a more important test. A young man wants to appear stronger and heavier, in keeping with the image that he has developed of manhood. A 27-year-old woman is anxious about being in shape for her swimsuit by the time the summer comes around. A 43-year-old wants to trim down his stomach for his twenty-fifth high school reunion. People have an idea of what they want to look like; and many make great efforts to achieve that look, even if only for a short time.

However, there is another element of equal or even greater significance. Looks and fashion are important for the present and can affect a person's self-concept and self-esteem, but there is an even more vital long-term issue. Overweight and underweight have been linked with chronic long-term medical problems, some of which are serious and even life-threatening.[2] This is especially true when a weight problem begins in childhood or adolescence[3] or lasts for a long time. Several life insurance companies publish tables which indicate ideal weights for men and women of different heights. These tables are compiled to help insurers assess the risk that a given person may die early, because the insurers have observed that, on average, people who are overweight have a shorter life span.

However, weight itself is not really the issue. People undergo weight changes all the time, both temporary and long-term. During a typical day a person's weight can vary considerably. Drink a glass or two of water and you may find that you are more than a pound heavier. Exercise for an hour and you will find that you have lost water weight—perhaps up to 3 pounds. Athletes can usually add a considerable amount of weight when they get into condition, as their muscle mass grows. And as people grow older, their bones frequently become more porous and lighter, even if overall body weight is increasing for other reasons. Yet none of these weight changes is considered a part of the "battle of the bulge."

Because weight is simple to measure, it has been the main focus of attention, even for the insurance companies; however, predictions from weight alone are not ideal. The more elaborate insurance tables include other factors—for example, age and body frame type—acknowledging that the relationship between weight and longevity is not simple. The real issue for health—and for appearance too—is not weight but body composition.

body composition—the proportion of fat in comparison with lean body tissue (muscle and bone) within the human body.

Body composition refers to the proportion of different substances within the body, in particular the proportion of body fat to other body tissues. It is the body's fat content—perhaps even, according to some recent studies, its fat distribution—that poses the main health problem. While weight can be an indicator of the amount of fat, it can be misleading because of the variable weight of other tissues, such as bone and muscle.

Weight, Body Composition, and Health

Body composition, particularly the proportion of fat in the body, can affect a person's total being. Physically, it affects cardiovascular fitness for the long term, and it also affects energy levels, stamina, and endurance in the present. Psychologically, it may affect self-image and self-esteem. Socially, of course, it affects a person's relationships with others.

Body Composition and Physical Health

Challenging evidence has come from recent laboratory research which showed that certain species of animals benefit greatly from reduced-calorie diets: a 50 percent reduction in calories appeared to add 50 percent to life expectancy. The applicability of these findings to human beings is unclear at this time.

One of the best documented health risks of excessive fat in body composition is heart disease (Chapter 11). In the Framingham study, a classic long-term study of the health of the residents of a town in Massachusetts, death from heart disease—and sudden death in particular—was found to occur more often among overweight people.[4] (For simplicity, the terms *weight, overweight,* and *underweight* will be used in this chapter, but they should be understood to indicate proportion of fat rather than weight alone.)

Obese persons (defined as 20 percent or more over ideal body weight) are also at increased risk for developing hypertension (high blood pressure), cancer, stroke, and adult-onset diabetes. Together, these four conditions account for 70 percent of all deaths in the United States every year.[5] Extreme underweight can also be a threat to health: the Framingham study found that the thinnest subjects had a lower life expectancy than those who were overweight.

In addition to the health risks noted above, body composition affects people's physical health and well-being in other ways. Both overweight and underweight can impair the body's stamina and endurance. This frequently leads to reduced participation in physical activities and sports. Such inaction not only deprives people of the enjoyment of physical activity, it also can aggravate the health risks of their body composition by depriving them of one means of managing it: exercise.

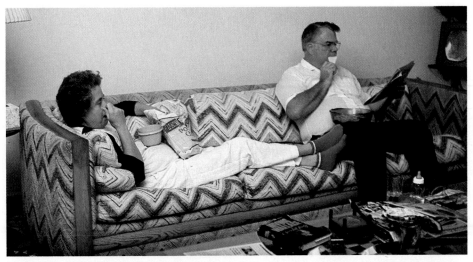

Individuals with an inactive lifestyle are more likely to become overweight than are those who exercise regularly. (Tony Freeman/PhotoEdit)

Body Composition and Emotional Health

There is a two-way relationship between emotional problems and problems of body composition. For years experts have observed that people who are depressed often have depressed appetites as well or, conversely, that they eat excessively to comfort themselves. Researchers have also found that problems of body composition can contribute to emotional and psychological problems.

The principal factor here is body image—how a person views his or her body—rather than the amount of fat itself. For example, a negative body image (regardless of whether a person is in reality too fat, too thin, or just right) may result in problems such as depression and feelings of guilt or poor self-esteem. These emotional problems can be compounded if a person attempts to lose weight and fails.

Paradoxically, the bad feelings people have as a result of body composition and body image often make it harder for them to deal with a body composition problem. Self-acceptance may be necessary *before* the problem is addressed. By realizing that weight is not a measure of self-worth, a person may be able to approach body composition management more objectively. Such self-acceptance, combined with a desire to improve, creates a positive emotional attitude; this can enable an individual to achieve easier and more effective body composition management. Instead of losing or gaining weight to feel better, the equation is reversed: feeling better enables people to develop self-efficacy and manage their weight more confidently.

Body Composition and Social Health

Social health is closely related to emotional health. People often fear that their bodies announce to others who they are and what they are and are not doing. As a result, a person's weight and body image may influence that person's social interactions. Whatever their appearance, people with a positive self-image can project a friendly, outgoing, and confident demeanor which helps them in social situations. Those with a more negative self-image may feel shy, aloof, or withdrawn, feelings that obviously inhibit social interaction.

While body composition may affect the first impressions one makes, it is only one aspect of a person. In fact, if one can temporarily accept one's weight and be at ease with other people, other facets of character—kindness, humor, enthusiasm—are more likely to be revealed, making for a richer and more

Scientists distinguish between **hunger** *and* **appetite.** *Hunger is an inborn, physiological need to eat; appetite is a learned response that is not always related to need.*

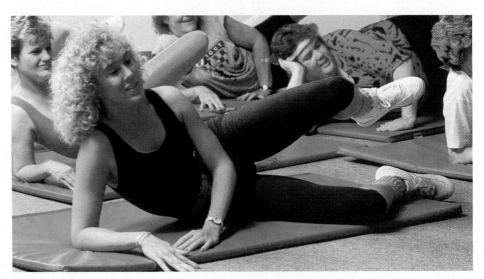

Getting involved in active pursuits can bring an overweight person benefits besides weight loss: social life and self-esteem may also improve. (Kevin Beebe/Custom Medical Stock Photo)

rewarding social life. This in turn helps a person develop a more positive self-image, once again making it easier to succeed in a program of body composition management.

Body Composition and Fat

As indicated in Chapter 5, fat is unique among the major nutrients: proteins and carbohydrates are used in the body only to cover immediate metabolic needs, but fats are available as an energy reserve for the future. This means that the fat content of the human body can vary far more readily than can that of other tissues. In fact, when other nutrients are not required for the body's needs, they can be converted to fat for additional energy storage.

However, stores of fat are maintained at a price. Not only does additional fat make exertion more difficult; it also requires more blood vessels to keep it nourished, putting a greater strain on vital organs such as the heart and arteries. Understanding and knowing how to measure fat therefore provides important background knowledge for weight control.

The Nature and Types of Fat

The human body is made up of many tissues, including muscle, bone, cartilage, connective tissue, skin, and the nerves. There is also fatty tissue, which includes fat cells and various other tissues such as cell walls and streaks of fat in the muscles.

essential fat—*fat that is necessary for the body's normal physiological functioning; it is involved in the storage and use of nutrients.*

The body needs some fat for survival. One type, called **essential fat,** forms part of the chain of chemical reactions by which the body stores nutrients from food and burns, or metabolizes, those nutrients to get energy. Essential fat is stored in the bone marrow, heart, lungs, spleen, and kidneys. A certain amount of essential fat is necessary for optimal health; without it, the body would be unable to metabolize nutrients effectively. The minimum essential proportion of fat for men is about 3 percent of total body weight; for women, it is about 12 percent.[6]

storage fat—*fat deposited under the skin and around the internal organs to protect them; some storage fat is used for heat production and energy.*

Another type of fat in the body is called **storage fat.** Some of this fat is brown and seems to be used for heat production, but most is white storage fat and is used for energy. This fat is found underneath the skin and around the internal organs; it helps cushion the body and protect the internal organs from injury.

Body Composition: A Ready Reckoner

Body composition is an important measure of health. The most direct way of assessing it would seem to be appearance—do you look too fat or thin?—but people's judgments are often distorted by ideas about fashion and other concerns. For years the objective method involved a simple ratio between weight and height, but this relationship can be misleading. Many other factors should be considered, including frame size and muscular development.

The most accurate measures used today come from hydrostatic weighing, bioelectrical impedance, and skinfold tests, as described in this chapter. However, these tests all require specialized equipment. Can one decide by oneself whether one has a body composition problem?

Medical researchers have recently focused attention on other body ratios that may provide more accurate clues than the weight-height ratio does. One is the waist-hip ratio. Because fat in the upper body is associated with greater health risks than is fat lower down, a simple comparison of waist and hip circumference provides an easy reckoning tool. Divide your waist measurement at the navel by your hip measurement at the hipbone. For women, the ratio should be 0.8 or less; for men, it should be 1.0 or less. If it is greater, you might consider a diet and exercise regimen or at least try some other tests.

Two other ratios which fit rather well with the waist-hip ratio are the weight-waist ratio for men and the hip-height ratio for women. The two charts included here provide a simple way of using these measures to estimate body composition. Lay a straightedge across the appropriate chart, from your weight to your waist girth if you are a man or from your hip girth to your height if you are a woman. Read off your percentage of fat on the center scale.

A healthy range for men is 12 to 15 percent; for women, 22 to 25 percent. If you are outside your healthy range in either direction, consider the benefits of weight management through exercise, diet, or both. Men who check out at above 25 percent and women who score above 30 percent should definitely take notice.

If you "failed" one of the ratio reckoner tests presented here, watch your weight. If you failed two, it may be wise to consult a physician. If you failed all three, perhaps you should read this feature more carefully.

Adapted from "Win the Weight War," *Prevention* (June 1990): 46; David Higdon, "Lean Measure: Estimating Body Fat," *American Health Magazine* 6, no. 6 (July 1987).

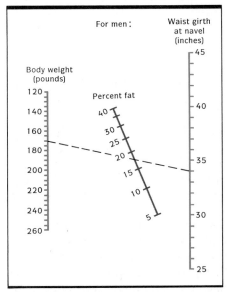 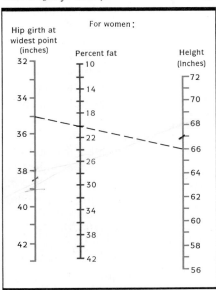

Source: David J. Higdon, *American Health* (1987). Used with permission.

Women have an extra layer of fat under the skin and greater fat deposits on the breasts and lower body. This extra fat is probably important for healthy childbearing and other functions that rely on hormones stored in fatty tissue, such as estrogen. However, recent evidence has suggested that the distribution of storage fat in the body may be related to disease. In overweight men, for example, excess fat often is distributed primarily in the abdominal area, and this has been associated with an increased risk of developing high blood pressure and heart disease. In women, abdominal fat distribution has been associated with diabetes.[7]

It is clear that too much fat in the body can be unhealthy. The average American woman carries 25 to 28 percent of her body weight as fat, and the average man carries 15 to 18 percent. Health and medical experts suggest reducing this to 22 to 25 percent for women and 12 to 15 percent for men.[8]

Measuring Fat and Body Composition

Calculating actual body composition can help people determine whether they really need to change their weight and what type of change would be best. As indicated earlier in this chapter, insurance company weight tables, while convenient, are not necessarily the most accurate tool for such calculations. There are several more direct ways to measure body composition, or the percentage of body fat. The three most popular methods—hydrostatic weighing, bioelectrical impedance, and skinfold measurements—do, however, all have limitations.

hydrostatic weighing method—*underwater weighing; a technique for measuring the proportion of lean tissue to fat tissue in the body. It involves weighing a person out of the water and then in the water and then calculating body density.*

Hydrostatic Weighing In the **hydrostatic weighing method,** also called underwater weighing, a person is weighed on a scale and then reweighed while totally submerged in water (Figure 6.1). This method is based on the principle that fat is lighter and more buoyant than lean tissue; thus, a person who is fatter will tend to float and appear less heavy when weighed underwater. After the dry and underwater weights are measured, technicians can use those numbers to construct a mathematical formula that calculates the body's density and determines the proportion of fat to lean tissue.

However, studies have shown that the results of hydrostatic weighing can be in error by as much as 5 percent because of the buoyancy of some parts of the body. For example, although people are told to exhale the air from their lungs, there will always be some air remaining—different amounts in different people—which adds to their buoyancy. Measurements may also be more inaccurate among older people because their bones sometimes are more porous and therefore more buoyant.[9]

bioelectrical impedance—*a method of determining body composition in which a weak current is used to measure the body's water content.*

Bioelectrical Impedance Another method of determining body composition is **bioelectrical impedance,** in which a weak electric current is used to measure the body's water content. This method is based on the fact that water can promote electrical conductance and that fat contains almost no water whereas lean tissue does. Small electrodes are clipped to a person's wrist and ankles, and a small electric current is sent through the person's body. A computer measures the amount of electric current that is lost and uses that measurement to calculate the percentages of lean and fat body weight. This method, however, may also produce inaccurate results because of the size and content of recent meals and the level of body dehydration.

skinfold measurement—*a method of measuring body composition using calipers to measure the fat under the skin.*

Skinfold Measurement A third method, **skinfold measurement,** uses calipers to measure the fat under the skin, where about half the body's fat is located. Measurements are taken on areas of the body such as the front of the thigh, the shoulder blade, the abdomen, the calf, and the back of the upper arm (Figure 6.2). From these measurements, the ratio of body fat to other tissues can be estimated. The primary limitation of this method is that the measurements must be very precise to yield reliable results.

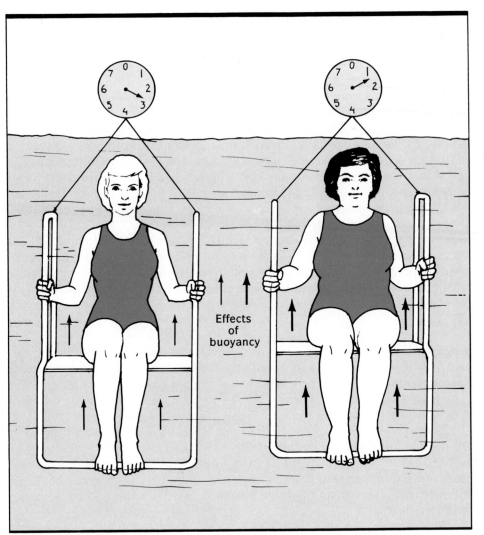

Figure 6.1 Underwater weight is always much less than weight in air: body fat gives people a tendency to float which counteracts their usual weight. This fact is used in hydrostatic weighing. Two people weighing the same in air may differ in their underwater weights: the person with more fat will appear lighter. Such differences in apparent weight show differences in body composition.

Effects of buoyancy

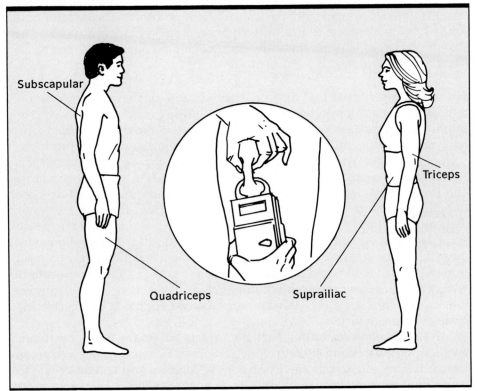

Figure 6.2 The skinfold measurement technique could better be called fat-fold measurement. An estimate of the body's percentage of fat is made by measuring key areas of subcutaneous fat, or fat under the skin. Because the sexes differ in their typical fat distribution, skinfolds are measured at the thigh and shoulder blade for men and near the hip and behind the arm for women.

Subscapular

Quadriceps

Suprailiac

Triceps

Common Approaches to Body Composition Management

Only 3 to 4 percent of adults who take off weight keep it off permanently.

Despite the time, money, and effort spent on body composition control, studies show that Americans lose and then regain weight with predictable regularity. While this may help their social lives and self-esteem for a while, it does little for their long-term health and life expectancy. In fact, continual weight change of this sort has been shown to be harmful in and of itself.[10] To achieve the kind of permanent weight management that can benefit health, a permanent change is usually needed in a person's lifestyle. Steps must be taken that people can feel comfortable with and feel they can maintain. Nevertheless, people keep using extreme methods to lose weight on their own, under the supervision of a physician, or by signing up with a commercial program.

According to a recent survey, the last decade has witnessed almost 30,000 theories, treatments, and programs for controlling weight, including diets, exercise programs, drugs, and even surgery. Unfortunately, many of these methods have been unsuccessful, inappropriate, and even dangerous.[11]

Diets

Fasting can be dangerous. It can result in a loss of lean body tissue, fluids, and electrolytes and can cause vitamin deficiencies and acidosis.

Almost certainly, the most common approach to controlling body composition is to go on a diet. Most people think of a diet as consisting of eating smaller portions and cutting out particular danger foods, such as foods laden with high-calorie fats and sugars. There are, however, a great many different types of diets, some of which are highly unusual in their approach.

The average American goes on one and a half diets a year—and also goes off them. Most often people are looking for a diet that is fast, because they want to lose weight for a specific occasion, and easy, because they have found from previous experience that dieting is difficult. Therefore, people are lured by diets that offer fast and painless results; many are willing to try anything that sounds simple.

Unfortunately, this goes against the standard advice of dietitians, who state that a 1- to 2-pound weight loss per week is realistic and healthy. Anything faster is unlikely to work and may cause health problems. The director of the Johns Hopkins University health, weight, and stress clinic warns that "less than 6 percent of existing diets are effective and an amazing 13 percent are downright hazardous."[12]

While Americans are being urged to cut their calories and dietary fat intake, experts agree that such restrictions should not apply to children under age 2 years. At this age, the extra calories and fat are needed for the body's development and energy needs.

Diet Concerns   Diets that may be detrimental to health and promote only temporary weight loss often include the following characteristics: very low caloric intake, extreme restriction of one or more of the macronutrients (protein, carbohydrate, and fat), and reliance on formulas or special products.[13]

Concern about widespread dieting prompted the American College of Sports Medicine (ACSM) to issue a paper titled "Position Statement on Proper and Improper Weight Loss Programs."[14] In particular, the ACSM described the adverse health consequences that may result from the very low calorie diets followed by many people. A person on a very low calorie diet may lose a great deal of water and minerals from the body and suffer dehydration, weakness, faintness, anemia, and a number of other medical problems as a result. Ironically, such a diet does not generally help a person shed fat; most of the weight lost is water from bodily fluids such as blood. People following very low calorie diets are thus taking a questionable approach to effective and lasting weight reduction.

Several diets involve cutting back not on fats but on the other macronutrients: carbohydrates and protein. Low-carbohydrate fad diets are not recommended. They cause your energy level to be lowered and will make you feel weak, light-headed, and fatigued; these conditions will not keep you operating at peak performance. Like low-calorie diets, they cause more water loss than fat loss; as a result, they do not promote true weight loss and may be dangerous. In addition to making the body use fats for energy, they also force it to deplete its supplies of protein, because the energy from fats cannot be used to power the main control center of the body: the brain. Such fad diets often result in short-term dietary deficiencies; they are particularly hazardous to pregnant women, children, and adolescents.

Low-protein modified fasts that allow dieters to take in less than 800 calories a day may cause serious physical and psychological health problems and are intended only for those who are seriously obese and under a doctor's supervision. It is also possible to consume too much protein while dieting. People who wish to lose weight may be handicapped in their efforts if they consume too much protein, because it is likely that fruits, vegetables, and grains will be crowded out of the diet.[15] The key to good nutrition is to balance the amount of protein consumed with the other important food components.

Finally, many formula diets involve limiting one's intake to a specially prepared product. These diets usually seek to provide all the essential nutrients, a minimum of calories, and something to satisfy the appetite. Although such diets may promote weight loss, they are usually followed by rapid weight gain and are associated with the same health risks as very low calorie diets. Formula diet products have also been promoted for use in addition to one's regular eating to help a person gain weight. Weight gain can be achieved, however, through increasing one's intake of any kind of food and is also enhanced if exercise is increased.

Criteria for Evaluating Diets   To help people choose wisely from the wide variety of weight control programs available, the California Dietetic Association has issued guidelines for evaluating the health and safety of diets. According to these findings, a diet should meet the following criteria:[16]

- It should satisfy all nutrient needs except energy.
- It should be tailored to individual tastes and habits.
- It should be sufficient to minimize hunger and fatigue.
- It should be readily obtainable and socially acceptable.
- It should lead toward the establishment of a changed eating pattern.
- It should be conducive to the improvement of overall health.

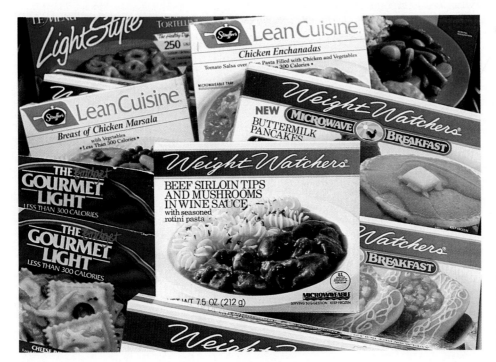

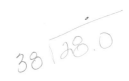

Commercial diet foods are nutritional and low-calorie, but if you eat more than the recommended servings, they will contribute little to weight loss. (Tom Dunham)

Exercise

Exercise plays an important role in physical health; one of its values is the contribution it can make to control of one's body composition. Many exercise products are said to remove if not pounds from your weight, then at least inches from your waistline. Clearly, health spas play an important role in sustaining the hopes of people who seek to lose, or to gain, bulk.

However, some researchers believe that not all exercise is equally good for controlling body composition. Specifically, they argue that anaerobic exercise (Chapter 4), which is defined as strenuous exertion that uses up energy faster than the blood's oxygen can supply it, may cause a considerable increase in appetite because it consumes glycogen, the substance used by the body to store carbohydrates, which must be replaced. Aerobic exercise—regular repetitive motions such as walking, swimming, and running—tends to consume fat to produce the needed energy, creating less of a craving for food.[17]

This is not to say that exercise is undesirable for body composition control. On the contrary, it is vital to a successful program. However, according to these researchers, the type of exercise chosen can materially affect the results: aerobic exercise may be better for weight loss, and anaerobic exercise may be helpful to a person who seeks to gain weight.

As suggested earlier in this book, any serious change in exercise patterns should not be undertaken without first seeking medical advice. Major dietary changes should also be discussed with a physician.

Dieting alone is not the best way to control weight. When you exercise as well, you lose more fat and less muscle and are less likely to gain the weight back.

Drugs

Every year Americans spend over $75 million on appetite suppressant drugs in an attempt to lose weight. These drugs are designed to reduce an individual's appetite by increasing the feeling of satiety. The major components of most of these over-the-counter drugs are caffeine and phenylpropanolamine hydrochloride, which do have limited effectiveness in controlling appetite.

Laxatives and diuretics are also used to lose weight. However, their use can result in serious dehydration, electrolyte abnormalities, and organ dysfunction. None of these drugs provide a long-term solution to weight problems because they do not address the need to change one's basic eating behaviors.

When used to expedite weight loss, over-the-counter laxatives can lead to serious illnesses such as anorexia nervosa and bulimia. (Tom Dunham)

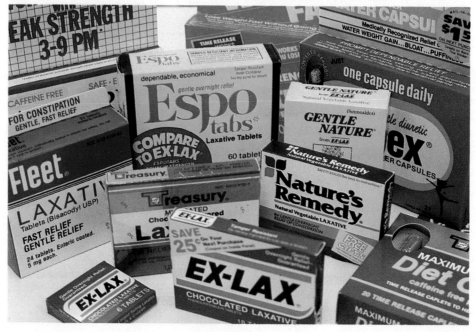

One group of drugs sometimes used by people in an attempt to gain weight, extra muscle mass in particular, is steroid drugs. Used primarily by athletes, though now banned by amateur athletic organizations—including the Olympic committee—these drugs contain special hormones that can help a person develop bulkier muscles.[18] Steroids are not safe. They can cause impaired liver function, permanent changes in the reproductive system, and possibly a higher risk of developing heart disease.[19]

Surgery

While surgical procedures for weight loss are less popular than other approaches, they are becoming increasingly available. The most common surgical approach today is **liposuction,** in which unwanted fat is sucked through a hollow tube after a surgical incision has been made. Liposuction was introduced in the United States several years ago and has become one of the most popular and controversial forms of cosmetic surgery. About 100,000 Americans undergo liposuction every year.[20] While liposuction may remove some unwanted fat, it does not cure obesity or deal with the underlying causes of a weight problem. Moreover, qualified surgeons have pointed out the potential dangers of misleading ads and untrained doctors performing the procedure.

A variation of liposuction aimed at changing body proportions is called fat recycling, or fat grafting. In this procedure fat is sucked from one part of the body and put back somewhere else, often on the breasts. Done primarily for cosmetic purposes, fat grafting is an unproven and perhaps dangerous method of changing body composition. One doctor has reported that it may lead to misdiagnosis of breast cancer.[21]

Other surgical approaches to the management of body composition include stomach stapling and intestinal bypass. While stapling the stomach may result in weight loss, it carries a risk of complications: stomach tissue is often damaged, and scar tissue may form. Bypass surgery, in which a portion of the small intestine is disconnected or removed, is seldom done anymore because of the potential complications and disappointing results. Not only do these procedures carry a risk of complications, the resultant weight loss is dependent on the individual's ability to limit food consumption after surgery.

liposuction—a surgical procedure in which unwanted fat is sucked from the body through a tube.

Sweating in steam baths, hot tubs, and plastic exercise suits is not effective for weight loss. You may lose water weight quickly, but you will gain it back when you drink water.

Group Weight-Loss Programs

Group weight-loss programs are big business. Each week over 1 million people participate in such programs, most of which include a dietary component and many of which encourage dieters to exercise (Table 6.1). Although rapid weight gain may result once these programs are discontinued, they have enabled many people to achieve a permanent change in their nutritional style and thus their body composition.

A key element in these programs is the external support provided by the group leader and the other participants. Other important features include exposure to successful role models, peer pressure, group solidarity, and healthy competition among participants. One of the best-known group programs, Weight Watchers, combines diet, exercise, and behavior modification and offers some of the latest techniques for controlling body composition. Various nutrition experts agree that group programs such as Weight Watchers are helpful for some people, particularly those who are only moderately overweight.[22]

Other commercial weight-loss programs include the Diet Center and Nutri/System. These programs differ from Weight Watchers in that individuals are counseled on a one-to-one basis rather than exclusively in group sessions.

Particular care must be taken if a weight-loss program involves a very low calorie intake. Such programs may pose health risks for some people, and so independent medical advice should always be sought.

Table 6.1   Popular Group Weight-Loss Programs

Program name	TOPS	Weight Watchers	Diet Workshop	Diet Center	Nutri/System
Founded	1948	1963	1965	1970	1971
Description	Motivational program only; group meetings, pep talks, and expert lectures held weekly	Weekly meetings with private weigh-ins, discussions, and lectures	Weekly weigh-ins (private), then group meetings	Combines private counseling with group sessions	Weekly meetings with nutritional specialist; small group meetings with behavioral counselor
Exercise	No formal plan	Low to moderate plan offered	No structured plan; offers walking program audiotape	Will tailor personal plan with help of certified athletic trainer	Individual plans offered
Reducing diet	Requires members to work with a personal physician; 3 levels of calorie exchange diets optional	5 weeks on 1,000–1,450 calories a day	900 calories a day for first week; 1,000 a day for second week; then 1,200 a day until goal is reached	915 calories a day (may be more for a physically active person)	1,100–1,500 calories a day
Maintenance plan	Members should work with personal physicians	Based on individual maintenance requirements	4 weeks of maintenance (caloric intake suited to individual)	1,200–2,500 calories; depends on body composition, metabolic rate, and amount of physical activity	Instructs members how to plan nutritionally balanced meals from the 4 food groups; stresses more than caloric consumption
Percent carbohydrate calories	As advised by physician	50–60% of total	50% of total	47% of total	62% of total
Percent fat calories	As advised by physician	20–30% of total	20% of total	25% of total	15% of total
Percent protein calories	As advised by physician	20% of total	30% of total	28% of total	23% of total
Staff	Meeting leaders are elected by group for period of 1 year	Staff members have lost weight and maintained goal weight through program	Staff members have reached goal through program	Staff members have successfully completed program	Staff members are nutritional specialists, behavioral counselors
Available experts	Members turn to own doctors for professional guidance	Dietitians, exercise physiologists, psychologists, obesity experts	Doctor of nutrition as consultant	Each group has advisory board of local physicians as consultants	Doctors and nurses on staff in home office; advisers include well-known obesity researchers

Based on information in Trisha Thompson, *"Best Bet Programs,"* Health (May 1990): 56–86.

Understanding Body Composition Problems

With all the approaches offered for managing body composition, it seems odd that so few people succeed in losing weight and then keeping it off. A recent study reported that only 12 percent of the people in weight-loss programs lost as much as 20 pounds and that only 17 percent of that group kept the weight off for 2 years.[23] In fact, only about 3 percent of people who lose weight keep it off.

There is no single theory or set of factors that can fully explain why some people gain or lose weight more readily than others do. There are, however, two general schools of thought for explaining body composition problems.[24] One approach, called the **pull school**, sees weight problems as being greatly influenced by physiological factors. The other, known as the **push school**, sees such problems as being more the result of psychological or social factors.

The Pull School: Physiological Bases for Body Composition Problems

The pull school argues that overeating results at least in part from physical metabolic factors that generate false signals to the body; the desire to overeat is stimulated by the "pull" of these factors. The eating response in turn leads to behaviors that increase eating and sustain excess weight. Overeating behaviors, in other words, are developed as a result of physiological stimuli rather than psychological needs. A number of physiological factors are known or thought to contribute to body composition problems.

Genetic Factors It is taken for granted that hair and eye color, facial features, and height are inherited traits. No one is surprised when a 6 foot, 2 inch father has a taller-than-average son or daughter. Evidence suggests that the genes a person inherits may influence that person's body composition just as they influence other physical traits. Data from genetic analyses strongly indicate that patterns of fat distribution within the body may be inherited. In addition, data on the body weight and body composition of adopted children and their biological parents show an impressive correlation, indicating a strong genetic influence rather than an environmental one. To some extent, therefore, body composition problems may be inherited.[25]

Regulatory Factors Body composition problems are thought to be caused in part by disorders of certain regulatory mechanisms in the body. The body's need for food is caused by the interaction of two regulatory mechanisms, one short term and the other long term. The **short-term regulatory mechanism** signals the body when to eat and when to stop eating. This mechanism includes neurotransmitters in the brain, peptides in the digestive system, hormones in the blood, and glucose in the liver.

The **long-term regulatory mechanism** monitors the body's nutrient levels over extended periods and controls food intake so that body weight is maintained within a relatively narrow range. This long-term mechanism is believed to arise from the fatty tissue itself, which sends signals to the brain through fatty acids in the blood. The concentration of fatty acids increases as fat cells enlarge.[26] When these existing fat cells reach their maximum size, new fat cells are produced. The tendency for fat cells to enlarge and increase in number may result not only in a permanent increase in weight but also in maintenance of that weight. The phenomenon, known as the *yo-yo effect*, which occurs when people who have reached a certain weight seem fated to return to that weight, is now thought to be a result of this physiological mechanism. The setpoint theory described below helps explain this phenomenon.

Setpoint Theory Many people have had the frustrating experience of going on a diet, losing a few pounds in a week or two, and then hitting a plateau at

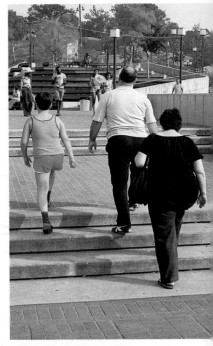

Obesity is known to have a genetic component, but learned eating habits also contribute to excessive weight. (Van Bucher/ Photo Researchers, Inc.)

pull school—*a school of thought for explaining body composition problems; sees weight problems as primarily resulting from physiological factors.*

push school—*a school of thought for explaining body composition problems; sees weight problems as primarily resulting from psychological or social factors.*

short-term regulatory mechanism—*a mechanism that signals the body when to eat and when to stop eating.*

long-term regulatory mechanism—*a mechanism that monitors the body's nutrient levels over extended periods and controls food intake so that body weight is maintained within a relatively narrow range.*

Weight Management: Is the Why Important?

Some 65 million Americans go on diets every year; on any given day 20 million are trying to lose weight. Some diet to prevent or reverse medical problems. Many dieters, however, are concerned primarily about their appearance. Does the reason why a person is dieting make any difference? The first speaker stresses that any reason for losing weight is beneficial because of the risks of being overweight. The other speaker says that many pitfalls lie in wait for dieters who focus on appearance rather than health.

Society's Emphasis on Thinness Is Desirable

More than 39 million adult Americans are obese, or dangerously overweight. Obesity means unhealthy body composition. It contributes to many conditions that lead to heart disease, including hypertension and high cholesterol levels.

In an ideal world people might be sufficiently motivated by health concerns to eat sensibly, get enough exercise, and keep their weight under control. But the fact is, people are more powerfully driven by social pressures and other considerations than by the desire to stay healthy; otherwise, no one would use tobacco or engage in other forms of behavior that endanger health.

When people keep their weight under control mainly because they want to look slim, the effort is beneficial to their health: they are lowering their risk of contracting heart disease. Without the pressure society exerts in favor of thinness, such people might not make that effort. And the effort benefits not only individuals but society as a whole.

The slimmer the population, the fewer doctors' bills for treating diabetes and other health disorders associated with overweight and the lower the cost of medical insurance. Conversely, fat-related heart diseases cause many people to drop out of the work force and collect disability payments from the federal government. These costs—and the taxes required to pay for them—might be lower if social pressures to be thin were even more influential.

A greater trend toward managing pounds might even increase American productivity: researchers have found that the overweight are absent from their jobs more frequently than are those whose weight is in the normal range.

---

setpoint theory—*a theory in which the basic idea is that each person has a given weight range, or setpoint, that is natural to his or her body. Depending on their setpoints, some people stay thin and others stay fat regardless of what they eat.*

basal metabolism—*the number of calories burned when the body is at rest but not sleeping.*

which their weight seems to stay the same no matter how little they eat. The **setpoint theory** has suggested an explanation for this phenomenon. The basis of this theory is that each person has a given weight range—the setpoint—that is natural to his or her body.[27] Depending on their setpoints, some people stay thin and others stay fat regardless of what they eat. People who have a high setpoint are going to have problems trying to lose weight: their bodies simply "want" to be fat.

The number of calories burned at rest (but not while sleeping) is called **basal metabolism.** Setpoint theorists argue that the body can change its basal metabolism to keep weight at the setpoint. The body reacts to a strict diet as if preparing for a prolonged famine: it hoards fat reserves to keep from starving to death. Suppose a person with a high setpoint tries to lose weight by means of stringent dieting. Setpoint theorists hypothesize that this person's brain "senses" what is happening by means of a special feedback system operating between the hypothalamus in the brain and fat cells throughout the body. The body responds by slowing its metabolism—burning food more slowly—to keep its weight stable. If the setpoint theory is correct, dieting will always be difficult because no matter how hard a person tries to cut back on food, that person's body will fight back by burning food more efficiently.

Although this theory is attractively simple and makes a good deal of sense, there is not much scientific evidence to support it in humans. Even if the theory is ultimately confirmed, this does not mean that people cannot lose

The National Obsession with Thinness Can Undermine Health   The average American starts on a diet more than twice a year. But many of these diets are not necessary to good health; in fact, some people actually harm themselves by dieting. Many dieters are not excessively overweight; in fact, some are not overweight at all. An obesity research group found that most women who are not overweight believe nonetheless that they should lose a few pounds.

Advertising, films, and television shows put pressure on everyone to be thin: they imply that we should all look like the reed-thin stars and models they present as ideals. Businesses that sell weight-loss products and services—such as clinics and spas, diet pill manufacturers, and low-calorie-soda bottlers—spent more than $250 million per year on advertising in the late 1980s to tell people that they should lose weight.

Furthermore, people who diet primarily out of concern for their appearance often follow fad diets or use products that promise rapid weight loss. These slim-down-quick plans can endanger a person's health. Doctors have expressed concern about the use of very low calorie liquid diets by people who are only mildly overweight; such people run the risk of losing muscle tissue instead of fat, which can lead to heart problems and damage other organs.

People who diet because of social pressure may be responding to an unhealthy lack of self-esteem, especially if their body composition is normal but they believe they are overweight. Dieting may lower their self-esteem still further: they may fail to reach their weight goals or—as many people do—regain the lost pounds within a year. People whose weight does not threaten their health would benefit more by accepting themselves as they are than they would by striving for slimmer bodies.

Do you agree that more people would be better off if they dieted for their health rather than their looks? Or do you think that the reason why people diet makes no difference so long as they manage to lose weight? Which reason for managing weight do you personally find more compelling, and which do you think would be more beneficial?

Statistics and ideas from Nancy Stedman, "Desperately Seeking Slimdom," *Health* (November 1985): 56–62; Erica Goode, "Getting Slim," *U.S. News and World Report* (May 14, 1990): 56–65.

---

weight. There are ways to speed the basal metabolism and thus lower the setpoint. The safest way is to increase physical activity in order to raise the body's overall metabolic rate.

The Push School: Psychological Bases for Body Composition Problems

Before the pull theory gained currency, programs for body composition management concentrated more on behavioral and dietary change, on the theory that if people can control their eating behavior and limit themselves to particular foods, they can successfully control their body composition. Although most people accept the idea that body composition is affected by a variety of factors related to behavior, attitudes, and values, the push school argues that obesity is primarily a behavioral disorder. The urge to eat is caused not so much by physiological signals from the digestive and metabolic systems but more by psychological needs. In effect, people are driven by behavioral habit to "push" food into their digestive systems, perhaps because they associate food with happiness or love or because they have been taught not to waste food.

Proponents of the push school feel that people need to change their attitudes and behaviors about food in order to change their body composition. Such an approach can be difficult, as anyone who has tried to change an attitude or behavior can attest. Nevertheless, it remains an important approach to body composition management.

Behavioral Factors One of the earliest approaches to the relationship of behavior to obesity was called the **externality theory.** Proponents of this theory argued that overweight people eat primarily in response to external food-related cues. Thus, it is the sight and smell of a steak more than internal hunger caused by metabolic needs that make such people eager to eat.

Several studies have suggested that overweight persons do not in the long run eat much more per unit of lean body mass than do nonoverweight persons.[28] (This is to be expected given the ideas of setpoint theory.) However, many experts maintain that the eating behaviors of people with body composition problems are different from the behaviors of people who do not have these problems. One researcher has identified four behavioral differences between thin and fat people.[29]

externality theory—*the theory that overweight people eat primarily in response to external food-related cues rather than only to internal hunger caused by metabolic needs.*

1. Thin people do not think about food and hardly ever eat unless they are hungry. Their lives do not revolve around food, nor do they relate food to depression or sadness or use it to replace love, comfort, or companionship.
2. Thin people eat exactly what and when they want. They eat not just to be eating but because a particular food appeals to them at a particular moment.
3. Thin people eat consciously. They know what and how much they are eating and eat only enough food to satisfy hunger.
4. Thin people stop eating when the body is no longer hungry. They will ignore food, leave it on the plate, and even throw it away if they do not want it.

The Impact of Habits, Ideas, and Values Push school theory emphasizes that the ways in which people think and behave in regard to food are rooted in a variety of habits, ideas, and values developed throughout their lifetimes. The quality of food you eat, how often you eat, and how much you eat are all based on simple habits. These habits, like all others, are automatic responses that are learned and then generated by the subconscious. Rather than the brain determining the body's *need* for food from internal physiological signals, life experiences have shaped the mind's *desire* for food.

Many body composition problems result at least partially from the ways in which such habits direct people's behavior and affect the way they use food. When programs for body composition management do not work, it is often because they do not address this issue effectively. Quite simply, a person cannot achieve and maintain a desirable weight and body composition without replacing habits that encourage overweight or underweight with other, more appropriate habits and behaviors.

Ideas and values formed early in life may also contribute to body composition problems. As children, people learn values, attitudes, and beliefs from their experiences and their parents, teachers, friends, and other role models. For example, children may have learned that "food is love," that "you'll feel better if you eat something," or that "you should eat everything on your plate because there are starving children all over the world." Such attitudes teach people to eat for reasons other than hunger and bodily requirements. Moreover, many people retain into adulthood views which continue to affect their eating behaviors. When people can recognize the views, attitudes, and behaviors that lead them to gain weight, they are in a better position to alter those habits and change their body composition.

Some of these attitudes and beliefs may have a great impact on a person's ability to achieve and maintain ideal weight and body composition. They may relate to a person's body image and attitudes toward proper nutrition and exercise: someone may feel that to look intellectual, one needs to be thin, and that it is better to eat only once or twice a day. For many people, achieving and maintaining ideal body composition requires replacing health-destructive ideas, attitudes, and self-images with positive, health-enhancing ones.

Compensatory Overeating Many scientists have suggested that people may overeat to compensate for something missing in their lives.[30] Eating gives them a feeling of satisfaction that cannot be obtained in any other way. For example, people often use eating to compensate for a lack of social interaction with others, unhappiness, loneliness, frustration, boredom, and depression. The question people should ask themselves in such cases is: What do I really need that I am substituting this food for? By identifying the real need, a person can strive to fulfill it rather than to compensate for it.

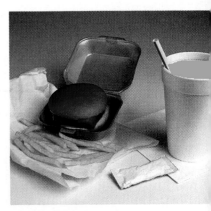

Junk foods are appetizing for the same reasons that they are not recommended: they contain considerable amounts of salt and fat. But people also eat them because they fit in with their lifestyle habits—always in a hurry and with no time to prepare meals. (Felicia Martinez/PhotoEdit)

Successful Control of Body Composition

Unfortunately, it is not advisable to try to alter quickly what took months or years to develop. Techniques for weight change that promise quick and easy results are usually ineffective and can be dangerous. The most successful programs for body composition management promote long-term changes in lifestyle—modifying unhealthy attitudes, beliefs, and habits—that lead to effective weight control. Body composition problems can best be overcome by combining proper nutrition, appropriate exercise, and appropriate eating behaviors.

Regulating Body Composition

Before looking at the components of a successful program for body composition management, it is useful to understand how the body regulates weight. The basic principle of weight regulation is the energy-balance equation:

Change in energy stores   = energy intake − energy expenditure
(body composition change)   (food/drink)   (activity/exercise)

The energy-balance equation suggests that body weight can be maintained at a stable level when the energy intake (calories from food and drink) equals the amount of energy expended (calories burned as a result of metabolism, activity, and exercise). If energy intake and expenditure are not equal, the result will be a gain or a loss of weight. For each 3,500 calories consumed in excess of energy expenditure, the body stores an additional pound of fat. Each time 3,500 calories are eaten below the level expended, the body loses a pound of fat (Figure 6.3).

The body is a good mathematician; it adheres strictly to the energy-balance equation. While it can apparently (in setpoint theory) change the amount of calories that a particular exercise will burn, it *never* loses track of the excess calories consumed. As a result, weight gain often results from a slow and insidious process in which the body gradually accumulates excess calories and stores them as fat.

Natural Body Composition Management

Since the body regulates energy intake and expenditure so carefully, it is not realistic to try to lose weight by dieting for a while and then going back to old eating habits. Excess calories will accumulate again and lead to weight gain. Nearly everyone who goes on periodic diets gains back all the weight lost—often even more.

Effective body composition management requires a long-range program that includes behavioral change, proper nutrition, sensible eating, and exer-

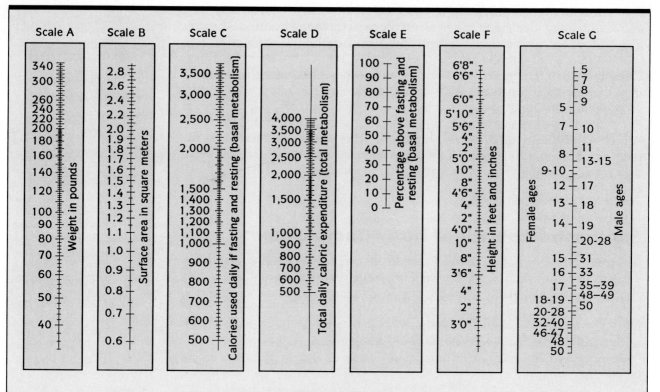

To use this calculator, you will need a pin and a ruler.

1. Position pin at your weight in pounds on scale A.

2. Pivot edge of ruler against pin, swinging other end of edge to your height on scale F.

3. Hold ruler firmly and move pin to where ruler crosses scale B.

4. Pivot ruler against pin and swing other end to your age on scale G (male or female).

5. Move pin to where ruler crosses scale C (your basal metabolism).

6. Pivot and swing ruler to percent on scale E that represents your average activity level (see below*).

7. Read where ruler crosses scale D. This is the caloric intake that maintains your present weight.

*Average daily physical activity as percent of basal metabolism
40% if your only regular exercise is walking between classes
50% if you must stand or walk more than 2 hours a day
60% for regular moderate exercise (volleyball or softball)
70% for heavy exercise (construction job, daily exercise program)
80–100% for especially strenuous physical work or the most strenuous intercollegiate sports—basketball, track, etc.)

Figure 6.3 This calculating chart will indicate the number of calories your body is using to maintain your present weight.

Source: Adapted from George A. Bray, *The Obese Patient* (Philadelphia: WB Saunders, 1976): 305.

cise—a "natural" plan for body composition management. The ACSM is clear in its recommendations for a successful weight management program:

When dieting, you may want to put the food onto your plate in the kitchen rather than place serving dishes on the table, where you may be tempted to overindulge.

A nutritionally sound diet resulting in mild caloric restriction coupled with an endurance exercise program along with behavioral modification of existing eating habits is recommended for weight reduction. The rate of sustained weight loss should not exceed 1 kg (two pounds) per week. To maintain proper weight control and optimal body fat levels, a lifetime commitment to proper eating habits and regular physical activity is required.[31]

Exercising Right for Body Composition Management Over the long term exercise is an essential tool in an effective weight management program. It has a cumulative effect on the body's caloric expenditure. Even if one's eating habits remain the same, beginning a program of regular physical exercise will start to shrink the body's fat tissues. A pound of fat can be lost in 7 to 12 exercise sessions (Table 6.2).

Reducing the consumption of high-fat foods will also lead to a substantial loss of fat over time. One expert has estimated that an exercise program consisting of a brisk 1-hour walk three times a week plus a reduction of 100 calories a day in food consumed will produce a weight loss of 20 to 30 pounds in a year.[32]

Table 6.2 Exercise and the Energy-Balance Equation[a]

Activity	Per Pound Every 10 Minutes	Calories used[b] By a 120-lb Person Every 10 Minutes	By a 190-lb Person Every 10 Minutes
Bicycling			
Slow (5 mph)	0.25	30 (0.25 × 120)	48 (0.25 × 190)
Moderate (10 mph)	0.5	60	95
Fast (13 mph)	0.72	86	137
Calisthenics	0.45	54	86
Canoeing (4 mph)	0.4	56	90
Football (touch)	0.40	48	76
Golf	0.29	35	55
Handball	0.63	76	120
Hiking	0.42	50	80
Judo and karate	0.87	104	165
Mountain climbing	0.86	103	163
Running			
6 mph (10 min/mile)	0.79	95	150
10 mph (6 min/mile)	1.00	120	190
Skiing (snow)			
Downhill	0.59	71	112
Cross-country	0.78	94	148
Soccer	0.63	76	120
Stationary run (70–80 counts/min)	0.78	94	148
Swimming (crawl)			
20 yds/min	0.32	38	61
50 yds/min	0.71	85	135
Tennis			
Moderate	0.46	55	87
Vigorous	0.60	72	114
Volleyball	0.36	43	68
Walking			
2 mph	0.22	26	42
5 mph	0.64	77	122
Basal metabolism[c]			
Man	0.076	9.1	14.4
Woman	0.068	8.2	13.0

[a] Compare the caloric consumption shown here with the 1,200 calories which might be gained from a typical hearty steak dinner or the 500 calories which might come from a peanut butter and jelly sandwich with milk.

[b] To calculate your own calorie use for each 10 minutes of an activity, multiply the figure in the "Per Pound" column by your weight in pounds.

[c] Do not forget to include calorie use by the basal metabolism, which functions not only when one exercises but 24 hours a day. Thus, every hour a 140-pound woman, even without exercise, uses 0.068 × 140 × 6 = 57 calories, or about 1,368 calories a day.

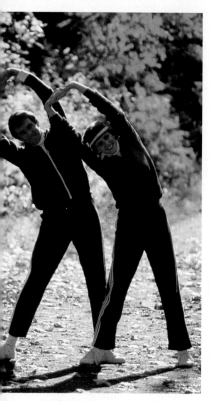

Make exercise enjoyable and it will be much easier to maintain it as part of your weight management program. (Michael Philip Manheim/Southern Light)

If you have doubts about the importance of exercise in a weight-loss program, consider this: a reduction in caloric intake alone will result not only in the loss of a great deal of water weight by means of dehydration (very dangerous in large quantities!) but also in the loss of other types of lean tissue, including muscle mass. People who diet without exercising regularly are also more likely to fall victim to the yo-yo syndrome, with the regained weight being mostly in the form of fat.

Some people may wonder whether an increase in physical activity is likely to make an individual eat more. While vigorous exercise may cause a person to consume more calories over the long run, the calories consumed do not equal the calories burned while exercising. Exercise helps tip the energy-balance equation in your favor.[33]

People might also question whether the muscle mass developed through exercise will result in regaining lost weight. While some pounds may come back, exercise helps ensure that they are pounds of muscle, not fat. Remember that muscle is heavier than fat. When a person gets heavier because the body has more muscle, that person is still leaner and thinner (and healthier) than he or she was when the body weighed less but had more fat. Of course, this is also good news for underweight people, who have little fat to lose but will still gain muscle.

What is the best exercise program for successful body composition management? The ACSM recommends the following program:

1. Exercise at least 3 days a week, although 4 or 5 is even better.
2. Exercise for at least 20 minutes at each session.
3. Exercise should be a continuous and rhythmic aerobic type, such as walking, jogging, swimming, or bicycling.
4. People over age 35 should not start a strenuous exercise program without first getting a checkup from a doctor.[34]

People of any age can hurt themselves by starting a vigorous exercise program too quickly, especially if they have not previously been active. Therefore, as noted in Chapter 4, an exercise program should start out slowly and include lighter, less strenuous exercise at first. This gives the body time to adjust to the demands of a new level of activity and prevents muscle soreness and more serious injuries. As the exercise program progresses, it can gradually include more strenuous activities. The important goal, however, is not to exercise strenuously but to exercise regularly. Every exercise program should be realistic, regular, and right for the individual.

Eating Right for Body Composition Management A successful weight management program must of course also deal with what one eats. The key to achieving and maintaining a desired weight loss is a high-carbohydrate, adequate-protein, low-fat diet. The term *diet* here does not mean a temporary change in how a person eats. It means a lifelong commitment, taken one day at a time, to eating more whole grains and fresh fruits and vegetables and fewer fast foods, processed foods, fatty meats, and rich desserts. It means putting into practice the recommendations presented in Chapter 5. Similarly, permanent changes in eating as well as exercise habits are required to achieve weight gain. An important step in any program for body composition management is to change the quality but not necessarily the quantity of the food consumed. Eating more low-fat, high-carbohydrate foods will in all likelihood decrease the number of calories consumed as well, since fats have more than twice the calories of carbohydrates and proteins.[35]

The body metabolizes carbohydrates faster than it does fats, which are burned slowly and stored in the body until needed. Thus, when the consumption of high-fat foods is decreased, there is a reduced accumulation of

The caloric "density" of different foods demonstrates the particular dangers of fat:

Nutrient	Calories per gram
Carbohydrate	4
Protein	4
Fat	9
Alcohol	7

excess fat in the body. Recent studies have reinforced the idea that low-fat diets are an effective approach to body composition management.[36] It is therefore important not to just count calories—all calories are not created equal. The most fattening macronutrient is fat.

Since the body needs proper nutrition, care must be taken if a person decides to decrease the quantity of food consumed. Nutrition surveys suggest that the American people, especially women, young children, and teenage girls, already are at the low end (less than 80 percent) of the estimated daily requirements of calcium, magnesium, iron, zinc, and manganese.[37] For this reason, it is important to improve the overall quality of food consumed before reducing the size of portions. Most people can accomplish their weight-loss goals through a combined program of increased exercise and improved diet. Improving the quality of the diet not only ensures better nutrition but also results in caloric reduction without decreasing the size of the portions eaten.

One way to fulfill your nutritional requirements is to eat high-quality snacks throughout the day. Frequent eating of nutritious foods also promotes feelings of satiety that help control the appetite. As a general rule, eating five smaller meals a day is better than eating two or three large ones.

Surprisingly, eating frequent small meals that include starchy foods such as corn, rice, and potatoes will also help people who are underweight. For these people, the problem is to *increase* caloric intake, which may be difficult if they are unused to eating large meals. Ideally, they should consume 1,000 to 1,500 calories more than they use each day, at the same time exercising so that these calories do not turn to fat. They should *not* attempt high-protein or high-fat diets, as these diets can be hazardous.

Proper nutrition is the cornerstone of a successful program for body composition management. The following guidelines should be considered when you are developing or evaluating a nutritionally sound food plan for weight management.[38]

1. Eat a quantity of food that will help you achieve a safe, progressive weight loss of 1 to 2 pounds a week.
2. Consume macronutrients (proteins and carbohydrates) in the amounts recommended in the U.S. Dietary Goals.

Though not the favorite food of many children, apples and other fruits have a high nutritional value and are available in enough varieties to satisfy almost everyone's taste. (Tom Dunham)

When buying a diet book, keep in mind the following factors:

- *Make sure the program incorporates balanced diet, exercise, and behavior modification.*
- *Avoid plans that are based on fewer than 1,000 to 1,200 calories a day.*
- *Check to see that average weight loss will be about 2 pounds a week.*
- *Be cautious about inflexible plans in which certain foods have to be eaten at certain times.*
- *Beware of the diet if you need to buy vitamins, special foods, gadgets, or gimmicks in order to follow it.*
- *Check to see how the book was received by nutrition experts.*
- *Do not buy a book that sounds too good to be true, with promises of significant weight loss in a short time.*

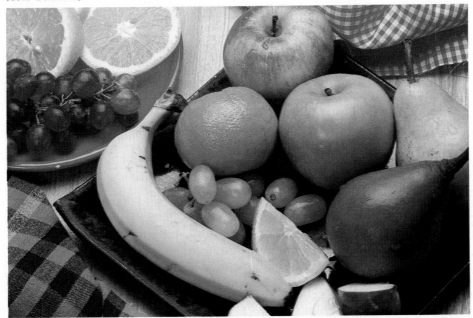

A reminder from Chapter 5: people seldom think about the importance of water in their diets. Drink six to eight glasses of water a day for optimal health. This does not include coffee, tea, and soft drinks.

3. Consume micronutrients (vitamins and minerals) in amounts recommended in the RDAs.
4. Be aware of and avoid excessive amounts of cholesterol, sodium, and fat.
5. Eat a wide variety of high-quality foods in moderation.
6. Be sure to include in your diet foods that can provide fiber—fruits, vegetables, or breads—and an adequate amount of water or other liquids: at least 1 pint but preferably more.

Weight Disorders and Eating Disorders

In addition to the body composition problems experienced by so many Americans, there are specific weight and eating disorders that afflict smaller proportions of the population. Before you embark on a program for weight gain or loss, it is wise to consider whether you have a more atypical problem. For some people, obesity may result from more than simple overeating; for others, extreme thinness seems to be more of a psychological than a physiological problem; and some people who look normal may have a strange and potentially damaging eating pattern.

Extreme Obesity

Although most people who become obese do so as a result of the eating and exercise habits of American society, there are a few whose excess weight seems to have been caused by other factors. Most frequently blamed is the thyroid gland, which controls the rate and efficiency of the metabolism, but research seems to show that malfunctioning of this gland is only rarely responsible for obesity. In some cases extreme obesity may in fact be caused by lesions in the brain, particularly in the hypothalamus, the part which receives energy signals from the body and controls hunger. Perhaps more common is obesity that is associated with diabetes (Chapter 2). While some theorists maintain that the development of obesity is a factor that causes diabetes, others argue that diabetes and obesity may both be caused by the same insulin abnormality.

Cases of extreme obesity, whether resulting from simple overeating or from other causes, are best treated similarly to overweight problems—with a slow, deliberate weight loss rather than a crash diet. Exercise is clearly more of a problem, but it is still recommended: one reason why people remain overweight is that even when they do the same activities as thinner people, they use less body motion.

Anorexia Nervosa

anorexia nervosa—an eating disorder in which people severely limit the amount they eat, in effect starving themselves.

At the other extreme is a disorder in which people severely limit the amount they eat, in effect starving themselves. This condition is called **anorexia** (loss of appetite) **nervosa** (nervous or psychogenic). The great majority of people with anorexia are teenage girls and young women; only about 10 percent are men. Most people with anorexia come from upper-class or middle-class homes and often seemed like model children before developing the disorder.

Description In a typical case of anorexia, the victim mysteriously becomes increasingly obsessed with the idea that he or she is fat. This leads to continuous and extreme dieting in an attempt to lose weight.

About one-third of those suffering from anorexia are mildly overweight before developing the disorder. Simple dieting to lose weight leads to a life characterized by a repetition of the same meal day after day, coupled with exhausting exercise, personal isolation, and social withdrawal. For some rea-

My Story

Losing Weight and Keeping It Off

I don't know which was tougher, dieting or staring at my obese figure in the mirror. How did I allow myself to get like this? When I was happy, I ate to celebrate. When I was sad, I ate to drown my sorrows. Any excuse was enough: I would use food to fill the void.

From the age of 12 I was an obsessive overeater. I would binge and gain weight dramatically. Then I would nearly starve myself to get the pounds off again. It didn't seem like a problem then, but it's been a really difficult habit to get rid of. It wasn't till my late teens and early twenties that I began to realize how difficult.

I had always thought of myself as a slim person who sometimes had to fight off fat, but when I was 19, I got a part in a TV commercial as a lovable but plump teenager. I saw it over and over again, and I thought to myself, "This girl is me." That was when I became determined to control my weight.

However, though I managed to bring my weight down somewhat, my battle of the bulge continued for 10 long years. I tried every diet imaginable. I even tried not eating at all. When that was a disaster (I was hospitalized), I tried one meal a day, but with many lapses when I felt sorry for myself. I averaged about 25 pounds less than my weight in the commercial, but that was an average: it was up one month and down the next.

What forced me to get serious was the birth of my youngest daughter. After I stopped nursing her, I was horrified that my weight was back up—in fact, it was 17 pounds higher than ever before. That's when I joined a group diet program.

This was not the hardest diet I had ever been on. It was a three-meal schedule, and I could design menus with a wide range of food choices. The diet, attendance at group meetings, and regular exercise helped me lose 40 pounds. It took longer than some other times—but I've kept it off!

Maintaining my weight means making an effort. I juggle things a bit to stay on the diet, but I can live with the way I arrange things. I try to recognize the times of day or situations in which I am likely to feel hungry. Then I plan snacks and meals for those times so I'm not taken by surprise and can control what I eat. When I go out to eat, before I arrive at the restaurant, I plan what my entrée will be. I usually ask for fish or chicken and order it plain or with sauce on the side.

I make every meal an occasion but eat sensible portions. Instead of eating beyond the point of fullness, I eat slowly and stop as soon as I begin to feel satisfied. And believe me, when you are as motivated as I am now to keep the weight down and when you feel the results, it's quite easy to stay "good."

In my cooking at home I follow healthful, diet-conscious tips that reduce calories. For example, I roast all meats on a rack so that the fat drips away. I remove the fatty skin from chicken. Vegetables at my house are steamed or boiled. At least, they are for me.

My family also eats far more healthily now than it did before. There's been a greater variety of foods in the house since I really took control of my diet, and that has pleased them as well as me. And I now know that I'm unlikely to fall back into my old ways, because I sometimes (not too often) cook fried foods for the family and don't even feel tempted.

It's a little more effort for me, because I have to plan my shopping and cooking more carefully, but I've really found what works for me. The most important thing is that I can eat and live like a normal person. I'm not obsessed by food. At 5 feet 6 inches and size 8 I look much better and feel fabulous. Best of all, I can sometimes daydream back to that teenager in the commercial—and feel really happy for her.

Loosely based on Elizabeth Meade Howard, "Lynn Redgrave's Diet Tips," *McCall's* (February 1988): 88–90.

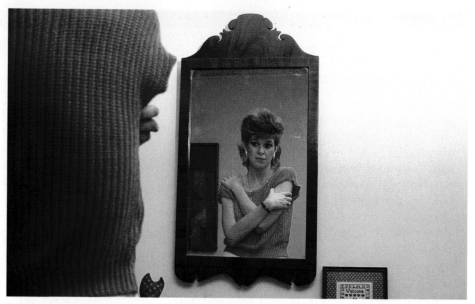

It is hard to believe that someone this thin can believe that she is overweight, but victims of anorexia nervosa not only believe it, they diet to lose still more weight. (Visual Education Corporation Archives)

son, a person with anorexia feels fat even after losing weight and continues dieting to the point of starvation, sometimes losing more than one-third of his or her total body weight.

In the United States 1 in every 250 women aged 12 to 18 develops anorexia nervosa. An estimated 9 percent of these women die of starvation; between 2 and 5 percent more commit suicide.[39] According to the *Diagnostic and Statistical Manual of Mental Disorders,* a diagnosis of anorexia nervosa requires evidence of the following: an intense fear of becoming obese that does not diminish as weight loss progresses, a disturbance of body image (for example, claiming to "feel fat" even when emaciated), a loss of at least 25 percent of original body weight, and a refusal to maintain normal body weight.[40]

Some experts have suggested that young women with anorexia may have abnormal fears of approaching womanhood. In losing so much weight, they lose their feminine curves, stop menstruating, and begin to look like little girls again. Specialists in treating anorexia feel strongly that both psychological counseling and medical treatment are necessary. Tube feeding and a high-calorie diet may be necessary at the start; not only is the patient's weight dangerously low, it is also difficult for the patient to reason effectively when his or her thinking processes have been disrupted by chronic malnutrition.

Medical Effects In addition to amenorrhea, or loss of menstruation, the most common medical consequence of anorexia in women is estrogen deficiency. This deficiency may contribute to osteoporosis, which is common among women with anorexia. In men with anorexia, testosterone levels may diminish, and this can contribute to impotence.[41]

Anorexia can also cause a slowed heart rate, slowed reflexes and respiratory rate, kidney problems, and cardiac arrest. The general malnutrition resulting from anorexia may cause lethargy, memory lapses, and even hallucinations and feelings of paranoia.

Bulimia

bulimia—*an eating disorder characterized by eating binges followed by purges.*

Bulimia, a disorder characterized by eating binges followed by vomiting, may occur with anorexia nervosa or as a separate illness with different psychological roots. According to the U.S. Food and Drug Administration, the symptoms of bulimia are found in 40 to 50 percent of people with anorexia nervosa.[42] As with anorexia, the majority of bulimia victims are women, typically in their early twenties, college-educated, single, and white. Unlike those with anorexia, the victims of bulimia tend to be of nearly normal weight and have healthy, outgoing personalities. The greatest difference is that a person with anorexia turns away from food while a person with bulimia is obsessively drawn to it.

Description   There is a distinct pattern to the eating binges of people with bulimia. An individual with this disorder typically eats secretly, consuming an enormous amount of food at one sitting. The urge that drives such eating is clearly something beyond simple hunger. After the eating binge comes the need to vomit or take laxatives to make sure the food does not stay in the body and produce a weight gain.

An occasional eating binge does not necessarily signal bulimia; most people overeat to the point of discomfort at one time or another. However, the following signs may indicate that a person is suffering from bulimia:

- Recurrent eating binges that the person realizes are abnormal but cannot stop voluntarily
- Eating binges followed by abdominal pain, sleep, or self-induced vomiting
- Repeated attempts to lose weight by severe dieting, self-induced vomiting, or an excessive use of laxatives and/or diuretics
- Regular fluctuations of more than 10 pounds in weight because of binge-and-fast episodes
- Feelings of depression after binge eating[43]

Medical Effects   While fewer deaths result annually from bulimia than from anorexia nervosa, the medical effects of bulimia can be quite severe. The characteristic binge eating can cause an enlarged stomach and even stomach rupture. Repeated vomiting can cause chronic swelling of the salivary glands, rashes, swelling around the ankles and feet, and inflammation of or tears in the esophagus.[44]

Causes of Anorexia and Bulimia

Current theories about the cause of these eating disorders fall into three categories: physiological, sociocultural, and psychological. Certain physiological factors linked to depression may contribute to the development of these disorders. Seven of 10 persons with anorexia and/or bulimia are prone to depression, as are many of their relatives.[45] The setpoint theory has also supplied a possible causal factor.

Sociocultural factors that contribute to these disorders may include the undue significance attached to slimness and physical appearance in American culture, particularly among adolescent girls. In a study by the Center for the Study of Anorexia and Bulimia, 89 percent of the 17-year-old girls questioned were on a diet, yet only 17 percent of them were actually overweight.[46]

There is also evidence to support a psychological cause of anorexia and bulimia. A report in the *New England Journal of Medicine* indicated that many people with these conditions have distorted attitudes and concepts that affect most areas of their lives. These attitudes include the idea that one should strive for perfection, that asceticism is superior to self-indulgence, that thinness is admirable while fat is disgusting, and that weight gain is a sign of lack of control.[47]

Whatever their cause, anorexia nervosa and bulimia are difficult to treat; the patterns associated with them are not easily disrupted. Moreover, many people with anorexia deny having the illness and refuse treatment. Those with bulimia, though frequently more inclined to seek treatment, often become easily frustrated and drop out of treatment.

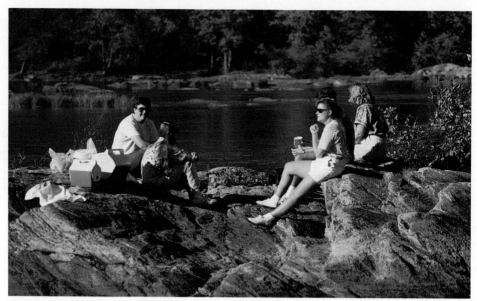

A social life shared with active, health-conscious friends can help engender a wholesome, vivacious lifestyle. (Richard T. Nowitz)

Achieving Your Goals

Even people who suffer from problems such as extreme obesity, anorexia, and bulimia can often make progress if they receive good advice and are able to make the effort. Body composition problems do require knowledge and determination, but in most cases they *can* be alleviated. As was noted earlier in this chapter, people's food habits are influenced by a variety of factors. People learn to eat as they do from family members, friends, and other role models as they are growing up. They develop a number of emotions relating to food, some of which—fear, insecurity, and guilt, for example—may cause negative attitudes or thoughts that affect their responses to food.

An important part of a successful program for body composition management must therefore involve identifying unproductive attitudes toward food and replacing them with positive, healthy, esteem-building thoughts and beliefs. Doing this is an essential part of achieving successful weight management.

While short-term progress may result from either a change in diet or an increase in exercise, long-term success requires that psychological changes be made. Fortunately, short-term progress can increase one's feelings of self-efficacy—confidence in one's power to succeed at one's goals—and such confidence can provide support in the long term. A real victory over body composition problems awaits those who make a lifetime commitment to good food, good exercise, and good thoughts.

Chapter Summary

- The American obsession with weight control could more accurately be described as a concern about appearance and health. This makes body composition a more crucial factor than weight itself.

- Body composition, specifically the proportion of fats to other tissues in the human body, can have long-term as well as short-term physical effects. It is a major influence in the development of heart disease and other chronic complaints later in life.

- Because of the effects of body image on self-concept, the fat content of one's body composition can have a profound effect on one's emotional and social life.

- Fats, while vital for human health and activity, are easily stored in excessive quantities and may be distributed in ways that are harmful to health. Americans in general have too much fat in their body composition.
- Techniques used to estimate body fat include the hydrostatic, electrical impedance, and skinfold methods.
- Diets are the most common approach to body composition management in the United States. There are many types of diets, some beneficial and others harmful. Crash diets, very low calorie diets, and diets that severely limit proteins and carbohydrates are not recommended.
- Exercise is a vital part of most weight control programs, though some researchers believe that the type of exercise taken is crucial.
- Appetite suppressant drugs, surgery, and group programs employing social pressure are other techniques for losing weight, but to keep weight off, diet and exercise are the most important factors.
- Altering body composition has proved to be difficult for most Americans.
- One explanation for this difficulty comes from the pull school, which argues that there are compelling physiological reasons why people gain and maintain weight, including genetic factors, disorders of the regulatory systems, and the development of a setpoint for body composition.
- Additional explanations for the difficulty of weight change are provided by the push school, which maintains that ingrained psychological habits of eating and food choice help maintain harmful eating behaviors.
- Today the theories of both schools are accepted as valid, and so programs for successful body composition control involve understanding both the internal physiological mechanisms of the appetite and personal psychological habits and motivators.
- The energy-balance equation of food and drink taken in versus energy consumed by exercise, activity, and basal metabolism is fundamental to all programs for the loss or gain of weight.
- Adequate exercise is the first requirement for body composition management; it may be enough by itself to produce the slow weight change that experts recommend.
- A change of diet to nutritious foods rich in vitamins and minerals is the second important step for control of body composition. More complex carbohydrates (fruits and vegetables) and fewer fats should be included in the diet, though fats may be desirable to achieve weight gain.
- Calorie-controlled diets may be necessary, but only if the other two steps have already been taken.
- Even in potentially destructive eating and weight disorders such as severe obesity, anorexia nervosa, and bulimia, the energy-balance equation is important. However, in these cases medical and psychological help are almost certainly indicated as well.
- If a person has understanding and a willingness to work, body composition problems can usually be controlled. These are goals which *can* be reached.

Key Terms

Body composition (page 140)

Essential fat (page 142)

Storage fat (page 142)

Hydrostatic weighing method (page 144)

Bioelectrical impedance (page 144)

Skinfold measurement (page 144)

Liposuction (page 149)

Pull school (page 151)

Push school (page 151)

Short-term regulatory mechanism (page 151)

Long-term regulatory mechanism (page 151)

Setpoint theory (page 152)

Basal metabolism (page 152)

Externality theory (page 154)

Anorexia nervosa (page 160)

Bulimia (page 162)

References

1. "A Nation of Healthy Worrywarts," *Time* (July 25, 1988): 66–67.

2. A. L. Stewart et al., "Conceptualization and Measurement of Health Habits for Adults in the Health Insurance Study: Vol. 11," in *Overweight* (Santa Monica, Calif.: Rand Corporation and HEWS, 1980); George E. Schauf, "Is the Caloric Theory Valid?" *Nutrition Today* (January–February 1979): 29–31.

3. Artemis P. Simopolous, "Characteristics of Obesity: An Overview," in *Human Obesity,* Richard J. Wurtman and Judith J. Wurtman (eds.), *Annals of the New York Academy of Sciences* (New York, 1987): 7.

4. W. B. Kannel and T. Gordon, "Obesity and Cardiovascular Disease: The Framingham Study," in *Obesity,* W. L. Burland, P. D. Samuel, and J. Yudkin (eds.) (London: Churchill-Livingstone, 1974): 24–51.

5. Simopolous, op. cit., p. 11.

6. Frank I. Katch and William D. McArdle, *Nutrition, Weight Control and Exercise,* 3d ed. (Philadelphia: Lea & Febiger, 1988).

7. Reva Frankle and Mei-Uih Yang, *Obesity and Weight Control: A Health Professional's Guide* (Rockville, Md.: Aspen, 1988): 7–8.

8. Trish Ratto, "The New Science of Weight Control," *Medical Self Care* 39 (March–April 1987): 25–30.

9. Alice Madar, "Heavy Facts about Body Fat," *Walking* (February–March 1988): 48.

10. Kelly Brownell, "The Yo-Yo Trap," *American Health* (March 1988): 82.

11. Marian Burros, "Diet Game, Where Chances of Winning Are Slim," *New York Times* (July 16, 1986): C1–C8.

12. Ibid.

13. Cheryl Rock and Ann Coulston, "Weight Control Approaches: A Review by the California Dietetic Association," *Journal of the American Dietetic Association* 88, no. 1 (January 1988): 44–48.

14. American College of Sports Medicine, "Position Statement on Proper and Improper Weight Loss Programs," *Medicine and Science in Sports and Exercise* 15, no. 1 (1983): ix–xiii.

15. "Dietary Protein and Body Fat Distribution," *Nutrition Review* 40 (1982): 89–90.

16. Rock and Coulston, op. cit.

17. Martin Katahn, *The T-Factor Diet* (New York: W W Norton, 1989): 205–226.

18. Charles Yesalis, "Winning and Performance Enhancing Drugs—Our Dual Addiction," *The Physician and Sports Medicine* 18, no. 3 (March 1990): 161–167.

19. C. Everett Koop, *Anabolic Steroids* (Washington, D.C.: U.S. Public Health Service, Department of Health and Human Services, 1987).

20. Carrie Dolan, "Fat-Cutting Surgery Gains Wide Popularity but Can Be Dangerous," *Wall Street Journal* CCIX, no. 1245 (June 26, 1987): 1, 10.

21. Jaroy Weber, quoted in Dolan, op. cit.

22. Patricia Hodgson, "Review of Popular Diets," in *Nutrition and Exercise in Obesity Management,* J. Storlie and H. Jordan (eds.) (Laurel, Md.: Spectrum, 1984).

23. Paul Williamson et al., *International Journal of Obesity* (December 1988).

24. M. R. C. Greenwood and Virginia A. Pittman-Waller, "Weight Control: A Complex, Various and Controversial Problem," in Frankle and Yang (eds.), op. cit., pp. 4–5.

25. S. B. Roberts et al., "Energy Expenditures and Intake in Infants Born to Lean and Overweight Mothers," *New England Journal of Medicine* 318 (1988): 461–466.

26. Joseph R. Vasselli and Carol A. Maggio, "Mechanisms of Appetite and Body-Weight Regulation," in Frankle and Yang (eds.), op. cit., p. 19.

27. R. E. Keesey et al., "The Role of the Lateral Hypothalamus in Determining the Body Weight Setpoint," in *Hunger: Basic Mechanisms and Clinical Implications,* D. Novin et al. (eds.) (New York: Raven Press, 1976).

28. E. Ravussin et al., "Reduced Rate of Energy Expenditure as a Risk-Factor for Body Weight Gain," *New England Journal of Medicine* 318 (1988): 467–472.

29. Vasselli and Maggio, op. cit.

30. Clark Cameron, *How You Can Benefit Most from Permanent Weight Loss* (Chicago, Ill.: Nightingale Conant Corporation, 1982).

31. American College of Sports Medicine, op. cit.

32. M. L. Pollack et al., *Health and Fitness through Physical Activity* (New York: Wiley, 1978): 28.

33. P. D. Wood et al., "Metabolism of Substrates: Diet, Lipoprotein Metabolism, and Exercise," *Federation Proceedings* 44 (1985): 358–363.

34. American College of Sports Medicine, op. cit., pp. vii–x.

35. Ratto, op. cit., p. 30.

36. Lauren Lissner et al., "Dietary Fat and the Regulation of Energy Intake in Human Subjects," *American Journal of Clinical Nutrition* 46 (1987): 886–892.

37. _____ , "Eating Management," in Frankle and Yang (eds.), op. cit., p. 169.

38. Reva T. Frankle, "Weight Control for the Adult and Elderly," in Frankle and Yang (eds.), op. cit., p. 376.

39. Karen Lehrman, "Anorexia and Bulimia: Causes and Cures," *Consumers Research Magazine* 70, no. 9 (September 1987): 29–32.

40. American Psychiatric Association, *Diagnostic and Statistical Manual of Mental Disorders,* 3d ed. revised (Washington, D.C.: American Psychiatric Association, 1987).

41. Lehrman, op. cit.

42. Ibid.

43. Craig Johnson et al., "Incidence and Correlates of Bulimic Behavior in a Female High School Population," *Journal of Youth and Adolescence* 13, no. 1 (February 1984): 15–26.

44. Ibid., p. 29.

45. Ibid.

46. Ibid.

47. Ibid.

Sharing Intimacy: Health and Relationships

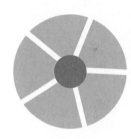

Part 3 of *Life and Health* moves on to the world of relationships, the social dimension of our lives. The emotional as well as the physical bases of intimacy are explored, the responsibilities as well as the joys. The part ends with an account of the creation of new life.

Chapter 7 covers close relationships, focusing on marriage and its alternatives and on parenthood. It discusses the vulnerability of relationships and provides rational ideas for improving our chances of successful intimacy.

Chapter 8 concentrates on our sexuality, explaining some of the psychology as well as the physiology of sex. It also looks at different types of sexual expression and sexual dysfunction.

Finally, Chapter 9 gives an overview of the reproductive function of sex, with information about the effectiveness of different techniques for preventing pregnancy and about the miracle of the reproductive process itself.

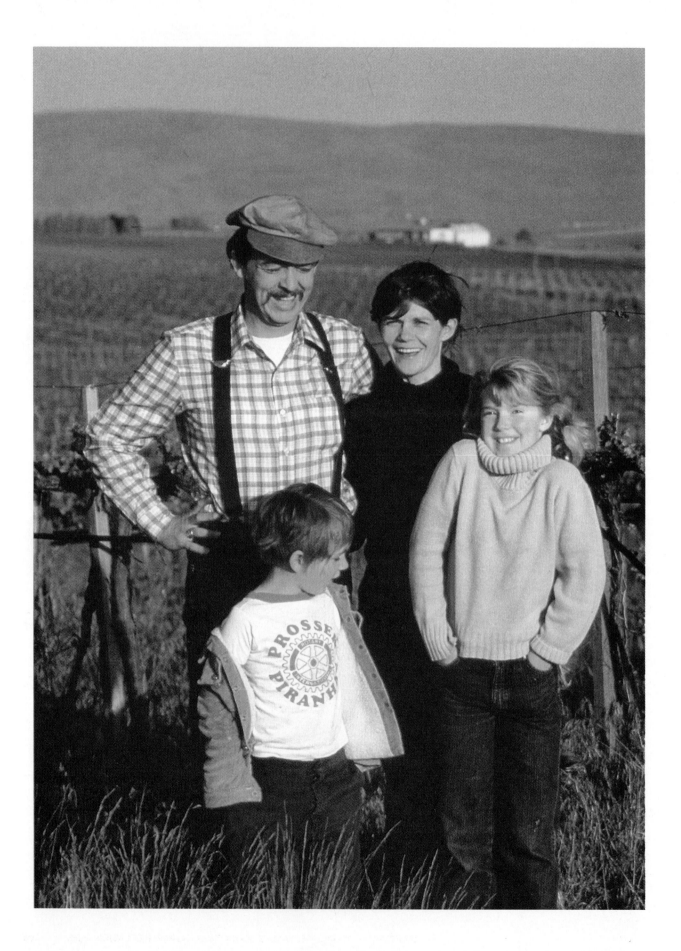

Chapter 7

Marriage, Family, and Other Intimate Relationships

To Guide Your Reading

When you have studied this chapter, you should be able to:

- Explain the importance of intimate relationships, identify some barriers to forming intimate relationships, and discuss ways to overcome those barriers.

- Identify and describe alternatives to marriage.

- Explain why divorce is on the increase and discuss some of its potential effects on a couple and their children.

- Discuss how the role of parenthood has changed in recent years and describe how parents can foster healthy physical, emotional, intellectual, social, and spiritual development in their children.

- Identify some of the factors associated with the incidence of domestic violence and describe various characteristics of battering by abusive parents.

- Discuss the nature of child abuse in the United States today and explain the effects of abuse on children.

Although American popular culture has always valued "rugged individualism" and "going it alone," most people develop and maintain intimate relationships with others: parents, children, relatives, friends, and sex partners. Such close ties help an individual develop a sense of worth as a human being and help satisfy a number of human needs.

Forming and maintaining successful long-term relationships is not always easy, however; at times it requires skill in coping with misunderstandings and other problems. Nevertheless, the learning and changing that are necessary to make a relationship work can foster personal growth, and people become healthier as they strive to achieve stronger ties with others.

Two of the most common types of intimate relationships are marriage and parenthood. There is a very good chance that most of you will be married at some point in your lives; by age 45 about 95 percent of Americans have been married.[1] Yet those of you who marry will probably wait longer than your parents did; you will also be more likely to get a divorce. Among people who decide to become parents, many choose to wait longer to have children than their parents did, and child rearing may involve different concerns than those held by the parents of earlier generations. Clearly, the changes in American society over the last few decades have altered the basic institutions of marriage and parenthood. Society is still struggling to come to terms with these changes.

Marriage rates over the past 50 years: number of marriages per thousand persons

Year	Marriage rate
1950	*11.1*
1960	*8.5*
1970	*10.6*
1980	*10.6*
1990	*9.7*

Marriage and Its Alternatives

Marriage is one of the basic institutions of society. Most people still choose to marry, but the institution of marriage is facing a greater challenge than ever before. No longer does everyone assume that heterosexual marriage is the only natural and vital adult lifestyle. Some people acknowledge other alternatives, many of which are becoming increasingly accepted as a normal part of

American life. Yet whether a person chooses to marry or to pursue an alternative to marriage, the goal is the same: to develop a strong intimate relationship with another person.

The Need for Intimate Relationships

Close relationships with others satisfy a number of emotional needs. Everyone needs *intimacy*—a close, loving relationship that allows two people to share their deepest feelings and thoughts in an atmosphere of trust and acceptance. A close relationship can also help by providing *reassurance of worth*—the feeling that individuals are valued and considered special by the important people in their lives. When people need it, such a relationship can provide a sense of *support*—the knowledge that there are people one can turn to for help—and *nurturance*—the feeling that one can care for and be cared for by others. The lack of an intimate relationship, by contrast, can lead to feelings of loneliness and distress which can contribute to more severe problems, such as alcoholism, drug abuse, and suicide.[2]

As people grow from childhood to adulthood, their emotional needs are met through different types of relationships. Young children's most intimate relationships are with their parents. Children are dependent on their parents' nurturance for their very survival. The support they get from their parents also gives them the security they need to take the first steps toward independence, and parental love gives them a sense of self-worth as well. As children grow, other close relationships become increasingly important. At first children develop more intimate relationships with their siblings and friends. Then, as adolescents and young adults, they begin to form romantic relationships as well. For many adults, marriage becomes the most important intimate relationship and friendships, while still important, are relegated to second place.[3] Although intimate relationships change as people grow, the need for intimacy remains strong at all ages.

A person's ability to form intimate relationships depends on several factors, including self-knowledge, self-esteem, self-efficacy, and feelings of caring, sharing, trust, commitment, and tenderness toward another person. Honesty and empathy are also essential components of interpersonal intimacy, and effective communication is an important catalyst in establishing intimacy and nurturing its growth.[4]

The fact that some people do not develop intimate relationships suggests that certain barriers prevent them from doing so. One study identified several barriers to the start of intimate heterosexual relationships, including physical unattractiveness, fear of rejection, shyness, and clinging to traditional sex-role norms.[5] The study also suggested, however, that such barriers can be overcome. People can begin to deal with unattractiveness, for example, by altering their appearance with new hairstyles or clothing styles or by modifying their body composition through exercise and diet. Learning effective social skills and better means of communication can help people overcome shyness and fear of rejection, as can efforts to boost their self-esteem, perhaps through improved appearance. Finally, although traditional sex roles are more difficult to alter, people can become more aware of their attitudes and attempt to learn new role behaviors that are more favorable to the development of intimate relationships.

The Decision to Marry

Marriage is an institution in a state of transition. Traditionally, marriage has been an economic arrangement in which husbands have worked outside the home to provide financial security for their families, while wives have cared for the children and run the home. Today, however, this traditional arrangement is changing. The roles of husband and wife are not as clearly defined as

Marriage fulfills various needs. These needs can be categorized as physiological, psychological, social, sexual, and spiritual.

Physiological needs: survival and safety

Psychological needs: caring, affection, love, emotional support, security and stability, romance, and intimacy

Social needs: companionship, friendship, and social support

Sexual needs: sexual gratification and pleasure in a socially approved or sanctioned setting

Spiritual needs: perpetuating part of oneself through one's children, participation in religious life, commitment to life role and self-fulfillment, and becoming everything one is capable of becoming.

Communicating About

Handling Differences between Friends

Conflicts between people are inevitable. Whenever two people interact—whether they are coworkers, friends, roommates, or husband and wife—there will be times when they disagree. A healthy relationship allows for occasional conflict and also for conflict resolution.

Unfortunately, many people feel that if a relationship is good, things should always go smoothly. When they have a falling-out with a friend, they are not prepared to try to find a way past their differences. Conflicts that are not aired and resolved at least to some extent will fester and can destroy a relationship.

The way you communicate about differences can determine whether the conflict will promote healthy growth and change. First, it is important to understand where conflicts come from. Then you need to follow some basic rules for communicating about those differences.

One basic cause of differences is the natural human desire for change. When one person wants to make a change, it can upset the balance of a relationship. For example, two friends are used to spending time together each week. Then one friend decides to go back to school to get an advanced degree and has less time and money to spend on recreation. The other friend may feel neglected and resentful. Other conflicts arise from differences in styles and values. A husband's need for neatness in the house may conflict with a wife's more casual attitude toward housekeeping.

When it is time to resolve differences, perhaps the most important thing to remember about communicating is to listen as well as talk. Hear what your friends have to say, be willing to concede their points, and try not to become defensive. Listen for the feelings behind the words. Do you sense anger that is not being brought out into the open? Do you hear that your friend is very upset? When you reply, summarize what you heard and what you sensed. Say, for example, "I understand that you're angry about how I'm spending my time."

Also think about how you appear to your friend. Do you seem supportive and reasonable or intimidating? Do you seem strong enough to hear someone's anger or too fragile to handle it? The expression on your face and other nonverbal cues affect how you appear.

When it is your turn to talk, try to be very clear about how you perceive the problem but stay away from name-calling and accusations. Instead of saying to a roommate, "You're a slob. You leave dirty dishes all over the kitchen," say, "When the dishes aren't done, it takes me much longer than it should to get a meal together."

Eventually, after the problem and your feelings have been aired, it is time to reach a compromise. Be willing to concede points on which your friend is right. Remember that it is very important for most people to save face and not look incompetent or foolish. Do not push for an admission of guilt on your friend's part. Try to move on to solutions. Be ready to apologize if you feel that you are at fault.

One of the best ways to move toward a compromise is to be the first to offer a concession. Saying "Okay, I'll cut out watching football one day every weekend so we can spend time together" can cut through a disagreement on how to spend free time. Once you have made a concession, it is fair to ask for something in return: "I'd like us to spend some of that free time hiking together instead of housecleaning."

Keep in mind that you want to maintain a good relationship. Take the long view. Think about how important this one issue is to you. Can you trade giving in on this issue for getting what you want later? Once you and your friend are talking, be creative about solutions. Maybe together you can come up with a solution that neither one could come up with alone. Instead of working against each other, you will be working together.

Based on Jeffrey Rubin and Carol Rubin, *When Families Fight* (New York: William Morrow, 1989).

in the past, especially when both partners work and provide financially for the family. Many people today expect and get more from marriage than economic benefits; they look to their spouses for sharing, nurturance, emotional support, and intimacy. Happily married people often identify the spouse as their best friend, a person whose company they thoroughly enjoy, who is there in times of need, and who shares their joys and sorrows.

Why Do People Marry? The pressures for a couple to marry can be enormous. This pressure often comes from parents and other relatives as well as from the media and romantic literature, which often portray married people as the only healthy, fulfilled individuals in society. Sometimes the members of a family, ethnic group, or religious group may exert pressure on individuals to marry so that a new generation can be raised in the teachings and values of the group.

Aside from these pressures, people marry for a variety of reasons. Some still marry for economic reasons. For others, marriage is viewed as the only acceptable framework in which to enjoy sex freely. Many people marry for reasons that have little to do with the desire to develop a meaningful long-term relationship. They may be trying to forge a sense of identity by picking a spouse who represents what they would like to become (secure, popular, or whatever). They may be escaping from an unhappy home life, marrying on the rebound from another relationship, or attempting to avoid loneliness. Young men and women who are building their careers may see marriage as a way of creating a better balance in their lives, allowing them to share leisure activities and experience more affection, sympathy, and support than single people do. In terms of achieving a more balanced lifestyle, men may have the most to gain from marriage. Even when they are single, women have relationships with friends and relatives that tend to be more supportive and affectionate than those formed by men.[6]

Researchers have identified several patterns in "high-quality," or well-balanced, marriages. Some married people tend to focus their energies on joint activities; their strongest wish is to spend time together, yet they also strike an even balance between privacy and togetherness. Other couples focus their energies on being parents, nurturing and raising their children. Some dual-career couples, although they spend much of their energy on their individual careers, develop intimacy by sharing what is going on in their work.[7] It thus seems that the desire to spend time together, raise children, and share other aspects of life and career are all healthy reasons for marrying.

Love, Romance, and Attraction A basic element in most marriages is the love one person feels for another. There are many different types of love between persons, including parental love, fraternal love, and romantic love. Each requires two essential qualities: caring and respect. Romantic love includes the qualities of deep intimacy and passion and begins with a feeling of intense attraction between two people.[8]

Although most marriages are based on romantic love at the outset, few couples can sustain that romance as the years go by. Instead, romantic love often develops into a less intense and all-consuming type of love known as companionate love.[9] A companionate love relationship is steadier than romantic love; it is based on trust, sharing, affection, and togetherness. Maintaining the love in a marriage requires considerable effort and commitment. Married partners who succeed in communicating, giving physical warmth, sharing interests, and sharing responsibilities are more likely to remain in love.[10]

Researchers investigating the bases of love have found that physical appearance is related to romantic attraction.[11] In one study, both men and women looking at photographs rated good-looking people as more interesting, sociable, kind, strong, outgoing, and sexually warm than less attractive

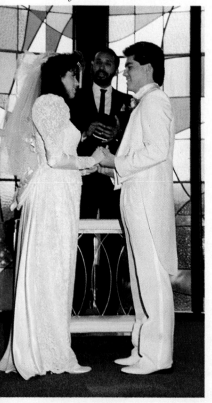

Since antiquity, the marriage ceremony has provided a formal setting in which a couple can publicly affirm their love for and commitment to each other. (Tony Freeman/PhotoEdit)

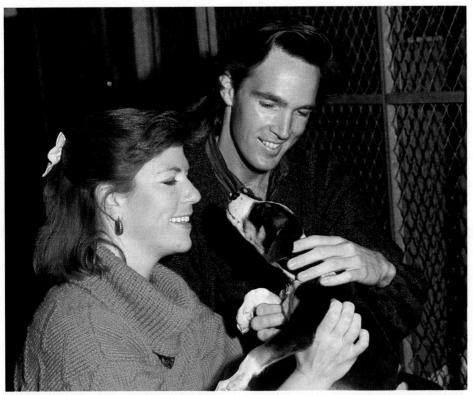

The sharing of mutual interests such as hobbies can help build solidity in a relationship; couples who have similar interests are more likely to sustain a long-term marriage than are those who do not. (Mary Kate Denny/PhotoEdit)

people.[12] Men especially rate a woman's physical attractiveness as important in a relationship, while women are likely to consider a man's occupational or financial status more important.[13]

Despite changes in society, people's views of attractiveness remain rather traditional. A young man's attractiveness to women seems to be enhanced by behavior that suggests he will achieve high social status and be a good provider. A woman is more attractive to men if she seems to have the qualities that will make her a good traditional wife and mother.[14] In addition, a recent study concluded that although norms of sexual behavior have changed, both men and women still prefer to date and marry people with little or no sexual experience.[15]

Assessing Compatibility When people are looking for a mate, they tend to gravitate toward potential partners whose ethnic, religious, economic, and educational background closely approximates their own; certain physical attributes are also significant factors.[16] Where they are least likely to match up with a similar person is in the area of compatibility of personality. Personality factors are not always easy to observe. Sometimes people do not reveal their true selves during courtship, when they are on their best behavior and eager to be accommodating. Moreover, people with opposite personality types often attract each other, perhaps with the notion that one personality rounds out the other.

Unfortunately, great differences in personality can often lead to conflict later on. One study found that a source of marital dissatisfaction among husbands was a feeling that their wives were too possessive, neglectful, and openly admiring of other men. Dissatisfied wives complained that their husbands were possessive, moody, and openly attracted to other women. The study also found that sex is a source of great difficulties for unhappy married men and women. It found that women see sex as following from emotional

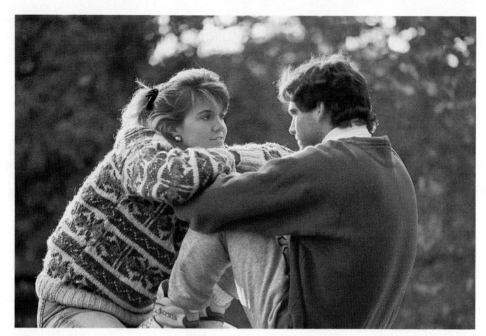

Assessing compatibility is an essential part of a serious relationship. (Rudi Von Briel)

intimacy, while men see it as a road to intimacy. As a result, men complain that their wives withhold sex from them and women complain that their husbands are too sexually aggressive.[17]

How can people be sure they are marrying people with whom they are truly compatible? One way is by taking plenty of time to get to know the other person. Researchers have found that couples seem to go through three stages in this process. First, each person tries to measure his or her good and bad qualities against those of the other person; people tend to be drawn to others who seem to have about the same assets and liabilities they themselves possess. Second, people look for compatible beliefs, attitudes, and interests to support the initial attraction. It is not until the third stage that people reveal to each other how they handle responsibility, react to disappointment, and cope with a wide variety of situations.[18] The key to compatibility is for the couple to be sure that they have arrived at this last stage before they think seriously about marriage. Such people are less likely to be unpleasantly surprised than are those who marry impulsively on short acquaintance.

Even the happiest partners in a marriage or other intimate relationship will encounter problems that create tension and discord. As an individual grows and changes, what he or she gives to a relationship may also change.

Alternatives to Marriage

Since the 1960s there have been real changes in society's views on marriage, divorce, parenting, gender roles, and premarital sex.[19] While the vast majority of young men and women still expect to marry, society no longer demands that people marry, stay married, or have children. Remaining single is now a widely accepted option; at any given time more than 50 million American adults age 18 and older are unmarried.[20] The restrictions and disadvantages of marriage are also an increasing concern for many people. In addition, there is a marked trend among both men and women toward marrying later in life.[21]

Single Living The annual percentage of people who marry in the United States has declined slightly every year from 1985 to 1988, when the marriage rate was the lowest it had been since 1967.[22] With increasing numbers of people choosing to remain single or becoming single through divorce, there is a new acceptance of singlehood as a fulfilling alternative. For example, studies have shown that negative attitudes toward remaining single declined dramatically between 1957 and 1976.[23] This seems to suggest that marriage is becoming less relevant as an institution for structuring intimate relationships.

Who are the people who choose to remain single? Some are men and women who have a new awareness about marriage and value their freedom and independence. Among women especially, greater career opportunities have brought more economic independence, and so marriage is no longer seen as the only route to economic security. In addition, many women no longer feel that marriage is necessary to achieve sexual expression and gratification. Studies have shown a strong trend toward less restrictive attitudes about premarital sex among both women and men since 1965.[24]

The single state can be comfortable and rewarding for many people. When a single person has a good income, he or she may be economically better off than is a married person who faces greater financial demands. Single people can buy houses or apartments and establish homes of their own without waiting for a partner to come along. Many singles also have more discretionary income that can be used to pay for vacations or buy luxury items and other products. Moreover, many people find that it is easier to meet the demands of a career when they do not have to consider another person's interests while scheduling their time and activities.

Singlehood is not without disadvantages, however. Single people may have more difficulty in meeting their emotional needs than married people do. It is often more difficult for those who live alone to satisfy their needs for intimacy, interdependence, sexual gratification, and parenthood. As a result, single people may have to make extra efforts to assemble the elements of a full and satisfying life.

Cohabitation   An increasingly common phenomenon in American society is **cohabitation,** an arrangement in which two unrelated people live together in a sexual relationship without marrying. Studies of cohabitation on college campuses indicate that 25 to 35 percent of students are living with a person of the opposite sex at any one time and that there are about 2 million cohabiting couples in the United States.[25] Although some groups still disapprove of cohabitation on moral or religious grounds, a majority of Americans now seem to accept the idea of two people living together without marriage.[26]

Why do people choose to live together instead of marrying? Some young people who are aware of the complexities of marriage prefer to try living together first so that they can find out whether they are mature enough to engage in a lifelong caring relationship. Often they also want to find out whether they are truly compatible. They reason that they can discover this better by living together than by seeing each other only on dates. Although many people feel this way, there is no evidence that living together increases the likelihood of a successful marriage.

Cohabitation is not limited to young people. A number of senior citizens live together but avoid formal marriage ties, often for economic reasons. Single, divorced, or widowed people who are retired sometimes lose their pensions or Social Security benefits if they marry or remarry; for these people, cohabitation makes good sense.

Researchers who study cohabitation are interested in finding the answers to a number of questions: Are cohabiting couples able to avoid the problems they might expect to encounter in marriage? Is there a greater degree of sexual equality among cohabiting couples? How does cohabitation affect the stability of a relationship? Does cohabitation erode the institution of marriage? The answers to some of these questions are becoming increasingly clear.

Couples who live together tend to face a number of problems, some of which are similar to the types of problems that confront married couples. In addition to the possibility of family disapproval and legal difficulties, cohabiting couples sometimes have conflicts over the purpose of the relationship; an

cohabitation—*an arrangement in which two unrelated people live together in a sexual relationship without marrying.*

Your Attitudes about Household Tasks

Whether people like it or not, certain household tasks must be performed regularly. Which marriage partner do you think should take responsibility for the following tasks? Check the response you feel is appropriate on the chart below.

Task	Only the Wife	Mainly the Wife	Shared Equally	Mainly the Husband	Only the Husband	A third party
Budgeting	☐	☐	☐	☐	☐	☐
Shopping	☐	☐	☐	☐	☐	☐
Household repairs	☐	☐	☐	☐	☐	☐
Auto maintenance	☐	☐	☐	☐	☐	☐
Paying bills	☐	☐	☐	☐	☐	☐
Banking	☐	☐	☐	☐	☐	☐
Child care	☐	☐	☐	☐	☐	☐
Housecleaning	☐	☐	☐	☐	☐	☐
Meal preparation	☐	☐	☐	☐	☐	☐
Laundry	☐	☐	☐	☐	☐	☐
Carrying out trash	☐	☐	☐	☐	☐	☐
Income earning	☐	☐	☐	☐	☐	☐
Disciplining children	☐	☐	☐	☐	☐	☐
Yard work and lawn care	☐	☐	☐	☐	☐	☐
Pet care	☐	☐	☐	☐	☐	☐
Other tasks	☐	☐	☐	☐	☐	☐

Which tasks did you assign to only or mainly the wife? Why?_____

_____

Which did you assign to only or mainly the husband? Why? _____

_____

Which did you assign to shared responsibility? Why? _____

_____

Does the set of tasks you assigned to the partner of the sex opposite to yours seem equitable in (1) responsibility and (2) amount of work? Why or why not?

_____

_____

What about the assignments you made to the person of your own sex? Why or why not? _____

_____

Do you think the division of tasks should be equitable in amount of work and responsibility?

Why or why not? _____

_____

Adapted from John Dorfman et al., *Well-Being: An Introduction to Health* (Glenview, Ill.: Scott, Foresman, 1980): 110. With permission.

inequitable division of labor and disagreements about sex roles; disagreements about spending money; incompatible goals, interests, and values; and violence (violence among cohabiting couples is three times higher than it is among married couples).[27]

Studies have suggested that the similarities between cohabitation and marriage are far more striking than the differences.[28] Cohabiting couples are not significantly different in regard to sex roles and division of labor; the way they tend to divide tasks closely mirrors the behavior of married couples of a similar age. Cohabiting couples also appear to be no less monogamous than married couples are. People who live together, however, are more likely to end an unsatisfactory relationship than married couples are to seek a divorce. This makes sense, because many cohabiting couples live together as a trial to see whether they are truly compatible. This does not mean that they are any less committed to the relationship. People who live together are often as deeply involved emotionally as a married couple, and a breakup can be just as painful as a divorce. Moreover, cohabitation has not displaced or eroded the institution of marriage, as many critics feared it might. Rather, it seems to have been incorporated into the courtship phase of a relationship for many young people, most of whom expect to get married eventually.

Divorce

One of the greatest changes that has occurred in interpersonal relationships during the last few decades has been the increasing unwillingness of people to remain in an unsatisfactory marriage. In part this reflects people's changing expectations of what marriage should be and what it should provide. For example, people today expect greater personal fulfillment in marriage than did the people of a few generations ago. Along with changing expectations have come changing attitudes toward divorce. The great majority of Americans now feel that married people should not stay together, even for the sake of the children, if they are not getting along.[29] The increase in divorce is also a reflection of the changing status of women. As women have become less economically dependent on their husbands, divorce rates have increased.[30]

Divorce rates over the past 50 years: number of divorces per thousand

Year	Divorce rate
1950	2.5
1960	2.2
1970	3.5
1980	5.2
1990	4.7

Divorce Today Between 1962 and 1981 the number of divorces per year in the United States tripled. Although the rate has decreased slightly since then, the number of divorces each year remains quite high. About one marriage in three now ends in divorce.[31]

Divorce is often financially difficult. To ease problems concerning the division of property, child custody and support, and alimony, all but two states have instituted some sort of provision for "no-fault" divorce, substantially reducing court costs. These divorce laws have backfired for many women, however. The provisions for equitable distribution of resources do not take into account the fact that most children live with the mother after a divorce. As a result, the income of women and their children one year after divorce is only about 67 percent of the predivorce income, while the income of divorced men is about 90 percent of the predivorce level.[32]

Changes have also taken place in the area of child custody, which is currently determined according to the best interests of the children. The laws in most states have been rewritten so that fathers now have a better opportunity to gain custody of their children.

The Effects of Divorce Even though current divorce laws may ease some of the problems of divorce, the dissolution of a marriage is painful for everyone involved. Divorced people are suddenly on their own, attempting to deal with feelings of loneliness, anger, rejection, failure, panic, and self-doubt. Despite these negative feelings, there is optimism as well. Divorce can represent a new beginning, a chance to rebuild one's life, and an opportunity to

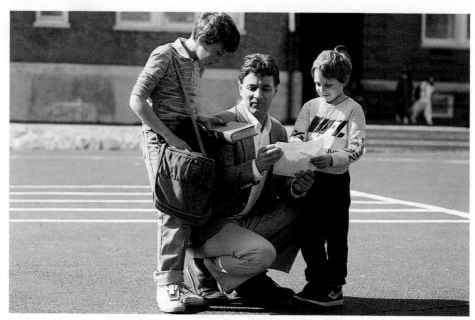

Parents who do not gain custody are usually given visitation rights not only for their own benefit but for the sake of the children, who will know that both parents are always there to provide care and support. (Richard Hutchings/InfoEdit)

seek a more fulfilling relationship than the one left behind. Most people who divorce do eventually remarry. Some studies have shown that these remarried people report high levels of satisfaction, love, and trust in their new relationships. Children from a previous marriage, however, may place added strains on the new relationship. Dealing with the ambiguous role of stepmother or stepfather may have a negative effect on a new marriage.[33]

What effect does divorce have on the children? For most children, the separation of their parents is a very traumatic experience. Extreme anger, regression to earlier forms of behavior, and physical symptoms such as asthma are not uncommon. For the first few months most children wish the couple could be reconciled so that the father or mother could rejoin the household. Children often feel that they did something to divide their parents. Younger children especially seem to blame themselves for the divorce; older adolescents, by contrast, are more often angry or ashamed.[34] It helps if parents explain to the children that they are not at fault and that the problems are between the mother and father. Although children do suffer from the divorce of their parents, most of them adjust as time goes by.

Parenthood

Parenthood is the ultimate responsibility a couple or individual can assume. Twenty-four hours a day, 7 days a week, 52 weeks a year, a small, weak, vulnerable, impressionable human being looks to his or her parents for food, clothing, shelter, love, and encouragement. It is more than a job: the parents cannot quit. It is more than a marriage: the parents cannot divorce the child. Parenthood is the supreme commitment, and for many parents it is the supreme joy—if they are ready to assume the responsibility.

The Decision to Have a Child

In the past people married to sanction sexual activity and to have children. Although there were other reasons to marry—love, companionship, money, family connections—the most common reason was the creation of a family. In fact, every married couple was expected to have children. The reasons for having children varied. One was to carry on the family name. Another was to have someone to help in the house or in the field or to provide additional income for the family. Still another was to have someone to help care for the couple in their later years. Of course, many people became parents because they loved children.

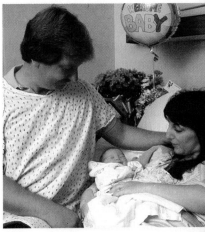

In recent years attitudes have been changing. Today a majority of people accept the notion that a couple can remain childless by choice.[35] There is an increased recognition that although having children can be a wonderful experience, it can also have a negative and restricting effect on one's lifestyle. Certainly people are aware of the economic impact of having children. The cost of rearing a child can be staggering, especially when college tuition is included. In addition to the financial strains of raising a child, parenthood may cause emotional and physical stress that sometimes results in depression, guilt, fatigue, and marital difficulties. Despite this new and perhaps more realistic assessment of parenthood, most people still expect to become parents, although they may have children somewhat later in life.[36] While the U.S. birthrate declined rapidly in the 1960s and early 1970s, it increased slightly after that period and has held steady since about 1975.[37]

For new parents, the birth of a child can be the embodiment of a dream; it is also the beginning of the most creative challenge of a couple's relationship. (Stephen McBrady/ PhotoEdit)

What are some of the reasons people decide to have children today? Children help fulfill various interpersonal, psychological, and social needs. They provide love and companionship and can bring stimulation and happiness to their parents' lives. They may help fulfill a need to find a meaning and purpose in life; watching children grow contributes to a feeling of accomplishment. Having children may also help parents feel more secure about their old age. Some of the reasons for having children arise out of a person's unique personality and upbringing—such as the desire to love, nurture, and care for a child. Others arise out of social and cultural situations—such as pressure from family members and friends and pressure to continue the family line.

Some of the reasons for having children may be more sound than others depending on how well people assume the responsibilities of parenthood. Many couples decide to become parents because they have developed a strong, secure relationship and would like to extend and enrich it with children. If these people are willing to accept the responsibilities of parenthood and can meet a child's physical and emotional needs, they will probably be happy with their decision. However, if a couple decide to become parents to try to "save" a marriage or relationship, because of pressure from others, or for other unsound reasons and are not ready to accept parental responsibilities, they may regret their decision.

Meeting Children's Health Needs

Parents are probably the most important single factor in determining whether a child is healthy at birth and will maintain healthy growth and development. They have a significant effect on the child's physical, emotional, intellectual, social, and spiritual development. Healthy child development is fostered by a number of factors, including nurturance, love and acceptance, competence and self-confidence, appropriate role models, and a stimulating and responsive environment.

Throughout history there have been books on raising children, but beginning with the publication of Benjamin Spock's Baby and Child Care in 1945, how-to books for parents have achieved wide popularity. Today the market for parenting handbooks is booming.

Physical Development Children have a better chance of enjoying good physical health if they receive optimal care beginning before birth and continuing throughout infancy, childhood, and adolescence. The first consideration is to prevent retarded growth, especially in the first year of life: growth that is too slow may produce developmental deficiencies that are never completely overcome in the adult years. Good prenatal care of the expectant mother gives the newborn an excellent start (Chapter 9). Providing a well-balanced diet, with restricted sugar and food additives, is important for ensuring healthy growth and development in the childhood and teenage years.

To promote optimal physical health, parents need to be sure that their children have regular medical checkups and all necessary immunizations against disease. They also need to provide their children with sufficient opportunities for exercise, rest, and relaxation. Since accidents are the major cause of death for people up to age 40, parents need to keep their children's environment as safe as possible.[38] In a car they should use approved safety seats for infants and seat belts for older children. At home they should make sure that children are not exposed to dangers such as open stairways, medications or toxic substances, and dangerous implements.

Emotional Development

Every child needs love and acceptance; only if a child feels deeply, basically loved can his or her emotional development proceed. To meet this need, parents must begin by helping the baby develop what psychoanalyst Erik Erikson called *basic trust*. If the parents can convey a sense of relaxation and enjoyment—rather than anxiety—as they feed and hold the baby, the baby will get the idea that the world is a friendly place and begin to feel that he or she can depend on the parents.[39]

Self-esteem in children largely results from parental support. When parents praise a child, show affection, and pay attention, this communicates approval to the child.

When early dependency needs are met, a child is free to grow toward security and independence. Eventually, just as the parents freely gave the child love, they must freely let him or her go. Love that is too possessive may prevent a child from developing independence and autonomy.

A feeling of security within the home environment is important for a child's emotional development. This does not mean that children suffer emotionally every time there is a parental conflict or the family encounters a problem; conflicts and problems are a part of life, and most children do well if their parents try to deal with such situations maturely. Researchers have found, however, that in homes where there is physical aggression between the parents, children tend to have a wide variety of emotional problems.[40]

Intellectual Development

Parental care is also a crucial factor in intellectual development and the key period is the child's first 5 years. One expert believes that about half of an individual's intellectual capacity has developed by age 4, about three-fourths by age 8, and the remainder by age 17.[41] Parents can help stimulate intellectual growth by singing and talking to an infant, offering choices (red or green shirt? peas or carrots?) to even very young children, explaining family rules, answering questions, and encouraging children to try new experiences and tasks even though they may fail the first few times. The best home environment for intellectual development is one in

Honest and open communication between parent and child builds trust, which is a basic element in proper emotional development. (M.C. Wallace/PhotoEdit)

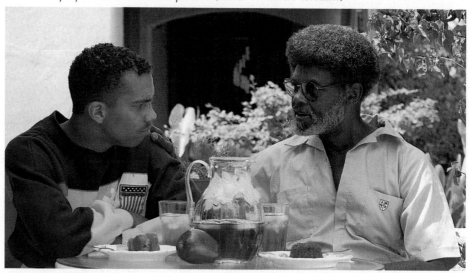

which the parents are warm and loving, take time to explain their actions, encourage creativity and problem-solving, and show concern for the development of the children's competence.

Social Development   A child's ability to deal with other people develops primarily from his or her early relationship with the parents.[42] Parents have the main responsibility for the *socialization* of their children—teaching them how to behave with other people. In part, children learn how to behave with others by watching how their parents act and then modeling their behavior on that of the parents. They also learn through *discipline*—the process by which parents communicate rules to them.

Parents often find that disciplining their children is the hardest task of parenthood.[43] Parents may use several modes of discipline. Some parents are authoritarian in their style of discipline. These parents lay down the law to their children; they demand mature behavior and exercise authority harshly. Authoritarian discipline often produces children who are dependent and rather aggressive. Other parents are permissive. These parents tend to have few rules for their children and often do not enforce the rules that do exist. The children of such parents tend to show little self-control and self-reliance. The best style of discipline seems to be one in which the parents demand high standards of mature behavior but also explain the rules and punishments. These parents respond to their children's individuality and set standards of behavior that are appropriate to a particular child's age and maturity. The children of this type of parent tend to be independent and self-controlled and to have good social skills.[44]

Spiritual Development   Parents also play an important role in a child's spiritual development. This may include various elements, such as the development of a child's value system, a sense of self-efficacy, and a feeling of purpose or meaningfulness in life. Values such as honesty, compassion, empathy, and tolerance for others are instilled in children in part by their parents. Parents can also help instill a sense of self-efficacy—a feeling of power to control one's own destiny—by encouraging their children to have confidence in themselves and make full use of their potential.

Being human also entails reaching out for a meaning so that one is fulfilled and connected to something or someone other than oneself. The people who are happiest and healthiest appear to be those who are connected to others by mutual need, who have a sense of identity and know and respect themselves, and, perhaps most important, who see a purpose in life and work actively toward it.[45] By encouraging their children to believe in or have faith in some force greater than themselves, many parents have helped the children find meaning and happiness in their lives.

The Child's Contribution to the Parent-Child Relationship

Parent-child interactions are not a one-way street from parent to child; children are active participants in this process.[46] Researchers think that even during the first 2 months after birth infants use signals—such as gazing eye to eye with the parent, smiling, crying, thrashing around, cooing, or appearing particularly helpless—to guide their parents in giving them the care they need.[47] They can often induce a parent to play with them when they are in the mood for amusement or help them when they are hungry, wet, or uncomfortable. Tiny as they are, they can exert a tremendous amount of power over an adult. One expert has even suggested that with a first baby, the infant "knows" more about infant care than the parent; the parent learns by interacting with the baby.[48]

While children get a great deal from their parents, parents gain something from their children in return. The warm and pleasant interactions with children that are part of parenting can have a powerful effect on a parent's psy-

Parent Effectiveness Training (PET) is a course that was developed by Dr. Thomas Gordon. It offers parents strategies for resolving problems with their children without either party feeling like a loser. Check your library or bookstore for more information.

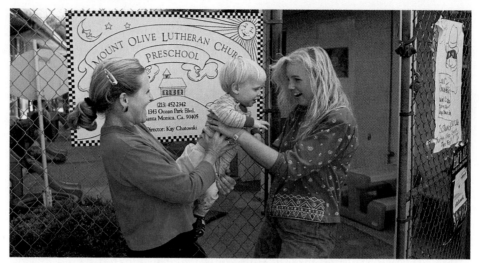

As more women join the full-time work force, children are spending increasing amounts of time with child care professionals. (David Young-Wolff/PhotoEdit)

chological well-being.[49] Although being a parent is a demanding task and is often tedious and frustrating, most parents feel that children bring a sense of purpose, fulfillment, commitment, and value to their lives.[50]

Who Cares for Children?

In recent years there has been a dramatic increase in the number of mothers who work outside the home. In 1988, 56 percent of mothers with children under age 6 and 73 percent of mothers with children between ages 6 and 17 were employed outside the home. In 1975 the comparable figures were 39 percent and 55 percent, respectively.[51] While these women sometimes work for self-fulfillment, more often than not they work because their families need the income. This change in the number of mothers in the work force has affected the way child care tasks are divided between mothers and fathers and has meant that many children have care givers other than their parents at some time in their lives.

The Mother's Role Traditionally, mothers have provided the majority of child care. They have been the ones to deal with the minute-to-minute demands of babies and young children and have been the primary source of care and comfort for older children. Even when mothers work, they usually still take primary responsibility for managing the work done by substitute care givers and for providing care when they are home. Mothers, more often than fathers, are also the ones who arrange their work schedules to meet their families' needs.[52]

Mothers who are employed often find balancing two major jobs—working and parenting—quite stressful and feel a conflict between the two responsibilities. However, working outside the home may confer benefits, such as greater intellectual stimulation, more social contacts with adults, and, of course, greater income. These benefits may outweigh the negative effects of stress, particularly if a woman is working by choice and not by necessity.[53] Furthermore, being happier may make a working woman a more effective mother when she is at home. Recent studies have shown that having a mother who works is not harmful even to young children. Children can form secure bonds both with their parents and with substitute care givers. Moreover, working outside the home does not appear to affect the commitment of either parent to parenting or to the children.[54]

Mothers who choose not to work may find staying home to raise children a rewarding experience in itself. Many women still prefer to remain at home to provide care and early learning experiences for their children. These women may find joy in watching the child's development and responding to the child's needs for security, love, and affection.

The Father's Role Most fathers still consider their most important role to be that of providing financial security for their families.[55] However, while today's fathers do not share parenting equally with their wives, they are very different from the fathers of a generation ago. Fathers today are much more involved in the day-to-day responsibilities of child care—changing diapers, feeding and bathing their babies—than were fathers in the past. They attend conferences at their children's schools and sometimes stay home with a sick child. There is some evidence that men feel proud of these new child care responsibilities but guilty that they still do not do as much as they feel they should.[56]

A father's contribution to child care is often of a different nature from a mother's. Fathers tend to be more playful, stimulating, and physically active with their children, who find them exciting. They are often a child's preferred playmate.[57] Such active play is important in helping children develop a kinetic sense of movement and balance, self-confidence, and social awareness. With older children, fathers are usually more directive in establishing discipline and instructive in dealing with issues such as plans for college or career. However, modern fathers are less likely to impose their own ambitions on their children and less likely to be authoritarian, arbitrary, austere, and unapproachable than were fathers in the past.[58] Since the father's role in child care usually complements and supports the mother's role, it is vital in raising well-adjusted children.

Other Child Care Possibilities For many new mothers today the question is not "Should I go back to work?" but "When should I go back to work?" Many women return to their jobs only days or weeks after a child is born or adopted. Others may wait 6 months, a year, or until the youngest child is in school. Some mothers or fathers work part-time and arrange their hours to coincide with the child's school hours or with the time when the other parent is home to care for the child. Parents must decide when to return to work and how many hours to work; the decision should be a practical one with which they are comfortable.

One factor parents should consider in making such decisions is that during the first 6 months infants do not become too upset at being separated from the mother. A child may begin to cry when the mother leaves, but this crying will stop a few minutes after she has gone. From about 6 months to 1 year, however, many children begin to develop "stranger anxiety" and become upset if the mother leaves. Infants can do well if left with a substitute care giver, especially if they have had a chance to form an attachment to that person.[59]

Some experts believe that during the first 3 years of life a child is better off with an individual adult care giver than in a group care situation. After age 3 children can benefit more from being in a group situation with other children. If a younger child must be placed in a group care setting, it is best if the same adult cares for the child every day.

In choosing a care giver, parents should look for a person whom they feel they can trust and whose child-rearing philosophy is similar to their own. Some things parents should consider include the following.

- Will the child be in a safe physical and emotional environment?
- Will the care giver provide affection and intellectual stimulation, not simply put the child in front of a television set?
- How many other children will the care giver be caring for?
- Can the parents communicate well with the care giver?
- Does the care giver plan to continue caring for the child for a long period of time so that the child will not have to become accustomed to a succession of new people?

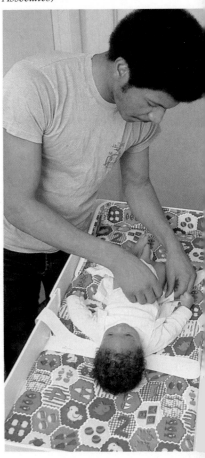

When the father participates actively in child care, both he and the child benefit. (Michal Heron/Woodfin Camp & Associates)

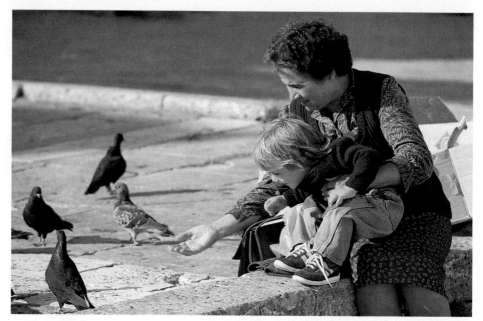

Many grandparents are eager to assume the role of care giver, devoting hours each day to the raising of their grandchildren. (Alan Oddie/PhotoEdit)

In the case of school-age children, some parents do not provide for substitute care giving while they are absent from the home. It is estimated that about 4 million school-age American children today come home to an empty house. There is concern among experts on child development that these latch-key children may be getting independence before they are mature enough to cope with it. Such children may develop behavior problems because they have not been socialized. They have not yet learned responsibility and consideration for others—concepts that they learn primarily from adults. They may also suffer from loneliness and fear, and this can affect their emotional development.[60] A better choice might be to have the child attend an after-school day care center or stay with a neighbor or baby-sitter until the child is old enough to act responsibly alone.

Single Parenthood

With the current rate of divorce, many people find themselves raising children alone. While some of these single parents are fathers, the great majority are mothers. It has been estimated that if present trends continue, nearly half of all children born since 1975 will live in a mother-only family at some point before reaching age 18.[61] Single-parent families also result from desertion, the death of a spouse, and the decision by some women to have children without marrying.

Single parents face special stresses beyond those which married parents normally confront. Single-parent families usually have incomes lower than those of two-parent families. In 1987, for example, the median income of families headed by a single mother was $14,620; for families headed by a single father it was $24,800; and for married-couple families it was $34,700.[62] One reason for this disparity is that women are generally paid at a lower rate than men are; another is that women often work fewer hours so that they can care for their children. Single mothers and fathers sometimes try to arrange "flextime" so that their work hours are more variable, giving them an opportunity to attend to their children's needs. Since raising children is expensive, the reduced income of a single parent puts a great strain on the budget. As a result of these financial pressures, roughly half of all single mothers live below the poverty line.[63]

According to the U.S. Bureau of the Census, in 1960, 9 percent of families with children were headed by a single mother. By 1985 the figure had climbed to over 20 percent. If present trends continue, nearly half of all children will live in mother-only families at some point before reaching age 18.

Single parents also face the stress of having to deal with changes and problems alone. They may need to deal with a new job, a different house, or even a move to a different part of the country. They have to juggle work and child care responsibilities and must cope with the everyday problems of child rearing without the help and support of a spouse. Single parents must also try to make a new social life for themselves in a world that is still geared to married couples. No wonder single mothers report feeling more stressed than married ones do.[64]

Although things can be difficult in a single-parent family, there is evidence that the situation is not necessarily harmful to the children. Some research has indicated that it is conflict between parents, not divorce, that causes children to develop problems.[65] One study found that teenagers living in families with high levels of conflict were more depressed, had higher levels of anxiety, and showed more physical symptoms related to stress than did teenagers in divorced families with low levels of conflict.[66] If parental conflicts are resolved by divorce and a single parent builds a good relationship with his or her children, the children may be better off.

Problems in Child Rearing

Research on families has shown that problem behavior in children can be fostered by certain maladaptive family patterns involving the general family environment as well as the child's relationship with one or both parents. Five family patterns in particular have been identified as being detrimental to the healthy development of a child. The first is a family environment characterized by inadequate methods for coping with the physical and psychological demands placed on the family. The second is a family environment characterized by a number of pathological behavior patterns on the part of the parents, including continual fighting and the inability to give a child love and guidance, along with exposure to negative and dysfunctional parental models. A third pattern is one in which the parents espouse antisocial values and engage in behavior that violates acceptable societal norms. Families disrupted by a parent's desertion constitute a fourth pattern that can produce problem behavior in children. A fifth pattern that can lead to problem behaviors is one in which the parents demonstrate a lack of caring and engage in harmful behavior, including various forms of child abuse, neglect, rejection, and a devaluation of a child's worth.[67]

Domestic Violence and Family Vulnerability

The ideal of a happy, healthy, and fully functioning family is all too often shattered by problems and negative behaviors which can be very harmful to family members. Domestic violence is a very real problem in American society today, one which poses a great threat to family viability. Besides physical violence, domestic violence can include other forms of abuse, such as forced isolation, belittling verbal abuse, threats, and intimidation.

Statistics have shown that domestic violence affects an alarming number of American families. Based on a national sample of family members, it has been estimated that 2 million to 3 million women and over 250,000 men are physically abused by their spouses.[68] Sometimes violent abuse escalates into murder. About 25 percent of all murders in the United States stem from domestic violence, and more police officers are killed or injured while trying to deal with family fights than in any other kind of situation, including drug-related arrests.[69] Women tend to be the victims of such fatal violence, as well as nonfatal violence, far more often than men are.[70]

Domestic violence is not limited to spouses or cohabiting couples; children are frequently the target of domestic violence as well. The rate of child abuse

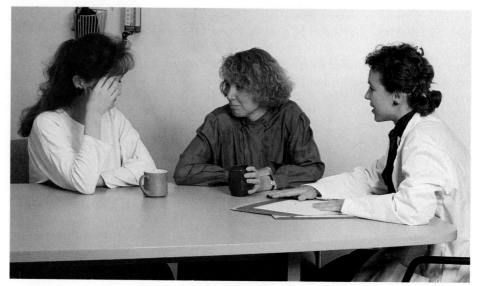

As a result of domestic violence, more than 400,000 women seek protection in shelters for battered women in a typical year. (Custom Medical Stock Photo)

in American society is appalling; in 1986 an estimated 2 million cases of child abuse and neglect were reported, and over the past 10 years reports of child abuse have increased 184 percent.[71] Moreover, one study has suggested that as many as 5,000 children die each year as a result of maltreatment.[72]

Why do family members abuse and commit violent acts against each other? Several factors have been found to be related to the incidence of domestic violence.[73]

- Persons who were victims of abuse and violence as children are more likely to become abusive adults.
- Domestic violence is more prevalent in families with low socioeconomic status.
- The incidence of domestic violence is related to social and environmental stressors such as unemployment and poverty.
- A lack of social support systems raises the risk of abusive behavior.

In general, domestic violence cuts across all racial, religious, and socioeconomic lines, frequently affecting otherwise "normal" people who are able to control their behavior at work and in other public settings. Within the privacy of their homes, however, abusive individuals leave their mark on their spouses or partners and their children.

Battered Partners

Battering is a continuum of violent and controlling behaviors that may lead to physical injury. In general, women are the ones most frequently battered among married and cohabiting couples. The man's abusive behavior is considered by most experts to represent an attempt to exercise control over his wife or partner—to silence defiance and show who is in charge.[74] A family in which domestic violence occurs may be a socially isolated one in which there are few outside social controls on the abusive behavior. In addition, it may be difficult for people outside the family to detect abusive behaviors. Abusive men often appear to be friendly, warm, outgoing, and helpful. Their controlling behavior tends to be focused on their partners and sometimes their children.[75]

Abusive individuals have often been victims of or witnesses to abuse as children and as a result consider such violence and abuse a normal part of family life, and the same may be true of their victims. Moreover, abused people often find it very difficult to leave an abusive situation. They may hope that things will get better or, among women in particular, find themselves in a precarious financial position that makes leaving virtually impossible.

Abusive behavior does not stop of its own accord. If both partners recognize the problem and seek professional counseling, it may be possible for them to work out their differences nonviolently and learn to express anger and frustration in ways that are not destructive. In many cases, however, battered partners and their children need to get out of an abusive situation, at least temporarily. Various community services are available for victims of domestic violence. Many communities have set up 24-hour telephone hot lines and shelters for victims of abuse. Support groups for both the abused and the abusers can also be found in some communities. Low-cost legal services are sometimes available to help victims file complaints, get restraining orders, and arrange for custody of children and financial support. Other services include vocational counseling, assistance in finding a job and a place to live, and referrals to social service agencies. The important thing is for the abused person to take action and get out of an abusive situation before worse injury occurs.

Child Abuse

Although most experts on child development do not recommend physical punishment of children, many parents discipline their children by spanking or verbally chastising them. A verbal dressing-down or occasional spanking does not make a parent a child abuser, especially when the parent is responding to a stressful situation in which the child seemed to be in danger. Some parents, however, lose control and seriously abuse their children. In a 1985 survey nearly 11 percent of the parents questioned admitted using severe violence against their children, including hitting, kicking, beating, threatening, and using knives or guns.[76] A 1989 study showed that about 15 percent of the children in America were the victims of violent abuse.[77] Many children are also victims of severe psychological or emotional abuse and neglect.

It is easy to label all child abusers as "sick" people, but a wide variety of people end up abusing their children when the stresses in their lives become intolerable. Some of the main risk factors have already been discussed in this chapter. There is, for instance, a strong relationship between poverty, unemployment, and violence toward children.[78] Other risk factors have also been associated with child abuse. For example, childhood health and developmental problems such as disability, congenital defects, and early childhood illnesses appear to increase the risk for maltreatment; families in which corporal punishment is sanctioned or encouraged also appear to be at greater risk.[79] Research has shown that over one-third of all cases of child abuse and neglect are associated with parental alcohol abuse.[80]

Everyone needs to be alert to the signs of child abuse. All states now have laws requiring health professionals to report suspected cases of child abuse to child welfare authorities. As a result, physicians as well as teachers, neighbors, and family friends are more likely to report signs of child abuse than they were a few years ago. Unfortunately, child welfare agencies are understaffed and are often unable to respond as they should.

When a family is under great stress, friends and neighbors can help reduce the potential for abusive behavior by offering to care for the children or trying to reduce the family's stress by other means. Parents can get help in a number of ways if they feel they are reaching the breaking point. Many communities have crisis intervention hot lines where parents who realize that they are losing control can call for immediate help. There is also a national self-help group—Parents Anonymous—in which abusive parents try to help one another overcome their tendencies toward violent behavior against their children.

The full extent of spousal violence is not known, but estimates include the following:

1. *Fifty percent of married couples experience violence at some time in their marriage.*
2. *Sixteen percent of married couples have at least one "violent" fight a year.*
3. *Ten percent of married couples have frequent episodes of violence.*
4. *Four percent of wives are severely beaten by their husbands, in many cases repeatedly.*

Another type of child abuse— sexual abuse—is even more widespread than violence. Some estimates suggest that up to one-third of all girls and one-sixth of all boys experience at least some molestation as they are growing up. Sexual abuse is discussed in Chapter 8.

Developing Successful Relationships

In all areas related to marriage, parenthood, and other close relationships, there have been changes in how people feel and live compared with the situation just 30 or 40 years ago. Moreover, marriage and other intimate relationships are still in a state of transition. Part of the challenge of developing and maintaining healthy and happy relationships today is learning to cope with these changes and deal with the problems and conflicts that arise.

Building a Lasting Relationship

One psychiatrist has written that "the quest for intimacy is fraught with difficulty."[81] Mutual caring and cooperation, communication about feelings, and commitment to another person often seem difficult to achieve. Nevertheless, many people manage to build successful and lasting relationships. There is no simple formula for building a healthy relationship; the people who are most successful ultimately find their own solutions to the challenges of intimacy. There are, however, certain qualities that one must bring to a relationship in order to make intimacy and emotional satisfaction possible. Among these qualities are the following.[82]

- A strong sense of identity. Lasting relationships are built by people who can say, "This is who I am, this is what I need, and this is what I have to offer."
- An ability to be mutually supportive and leave room for oneself and one's partner to grow emotionally and intellectually.
- A knowledge of how to give and accept love and an understanding that love must be worked for and earned.
- An accurate and realistic perception of one's partner.
- A willingness to loosen ties with one's original family.
- A capacity to take criticism, express and share emotions, and argue fairly and effectively.
- A willingness to share power. A relationship in which power is shared in a setting of cooperation, relaxation, and good humor creates an atmosphere in which love and trust can thrive.
- A commitment to keeping the lines of communication open and resolving differences together.

Lasting relationships develop over years of mutual exchanges and unselfish commitment. (Myrleen Ferguson/PhotoEdit)

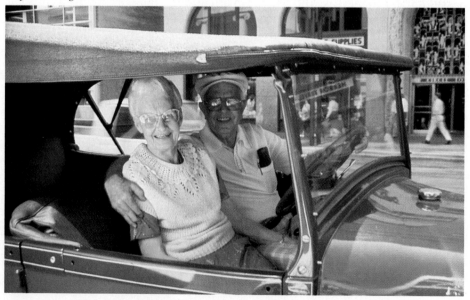

Relationships, Dependency, and Self-Efficacy

Just how concerned should people be with the needs of others? If people put their own needs first, are they exhibiting healthy self-efficacy or displaying selfishness that will prevent them from having strong, close relationships? Two points of view on these questions follow. The first speaker argues that in a healthy, satisfying relationship, people attend to each other's needs. The second says that relationships are better if people take responsibility for their own needs and help others take similar responsibility for theirs.

Meeting Each Other's Needs Builds Strong Relationships

Human beings need to feel wanted; people also need to feel that others care about them. These needs are the basis of any close personal relationship, whether the people involved are friends, relatives, or lovers. If two people are determined to be self-sufficient, what is the point of their relationship with each other?

Most people want to share in their marriages or other intimate partnerships as well as in their close relationships with family members and friends. Maintaining close relationships of all kinds requires sensitivity to each other's needs and preferences. This often means putting the other person's needs ahead of one's own plans. If all people felt that they should take care of their own affairs first, their emotional connections with other people would not be very strong.

Maintaining marriages, friendships, and other close relationships requires hard work and commitment, a willingness not only to stay together during good times but to help each other through hard times as well. Most people have more to give at some times than at others; this is true of emotional resources and time as well as material resources. If people have friends who need assistance or support, friendship dictates that they should give that help. Their needs may mean that they are unable to give back much in return. Later on, however, they may have more to give and may be able to meet major needs of your own.

Over time, in a healthy relationship, the giving and taking even out more or less. Without keeping score of who has done what for whom, partners in a successful relationship usually find that if they give when giving is needed, they are also cared for in their times of need.

Without Taking Care of Oneself, One Cannot Take Care of a Relationship

People who regularly sacrifice their own needs and plans to help others are destroying their lives, and they may be harming their friends, too. Such relationships are not healthy and have been described as codependent relationships. They can lead to dissatisfaction and resentment on both sides and help no one in the long run.

For example, if parents continually give money and other kinds of help to their adult offspring, the children may not learn to live independently of the parents; too much help from the parents may keep the "children" from growing up. Similarly, people's efforts to help their peers or even their spouses can backfire by making them less able to take responsibility for themselves.

Rather than strengthening the positive feelings in the relationship, such help may actually destroy it. People may come to resent those whom they have helped and blame them for their own problems if their needs go unmet. At the same time, the people on whom you have been focused may resent you for taking too much control over their lives. Thus, instead of strengthening relationships, focusing primarily on the needs of others may actually threaten them.

People will have more respect for each other and for themselves if each person in a relationship assumes full responsibility for his or her own well-being. This mutual respect makes for a stronger, healthier relationship.

What is your opinion? Do you think relationships are stronger when people can meet each other's needs? Would you agree instead that having one's needs taken care of by someone else is destructive in a relationship? If the truth is somewhere in the middle, can you explain when meeting others' needs is destructive and when it can enhance a relationship?

Includes ideas from Carol Tavris, "Do Codependency Theories Explain Women's Unhappiness—or Exploit Their Insecurities?" *Vogue* (December 1989): 220–226; Gail Rosenblum, "When Johnny Comes Marching Home," *New Choices* (October 1989): 54–57.

- An ability to have fun. Adult responsibilities can become oppressive if people are unable to retreat together occasionally into fun, fantasy, and laughter.
- A respect for and commitment to the other person, which requires a shift in focus from *me* to *we*.

Problems in Intimate Relationships

There are several potential problem areas in every marriage or other intimate relationship. Being aware of these possible areas of conflict can help people understand and resolve difficulties when they arise. Some of the most common problems are related to notions of intimacy, the division of labor, money, and sex.

Differing Ideas of Intimacy Many researchers have found that women and men today have differing ideas about what intimacy is and should be.[83] As a result, they often enter a relationship with differing expectations about what it should be like and what they will get from it. These conflicting expectations can lead to trouble.

In the United States women tend to be more expressive of their emotions than men are and look for greater emotional warmth and expressiveness in a relationship than many men are comfortable giving them. Men tend to express their sense of intimacy through practical help, shared activities, sex, and economic support. Such differences help explain why women complain that men do not deal with feelings and why men complain that they do not understand what women want from them.[84]

Division of Labor The increase over the last few decades in the number of women who work outside the home has made the division of labor a greater source of conflict in relationships. Couples often find that it is necessary for both partners to work, yet the woman most frequently retains the responsibility for housework and child care. Studies have shown that women normally do two to three times more household work than their husbands do, while for the most part men have taken on only slightly more of the domestic responsibilities even when their partners are employed full-time. Also, men still tend to do the more occasional and nonroutine tasks, such as trash removal, yard work, and repairs, while women do the more repetitive, routine, and never-ending tasks, such as cleaning, shopping, child care, and laundry. Thus, working outside the home has become a major source of stress for many women, except when they feel their partners are doing a fair share of the routine domestic tasks.[85]

Money Money can be an explosive issue in any relationship, especially a marriage. The amount of money a couple has may not be a problem. How they arrive at decisions on how money should be spent, however, can be major sources of conflict. Unresolved differences about spending and saving habits can cause real troubles in a relationship. The issue of how much each partner makes is also a potential problem area. Despite society's changing ideas of sexual equality, most men are still very uncomfortable if their wives make the same amount of money they do or more. Even many women tend to minimize their financial contributions to a relationship, although a growing number are bothered by the view that the wife's contribution is less important.[86]

This situation is made more extreme because gender discrimination still exists in the American job market. Women are concentrated in lower-paid service jobs; and those who work full-time are paid only about 60 percent of what men are paid.[87] Political pressures are causing a change in this situation, but couples should recognize that though a woman may not earn as much money as her partner, that does not mean she is working less hard to support the family unit.

Sex   The greater openness about and emphasis on sex in American society may be putting more strain on intimate relationships: couples may feel a conflict between the traditional standards of behavior they learned long ago and pressure to achieve the level of sexual satisfaction suggested by the media and other sources. Although many people now feel that sex is acceptable before or without marriage, in recent years there has been a greater stress on faithfulness within a marriage or other type of relationship.[88] When a couple do not agree on the sexual issues that are troubling them, their relationship is headed for trouble.

Coping with Problem Areas   Wherever the difficulty lies in a relationship, the key to resolving the problem is good communication. Partners must be aware of their problems, be willing to confront them, and be willing to work out a plan together to cope with them. The more a couple work on a problem through give-and-take discussion, the more likely they will be to reach a decision that both can accept.[89] This means that neither partner tries to coerce the other into reaching a decision. Rather, they present their own ideas, listen carefully to the other, and try to reconcile their differences.

Learning to Argue Constructively   Most counselors consider the statement "We never fight" as a sign that a relationship is in jeopardy. It is both human and healthy to disagree occasionally. Strong relationships are built by working through problems, not by avoiding them.[90] Although arguments may be uncomfortable in the short run, the end result is often greater satisfaction in the relationship.

The way in which a couple argues may be the determining factor in whether their arguments produce positive or negative results. For example, expressing anger in an argument is productive, but being stubborn, withdrawn, or whiny can be harmful to the relationship.[91] Researchers have identified three basic types of quarrels—acute, progressive, and habituated—which have practical implications for learning how *not* to fight.[92]

Acute quarrels are usually sharp and loud disagreements; they are common in new relationships when each partner is jockeying for position. Ominously, when the partners are genuinely in love, they may hide their anger and resentment to avoid hurting each other. Built-up resentments may then explode unpredictably and with force. The point is that couples should try to ventilate their anger early, when it will do less damage.

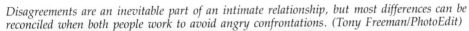

Disagreements are an inevitable part of an intimate relationship, but most differences can be reconciled when both people work to avoid angry confrontations. (Tony Freeman/PhotoEdit)

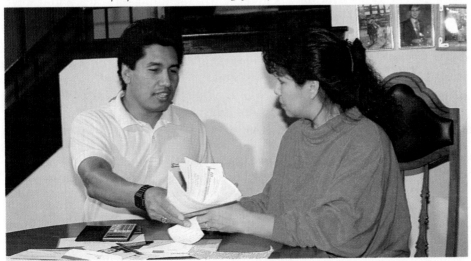

Quarrels become *progressive* when couples fail to focus on their differences and make the necessary adjustments. Conflicts blend into one another and ultimately snowball into a verbal brawl in which each partner points out the other's weaknesses. Even after the quarrel ends, scars remain. To safeguard a relationship, it is best to try to keep conflicts from festering in this way.

Habituated conflict results when couples recognize that there are some areas in the relationship on which they will never agree. It is often best to sidestep these problem areas as much as possible and try to avoid becoming overly emotional when they arise. If there are not too many of these unresolved areas of disagreement and if they are not important ones, the relationship may not suffer at all.

Moving toward Better Relationships

Most people today would prefer to have a fair, equitable relationship that produces satisfaction and happiness. A vital element in building a good relationship is accepting responsibility. People need to recognize what they are doing, how it affects the partner, and whether it is good or bad for the relationship. One study showed that when spouses took greater responsibility for the negative things in a marriage than their partners attributed to them, their marriages were more satisfying.[93]

Another important factor in a successful relationship is that the partners be aware of and responsive to each other's expectations and needs. For example, to develop greater intimacy in a relationship, some partners may need to express more warmth and tenderness, while others may need to participate more actively in the spouse's interests and activities. Couples may also need to talk more about their sexual needs and desires and be willing to compromise about sexual matters. While such actions may go against what people have learned, change and compromise are necessary to make relationships work.[94]

Compromise and adaptation are also needed as relationships change and mature. As relationships season with time and experience, expectations may change. People may find that their sexual needs, their relationships with their children, and their intellectual, emotional, and social needs are different as well. To maintain healthy and successful relationships over time, it is necessary to reevaluate a relationship continually to determine where it is, where it is going, and how it can be improved or maintained.

In a time when marriage and other intimate relationships are in a state of transition, it may take a little more work to build a healthy, satisfying long-term relationship. The end result, however, can be a relationship that is as happy and rewarding as the more traditional ones of the past, perhaps even more so. The important thing is to recognize the difficulties, work to resolve them, and remain optimistic about the possibilities.

Chapter Summary

- Intimate relationships satisfy a number of emotional needs, including intimacy, reassurance of worth, a sense of support, and nurturance.
- Barriers to intimate relationships include physical unattractiveness, a fear of rejection, shyness, and clinging to traditional sex-role norms.
- The roles of husband and wife are not as clearly defined as in the past; many husbands and wives are exhibiting greater flexibility in their roles.

- People today marry for a variety of reasons, such as financial security, an acceptable framework for sexual relations, escape from an unhappy home life, and avoidance of loneliness.
- In assessing compatibility, people try to measure their own qualities against those of the other person, look for compatible beliefs and interests, and evaluate how the other person handles responsibility, reacts to disappointment, and copes with problems.

- Some people choose to remain single because they value freedom and independence and do not view marriage as essential for financial security or sexual gratification.
- Cohabitation may help people discover whether they can handle a mature relationship and are compatible; people who live together, however, may experience many of the same problems that confront married couples.
- Many people see divorce as a viable alternative to an unsatisfactory marriage, but divorce may be financially and emotionally difficult for the family.
- In recent years more couples have chosen to remain childless, feeling that life can be rewarding and rich without children; nonetheless, most couples choose to have children.
- Parents have the primary responsibility for fostering their children's healthy development. Prenatal care and the provision of adequate nutrition, exercise, and medical attention are essential for children's physical health. Love, acceptance, trust, and autonomy also are important for emotional health. Parents stimulate their children's intellectual growth by offering choices, providing stimulation, and encouraging new experiences and discoveries. Children learn socialization skills by watching their parents and abiding by parental rules. Spiritual development is fostered when parents encourage the development of a value system, a sense of self-efficacy, and a feeling of purpose in life.
- Although mothers have traditionally provided the majority of child care, some fathers are taking increased responsibility in this area.
- When they investigate child care alternatives, parents should consider the safety of the environment, the care giver's ability to communicate with and provide adequate supervision and stimulation for the child, and the care giver's reliability.
- Single parents often face financial pressures, have to deal with child problems alone, and must juggle work, child care, and their own emotional needs.

- Domestic violence is associated with a pattern of abuse in the abuser's background, low socioeconomic status, social and environmental stressors, and a lack of social support systems.
- Women are the most frequent victims of battering; a man's abusive behavior represents an attempt to exercise control and silence defiance. Battering often occurs in socially isolated families and is sometimes difficult for outsiders to detect. Abused people often find it difficult to leave such a situation because of insecurity and fears of financial problems.
- Child abuse is a significant problem today; it is sometimes associated with poverty and unemployment, and child abusers were often abused as children themselves. Child abuse may be physically and emotionally traumatic for the victim.
- Lasting relationships are enhanced by a strong sense of identity, mutual support and flexibility, a capacity to take criticism and share emotions, a willingness to share power, open lines of communication, respect and commitment, and an ability to have fun.
- Different ideas about intimacy, conflicts over the division of labor, decisions about spending money, and sexual conflicts may all put great pressure on a relationship.
- Acute quarrels, in which disagreements are sharp and loud, are not unhealthy unless the partners hide their anger and keep their feelings pent up. Progressive quarrels, in which couples fail to focus on differences and make adjustments, can fester and endanger a relationship. Habituated conflicts are based on areas of conflict about which couples can never agree; these areas should be avoided, and the partners should not become overly emotional when they arise.
- As relationships change over time, people need to compromise and adapt to new situations and expectations; healthy relationships involve continual reevaluation and give-and-take on the part of both partners.

Key Terms

Cohabitation (page 175)

References

1. *1990 Information Please Almanac* (Boston: Houghton Mifflin).
2. Susan Sprecher and Kathleen McKinney, "Barriers in the Initiation of Intimate Heterosexual Relationships and Strategies for Intervention," *Journal of Social Work and Human Sexuality* 5, no. 2 (Spring–Summer 1987): 97–110.

3. Judith L. Fischer et al., "Marital Status and Career Stage Influences on Social Networks of Young Adults," *Journal of Marriage and the Family* 51 (May 1989): 521–534.

4. James C. Coleman, *Intimate Relationships, Marriage and Family* (Indianapolis: Bobbs-Merrill, 1984).

5. Sprecher and McKinney, op. cit.

6. Fischer et al., op. cit.

7. Based on Stephen R. Marks, "Toward a Systems Theory of Marital Quality," *Journal of Marriage and the Family* 51 (February 1989): 15–26.

8. William H. Masters et al., *Human Sexuality*, 3d ed. (Glenview, Ill.: Scott, Foresman, 1988).

9. Ibid.

10. Ibid.

11. G. R. Adams and T. L. Huston, "Social Perception of Middle Aged Persons Varying in Physical Attractiveness," *Developmental Psychology* II (1975): 657–658.

12. Karen K. Dion et al., "What Is Beautiful Is Good," *Journal of Personality and Social Psychology* 24 (1972): 285–290.

13. Elaine Walster and G. W. Walster, *A New Look at Love* (Reading, Mass.: Addison-Wesley, 1978).

14. S. B. Ortner and H. Whitehead (eds.), *Sexual Meanings: The Cultural Construction of Gender and Sexuality* (New York: Cambridge University Press, 1981).

15. John D. Williams and Arthur P. Jacoby, "The Effects of Premarital Heterosexual and Homosexual Experience on Dating and Marriage Desirability," *Journal of Marriage and the Family* 51 (May 1989): 489–597.

16. Bernard I. Murstein, "Mate Selection in the 1970s," *Journal of Marriage and the Family* 42, no. 4 (November 1980): 777–792.

17. Daniel Goleman, "Study Defines Major Sources of Conflict between Sexes: Differences Are Found in What Disturbs Men and Women," *New York Times* (June 13, 1989): C1, C14.

18. Bernard I. Murstein (ed.), *Theories of Attraction and Love* (New York: Springer, 1971).

19. Discussion of changing attitudes in this section taken from Arland Thornton, "Changing Attitudes toward Family Issues in the United States," *Journal of Marriage and the Family* 51 (May 1989): 873–893.

20. Coleman, op. cit.

21. "Americans Are Marrying Later Than They Used To," *NCHS Monthly Vital Statistics Report* 38, no. 2 (Supplement) (April 3, 1990): 4.

22. National Center for Health Statistics, "Annual Summary of Births, Marriages, Divorces, and Deaths: United States, 1988," *Monthly Vital Statistics Report* 37, no. 13 (Hyattsville, Md.: U.S. Public Health Service, 1989).

23. Thornton, op. cit.

24. Ibid.

25. M. Sheils et al., "A Portrait of America," *Newsweek* (January 17, 1983): 20–32.

26. Thornton, op. cit.

27. Coleman, op. cit.

28. Eleanor D. Macklin, "Nonmarital Heterosexual Cohabitation," in *Marriage: Creating a Partnership*, 2d ed., Chesser and Gray (eds.) (Dubuque, Iowa: Kendall-Hunt, 1979): 67.

29. Thornton, op. cit.

30. Katherine Trent and Scott J. South, "Structural Determinants of the Divorce Rate: A Cross-Societal Analysis," *Journal of Marriage and the Family* 51 (May 1989): 393.

31. National Center for Health Statistics, op. cit.

32. Sara McLanahan and Karen Booth, "Mother-Only Families: Problems, Prospects, and Politics," *Journal of Marriage and the Family* 51 (August 1989): 557.

33. Lawrence A. Kurdek, "Relationship Quality for Newly Married Husbands and Wives: Marital History, Stepchildren, and Individual-Difference Predictors," *Journal of Marriage and the Family* 51 (November 1989): 1053–1064.

34. Judith Wallerstein and Joan Kelly, *Surviving the Breakup: How Children and Parents Cope with Divorce* (New York: Basic Books, 1980); Wallerstein and Kelly, "The Effects of Parental Divorce: Experiences of the Child in Later Latency," *American Journal of Orthopsychiatry* 48 (1979): 256–269; Wallerstein and Kelly, "The Effects of Parental Divorce: The Adolescent Experience," in *The Child in His Family: Children at Psychiatric Risk*, vol. 3, A. J. Koopernik (ed.) (New York: Wiley, 1974).

35. Thornton, op. cit.

36. Thornton, op. cit.

37. National Center for Health Statistics, op. cit.

38. Ibid.

39. J. Evoy, *The Rejected: Psychological Consequences of Parental Rejection* (University Park: Pennsylvania State University Press, 1982).

40. Ernest N. Jouriles et al., "Interspousal Aggression, Marital Discord, and Child Problems," *Journal of Consulting and Clinical Psychology* 57, no. 3 (1989): 453–455.

41. Benjamin Bloom, *Stability and Change in Human Characteristics* (New York: Wiley, 1964): 68.

42. Willard W. Hartup, "Social Relationships and Their Developmental Significance," *American Psychologist* 44, no. 2 (February 1989): 120–126.

43. Discussion of discipline styles based on Ellen Greenberger and Wendy A. Goldberg, "Work, Parenting, and the Socialization of Children," *Developmental Psychology* 25, no. 1 (1989) 22–35.

44. Ibid.

45. Victor Frankl, *Man's Search for Meaning*, 3d ed. (New York: Touchstone, 1984).

46. Richard B. Felson and Mary A. Zielinski, "Children's Self-Esteem and Parental Support," *Journal of Marriage and the Family* 51 (August 1989): 727–735.

47. Jerome Kagen and Howard A. Moss, *Birth to Maturity* (New York: Wiley, 1962).

48. Richard Q. Bell, "Parent, Child, and Reciprocal Influences," *American Psychology* 34, no. 10 (October 1979): 821–826.

49. Debra Umberson, "Relationships with Children: Explaining Parents' Psychological Well-Being," *Journal of Marriage and the Family* 51 (November 1989): 999–1012.

50. Linda Thompson and Alexis J. Walker, "Gender in Families: Women and Men in Marriage, Work, and Parenthood," *Journal of Marriage and the Family* 51 (November 1989): 845–871.

51. *1990 Information Please Almanac*, op. cit.

52. Thompson and Walker, op. cit.

53. Pamela Kotler and Deborah Lee Wingard, "The Effect of Occupations, Marital, and Parental Roles on

Mortality: The Alameda County Study," *American Journal of Public Health* 79, no. 5 (May 1989): 607–612.

54. Ellen Greenberger and Wendy A. Goldberg, "Work, Parenting, and the Socialization of Children," *Developmental Psychology* 25, no. 1 (1989): 22–35.

55. Thompson and Walker, op. cit.

56. Ibid.

57. Ibid.

58. David Lynn, "Father and America in Transition," in *Family in Transition,* 2d ed., Arlene S. Skolnick and Jerome H. Skolnick (eds.) (Boston: Little, Brown, 1977): 380–384.

59. Hartup, op. cit.

60. S. N. Wellborn, "When School Kids Come Home to an Empty House," *U.S. News and World Report* (September 14, 1981): 42–47.

61. Sara McLanahan and Karen Booth, "Mother-Only Families: Problems, Prospects, and Politics," *Journal of Marriage and the Family* 51 (August 1989): 557.

62. *1990 Information Please Almanac,* op. cit.

63. McLanahan and Booth, op. cit., pp. 558–559.

64. Carolyn Webster-Stratton, "The Relationship of Marital Support, Conflict, and Divorce to Parent Perceptions, Behaviors, and Childhood Conduct Problems," *Journal of Marriage and the Family* 51 (May 1989): 417–430.

65. McLanahan and Booth, op. cit., p. 563.

66. David Mechanic and Stephen Hansell, "Divorce, Family Conflict, and Adolescents' Well Being," *Journal of Health and Social Behavior* 30 (March 1989): 105–116.

67. J. C. Coleman and A. L. Glaros, *Contemporary Psychology and Effective Behaviors,* 5th ed. (Glenview, Ill.: Scott, Foresman, 1983); Coleman, op. cit.

68. M. A. Strauss, *Behind Closed Doors: Violence in the American Family* (Garden City, N.Y.: Doubleday, 1980).

69. T. W. Coleman and D. R. Cressey, *Social Problems* (New York: Harper & Row, 1980).

70. James A. Mercy and Linda E. Saltzman, "Fatal Violence among Spouses in the United States, 1976–1985," *American Journal of Public Health* 79 (1989): 595–599.

71. D. Daro and L. Mitchel, *Deaths Due to Maltreatment Soar: The Results of the 1986 Annual Fifty State Survey* (Chicago: National Center on Child Abuse Prevention Research, National Committee for Prevention of Child Abuse, 1987), cited in National Committee for Injury Prevention and Control, "Child Abuse and Sexual Assault, Injury Prevention: Meeting the Challenge," *American Journal of Preventive Medicine* (1989): 213–222.

72. M. Meyers and J. Bernier, *Preventing Child Abuse: A Resource for Policymakers and Advocates* (Boston: Massachusetts Committee for Children and Youth, November 1987), cited in "Child Abuse and Child Sexual Assault, Injury Prevention," op. cit.

73. Richard Gelles, "Violence in the Family: A Review of Research in the Seventies," *Journal of Marriage and the Family* 42 (November 1980): 873–885.

74. Thompson and Walker, op. cit.

75. D. Adams, "Stages of Anti-Sexist Awareness and Change for Men Who Batter," presented at the 92d annual convention of the American Psychological Association, Toronto, Canada, 1974, cited in National Committee for Injury Prevention and Control, "Domestic Violence, Injury Prevention: Meeting the Challenge," *American Journal of Preventive Medicine* (1989): 223–232.

76. P. A. Langan and C. A. Innes, "Preventing Domestic Violence against Women," (Washington, D.C.: U.S. Department of Justice, Bureau of Justice Statistics, 1986), cited in "Domestic Violence, Injury Prevention," op. cit.

77. Robert L. Hampton et al., "Is Violence in Black Families Increasing? A Comparison of 1975 and 1985 National Survey Rates," *Journal of Marriage and the Family* 51 (November 1989): 970.

78. Ibid., p. 972.

79. "Child Abuse and Sexual Assault, Injury Prevention," op. cit., p. 216.

80. Louis J. West, *Alcoholism and Related Problems* (Englewood Cliffs, N.J.: Prentice-Hall, 1984).

81. Theodore I. Rubin, "Intimacy and Cultural Pressures," *American Journal of Psychoanalysis* 49, no. 1 (1989): 1.

82. Arthur Burton, "Marriage without Failure," in *Marriage: Creating a Partnership,* 2d ed., B. J. Chesser and A. A. Gray (eds.) (Dubuque, Iowa: Kendall-Hunt, 1979): 81–86; Edward Waring et al., "Dimensions of Intimacy in Marriage," *Psychiatry* 44 (May 1981): 169–175; W. R. Beavers, "A Theoretical Basis for Family Evaluation," in *No Single Thread: Psychological Health in Family Systems,* J. M. Lewis et al. (eds.) (New York: Brunner/Mazel, 1976): 46–82.

83. Thompson and Walker, op. cit., pp. 846–847.

84. Ibid.

85. Ibid., p. 858.

86. Ibid., p. 864.

87. McLanahan and Booth, op. cit., p. 559.

88. Thornton, op. cit., p. 889.

89. Deborah D. Godwin and John Scanzoni, "Couple Consensus during Marital Joint Decision-Making: A Context, Press, Outcome Model," *Journal of Marriage and the Family* 51 (November 1989): 943–956.

90. John M. Gottman and Lowell J. Krokoff, "Marital Interaction and Satisfaction: A Longitudinal View," *Journal of Consulting and Clinical Psychology* 57, no. 1 (1989): 47–52.

91. Ibid.

92. G. R. Leslie and E. M. Leslie, *Marriage in a Changing World* (New York: Wiley, 1977): 154–156.

93. Frank D. Fincham and Thomas N. Bradbury, "Perceived Responsibility for Marital Events: Egocentric or Partnercentric Bias?" *Journal of Marriage and the Family* 51 (February 1989): 27–36.

94. Thompson and Walker, op. cit., p. 847.

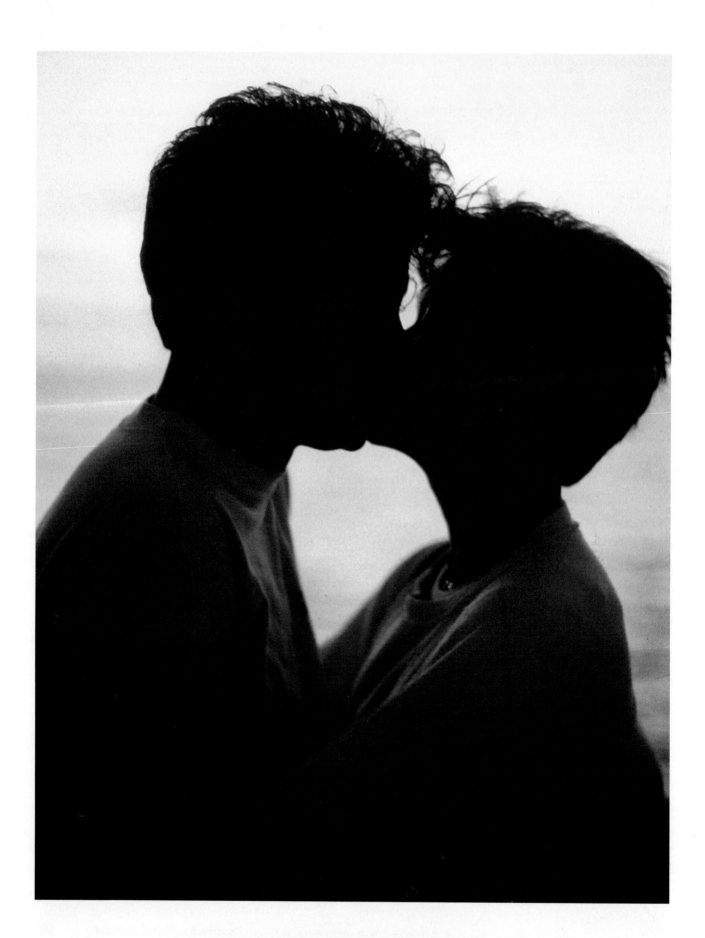

Chapter 8

Human Sexuality

To Guide Your Reading

When you have studied this chapter, you should be able to:

- Distinguish between sex and sexuality and discuss the basis of sexuality and sexual behavior.

- Discuss the origin of attitudes toward sex and explain how those attitudes may change over time.

- Identify and describe the erogenous zones and the major external structures of the male and female anatomy.

- Describe the four general stages of human sexual response and explain any differences between male and female responses.

- Explain the various forms of sexual expression and discuss why responsible sexual expression is important.

- Identify and explain various male and female sexual dysfunctions and discuss methods for dealing with sexual dysfunction.

From commercials on television to romance novels to appreciative glances on the street, people are bombarded by messages about sex and sexuality. The way people think and feel about sex and sexuality is woven into the fabric of their daily lives and has a profound impact on their personalities and their relationships with other people.

What exactly is the difference between sex and sexuality? Essentially, **sex** usually refers to either gender or the way in which people physically express affection or erotic feelings, sometimes culminating in sexual intercourse. **Sexuality** refers to the ways in which people's gender—male or female—is integrated into their emotional, intellectual, social, and spiritual lives, in other words, what it means to be a man or woman in society.

Sexuality includes not only actions and attitudes directly connected with sex but also behaviors quite removed from it, such as assertiveness versus submissiveness in work or other activities. Gender is not the only factor in sexuality; sexuality also derives from what people have been taught in the past to think and feel about being male or female and how they react to the expectations of others.

sex—*gender (maleness or femaleness); the physical expression of affectionate or erotic feeling which sometimes culminates in sexual intercourse.*

sexuality—*masculinity or femininity; the ways in which gender—male or female—is integrated into a person's personality and behavior.*

The Basis of Sexuality

People tend to act in certain ways because of a variety of factors, some biological and others learned. In men, the sex hormone testosterone may be a factor in an increased competitiveness toward other men. However, men may act in certain other ways because of what they have learned since childhood: they may, for example, feel particularly drawn to physical sports and other active pursuits rather than more passive activities. There are still other ways in which men behave because of social pressure, such as acting in accordance with certain masculine roles.

The biological symbol for male ♂ represents the spear and shield of Mars, the god of war. The symbol for female ♀ represents the hand mirror of Venus, the goddess who represents love and fertility.

These types of behavior reflect aspects of men's personalities that are related to gender. It is often difficult, however, to tell whether a particular "male" behavior comes from a man's biological makeup, childhood upbringing, or response to social expectations.

Similarly, women may act in certain ways because of the sex hormones estrogen and progesterone, so-called feminine behaviors learned since childhood, and adherence to societal expectations. Once again, it may be difficult to determine whether an aspect of women's sexuality is a result of being "born that way," being brought up that way, or feeling pressured by other people to act in a certain manner. For example, the traditional view is that women do not express anger through physical aggression, but there is still disagreement about how much of this is biological, how much is learned, and how much results from societal or cultural expectations. In fact, it is most likely that these are all significant factors—depending on the individual woman.

Some inborn differences in the way male and female babies behave are noticeable shortly after birth, although these differences are not as great as people once assumed.[1] Such sexual differentiation, which begins during prenatal development, is largely controlled by genes and hormones.[2] But then, from the first announcement of a baby's gender, society imposes different expectations that depend on which gender the baby is. The baby gets a girl's name or a boy's name, a pink blanket or a blue one. The parents tend to talk more with a baby girl and roughhouse more with a baby boy. In most instances *core gender identity*—the fundamental sense of oneself as a male or female—is established by age 3, and children behave in ways appropriate to their sex.[3]

Although core gender identity is established at an early age, sexuality should not be thought of as something which is set unchangeably when people are young. Teenagers express their sexuality very differently from people who are middle-aged, and the sexuality expressed in middle age is different from the sexuality of older individuals.

The tradition of treating male and female babies differently may start with different colored outfits, but by the end of the first year of life it may contribute to marked differences in behavior. (Wayne Floyd/Unicorn Stock Photos)

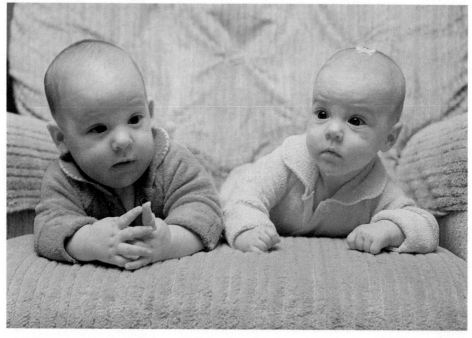

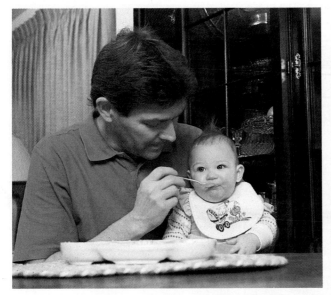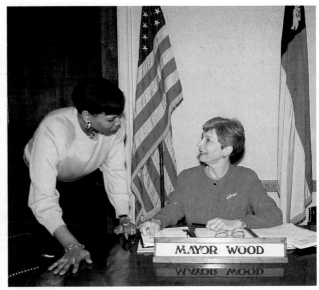

While many people are still surprised and even threatened by changes in sex roles, society as a whole is beginning to accept that men can be nuturing, and women can make tough decisions. This enriches the lives of both sexes. (Barry Levy/Profiles West; Tyler Cox)

Today the social conditioning that shaped the "typical" man and woman of the past has changed somewhat. More mothers are working, and they provide different role models than did the homemakers of several decades ago; children can now see that women have careers, and many little girls are encouraged to become physically active, assertive, and achievement-oriented. Many children also see that their fathers often help with the housework; they do not always have to fit a macho stereotype but can be loving and tender.

These changes have affected the approach of many Americans not only to work and family but also to sexual experience. Some women now feel more free to be sexually assertive, and some men feel more free to express their emotional needs in a relationship. Men and women are also becoming better able to communicate their needs and desires to each other in an honest and open manner.

Such changes, however, are also leading to tensions both within society and for individuals. While some people feel at ease with changing gender roles, others feel considerable discomfort. When behavior conflicts with what was learned in childhood or adolescence, acting according to new expectations may not seem to come naturally. People must decide for themselves what they feel comfortable with and act accordingly. Sexual expression can be an enriching and fulfilling experience, but only if people are fully aware of their attitudes toward sex and sexuality and can make responsible choices based on their individual needs.

Attitudes toward Sex

Like all human behavior, sexual responses are not based on biology alone. People have what might be called a *psychosexual response* that integrates their physical and psychological reactions. The way people feel about themselves and their sexuality also influences how they relate to other people through sex. Thus, sexual behavior is shaped by what people have learned—starting as young children and continuing throughout life—from family members, friends, previous sexual encounters, religious training, and even the mass media with their numerous messages about and images of gender and sexuality.

Figure 8.1 There is still quite a gap between the content of today's sex education curriculum and what teachers feel ought to be included. This graph compares the percentage of teachers who think particular topics should *be taught by the end of the seventh grade and the percentage who are in school districts where the topics* actually *are taught at that level. Overall, however, sex education is gaining support. Eighty-five percent of Americans now approve of having sex education taught in schools, up from 69 percent 25 years ago.*

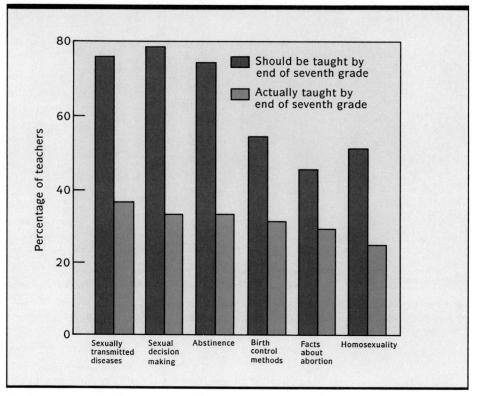

Source: Alan Guttmacher Institute, *Risk and Responsibility: Teaching Sex Education in America's Schools Today,* 1989. With permission.

A major source of sexual learning is sex education classes in school (Figure 8.1). Although still controversial, sex education is generally accepted by a majority of the population, and courses are offered in over three-quarters of the nation's school districts. Recent investigation has shown that such programs do *not*, as once feared, promote early sexual behavior. In fact, some sex education programs are reported to have lessened the incidence of teenage pregnancies in their school districts.[4] Coupled with school-based clinics, therefore, the information-based approach of sex education has had dramatic effects in certain areas of the nation.[5]

So far as feelings are concerned, however, most people do not learn about sex or sexuality directly. Instead, they receive indirect messages from other people—starting with their parents—while observing the way those people act toward each other and the way they feel about their own sexuality. A person may feel ashamed of his or her body, for example, if that person's parents showed extreme embarrassment and anger about nudity, insisting that their children's bodies be well covered and hidden from others. As people grow older, they also learn about sex and sexuality from a variety of sources, including friends; magazines, books, and movies; and advertisements.

Using what they have learned, people begin to shape their own ideas about how men and women should behave sexually, what is right and wrong, and the correct and incorrect way to handle sexual encounters and sexual feelings. Rarely, however, do people talk about how they feel about their bodies and about sex and sexuality: despite the fact that feelings play a crucial role in sexual activity, people often ignore them, almost denying that they exist. This denial may be based on a conflict between sexual activity and feelings and deeply held beliefs and values.

Feelings of guilt may result and cause some people to be uncomfortable about having sex, preventing them from enjoying the experience. Others may deal with this conflict by repressing sexual behavior or feelings completely. Some people reduce their guilt by redefining their behavior; it is common to

Comfort Level

Sex Roles

People's self-esteem is very much affected by their success in measuring up to role expectations—their view of how others think they should behave. Some of the strongest role expectations are connected with sexuality. People want others to admire them as sexual beings and members of their gender—however members of their gender are expected to be.

For example, people often think they are supposed to feel strong attractions to others. The fact is, however, that people of both genders have varied levels of interest in sex: some people put a high priority on sex for its own sake, others value sex primarily for its emotional associations, and some people have relatively less interest in sex. Role expectations are nearly always narrower than the range of real human behavior.

People whose real nature fails to match sex-role expectations often suffer greatly. Having a low interest in sex may cause them to worry that they are homosexual; effeminate behavior in a man or aggressive behavior in a woman may also lead to fears of homosexuality. Homosexuality still carries a major stigma in American society. People not only tend to view it as opposite to their expectations about sexual preference, they also associate it with confusion involving other aspects of sexuality.

Is a man with predominantly feminine interests or a woman whose behavior is masculine necessarily homosexual? Certainly not. Some extremely macho men are gay, and some ultrafeminine women are lesbians. In a study of homosexual and heterosexual men by the Kinsey Institute, 18 percent of the gay men said they had been "very masculine" children. Most had not particularly enjoyed typical girls' games as children. By contrast, 11 percent of the straight men said they had enjoyed typically feminine childhood activities such as playing with dolls.

The way in which parents raise children has little effect on how masculine or feminine the children are or on whether they are straight or homosexual. However, stifling masculine or feminine traits in children may have the unfortunate effect of narrowing and reinforcing the children's expectations about sex roles. When parents reject parts of a child's personality, the child may come to undervalue and try to hide those traits. In fact, the family is one place in which sex-role expectations are developed.

The roots of these expectations are doubtless complex, based in the history of society and its traditional division of labor. But such expectations survive so strongly because the popular media—television, movies, literature, and other sources—bombard people with information about so-called masculine and feminine behavior. The message is that men and women should conform to opposite roles: men should be aggressive, and women should be passive; men should be interested in business and sports, while women should be concerned primarily with caring for their homes and families. Other expectations—for example, the intense part sex should play in people's lives—are also supported by the media.

However, sexuality is, after all, only one component of a full life. A person who has less interest in sex than others have may take greater pleasure in many other aspects of life. A relatively low sex drive is by no means a sure sign of emotional disturbance. Similarly, sexual orientation is only one part of the human personality. Although homosexual people and straight people differ in terms of sexual attraction, people in both groups can be valued for strengths and qualities—such as integrity, sensitivity, and generosity—that have little or nothing to do with sexual orientation.

All people need to know that other people can accept them and love them as they are, regardless of their sexual orientation or whether they conform to the stereotypes of male and female roles. More important, people need to accept themselves as they are and feel comfortable with their sexual personalities rather than judging them against narrow role expectations.

Includes ideas from David Bjorklund and Barbara Bjorklund, "Straight or Gay?" *Parents* (October 1988): 93–98; Elizabeth Allgeier and Albert Allgeier, *Sexual Interactions* (Lexington, Mass.: D C Heath, 1984): 431–484.

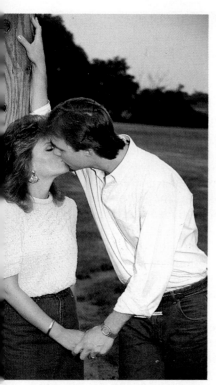
Everyone is sexually aroused in different ways, but kissing is a pleasure for most people. (Eric A. Wessman)

attribute sex to being "carried away at the time" and not really being responsible for one's behavior. Such an attitude may lead people to engage in hazardous sexual behaviors, such as risking pregnancy or disease by not planning for or using appropriate methods of contraception.

Sexual guilt and inner conflicts are not universal, however, and are in any case poor reasons for people to take major risks involving sexual matters. Knowledge, rational thought, and self-appraisal can help people make decisions about these matters that are both comfortable for them and sensible in regard to their lives and futures.

Sexual Anatomy and Arousal

An essential factor in developing a healthy sexuality is an understanding of sexual anatomy and physiology. This will contribute not only to a person's body awareness but also to enhanced communication between sexual partners. Effectively communicating to one's partner what does or does not feel good helps make the sexual experience more pleasurable and gratifying for both individuals.

Basically, of course, the sexual anatomy is the mechanism that enables human beings to reproduce. Chapter 9 presents a fuller account of the internal sex organs and explains how sexual intercourse can lead to reproduction. However, the reproductive aspect of sex is only one part of human sexual activity; another aspect involves the intense sensations and feelings that people experience during sexual activity. These sensations and feelings are part of the erotic qualities associated with the sexual anatomy. This chapter will focus more on the sexual organs that contribute most to the erotic and passionate experience of sex.

Erogenous Zones

erogenous zone—*any area of the body that is related to sexual desire or can be stimulated to produce sexual arousal.*

The human body has many areas called **erogenous zones** that are related to sexual desire or can be stimulated to produce sexual arousal. These erogenous zones include anatomic structures, mostly external, which will be described in the next two sections of this chapter. For men, they include the penis and scrotum; for women, the vulva and clitoris; and for both men and women, the breasts and perineum, a hairless area of skin between the anus and the vulva or scrotum.

The term *erogenous zone* is not very specific. Virtually any part of the body can become associated with sexual desire and produce sexual arousal, and individuals are different in terms of what areas are erogenous for them. For most people, the mouth area is especially reactive; hence the practice of kissing to achieve sexual excitation in this society. People may experience sexual arousal from stimulation of the breasts, the ears, the insides of the thighs, or any other part of the skin. So far as the body is concerned, people can learn to associate almost any part—or any activity, even thought—with sexual arousal. Thus, some people respond sexually to things they see, some to things they hear or even read, and some to touch. Most people react to a variety of stimuli that have an erotic quality, and they often develop a preference for stimulation of particular areas in specific ways. It is a mistake to think that everyone has the same patterns of sexual arousal and that gratifying sex results from merely learning the proper erogenous zones to stimulate. Sex is not—and should not be—just a mechanical process of stimulating the right areas; it requires a more sensitive exploration of the other person's body and a mutual sharing of the sexual experience.

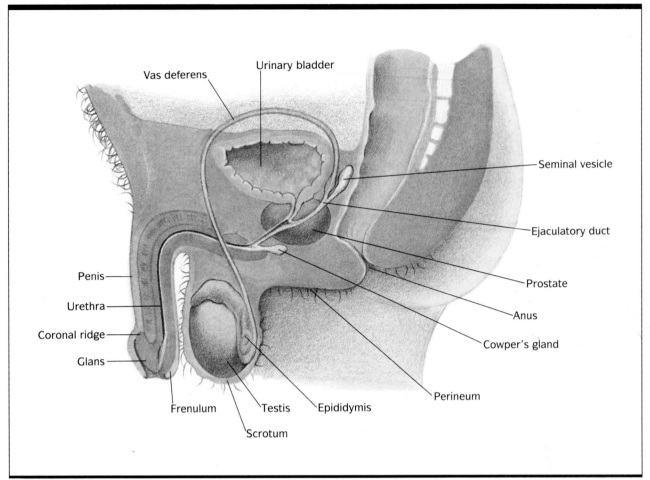

Figure 8.2 These are the anatomical features of the male sex organs. The testes, the male sex glands, are outside the main abdomen; this maintains a lower temperature which seems to favor sperm production.

The Male Sexual Anatomy

Several parts of the male sexual anatomy function not only reproductively but also as erogenous zones that can produce pleasure during sexual arousal (Figure 8.2). These sexual structures, especially the penis, normally respond readily to stimulation.

The Penis The most visible male sexual structure is the **penis,** the external organ of sexual intercourse (and urination). It is the outlet for the **urethra,** the passage through which male reproductive cells (sperm) and urine are discharged from the body. The penis is flaccid (limp) except when sexually aroused. As a man becomes sexually excited, blood rushes to the arteries that supply the penis and the surrounding tissue; the increased blood flow and pressure in the area cause the penis to become erect. The head of the penis—the **glans**—is particularly sensitive, as are the rim of tissue (the **coronal ridge**) between the glans and the shaft of the penis and the triangular region (the **frenulum**) on the underside of the penis.

The Scrotum The **scrotum** is the loose pouch of skin that hangs behind and under the penis. It contains two sets of important male reproductive organs: the testicles, or testes, where sperm are produced, and the epididymis, the long tube behind each testicle where sperm are held until they mature. The contents of the scrotum are so sensitive to touch that sometimes even light caressing can be irritating. Some men find gentle squeezing of the scrotum arousing.

penis—*the external male organ used in sexual intercourse and urination.*

urethra—*the tube from the urinary bladder through which urine is passed out of the body.*

glans—*the head of the penis.*

coronal ridge—*the rim of tissue between the glans and the shaft of the penis.*

frenulum—*the triangular region on the underside of the penis.*

scrotum—*the loose pouch of skin that hangs behind the penis and contains the testicles.*

The Male Internal Sex Organs   In addition to the testes and epididymis, several other organs make up the internal male reproductive system. These organs are all involved with producing sperm cells and transporting them out through the penis (Chapter 9). A connecting tube called the vas deferens leads from each epididymis to the seminal vesicles and the prostate gland, both of which supply fluids that nourish and transport the sperm. Ejaculatory ducts connect the prostate to the urethra in the penis. The Cowper's glands secrete a small amount of fluid which cleanses the urethra before ejaculation.

The Perineum   The virtually hairless area behind the genital organs and in front of the anus is called the **perineum.** Many men find that this area can be stimulated by touch, pressure, and temperature change.

perineum—*a hairless area of skin behind the genital area and in front of the anus.*

The Breasts   A man's breasts can also add to sexual arousal. Although a man's breasts are less sensitive to touch than a woman's, some men find that having their breasts caressed can increase sexual excitement.

The Female Sexual Anatomy

The female sexual anatomy also functions as both a reproductive system and a source of pleasure during sexual arousal (Figure 8.3). The major sexual structures of the human female anatomy are discussed below.

The Vulva   Most of a woman's most sensitive sexual areas are located in the external genital region called the **vulva** (which means "covering"). This area includes the mons veneris and labia. Over the pubic bone is the **mons veneris** (Latin for "mound of Venus"), a cushion of fatty tissue that is covered with skin and hair and contains a rich supply of nerve endings and sweat and oil glands. Many women find the mons extremely sensitive, and its stimulation can produce very pleasurable sensations.

vulva—*the external genital region surrounding the opening of the vagina.*

mons veneris—*a sensitive cushion of fatty tissue covered with skin and hair; it is in the female vulva over the pubic bone.*

labia—*soft, sensitive folds of skin at either end of the opening of the vagina. The outer broad folds are called the* labia majora; *the inner, hairless lips are called the* labia minora.

The two soft, sensitive folds of skin at either side of the opening of the vagina area are called the **labia** (Latin for "lips"). The outer broad folds of skin are called the *labia majora;* inside them are two hairless lips called the *labia minora.* These structures provide protection for the urethra (the tube from the urinary bladder through which urine passes out of the body) and the vagina. The labia have many sensitive nerve endings, and their stimulation can add to a woman's sexual arousal.

The Clitoris   The labia minora meet to form a hood over the **clitoris,** one of a woman's most sensitive sexual organs. For many women the clitoris is the primary focus of sexual arousal.

clitoris—*an extremely sensitive external female sexual organ located under a hood formed by the upper joining of the labia minora.*

vagina—*the canallike structure of the female body that extends from the bottom of the uterus to the vulva; it receives the penis during sexual intercourse and acts as a passageway for a baby during birth.*

The Vagina   The **vagina** is a canallike structure that extends from the vulva inward to the internal sex organs. The vagina receives the penis during sexual intercourse and also acts as a passageway for a baby during birth. The vaginal opening may be narrowed by a circular membrane called the **hymen,** which looks like the shutter of a camera. (This structure usually has a central opening large enough to admit a tampon.) It used to be believed that one could tell if a woman was a virgin by noting whether her hymen was still intact. It is now known, however, that physical activity or the passing of time can cause the hymen to tear even when intercourse has not occurred. If it is still present at the time of first intercourse, the hymen normally stretches or tears to accommodate the penis.

hymen—*a circular membrane that narrows the opening of the vagina in some women who have never had sexual intercourse.*

The vagina is much more than a simple opening: it is a responsive muscular organ that can widen or contract when necessary—a full-sized baby can pass through it at birth, yet during sexual arousal and intercourse it is narrow enough to produce friction with the penis. It is about 4 inches long and has an inner lining of moist membrane, much like the inside of the mouth. It has few

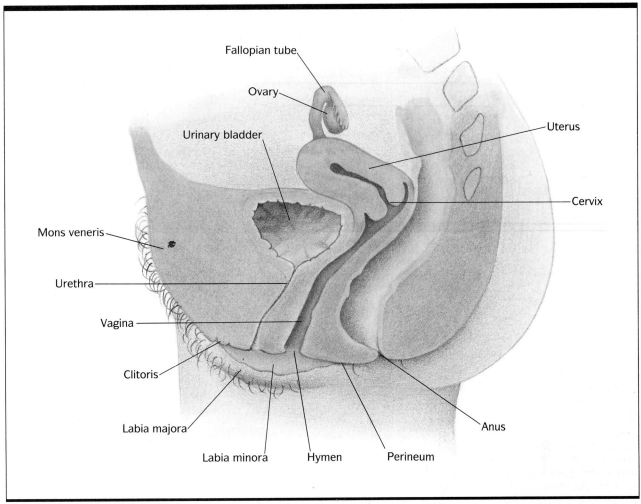

Figure 8.3 *The primary female sexual structures include many external sensory zones as well as the internal reproductive organs, such as the female sex glands (the ovaries).*

sensory nerve endings, except near its opening, so its inner two-thirds is relatively insensitive to touch or pain. During sexual arousal it also secretes a fluid which is visible at the vaginal opening. Researchers do not yet completely understand this fluid, but it seems to provide lubrication that makes intercourse easier and create a more appropriate environment for the movement of sperm into the internal sexual structures.

The Female Internal Sex Organs   At the internal end of the vagina is the uterus, or womb. This is a hollow muscular structure which holds and nourishes the fetus during pregnancy. Its narrow lower end—the cervix—is a firm, smooth knob that can be felt at the upper end of the vagina.

From either side of the uterus, the Fallopian tubes extend to the ovaries, two almond-sized glands that produce female hormones and eggs, or ova. Eggs produced in the ovaries travel through the Fallopian tubes on their way to the uterus (Chapter 9).

The Perineum   A woman's perineum is the hairless area of skin between the back end of the labia and the anus. As with men, this area is sensitive to touch, pressure, and temperature change.

The Breasts   A woman's breasts can also play a role in sexual response. When a woman is sexually excited, the breasts may actually expand slightly, and the nipples may grow firm and erect. Sometimes, however, the nipples may feel sore, bringing pain rather than pleasure.

The Physiology of Sexual Response

Although the male and female sexual responses are considerably different, there are also surprising similarities. Both men and women have the capacity to experience several general stages of sexual response and also to experience similar physiological changes when they are sexually excited.

The physiology of human sexual response was not well understood until the middle of this century, when William Masters and Virginia Johnson conducted extensive studies at their research institute in St. Louis, Missouri. Using human subjects under controlled laboratory conditions, Masters and Johnson produced specific descriptions of the typical physiological and behavioral responses involved in sexual activity. They used electrodes and other laboratory paraphernalia to gather precise quantitative data on bodily changes during coitus and other sexual acts.[6]

In their studies, Masters and Johnson measureed both standard physiological responses—blood pressure, respiration, heartbeat, and temperature—and the specific responses of various sex organs—the penis, scrotum, vagina, and uterus, for example—while "in action." Bodily changes that correlated with sexual activity were then documented.

Masters and Johnson's laboratory work lasted 11 years before they published their findings in Human Sexual Response *in 1966.*

Stages of Sexual Response

The work of Masters and Johnson helped establish a pattern of four general stages that most human beings go through in their sexual response cycle (Figure 8.4). The following is a brief summary of these four stages.[7]

The First Stage: Excitement   Poets have written about the palpitating heart, and Masters and Johnson have confirmed it: when a person is sexually stimulated, the heart beats faster and blood pressure rises. Blood flow to the genital organs increases, a condition known as **vasocongestion.** In addition, a response called **myotonia** causes muscles all over the body to tense with excitement.

vasocongestion—*the increase of blood flow to the genital region during the first stage of sexual excitement.*

myotonia—*a generalized sexual response in which muscles throughout the body have an increase in tension.*

spermatic cords—*muscular structures from which the testicles are suspended within the scrotum.*

In a man, blood congests in the pelvic organs, the spongy tissue in the penis fills with blood, and an erection begins to form. In this phase, the scrotum grows more sensitive and the testicles are drawn closer to the body: the muscles in the **spermatic cords** (the structures from which the testes are suspended within the scrotum) tighten and actually pull in the testes to prepare for eventual ejaculation. Late in the excitement phase the nipples may become erect, although not all men have this response. The intensity of all these responses varies between individuals and circumstances, and these reactions can reverse themselves quickly if circumstances change.

In a woman, muscles tense and the vagina begins to produce lubrication. The clitoris and the tissues around it swell as blood rushes into them. (This phenomenon is subtle; the difference may not be visible.) As sexual stimulation increases and continues, the vagina actually increases in length by 2 or 3 centimeters. At this stage the nipples may also become erect and slightly larger.

The Second Stage: Plateau   If sexual excitement continues, the next stage of response includes further muscle tension and even greater blood flow.

During the plateau stage a man's penis increases slightly in circumference, the coronal ridge deepens in color, and as the testicles continue to be drawn inward, they also swell because of increased blood flow. At this stage a small amount of clear fluid may leak out of the penis. This fluid may contain viable sperm even though ejaculation has not yet occurred.

In a woman at this stage, the heart beats faster and there is a marked change in the color of the tissue in the labia minora and labia majora—so much so that these tissues are sometimes called sex skin. Parts of the labia

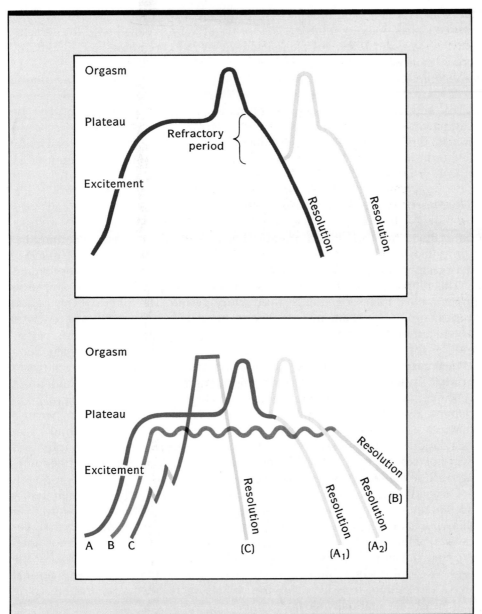

Figure 8.4 Masters and Johnson's graphs of male and female sexual response phases. Top: *A man's rise in sexual tension is shown diagrammatically. Once orgasm is achieved, there is usually a refractory period before the man can have another orgasm.* Bottom: *A woman can experience two or more orgasms in succession with no refractory period (line A). If she fails to experience orgasm, however, her resolution phase is longer (line B). Line C shows a rare kind of prolonged orgasm known as status orgasmus.*

turn bright red, and others become a burgundy color. (The color depends on whether the woman has had children.) The walls of the outer third of the vagina thicken to form what is called the orgasmic platform, and the clitoris engorges with blood and retracts upward toward the pubic bone. The uterus moves toward the spine. As the excitement continues, the pulse, respiration, and blood pressure increase.

The Third Stage: Orgasm   Immediately before **orgasm**—the stage of sexual response sometimes referred to as the climax—physiological reactions reach their most intense level in both men and women. The muscles are taut and will become even more tense in the contractions of the actual orgasm.

A man's orgasm begins with the contraction of the internal sex organs within the scrotum, near the base of the penis, and below and behind the bladder. These contractions release semen into the urethra, and the man reaches a point where ejaculation is about to happen and can no longer be controlled. A sense of impending orgasm is created as semen collects in the urethra before ejaculation. In **ejaculation,** contractions of the urethra, the penis, and some of the internal organs force semen out of the tip of the penis.

orgasm—*the climactic stage of sexual response.*

ejaculation—*contractions of the urethra, penis, and prostate gland that usually accompany orgasm in the male, forcing semen out of the tip of the penis.*

(At ejaculation, a band of muscle surrounding the exit from the urinary bladder contracts, making it impossible for urine to be expelled with the semen.) As the man ejaculates, muscle tension, heart rate, breathing, and blood flow reach their peak.

A woman's orgasm is characterized by rhythmic contractions of the uterine and vaginal muscles, a feeling of intense warmth, and an extreme awareness of the clitoral-pelvic area. As the contractions begin in the outer third of the vagina, an overwhelming sexual tension—a sense of total pelvic contraction—is felt. Orgasms are the peak of sexual pleasure and involve a total body response, not just a genital response; their length and intensity may differ greatly from individual to individual.

The Fourth Stage: Resolution   In the final stage of the sexual response, the partners begin to relax and the tension throughout their bodies starts to dissipate. Blood flow and blood pressure begin to slow to normal, breathing becomes more regular, and muscles relax. The return to normal will be quickest if orgasm has occurred; without orgasm, resolution usually takes longer.

The return to an unstimulated state occurs quickly in a man, and after orgasm most males experience a **refractory period.** The length of this period varies, and during it a man cannot be restimulated; in fact, efforts at renewed sexual stimulation may be irritating. The resolution of sexual tension begins even as the last contraction of the penile muscles completes the orgasm. Soon after orgasm normal heartbeat returns, muscles relax, and breathing slows to normal. In general, the refractory period lengthens as men grow older.

The refractory period in men seems to include a strong psychological component. Some men experience extended refractory periods, perhaps because they consider ejaculation the end of sexual relations. Others may think of an ejaculation as just one part of their script for a given sexual encounter and may not experience an extended refractory period. The keys to this phenomenon are sexual *desire* and physiology.

During the resolution stage the tension fades more slowly in women than it does in men. A woman may have strong feelings of well-being and warmth at this time as heightened physiological processes slowly return to normal. Because women do not experience a refractory period after orgasm, as most men do, they have the physical capacity to have additional orgasms soon after the first. Without further stimulation, however, the vagina returns to its normal size and position, muscles relax, the breasts decrease in size, and breathing and heart rate gradually slow.

Common Misconceptions about Sexual Response

Over the years a number of misconceptions and myths about human sexual response have arisen, primarily because of lack of communication about sexual issues. These misconceptions not only block a true understanding of sex and sexuality, they also may have a detrimental effect on sexual relationships.

The man's sexual response has been the subject of several myths and misconceptions. One is the idea that **circumcision**—the surgical removal of a flap of tissue called the **foreskin** from the head of the penis—influences sexual pleasure and behavior. Comparisons of circumcised and uncircumcised men have shown no differences in ejaculatory control, difficulty in achieving an erection, or sensitivity of the penis.[8] Another commonly held belief is that men have a greater sexual capacity than women do. The evidence does not support this misconception either.[9]

Perhaps the oldest myth of all is that the larger a man's penis, the better his sexual performance and the greater his partner's satisfaction. Research has not supported this myth. A small penis usually increases more in size during erection than does a larger one, so that the two are likely to be about the same size once they are erect.[10] Also, a woman's vagina can adapt to accommodate

refractory period—*a temporary state following orgasm during which most males cannot respond to renewed sexual stimulation.*

circumcision—*surgical removal of the foreskin from the head of the penis.*

foreskin—*the ring of tissue at the head of the penis.*

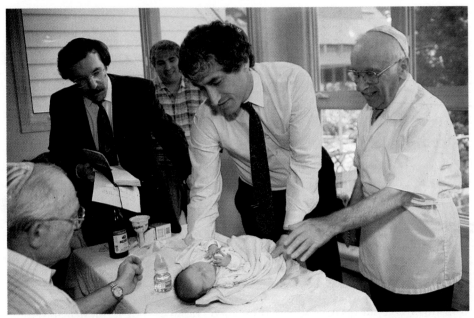

An ancient religious ceremony for Jews as well as other ethnic groups throughout the world, circumcision is also performed on most American males shortly after birth. (Richard T. Nowitz)

a penis of almost any size. Therefore, penis size is not believed to be a critical factor in sexual response.

There have also been many myths and misconceptions about the female sexual response. It was long believed, for example, that orgasms resulting from stimulation of the vagina—as in intercourse—are distinct from those resulting from stimulation of only the clitoris, which might occur during masturbation. Data from the studies of Masters and Johnson have refuted this view and revealed that orgasms are physiologically the same regardless of the source of stimulation.[11]

Misconceptions also exist concerning the nature of the clitoris. The characteristics of the clitoris show that it is the focal point in a woman's pelvic area. It has the unique function of responding to and sending out neural messages of sexual stimulation.[12] The size and position of the clitoris have not been found to affect the intensity of orgasm.

Many women do not respond to stimulation of the clitoris. They reach orgasm by means of stimulation of other sex organs, such as the vagina and the vulva, and need only indirect stimulation of the clitoris. Most women respond to direct stimulation of the clitoris in their pattern of sexual arousal, but the nature of the stimulation varies from woman to woman. Some find direct touching of the clitoris irritating rather than stimulating and prefer a more general stimulation of the clitoral area. Others respond well to clitoral stimulation by the penis during intercourse, although research shows that many more do not respond fully to such stimulation.[13] Since women respond to sexual stimulation in different ways, each woman needs to discover what works best for her and communicate this to her partner.

Another common myth is that sexual activity during a woman's menstrual period hurts the woman or causes other physical distress. Research has not proved this to be true; indeed, in some women just the opposite may be the case. In one study 10 percent of the women reported that masturbation relieved discomfort at the onset of menstruation: during orgasm, the uterus contracts and expels blood clots that can contribute to cramps. About 40 percent of the women in the study expressed no particular like or dislike for sexual activity during menstruation. About 50 percent wanted sexual activity during menstruation, and only the remaining 10 percent objected to it on religious or aesthetic grounds.[14]

Religious customs, *such as those of the Jews and Muslims, require circumcision. Because of* social customs *in countries such as the United States, about 90 percent of newborn boys are circumcised. Although it was once believed that circumcision reduces the risk of contracting cancer and venereal diseases, the American Academy of Pediatrics now maintains that there are no proven* medical *benefits to the procedure.*

Forms of Sexual Expression

People's knowledge and attitudes about sex influence and are reflected in the ways in which they express their sexuality. Sexual expression can take many forms, from sexual fantasies to sexual intercourse to a variety of other types of sexual expression and behavior.

Sexual Fantasies

Sexual fantasies arouse people just as much as does the real thing. People spend time wondering about, hoping for, wishing for, and even fearing different kinds of sexual experience. It is not unusual to dream of running off with a favorite singer or even to wish for a passionate love affair with a friend or a mysterious stranger. Fantasies are a safe way for people to explore their feelings about themselves and others.

Sexual fantasies are usually harmless—in fact, healthy—even when they involve what might be considered bizarre behavior. Many people fantasize, for example, about having sexual relations with someone of their own sex; this does *not* necessarily mean they have homosexual tendencies. Others dream of having sex forced on them. Such fantasies can be repulsive or frightening at times, and the person having them begins to wonder: Is that what I really want? For most people sexual fantasies are a safe way of working out fears, anxieties, or forbidden desires.

It is quite normal for fantasies to interject themselves spontaneously into a person's consciousness in the midst of daily chores and then vanish. Sharing these sexual fantasies with a partner may strengthen intimacy and enrich the sexual experience. Fantasies may be a problem, however, if they become too burdensome, monopolizing too much time and interfering with normal behavior.

A controversial issue associated with sexual fantasies is the use of pornography or erotica to stimulate sexual arousal. There is a great degree of disagreement over the effects of exposure to pornography. Some experts claim that erotic and pornographic materials provide a normal sexual outlet for individuals, especially those who might use other, perhaps unacceptable, means to satisfy their sexual desires if the materials were not available. Others argue that these materials stimulate people to engage in sexual acts they would normally avoid and may lead to criminal activity, sexual deviancy, and emotional disturbances. The issue is unresolved, although laws have been passed prohibiting the exploitation of children in pornography and erotica.[15]

Masturbation

masturbation—*sexual self-stimulation.*

Attitudes toward **masturbation**—sexual self-stimulation—have changed in recent years. For centuries people were discouraged from masturbating because of myths surrounding the activity. One myth was that masturbation is harmful to the body—that it saps a person's strength. Today, however, authorities on sexual behavior recognize masturbation as a legitimate way of exploring the body and finding out how it works. People start masturbating when they are infants, touching themselves all over to find out what feels good. In the same way, some adults find that masturbation can provide a release for sexual feelings or can help them learn what is sexually pleasurable. Many people reach orgasm more quickly and easily in masturbation than in intercourse.

In excess, masturbation may be a symptom of dissatisfaction or anxiety, a signal that other areas of one's sex life need fulfillment. However, unless it interferes unduly with daily life, masturbation can be considered a normal sexual behavior.

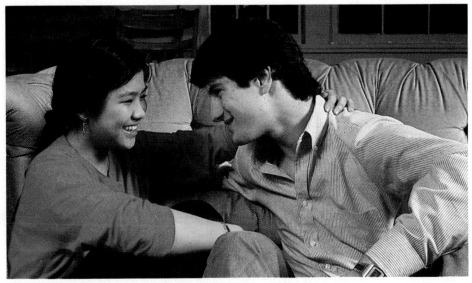

Good communication is an essential part of sexual expression between partners. (Harriet Gans/The Image Works)

Petting and Foreplay

There are many ways of showing affection and enjoying sex with another person besides sexual intercourse. Most people start out kissing and stroking each other and then move on to other types of petting as they get more excited. As they hug and kiss, a couple may explore each other's bodies, fondling and caressing genital areas, the breasts, and other erogenous zones. Petting techniques vary from person to person and from partner to partner depending on what the lovers enjoy and feel comfortable with. Many couples enjoy petting as much as intercourse and use it as a substitute when they want to feel close but intercourse is impossible or inconvenient. Quite often petting is also a form of **foreplay**—sexual activity leading to intercourse.

foreplay—*sexual activity leading to intercourse.*

American society tends to emphasize intercourse as the most important sexual act, and many people behave as if all emotional and moral issues connected with sexual behavior were linked to that single act. However, petting is where most people usually first encounter the emotional issues and conflicts that arise in sexual relationships.

Sexual Intercourse

The act of sexual intercourse is regarded by most people in most cultures as the culmination of a sexual relationship, yet people rarely discuss the experience of intercourse, which is as variable as sexual relationships themselves. Sexual intercourse can be passionate, the expression of the deepest love between two people, but it can also be awkward, playful, or even dull depending on the two people involved, their feelings for each other, and the circumstances.

Although there are many parallels between the sexual responses of men and those of women, there are also some significant differences in regard to sexual intercourse. Men are usually more easily aroused and can engage in sexual intercourse more rapidly than women can. The average woman requires more psychological and physical stimulation before she begins to respond. Men also tend to depend less on circumstances—such as romantic settings—to become aroused. Yet the differences between the sexes are not nearly as great as those between different individuals. There are women who respond very rapidly to sexual stimulation and men who respond quite slowly.

What Are Your Attitudes about Sex?

Indicate your reaction to each statement below by choosing a number from 1 to 5 according to the following scale. (The letters will help you interpret your responses.)

Agree Strongly	Agree Somewhat	Cannot Decide	Disagree Somewhat	Disagree Strongly
5	4	3	2	1

(P)_____ Premarital intercourse between consenting adults is acceptable.

(C)_____ Sexual intercourse is a kind of communication.

(O)_____ Oral sex can provide more effective sexual stimulation than does intercourse.

(H)_____ Homosexuals should be eligible for jobs where they may serve as role models for children.

(M)_____ Masturbation is acceptable when the objective is simply to attain sensory enjoyment.

(O)_____ Oral sex should be viewed as an acceptable form of sex play.

(C)_____ Communication barriers are the key factors in sexual problems.

(H)_____ Homosexuality should be regarded as a personal inclination or choice.

(M)_____ Relieving tension by masturbating is healthy.

(O)_____ Women should be as willing as men to participate in oral sex.

(P)_____ Women should experience sexual intercourse before marriage.

(P)_____ Many couples live together because the partners have a strong sexual need for each other.

(C)_____ The basis of sexual communication is touching.

(P)_____ Men should experience sexual intercourse before marriage.

(M)_____ Masturbation should be encouraged in certain circumstances.

(H)_____ Homosexual practices are acceptable between consenting adults.

Oral Sex

Oral stimulation of the female genitals (*cunnilingus*) or the male genitals (*fellatio*) by a sexual partner is a matter on which people—and even cultures—differ markedly. In some cultures oral sex is prevalent; in others it is rare. In the United States oral-genital contact is common, practiced by more than half of all married couples.[16] The religious beliefs of some communities and families, however, forbid any type of sexual activity except intercourse.

There are a wide variety of attitudes toward oral sex, ranging from pleasurable anticipation to disgust. In many ways oral sex is one of the most intimate types of lovemaking, for it involves exposing parts of the body that many feel most shy about to another person's view and touch. While oral sex is pleasurable for some people, not everyone enjoys it. As with any kind of sexual activity, it is best for each individual to decide whether to engage in oral sex and not to feel pressured if he or she does not enjoy the activity.

Now total your responses for each letter category and find your grand total.

Total	Category	Liberal	Undecided	Traditional
(C) _____	Sexual communication	15–12	11–7	6–3
(H) _____	Homosexuality	15–12	11–7	6–3
(M) _____	Masturbation	15–12	11–7	6–3
(O) _____	Oral sex	15–12	11–7	6–3
(P) _____	Premarital intercourse	20–12	15–9	6–4
_____	Grand total	80–60	59–37	36–16

Questions:

In which categories do you have the most extreme opinions, positive or negative?

Do any of your scores reveal an attitude that you might not have expected in yourself?

Would you be able to cope with sexual matters better if any of your expressed attitudes changed? Which ones?

Think about your sexual *behaviors* and sexual *attitudes*.
    Do you consciously make decisions about your sexual behaviors?
    Would it be better if you did?
    Are your decisions about sexual behaviors ever inconsistent with your attitudes?

Adapted from R. F. Valois, "The Effects of a Human Sexuality Program on the Attitudes of University Residence Hall Students" (Master's thesis, University of Illinois at Urbana-Champaign, 1980), in *Wellness R.S.V.P.*, S. G. Cox et al. (eds.) (Menlo Park, Calif.: Benjamin-Cummings, 1981): 9–65.

Homosexuality

Homosexuality is a sexual or emotional preference for persons of one's own sex. Few areas of human behavior have generated more theories or provoked more controversy than the sexual tendencies and behaviors of gay men and lesbian women.

    A number of ancient societies and some contemporary ones have sanctioned homosexual behavior and at times even made it an established practice. A comprehensive study of various cultures conducted several decades ago revealed that 49 of 76 preliterate societies either accepted or actually prescribed homosexual activity, although none practiced it exclusively.[17] Modern Western cultures, however, have encouraged only the expression of **heterosexuality**—a sexual or emotional preference for persons of the opposite sex. As a result, many men and women may repress their homosexual tendencies and behaviors.

homosexuality—*a sexual or emotional preference for persons of one's own sex.*

heterosexuality—*a sexual or emotional preference for persons of the opposite sex.*

No one knows for certain what factors cause a person to pursue a predominantly or exclusively homosexual behavior pattern. It is known that earlier psychological theories are overly simplistic. Previously accepted explanations, such as family environment or seduction by older individuals, have not withstood scientific scrutiny. The idea of a genetic basis for homosexuality is also inconclusive, although research has indicated that genes may have an indirect effect on sexual orientation by acting through hormones. Animal studies have suggested that prenatal exposure to sex hormones affects the formation of the genitals and also affects sexual orientation and behavior. These studies have led some researchers to assume that prenatal hormonal activity in humans may set the stage for later sexual development, including sexual attraction and orientation.[18]

Whatever the factors that lead to homosexuality, an awareness of sexual orientation (homosexual or heterosexual) generally occurs during late childhood and adolescence, before interpersonal sexual experiences have begun.[19] Moreover, researchers agree that incidental, experimental homosexual activity is rather common, especially in adolescence. In surveys of sexual behavior conducted by Alfred Kinsey in 1948 and 1953, one-third of the men and one-fifth of the women reported having had at least one homosexual experience.[20]

Contrary to some stereotypes, homosexuality does not constitute proof of emotional or mental illness. In fact, the American Psychiatric Association in its *Diagnostic and Statistical Manual of Mental Disorders* (DSM-III) removed homosexuality from its mental illness categories in 1980.

In recent years, homosexuals have formed organizations to help fight for equal rights, and society has become somewhat more accepting of homosexuality. Discrimination still persists and appears to have increased in some quarters as a response to the AIDS epidemic, but this epidemic has also brought public sympathy, and people increasingly recognize that gay individuals should have the opportunity to live openly without being penalized by society for their sexual preference.

Unacceptable Sexual Behavior

According to FBI statistics for 1988, there were 75,441 rapes and 17,049 attempted rapes, a total of 92,490 cases that were reported to the police.

Female activists take a powerful stand against violence directed at women; self-defense programs for women are representative of their efforts. (David Brownell)

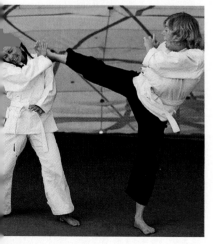

Sexual behavior is a very private affair, and what is considered acceptable or unacceptable depends a great deal on the people involved. What some people consider abnormal may be perfectly normal and acceptable to others, but certain behaviors can certainly be considered deviant and undesirable. Many of these behaviors involve sex as a result of coercion rather than a mutual act between willing and consenting individuals. One example of such behavior is rape. Another is the sexual abuse of children, including incest.

Rape Most states define *rape* as "sexual intercourse that occurs under actual or threatened forcible compulsion that overcomes earnest resistance of the victim." Though occasional cases are reported in which men are raped, the picture this commonly suggests is of the habitual rapist, who arbitrarily threatens younger and older women alike, attacking the unattractive as well as the attractive. Such rapes are thought to be motivated more by anger and violence than by sexual desire,[21] and they are relatively rare.

However, in recent studies of women on college campuses, one in six said they were the victim of rape or attempted rape during the preceding year.[22] Often it is not a stranger who is the offender but a man the woman knows— so-called acquaintance or date rape. A recent report revealed the disquieting fact that among males and females in the same college, only 25 percent of the men reported perpetrating sexually aggressive behaviors (including rape), whereas 54 percent of the women reported being sexually victimized. While it might be thought that many of the men, or many of the women, simply lied, the questionnaire was designed and tested in a way that minimized the likelihood of this occurring. Instead, the researchers suggest that the men, "although they used physical force and injured their victims, saw their behavior as congruent with consental sexual activity."[23] Apparently some men do not perceive accurately the amount of force and coercion they are using and fail to respect, or to interpret correctly, a woman's resistance and nonconsent.

In addition to the thousands of rapes reported each year, official estimates suggest that there may be 3 to 10 times as many cases that are committed but not reported.[24] In some of these cases it is men who are sexually assaulted, but women are the victims in the vast majority of cases. This suggests a problem of overwhelming proportions for women.

The problem has been worsened by the fact that rape is an area where the victim has sometimes been blamed for instigating the crime because of the clothes she wears, her actions, or even because she has walked alone late at night. Many times the law has looked at the behavior and reputation of the victim when putting a rapist on trial.

Conventional preventive measures have also been directed largely at women: they are advised to take extra caution in potentially dangerous situations. For example, when taking car trips alone, women are urged to have a good supply of gas, to lock the vehicle when leaving it, and to check both the front and the back before getting in. They are advised to drive with friends and not to pick up hitchhikers or hitchhike themselves. They are also warned that an empty home or apartment can be a potential danger, that they should take care to identify strangers before opening the door to them and should avoid entering themselves if they suspect someone is inside, and that they should avoid going to a date's home unless they know him well.[25]

All this is sound advice, but it still has the effect of suggesting that victims are responsible because they neglected to take care. However, society is slowly changing its views on rape. Rape hot lines are being made available to victims. Hospitals and police departments have specially trained personnel, often women, to help. Education is being seen as another important method for helping to prevent rape: there are courses and books that teach women the psychological and physical skills needed to help them take care of themselves, including how and when to fight an assailant.

Incest and Child Sexual Abuse   A serious misuse of sex also occurs in the case of incest and other child sexual abuse. Sexual abuse of children cuts across all socioeconomic boundaries and leaves great emotional scars on those who are molested.[26] It is estimated that as many as 40 million Americans may have been sexually victimized as children. These numbers are disturbing, especially when considered in light of the finding that children who are abused are more likely to become abusers when they reach adulthood.[27]

Studies have shown that most sexual abuse happens to children between the ages of 9 and 12, although abuse of children as young as 2 years old is not unusual. The vast majority of cases, from 85 to 90 percent, involve a person who is already known to the child, most frequently parents, other relatives, and family friends.[28] Moreover, rather than being an isolated incident, most cases of sexual abuse involve a situation that develops gradually over a period of time, with repeated incidents. In most cases the abuser uses bribery or intimidation rather than force to get the child to do what he or she wants.[29]

Children who are sexually abused are frequently traumatized and embarrassed and keep the painful experience to themselves. One newspaper poll reported that one-third of people who said that they had been sexually abused never told anyone about the experience.[30] Although experts have found that some victims of sexual abuse reach adulthood relatively unharmed, many others develop serious psychological problems. Women may be distrustful of men, feel unattractive, or be afraid of intimacy. Men may be confused about their sexual identity, deeply ashamed, or sexually aggressive. In general, people who were sexually abused as children have lower self-esteem than others and are often anxious, depressed, and guilt-ridden.[31]

If you are raped:

1. *Despite what you may have heard about police skepticism, you* **should** *report the attack even if it was unsuccessful. The information you provide may help protect other women. Give as much detail as you can. Describe the attacker's physical appearance, voice, clothes, and car.*

2. *Call the police immediately; do not take a bath or change your clothes. Semen, hair, and other materials may be aids to identification.*

3. *Most important, do not blame yourself for what happened. The person who raped you had* **no** **right** *to do so. If there is a rape counseling center in your area, contact the center as soon as possible or talk to a friend, guidance counselor, psychologist, or member of the clergy. It is essential that you get a chance to work through the emotional trauma of the experience with a supportive listener.*

An increasing number of groups and organizations are making people more aware of the problem of sexual abuse and giving parents reassuring commonsense guidelines for protecting their children from sexual abuse and dealing with it if it does occur. Special programs in schools teach young children to say no, to run away, and to tell another adult when they are threatened with any kind of sexual abuse. Books are available that explain these concepts to children in a nonfrightening manner. Parents should be alert to potential sources of danger and should take their children very seriously when they report an incident.

Sexual Problems and Sexual Dysfunction

At one time or another many people become concerned about difficulties with sex (Table 8.1), but for some people sexual problems occur repeatedly and cause great anxiety. Any problem that prevents a person from engaging in sexual relations or reaching orgasm is known as a **sexual dysfunction.**

sexual dysfunction—*a problem that prevents a person from engaging in sexual relations or reaching orgasm.*

While many forms of sexual dysfunction result from emotional or psychological disturbances, others develop from organic, or physical, causes. Anatomic variations, hormonal imbalance, and illness (heart disease, for example) are all organic conditions that have been linked to sexual dysfunction. Certain medical treatments (for high blood pressure or seizures) have also led to sexual problems.

It is important to be able to recognize a sexual dysfunction. Organically caused dysfunctions can be eliminated; in the case of conditions that cannot be treated medically, there are therapeutic techniques that help improve sexual functioning and satisfaction.

Sexual Dysfunction in Men

More information is available about sexual dysfunction in men than about that in women. Some of the more common difficulties experienced by men are premature ejaculation, retarded ejaculation, impotence, and inhibited sexual desire.

premature ejaculation—*unintentional ejaculation before, during, or immediately after insertion of the penis into the vagina.*

Premature Ejaculation   Among the most common male sexual dysfunctions is **premature ejaculation**—the expulsion of semen before the partners want it to occur, typically before or soon after insertion of the penis into the vagina. Premature ejaculation is a problem when it causes sexual difficulty for the couple. While it may be caused by a number of factors, it often has a psychological basis.

Consider the case of a 24-year-old man who went to a therapist because chronic premature ejaculation had disrupted his relations with his wife. (In his case, ejaculation typically occurred within 15 to 20 seconds of penetration into his wife's vagina.) It turned out that before marriage his sexual encounters had taken place in locations such as the backseat of an automobile, where he had to hurry and had little privacy. Thus he had never learned to slow down the time it took to ejaculate. Therapy helped him overcome these early experiences and learn better control.[32] Many men troubled by premature ejaculation find that they can train themselves to delay ejaculation by using techniques developed by sex therapists.

retarded ejaculation—*a condition in which a man takes overly long to reach the point of ejaculation, possibly causing pain to his partner.*

Retarded Ejaculation   Some men take overly long to reach the point of ejaculation, possibly causing pain to their partners. Such **retarded ejaculation** may have a physiological or a psychological basis. Ejaculation is controlled by a spinal reflex associated with the sympathetic nervous system. Any disease that interferes with this reflex, such as bowel or bladder dysfunction and diabetes, may impair or retard the ability to ejaculate. Stress and drugs also may interfere with this reflex.

Table 8.1 Sexual Satisfaction and Difficulties Reported by a Sample of 100 Married Couples without a Specific Dysfunction

	Women	Men
How satisfying are your sexual relations?		
Very satisfying	40%	42%
Moderately satisfying	46	43
Not very satisfying	12	13
Not satisfying at all	2	2
How do your sexual relations compare with other aspects of your married life?		
Better than the rest	19	24
About the same	63	60
Worse than the rest	18	16
Do the following difficulties interfere with your sex life?		
Partner chooses inconvenient time	31	16
Inability to relax	47	12
Attraction to person(s) other than mate	14	21
Disinterest	35	16
Attraction to person(s) of same sex	1	0
Different sexual practices or habits	10	12
Turned off	28	10
Too little foreplay before intercourse	38	21
Too little tenderness after intercourse	25	17

Source: From E. Frank et al., *New England Journal of Medicine* 299 (1978): 111–115. By permission.

Occasional difficulty with ejaculation should not be considered a symptom of sexual dysfunction. Such difficulty may be caused by fatigue, illness, stress, or the temporary effects of alcohol or other substances. Furthermore, the time from erection to ejaculation increases with age, and so an older man should anticipate taking longer to arrive at orgasm. This should not be considered a problem or thought to be a detriment to sexual satisfaction. Since women's sexual response peaks later in life than men's, the longer it takes for a man to ejaculate, the more gratifying it may be for the woman.

Impotence Psychologists use the term **impotence** to describe a man's inability to achieve or maintain an erection long enough to reach orgasm with a partner. The causes of the condition may be either organic or psychological. In the rare condition known as **primary impotence,** the man has never been able to achieve an erection. In most cases, however, the man has been able to have an erection in the past but is now unable to do so in some or all sexual encounters; this condition is termed **secondary impotence.**

Inhibited Sexual Desire Men, and women as well, may experience inhibited sexual desire, including reduced desire, absent desire with or without sexual response when stimulated, and an aversion to all or certain types of sexual activity.[33] Many researchers believe that inhibited sexual desire is usually a result of training or life experiences, although disease or factors such as chronic dieting, excessive weight loss, and surgery may temporarily or permanently impair desire as well.[34]

Sexual Dysfunction in Women

As with men, sexual dysfunctions in women may be caused by a variety of factors. Some of the more common difficulties experienced by women are anorgasmia, dyspareunia, and vaginismus as well as inhibited sexual desire, which is similar to that experienced by men.

impotence—*sexual dysfunction in which a man is unable to achieve or maintain an erection long enough to reach orgasm with a partner.*

primary impotence—*a sexual dysfunction in which a man has never been able to achieve an erection.*

secondary impotence—*a sexual dysfunction in which a man who has previously been able to achieve an erection is now unable to do so in some or all sexual encounters.*

Therapy Saved Our Relationship

Carl and I have been together for just over 2 years, and we're both very satisfied with every aspect of our relationship. However, a year and a half ago it was difficult to imagine this kind of happiness, because our relationship was seriously troubled by a sexual problem that caused concern and embarrassment for both of us.

I was attracted to Carl because he is great fun to be with, good-looking, and a tender and caring person, but our love life was a great disappointment. Whenever we made love, Carl would ejaculate very quickly, often within a minute of starting intercourse. At first I thought this might be related to excitement or nervousness about our new sexual relationship, but the problem continued. Worse, we couldn't seem to discuss what was happening, except for his embarrassed apology and my quick (and untrue) response that it was "okay." I think we both hoped that the problem would somehow resolve itself and simply disappear, but it didn't. He seemed humiliated, and I felt helpless about what I could do. The tension that came from not dealing with these feelings began to gnaw at me.

This might have signaled the beginning of serious trouble in our relationship, but I was determined to try to resolve this problem. I started by reading Masters and Johnson's *Human Sexual Inadequacy*, where I learned that premature ejaculation is fairly common. I was glad to find out that it's usually easily treatable and that there are a number of effective therapies in which a woman can participate to help her partner.

I knew that Carl was feeling upset and guilty about our disappointing lovemaking, and I hoped he would trust me and accept my help. One night, relaxing over after-dinner coffee, the time seemed right to talk. Although hesitant at first, Carl later said he was glad I had taken the initiative and was relieved we were finally taking steps to resolve a problem we'd been avoiding. He assured me that he loved me and that the problem wasn't with me or our relationship—

he'd had a similar experience with a previous partner. Carl admitted he'd tried everything to last longer, even reciting baseball statistics while making love!

Our decision to consult a sex therapist turned out to be an excellent move. At the first meeting Dr. Asherman diffused our nervousness by explaining that learning to last longer, like learning any skill, takes patience and practice. She counseled Carl not to get angry with himself or with me if he didn't make rapid progress, and she reminded us both to keep our sense of humor. We learned that Carl's technique of thinking of "other things" was counterproductive: instead of tuning his body out, he should have been making every effort to tune it in.

Since we wanted to work together, Dr. Asherman suggested we begin a couples program, which introduced sensual focusing techniques such as deep breathing, massage, and bathing together to help us to relax and feel in touch with each other. She gave Carl exercises to improve pelvic muscle tone and outlined a step-by-step therapy to help Carl learn the subtleties of his own sexual response cycle. We progressed together through the steps at home and had regular sessions with Dr. Asherman for guidance and encouragement. She counseled us to allow plenty of time to work on each step and not to rush from one step to another. As the therapy proceeded, Carl's feeling of control increased dramatically.

Our therapist had additional suggestions about how we could work together, including different lovemaking positions. For example, positions with the woman on top or sideways result in less tension for the man and can help increase ejaculatory control.

We are convinced that going through the couples program together was the ideal way to solve this problem. More important, we both feel that committing ourselves to working together strengthened our relationship and deepened our trust and love for each other.

Anorgasmia   The inability of a woman to experience an orgasm is called **anorgasmia.** Women who have never experienced an orgasm are described as having **primary anorgasmia.** Those who have lost the ability to have an orgasm are said to suffer from **secondary anorgasmia.** Women who are able to experience orgasm in certain situations but not in others are considered to have **situational anorgasmia.**[35]

For many women, "learning" to be orgasmic may be complicated by sociocultural or religious inhibitions that interfere with experimentation in which they learn how to get pleasure from sex. A lack of factual knowledge about sex and sexuality also may interfere with sexual development and learning to be orgasmic. Women who have primary anorgasmia sometimes achieve a relatively low level of sexual excitement and think of intercourse as "pleasant" but may get the most pleasure from touching, holding, kissing, caressing, attention, and approval.[36] A woman can learn to become orgasmic through self-stimulation or by experimenting with a trusted partner in a safe, private, and socially approved setting.

In women with secondary anorgasmia, a causal event—such as alcoholism, depression, grief, medication, illness, or estrogen reduction associated with menopause—usually occurs close to the time when the capacity for orgasm is lost. The causal event may also be linked to a violation of trust, love, respect, warmth, or other sexually associated values.[37] When the causal events pass or her emotional needs are satisfied, the woman's responsiveness usually returns.

Some women may experience orgasm through self-stimulation or oral sex but not through sexual intercourse. Others may experience orgasm only with a certain type or amount of foreplay. Such situational anorgasmia is within the range of normal sexual expression, although the woman may wish for a change in these modes of achieving orgasm. Sexual experimentation and the use of techniques to associate orgasmic experiences with nonorgasmic ones can be used to help a woman learn to experience orgasm in other situations.[38]

Dyspareunia   Some women experience physical pain during sexual intercourse, a condition known as **dyspareunia.** There are a variety of possible causes for this pain. Pain on penetration may be caused by inflammation, scarring, or trauma to the clitoris, vagina, or vulva; vaginismus (described below); urethritis; or inadequate vaginal lubrication. Painful intercourse may also result from cervical disease, bladder or bowel problems, and a vagina that is shorter than the erect penis being inserted, particularly if penile thrusting is forceful.[39] Medical treatment may reduce many of these factors and alleviate the pain. If the problem is caused by inadequate vaginal lubrication, dyspareunia can be treated by using medically approved lubricants and by engaging in sexually exciting experiences, such as showering together and mutual caressing, that tend to increase both natural lubrication and dilation of the vagina.

Vaginismus   Some women suffer from **vaginismus,** a condition in which involuntary muscle spasms cause the vagina to shut tightly so that it is impossible or painful for a penis to penetrate. Vaginismus may result from a reflex pattern that a woman has not yet learned to control or may occur as a protective reflex against the pain of dyspareunia. Women who have been genitally traumatized by rape or abuse may also develop vaginismus.[40]

Dealing with Sexual Dysfunction

The first goal in treating a sexual dysfunction is to rule out an organic cause for the problem. Recent advances have made the task of identifying organic causes of dysfunction much easier.[41] If an organic condition is found to be the

anorgasmia—*the inability of a woman to experience an orgasm.*

primary anorgasmia—*a sexual dysfunction in which a woman has never experienced an orgasm by any method.*

secondary anorgasmia—*a sexual dysfunction in which a woman frequently has difficulty achieving an orgasm.*

situational anorgasmia—*a condition in which a woman is able to experience orgasm in certain situations but not in others.*

dyspareunia—*a condition in which a woman experiences physical pain during sexual intercourse.*

vaginismus—*a sexual dysfunction involving involuntary muscle spasms that cause the vagina to shut so tightly that penetration by a penis is impossible or painful.*

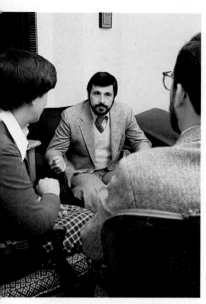

Though the setting looks very much like a psychotherapy consultation, sex therapy in fact represents a decidedly different—and often markedly successful—approach to sexual problems. (Freda Leinwand/ Monkmeyer Press)

cause, it often can be treated medically, perhaps through surgery or by treating related diseases, such as urethritis (an inflammation of the urethra caused by microbes or physical irritation).

If sexual dysfunction is found to be a result of psychological, social, spiritual, or developmental factors, the most effective treatment is sex therapy. A person's sexual partner is often included in the therapy; if the person is single, a surrogate partner may be provided. The prognosis is often very good, especially if no serious psychopathology is involved.

The aims of sex therapy are to sensitize individuals to their erogenous zones, make them more aware of their sexual needs and those of their partners, and help them to communicate more effectively with their sex partners. Through therapy, couples may learn sexual exercises and techniques that can help them learn gradually how to achieve satisfactory lovemaking. Sex therapy is often briefer and therefore relatively less expensive in the long run than psychotherapy.

It is important to determine the level of psychopathology in a person before deciding on a plan of treatment. People with relatively minor psychological problems may benefit most from brief sex therapy, whereas those with more serious problems may require extensive psychotherapy before, during, or instead of behavioral sex therapy.

Three levels of psychological causes of sexual dysfunction are often used to help determine the type of therapy used.[42] The *superficial* level is characterized by performance anxiety, fear of failure, passivity, and feelings of unattractiveness. Sexual dysfunction based on these causes is most effectively treated by short-term therapy—perhaps a month or two at most. *Midlevel* conflicts may originate in negative family messages and childhood traumas; such conflicts often include power struggles between partners. For midlevel problems, long-term psychotherapy in addition to or before sex therapy may be recommended. *Deep-level* conflicts may result from extreme religious or family negativism about sex and strong conflicts stemming from the first 5 years of life, including conflicts involving trust, dependency, and the need to control. Such conflicts may undermine a person's ability to form suitable romantic attachments in later years and lead to serious discord between partners. Deep-level conflicts are the most difficult to treat. In most cases psychotherapy must precede sex therapy.

Since organic causes can usually be identified and treated and psychosocial factors can be dealt with through counseling or therapy, people should not be disillusioned about the potential for successful treatment of sexual problems. In recent years many people have been helped to achieve their maximum sexual comfort level. With help and cooperation, men and women can be very successful in overcoming sexual problems and providing pleasure for a partner while obtaining sexual gratification for themselves.

Approaching Sex Responsibly

Sexuality is a very powerful force that influences many of the ways in which people act and behave. Many people view sexual experience as a peak expression of interpersonal relationships, but sex can also be misused and abused and can result in a great deal of pain and suffering. Responsible and healthy sexuality involves a consideration of the feelings and needs of others as well as one's own.

When approached responsibly, sexual expression adds a new dimension to relationships—a dimension that can add greater intimacy and understanding. Approached irresponsibly, however, it can lead to greater risk. Partners who communicate poorly with each other or treat each other badly may not

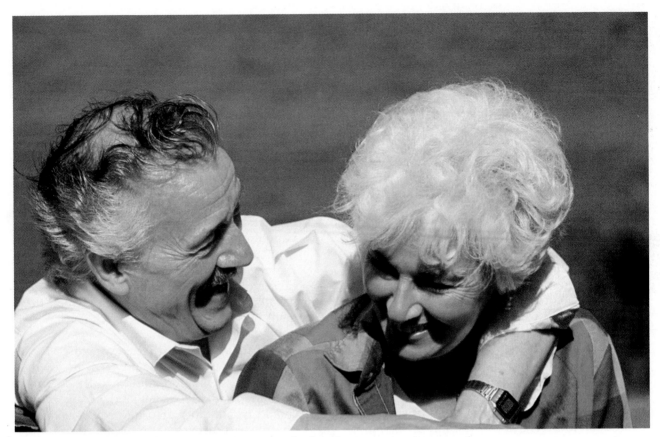

Long-lasting relationships are based not only on attraction but also on trust and a sense of caring and responsibility. (Focus Stock Photo)

enjoy sex, and their relationship may be jeopardized. Today, with the prevalence of AIDS and other sexually transmitted diseases, a greater responsibility between partners is also required to ensure that sex is safe and not detrimental to health.

Most people feel awkward and uncomfortable about sex, especially in first or new sexual encounters. Sexual feelings are exciting, even overwhelming, and acting on them can conflict with what a person has been taught by parents, friends, and cultural or religious leaders. Some people feel pressured to keep up with the sexual exploits and experiences of friends even if they have personal reservations about engaging in sex. Such conflicts and pressures can be puzzling; it is often hard to sort out what one feels about sex, one's partner, and oneself. There is nothing wrong with abstaining from sex if a person is not ready. Approaching sex responsibly and safely is a healthy approach to sexual behavior.

Sex as a means of intimate expression is obviously only part of the story. The reproductive function of sex is another major concern not only for the creation of children but also for the additional hopes, feelings, and fears that it awakens in any relationship. Sexuality therefore involves responsibility for life as well as for the needs and feelings of others.

Chapter 9 will look at the reproductive aspect of sex in more detail. In sex as in other activities, it is very important that the individual be able to feel comfortable with his or her actions and decisions. Sexual expression is most satisfactory when people carefully consider not only themselves and others but also the implications that sex, including its reproductive aspects, may have on their future.

Chapter Summary

- Essentially, sex refers to a person's gender and to types of sexual expression, while sexuality refers to the way gender is integrated into all aspects of life. Sexuality is based on a variety of factors, some biological and some learned.

- Attitudes toward sex and sexual behavior are shaped by the influence of other people and through experience and education. Often people learn about sex indirectly by observing the attitudes and actions of others, including their parents and friends.

- Many areas of the body can function as erogenous zones, which are related to sexual desire and can be stimulated to produce sexual arousal. Major erogenous structures of the male sexual anatomy include the penis and scrotum. Major structures of the female sexual anatomy include the vulva, labia, clitoris, and vagina.

- The four general stages of human sexual response are excitement, plateau, orgasm, and resolution. Each stage is marked by specific and different physiological changes in the male and the female.

- There are a great variety of types of sexual expression and behavior, including sexual fantasies, masturbation, petting and foreplay, sexual intercourse, oral sex, and homosexuality. Individuals may differ in the types of sexual expression with which they feel most comfortable and which they will accept and engage in. Each of these forms of expression has an important role in providing an outlet for sexual needs and desires.

- Certain sexual behaviors—those which result from coercion rather than mutual consent and caring—are considered unacceptable in society. Among these deviant behaviors are rape, incest, and child sexual abuse.

- People may suffer from a variety of sexual problems and dysfunctions. For men these include premature ejaculation, retarded ejaculation, impotence, and inhibited sexual desire. For women they include anorgasmia, dyspareunia, vaginismus, and inhibited sexual desire. If the causes of sexual dysfunction are organic, they usually can be corrected through medical treatment. Those which have a psychological basis are best treated with therapy.

- Responsible sexual expression requires a consideration of the feelings and needs of others as well as one's own. It requires good communication and mutual respect and caring. People should not be pressured into sex or engage in unsafe sex practices. Approached responsibly, sex adds greatly to a relationship; approached irresponsibly, it can result in pain and suffering.

Key Terms

Sex (page 197)
Sexuality (page 197)
Erogenous zones (page 202)
Penis (page 203)
Urethra (page 203)
Glans (page 203)
Coronal ridge (page 203)
Frenulum (page 203)
Scrotum (page 203)
Perineum (page 204)
Vulva (page 204)
Mons veneris (page 204)

Labia (page 204)
Clitoris (page 204)
Vagina (page 204)
Hymen (page 204)
Vasocongestion (page 206)
Myotonia (page 206)
Spermatic cords (page 206)
Orgasm (page 207)
Ejaculation (page 207)
Refractory period (page 208)
Circumcision (page 208)

Foreskin (page 208)
Masturbation (page 210)
Foreplay (page 211)
Homosexuality (page 213)
Heterosexuality (page 213)
Sexual dysfunction (page 216)
Premature ejaculation (page 216)
Retarded ejaculation (page 216)
Impotence (page 217)

Primary impotence (page 217)
Secondary impotence (page 217)
Anorgasmia (page 219)
Primary anorgasmia (page 219)
Secondary anorgasmia (page 219)
Situational anorgasmia (page 219)
Dyspareunia (page 219)
Vaginismus (page 219)

References

1. Elizabeth R. Allgeier and Albert R. Allgeier, *Sexual Interactions* (Lexington, Mass.: D C Heath, 1984): 155–156.

2. S. S. Wachtel, "H-V Antigen and Sexual Development," in *Genetic Mechanisms of Sexual Development*, H. Vallet and I. Porter (eds.) (New York: Academic Press, 1979): 271–277; F. Haseltine and S. Ohno, "Mechanisms in Gonadal Differentiation," *Science* 211, no. 4488 (1981): 1272–1278.

3. W. Masters et al., *Human Sexuality*, 3d ed. (Boston: Scott, Foresman, 1988).

4. M. D. Perlman et al., "Sex Education in the Inner City," *Journal of the American Medical Association* 255 (1986): 43–47.

5. Jeanne Brooks-Gunn and Frank F. Furstenburg, "Adolescent Sexual Behavior," *American Psychologist* 44, no. 2 (February 1989): 249–257.

6. William H. Masters and Virginia E. Johnson, *Human Sexual Response* (Boston: Little, Brown, 1966): 21.

7. Masters et al., op. cit., pp. 80–95.

8. Masters and Johnson, op. cit., p. 190.

9. Masters et al., op. cit.

10. Masters and Johnson, op. cit., p. 191.

11. Ibid., p. 45.

12. Ibid.

13. Ibid., pp. 58–60.

14. Ibid., p. 125.

15. Allgeier and Allgeier, op. cit.

16. Ibid., pp. 209–215.

17. Clellan S. Ford and Frank A. Beach, *Patterns of Sexual Behavior* (New York: Harper & Row, 1951).

18. David Bjorklund and Barbara Bjorklund, "Straight or Gay?" *Parents* (October 1988): 93–98.

19. G. T. McDonald, "Individual Differences in the Coming Out Process for Gay Men: Implications for Theoretical Models," *Journal of Homosexuality* 8 (1982): 47–60.

20. A. C. Kinsey et al., *Sexual Behavior in the Human Male* (Philadelphia: W B Saunders, 1948); A. C. Kinsey et al., *Sexual Behavior in the Human Female* (Philadelphia: W B Saunders, 1953).

21. Robert Crooks and Karla Baur, *Our Sexuality* (Menlo Park, Calif.: Benjamin-Cummings, 1980): 256–263.

22. Liz McMillen, "Colleges Urged to Set Up Efforts to Prevent Rape, a Major Menace to Students on Campuses," *Chronicle of Higher Education* 35 (September 1, 1988): 1.

23. Mary P. Koss et al., "The Scope of Rape: Incidence and Prevalence of Sexual Aggression and Victimization in a National Sample of Higher Education Students," *Journal of Consulting and Clinical Psychology* 55, no. 2 (1987): 162–170.

24. Ibid.

25. Domeena C. Renshaw, "Treatment of Sexual Exploitation," *Psychiatric Clinics of North America* 12, no. 2 (June 1989): 257–277.

26. Ibid.

27. Alfie Kohn, "Shattered Innocence: Childhood Sexual Abuse Is Yielding Its Dark Secrets to the Cold Light of Research," *Psychology Today* (February 1987): 54–58.

28. D. Schetky, "Emerging Issues in Child Sexual Abuse," *Journal of the American Academy of Child Psychiatry* 25 (1986): 490–492.

29. Kohn, op. cit.

30. Ibid.

31. Ibid.

32. C. D. Tollison and H. E. Adams, *Sexual Disorders: Treatment, Theory, Research* (New York: Gardner Press, 1979).

33. R. A. Hatcher et al., *Contraceptive Technology 1988–1989*, 14th rev. ed. (Atlanta: Printed Matter, 1988).

34. Ibid.

35. Ibid.

36. Ibid.

37. Ibid.

38. Ibid.

39. American Psychiatric Association, *Treatments of Psychiatric Disorders: A Task Force Report of the American Psychiatric Association* 3 (Washington, D.C.: American Psychiatric Association, 1989): 2237–2247.

40. Hatcher et al., op. cit.

41. American Psychiatric Association, op. cit.

42. Ibid.

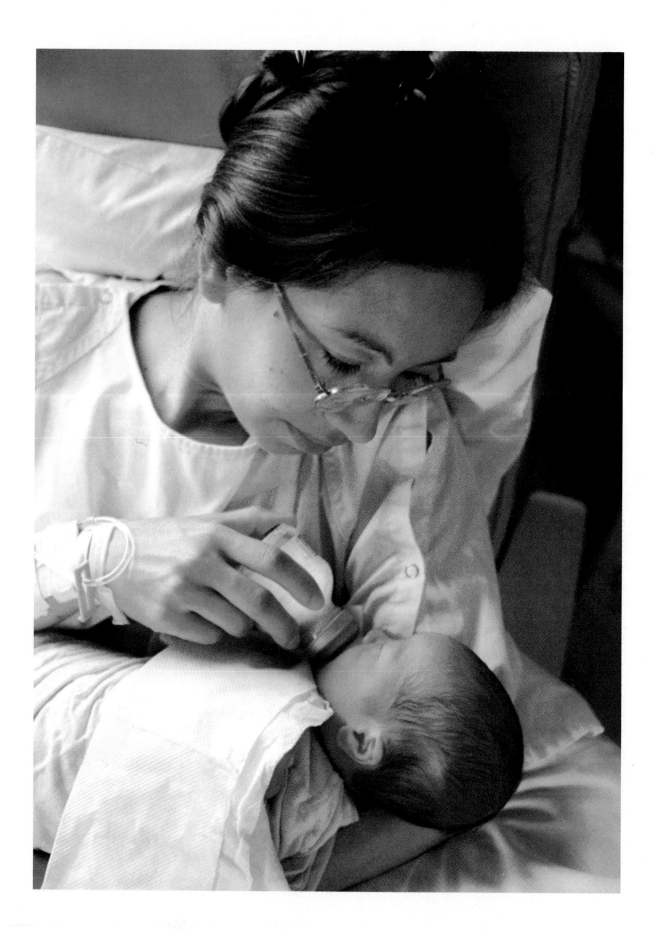

Chapter 9

Reproduction and Sexual Health

To Guide Your Reading

When you have studied this chapter, you should be able to:

- List the major parts of the female and male reproductive systems and describe their functions.

- Identify the various contraceptive methods, explaining the benefits and drawbacks of each, including the techniques used in natural family planning.

- Discuss the importance of planning for pregnancy and describe the beginnings of pregnancy and the development of a fetus.

- Identify and explain various techniques for terminating a pregnancy and discuss attitudes toward abortion.

- Discuss the choices parents must make in preparing for childbirth and describe the stages of labor.

Sexual activity plays an important role in many close relationships, but it has a much greater significance. As the beginning of the process through which new lives are formed, it is intertwined with some of the most important questions people face. While such questions have always existed, as the end of the twentieth century approaches, new technologies and medical advances have added new and challenging dimensions to reproduction and sexual health.

In regard to reproduction, at least three major issues touch on individual health and the health of society at large. The first is a fundamental concern—how to maximize the health and well-being of the child and the mother during the reproductive process.

The second issue concerns the dangers of infectious disease. Sexually transmitted diseases (STDs), as you will read in Chapter 10, have been very resistant to public health measures in the United States and throughout the world. These diseases include several types that can be transmitted from a mother to her developing fetus.

The third issue has to do with conflicting personal philosophies. For example, techniques for birth control have been a source of major disagreement in American society for some time. Some people believe that given the growing world population and the number of unwanted pregnancies, birth control is a viable and responsible course of action. Others believe that interrupting the natural link between sex and pregnancy or terminating a pregnancy once it has started goes against basic tenets of morality and ethical thought. Some people also believe that the availability of birth control has undermined traditional morality and the institution of marriage by removing "natural" penalties for sex before and outside of marriage. People on all sides of these issues may feel profound moral and ethical conflicts as they struggle to make choices and decisions concerning birth control and abortion.

This chapter will address these three issues by exploring mechanisms of reproduction, methods of birth control, the process of pregnancy, techniques of abortion, and finally the birth event itself. It will not attempt to answer philosophical questions, because that is the responsibility of the individual.

Before discussing the process of reproduction and the various methods of contraception, this chapter will complete the description of human sexual anatomy by describing the internal reproductive organs.

The Female Reproductive System

ovum (plural: **ova**)—*a female reproductive cell.*

The female reproductive system has three main functions: to produce egg cells, or **ova** (singular: **ovum**); to position an ovum where it can meet incoming sperm; and to provide a hospitable environment where, if fertilized, the ovum can develop into a fetus. All these functions are carried out in a woman's body by specialized organs—the ovaries, the Fallopian tubes, and the uterus (Figure 9.1)—in a process governed by a fairly regular monthly cycle in women of reproductive age.

The Ovaries

ovaries—*two small internal female sexual organs that produce ova and female hormones.*

menarche—*the first menstrual period.*

ovulation—*the process by which ova periodically ripen and leave the ovaries.*

The **ovaries** are two small organs, each about the size and shape of an almond. Each ovary is positioned close to the end of a Fallopian tube, which is the route the ovum takes when it leaves the ovary. Every normal woman is born with hundreds of thousands of unripened ova already present in her ovaries, but only about 400 will mature during her reproductive years.

Ovulation   At a point during puberty called **menarche,** a woman's ova begin to mature periodically and leave the ovaries in a process known as **ovulation.** This generally takes place at about the midpoint of a woman's

Figure 9.1 The female reproductive system has three main functions: expelling an egg cell each month (in the ovaries); positioning it in the Fallopian tubes, where it can be fertilized; and providing an environment in the uterus, where it can develop if fertilized.

The Fallopian tubes are not attached directly to the ovaries. They cover the ovaries like funnels. Long fingerlike projections called **fimbriae** *pull the mature eggs into the tubes by creating wavelike motions.*

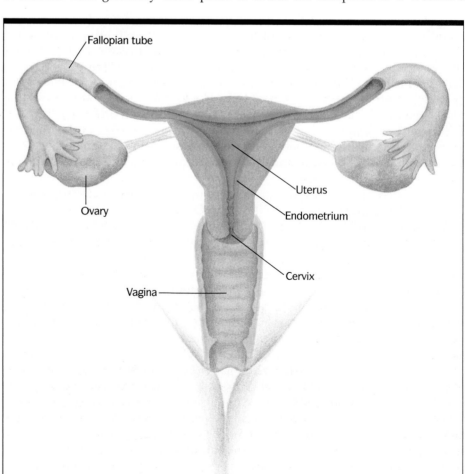

menstrual cycle. In normal cycles ovulation occurs approximately 13 to 15 days before the first day of menstrual flow, but in prolonged cycles it occurs later than the midpoint, and in short cycles it can occur earlier, even during menstruation—an important thing to know for practicing effective birth control. Certain factors, including stress, fatigue, and anorexia, may disrupt a woman's menstrual cycle.

A woman cannot always tell when she is ovulating. Some women do sense the moment, however: the pelvis seems heavy or they feel a mild ache on one or both sides of the abdomen for a few hours or days.

The Fallopian Tubes

The **Fallopian tubes,** or **oviducts,** are tiny muscular tunnels that connect the ovaries and the uterus. When a mature ovum enters one of the Fallopian tubes, it travels slowly down the tube toward the uterus. It is in the Fallopian tubes that fertilization usually takes place.

Fallopian tube (oviduct)— *one of two tiny muscular tunnels that transport ova from the ovary to the uterus.*

The Uterus

The **uterus,** or womb, is pear-shaped in appearance and rests on its small end (the **cervix**) in the center of a woman's pelvis. It protects and nourishes the fertilized ovum, allowing it to develop into a fetus. During pregnancy the uterus expands tremendously—from the size of a woman's fist into a large muscular pouch that almost entirely fills the woman's abdomen to accommodate the developing fetus.

uterus—*the womb; a hollow muscular internal female sexual organ that contributes to sexual response and shelters and nourishes the fetus during pregnancy.*

cervix—*the narrow lower end of the uterus; located at the upper end of the vagina.*

The Menstrual Cycle

Every month, if a woman is not pregnant, the inner lining of the uterus (the **endometrium**) goes through a process of renewal and preparation known as the **menstrual cycle.** Basically, the menstrual cycle is the way in which a woman's uterus prepares to receive and nourish a fertilized ovum.

The menstrual cycle begins when the pituitary gland secretes follicle-stimulating hormone (FSH). This hormone signals the ovary to ripen an ovum. At the same time, luteinizing hormone (LH) is also released from the pituitary gland, stimulating the manufacture of estrogen within the ovaries. This causes the uterine wall to thicken and become rich in blood vessels. Another substance is also secreted in the ovaries—progesterone, which causes the walls of the uterus to thicken further and to store nutrients in preparation for a fertilized ovum (Figure 9.2).

If an ovum in one of the Fallopian tubes becomes fertilized, it travels down to the uterus and implants itself in the uterine lining, which develops further and nourishes the growing fetus. If pregnancy does not occur, the uterus sloughs off the lining entirely and prepares a new one. The blood and tissues of the old lining pass through the cervix and vagina in a discharge known as **menstruation,** a term that comes from the Latin *mensis,* meaning "month." A woman's menstrual flow generally lasts 3 to 6 days, and the typical menstrual cycle lasts 27 to 34 days.

endometrium—*the inner lining of the uterus.*

menstrual cycle—*the monthly cycle in which the lining of the uterus first thickens and prepares to receive a fertilized ovum, then is discharged during menstruation if a pregnancy does not occur.*

menstruation—*the sloughing off of the thickened lining of the uterus that occurs about once a month if pregnancy does not occur.*

Physical Effects of the Menstrual Cycle   Many women experience very little if any physical discomfort during menstruation. Others may feel some physical effects immediately before or during the menstrual period. These women may feel bloated, their breasts may be tender, or they may have headaches, backaches, leg pains, or changes in energy level. A few women have abdominal pains, or cramps, that may be severe enough to interfere with their normal activities for a day or two. These effects result from a normal physiological process.

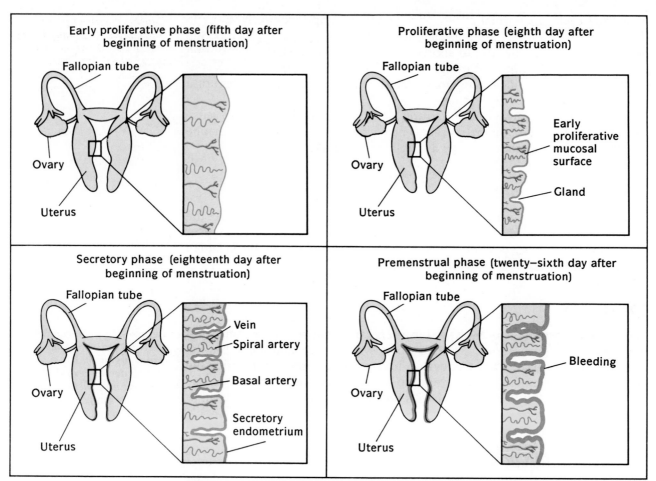

Figure 9.2 Changes in the uterine wall during a monthly menstrual cycle. On the fifth day after menstruation, bleeding has generally ended and the denuded surface is fed by short basal arteries. By the eighth day, estrogen is causing glands and arteries to proliferate and the uterine wall grows thicker. After ovulation, the lining swells as arteries corkscrew to the surface and glands secrete mucus. Finally, if fertilization does not occur, the spiral arteries constrict, the surface layers lose their nourishment, and the endometrium becomes ready to be sloughed off as menstrual discharge.

Occasionally women may experience problems that are more intense: painful menstruation (dysmenorrhea), excessive bleeding, and amenorrhea (the cessation of menstrual periods). It has been estimated that up to 50 percent of all women have such problems at some time in their lives.

Recently it has been discovered that women with severe menstrual pain often have an excess of hormonelike substances known as **prostaglandins** in their bodies when they menstruate. Prostaglandin levels can be reduced and other menstrual problems can be treated with ibuprofen or medications prescribed by a physician.

Psychological Effects of the Menstrual Cycle The menstrual cycle may also affect women psychologically. Some women experience mood changes at certain times during the menstrual cycle, typically just before the menstrual flow begins. This is not surprising, since the menstrual flow is brought on by dramatic changes in the levels of hormones which act on the whole body, including the brain.

The psychological effects of menstruation are still being studied. A condition known as **premenstrual syndrome (PMS),** which some—though not all or even most—women experience, can cause great distress. PMS can include symptoms such as irritability, lethargy, and depression in addition to the

prostaglandins—*hormonelike substances secreted by various parts of the body into the bloodstream; excessive amounts of prostaglandins are suspected to be a cause of severe menstrual pain.*

premenstrual syndrome (PMS)—*a pattern of physiological symptoms, irritability, lethargy, and depression that precedes menstruation in some women.*

Table 9.1 Problems of the Female Reproductive System

Condition	Known or Suspected Cause	Remedy
Irregular periods	Stress, fatigue, anorexia, hormonal imbalance, extreme exercise regimen (e.g., marathon training)	Medical consultation; hormone therapy
Ectopic pregnancy	Diseased or inflamed Fallopian tubes that leave scars and may cause blockage	Surgery
Infertility	Blocked Fallopian tubes, hormonal imbalance, sexually transmitted infection, glandular disorder	Surgery for blocked Fallopian tubes; hormone therapy; medical treatment for STD infection; in vitro fertilization

Causes of missed periods other than pregnancy include emotional stress, sudden weight loss, the onset of menopause, and medical problems such as tumors.

The average woman loses between 5 and 8 tablespoons of blood during menstruation.

physiological effects just mentioned. It has been suggested that these symptoms can even trigger violent behavior, although this has been disputed. Most doctors and researchers seem to agree that such a syndrome does exist in some women, and the American Psychiatric Association is considering a controversial proposal to classify severe PMS as a mental disorder. The syndrome is currently thought to be a result of a lack of the hormone progesterone, and some patients have been treated successfully with doses of progesterone.[1] A recent study indicated that the incidence and severity of PMS may be linked to high consumption (more than 4 ½ cups a day) of caffeine-containing beverages.[2]

Further research will probably help clarify the psychological changes that can accompany the menstrual cycle. It is interesting to note that some women may actually perform better in their premenstrual days. One study found that typists were more accurate during that time. Other research has found that women's senses of taste and smell, their identification of musical pitches, and the strength and steadiness of their hands vary slightly over the menstrual cycle.[3]

Menopause: Myths and Reality

Menopause is the gradual, permanent cessation of a woman's menstruation and cyclic reproductive activity, brought on by decreased production of female sex hormones. On the average menopause begins at about age 51, but it may begin as late as age 55.[4] At that time a woman's menstrual periods usually falter for a few months and then cease altogether, at which point the woman is said to have "gone through" menopause or had her "change of life." This change is also known as the **climacteric,** the time that marks the end of the reproductive phase of a woman's life.

During menopause the ovaries, after 30 or 40 years of activity, lose their ability to produce mature eggs. While a woman may welcome the end of fertility, the reduced production of female hormones in her body can create problems. Subtle changes may occur in the body as a result of hormone deficiency. The skin may gradually become drier and more wrinkled. The vagina may become drier, and its lining thinner and more tender. Throughout the body bones may lose calcium and become more brittle—a condition known as osteoporosis (Chapter 17). Doctors often recommend calcium supplementation to ameliorate this condition. Estrogen replacement therapy is another treatment prescribed for these changes, although its risks are still not completely understood.

It is not true, however, that a woman's sexual interest and activity decline after menopause. In fact, many menopausal and postmenopausal women, no longer concerned about becoming pregnant, actually feel more sexual desire and satisfaction.

*menopause—the gradual permanent cessation of a woman's menstruation and therefore of the reproductive phase of her life. Also known as the **climacteric**.*

climacteric—see menopause.

A lifelong plan for healthy living, including proper nutrition and exercise, helps minimize problems with osteoporosis after menopause.

The Male Reproductive System

The male reproductive system has two basic functions: to produce sperm and to transport mature sperm to the site of conception. These two functions are carried out by specialized organs in the male reproductive system (Figure 9.3).

The Testes

testes (testicles)—*the male organs that produce sperm and male hormones.*

sperm—*the male reproductive cells.*

spermatogenesis—*the continual process of sperm production.*

The **testes,** or **testicles,** are two walnut-shaped organs located in the scrotum. Within the testes, male reproductive cells—the **sperm**—are produced. Unlike women, who are born with a full set of ova in their ovaries, men are not born with sperm. Instead, their bodies produce new sperm cells every day after reaching puberty—at the rate of about 200 million daily in a normal man. This process of continual sperm production, called **spermatogenesis,** begins at puberty and can continue well into old age. The testes also produce the male sex hormone testosterone, which stimulates the development of the sexual organs in a human fetus and the secondary sexual characteristics in an adult male.

The Epididymis and Vas Deferens

epididymis—*a highly coiled network of tubing in the back of each testicle through which sperm cells travel as they mature.*

After sperm are produced in the testes, they mature while traveling through a network of several tubes—the **epididymis**—located in the scrotum behind each testicle. The sperm are stored and nourished in the epididymis before ejaculation. During ejaculation the walls of each epididymis contract, pushing

Figure 9.3 The male reproductive system has two basic functions: producing mature sperm in the testes and epididymis and transporting them alive to the site of conception.

For sperm to develop properly, the temperature of the scrotum should normally be 2 or 3 degrees below body temperature. Sweat glands in the scrotal wall and thin scrotal skin with no insulating fat also help regulate temperature. In addition, muscles in the scrotal wall raise and lower the testes as a response to outside temperature changes such as cold weather and hot baths.

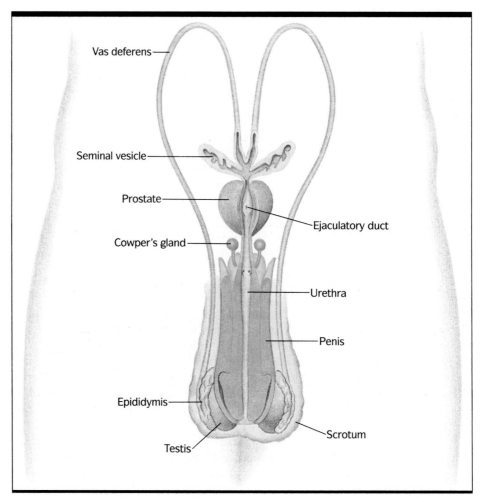

the sperm into a pair of conducting tubes called the **vas deferens,** which lead up into the man's body toward two other internal organs: the seminal vesicles and the prostate gland. In the vas deferens sperm become *motile,* or capable of moving spontaneously in preparation for their journey into the female reproductive system.

The Seminal Vesicles and Prostate Gland

The **seminal vesicles** and **prostate gland,** which are located behind the urinary bladder, play an important role in the male reproductive system. Both glands secrete fluids that combine with sperm to form a mixture called **semen,** or **seminal fluid,** the liquid that leaves the penis during ejaculation. This fluid provides the means for sperm to travel outside the body.

After linking with the seminal vesicles, each vas deferens constricts to form the **ejaculatory ducts,** which then join the urethra within the prostate gland. The urethra, which is the passageway for urine from the bladder, continues on to the opening of the penis. During ejaculation semen containing several hundred million sperm is discharged through the urethra and out the tip of the penis.

Cowper's Glands

During sexual arousal a few drops of fluid may appear at the end of the penis. This fluid is produced by the **Cowper's glands,** two pea-sized organs just below the prostate gland. This fluid may reduce the acidity of the urethra before ejaculation, but researchers remain uncertain about this. Knowledge about the Cowper's gland fluid, which may contain viable sperm, is important for effective birth control.

vas deferens—*long tubes that carry sperm from the epididymis to the seminal vesicles.*

seminal vesicles—*two small structures located at the base of the bladder that produce about 70% of the seminal fluid.*

prostate gland—*the male organ that surrounds the urethra and produces about 30 percent of the seminal fluid. Prostate problems are common as men grow older. Many men experience enlargement, or* **hypertrophy,** *a condition in which the prostate begins to enlarge and tighten around the urethra, often causing bladder and urination difficulties. This condition can usually be treated successfully.*

semen—*the sperm-carrying liquid expelled from the penis during ejaculation; also called* **seminal fluid.**

ejaculatory ducts—*two structures formed by the ends of the seminal vesicles and the vas deferens that in turn join the urethra.*

Cowper's glands—*two pea-sized organs just below the prostate gland that sometimes produce a few drops of fluid at the end of the penis during sexual arousal.*

Table 9.2 Problems of the Male Reproductive System

Condition	Known or Suspected Cause	Remedy
Sterility	Diseases of the testes and epididymis; testicular tumors	Radiation treatment for tumors; treatment for STDs to minimize certain diseases of the epididymis
Prostate disease	Inflammation of the prostate as a result of bacterial infection, history of STD, drug abuse, or habitual use of alcohol or tobacco; cancer; benign hyperplasia (a benign enlargement of the prostate gland)	Medical treatment; avoidance of drugs, alcohol, or tobacco; use of the synthetic female hormone stilbestrol for prostate cancer; surgical removal of the prostate for benign hyperplasia
Infertility	Obstructions and infections anywhere in the reproductive system; undescended testes (cryptorchidism); disorder of the penis (including hypospadias, in which the urethra opens on the underside of the penis); hormonal abnormalities; sexually transmitted diseases; consumption of tobacco, alcohol, or drugs	Surgery for obstructions, cryptorchidism, and penis abnormalities; hormone therapy for hormonal abnormalities; medication for STDs or surgery to correct scarring; avoidance of hazardous substances

Sexual Responsibility and Safer Sex

In sexual intercourse the male's penis deposits millions of sperm into the female's vagina. From there the sperm travel up into the uterus and then the Fallopian tubes, where they may encounter an ovum. If a sperm and ovum unite, the egg becomes fertilized and a few days later implants itself in the woman's uterine lining.

Frequently, however, a couple does not wish to conceive a child. They may be unable or unwilling to care for a child. Perhaps they are not economically ready or have several children already and do not want any more. Perhaps they are unmarried and do not want children or are married but wish to remain childless. In such cases they will want to avoid pregnancy.

In addition to pregnancy, another result of sexual expression and sexual intercourse may be the contraction of a sexually transmitted disease (STD). STDs can be very serious; they are covered in depth in Chapter 10. People who approach sex responsibly and safely are also concerned about not spreading an STD to their partners.

There are a variety of methods for avoiding pregnancy and reducing the possibility of contracting an STD. Knowledge about the different possibilities, how to use them, and how effective they are is vital for a safer and more responsible sex life. Decisions about contraceptive methods should be based on reliable information about their safety and effectiveness. Another factor, of course, must be the individual's personal beliefs. If a person has ambivalent feelings about sexuality and reproduction or has inner doubts about employing a contraceptive method, he or she may hesitate to use it. Clearly, this is an issue involving considerable personal responsibility.

In the past, workers in the field of family planning thought that the ultimate answer to effective birth control could be found in good, easy-to-obtain contraceptive methods, but this idea was only partly true. What these family-planning experts were ignoring was the human factor—the question of whether people would learn about contraceptive methods and then apply them correctly every time. It turns out that human error has a great deal to do with the effectiveness of any birth control method. As Table 9.3 shows, with many contraceptive methods there is a significant difference between how effective the method is in theory and how effective it is when people actually use it.

Contraceptive Methods Requiring No Medical Supervision

Of the various contraceptive and birth control methods available, those which do not require medical prescription or supervision include abstinence; condoms; spermicidal jellies, creams, and foams; vaginal sponges; and withdrawal.

Abstinence   The most effective means of avoiding pregnancy and controlling the spread of STDs (including AIDS) is abstinence from sexual intercourse. Abstinence, though unpopular, is possible. For some people it may mean avoiding all forms of sexual expression. For others it may mean engaging in alternative forms of sexual intimacy (Chapter 8), such as petting, mutual masturbation, and oral sex (though there is evidence that this does *not* remove the danger of disease).

condom—*a thin latex or natural skin sheath that is placed over the erect penis before intercourse to prevent conception.*

Condoms   A **condom** is a thin latex or natural skin sheath that is placed over the erect penis just before intercourse. If used correctly, it captures and holds the man's semen so that sperm will not be deposited in the vagina.

The condom is an effective contraceptive device. It is also the second most effective method, after abstinence, for protection against AIDS and other STDs. To achieve the best protection against disease, however, latex condoms must be used; natural skin condoms may have minute holes that allow some semen to pass through. Moreover, condoms must be applied at the appropriate time to ensure that any sperm carried by the Cowper's gland fluid does not impregnate the woman during foreplay. Care must also be taken during withdrawal to prevent semen from touching the female genitals.

The condom has been widely used throughout the world for centuries. With no harmful physical side effects, it is the leading barrier method of birth control. When used in combination with vaginal foam, it is one of the most effective birth control devices. The fact that it provides a physical barrier between the partners makes it effective against disease too.

Some people object to using condoms on the grounds that they diminish sensation. For others, however, the use of a condom results in pleasurable prolongation of intercourse. Some couples consider a condom an annoying distraction, while others consider it an integral part of the sexual experience.

Jellies, Creams, and Foams Nonprescription jellies, creams, and foams are spermicides that the woman inserts before intercourse, deep in her vagina against the cervix, with a plastic applicator; they act by destroying sperm, and are effective as additional protection when used with barrier devices such as condoms and diaphragms. In addition to killing sperm, spermicides are also effective in reducing bacterial and virally caused STDs. In fact, researchers state that if spermicides are used in addition to condoms, the risk of contracting AIDS can be further reduced.[5] (Spermicides should not be used alone for

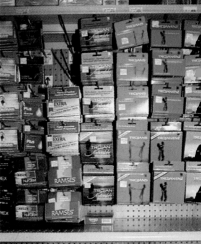

Readily available in most pharmacies, condoms are an efficient birth control method; they are also the most effective devices for lowering the risk of contracting sexually transmitted diseases such as AIDS. (David R. Frazier/Photo Researchers, Inc.)

Heat may cause latex to deteriorate, so condoms should not be carried in a pocket wallet.

Douching seems to be a popular practice among many American women, but it is not necessary for good health. The normal vaginal environment is acidic, which keeps it free from harmful bacteria. Douching does no particular harm provided that a mild acidic solution such as vinegar and water is used, but it is not a good idea to use alkaline or commercial chemical douches because they may neutralize the vagina's protective acids, allowing harmful bacteria to multiply. Douching is not a means of birth control.

Table 9.3   Contraceptive Methods and First-Year Pregnancy Rates

Method	Percent of pregnancies within the first year for couples using method	
	Lowest expected[a]	Typical[b]
No medical care required		
No precaution	89	89
Douching	89	89
Natural methods:		
Withdrawal	4	18
Calendar	10	14–47[c]
Temperature	n/a[d]	n/a
Mucus evaluation	3.5	19–24[e]
Sympto-thermal	6	11–20
Condoms	2	12
Foams, creams, and jellies	3	21
Vaginal sponge	5	18
Medical care required		
Oral contraceptives	0.1–0.5	3
Contraceptive implants	0.3	0.3
Intrauterine device (IUD)	1.5	6
Diaphragm (with spermicide)	3	18
Cervical cap	5	18

[a] Pregnancies resulting from failures in the method.

[b] Pregnancies resulting from incorrect application or discontinuation of the method and failures of the method itself.

[c] Most pregnancies resulted from failure to abstain.

[d] Method not commonly used because of long periods of abstinence required.

[e] Most pregnancies resulted from conscious deviations from the rules of the method.

Sources: R. A. Hatcher et al., *Contraceptive Technology 1988–1989*, 14th ed. (New York: Irvington, 1988); Daniel R. Mishell, Jr., M.D., "Contraception," *New England Journal of Medicine* (March 23, 1989): 777. With permission.

this purpose, however.) In addition, women who use spermicides are only one-third as likely to develop cervical cancer and other diseases that are linked to sexual infection.[6]

The Vaginal Sponge In 1983 the U.S. Food and Drug Administration (FDA) approved the vaginal contraceptive sponge for over-the-counter sale. It was the first nonprescription contraceptive to undergo safety and effectiveness tests as stringent as those required for prescription contraceptives. The sponge, which must be moistened to release its spermicidal chemical, fits into the vagina and covers the cervix; it must be left in place for at least 6 hours after intercourse and can work effectively as long as 24 hours. A loop is attached to the sponge for easy removal.

Convenient, comfortable, and easy to use, the vaginal sponge does not provide protection against AIDS or other STDs. However, it appears to prevent pregnancy as reliably as the diaphragm, though not as dependably as the pill and the intrauterine device. In some women the sponge may cause irritation or an allergic reaction, and problems with removal have been reported. There is some concern that use of the sponge may carry a risk of toxic shock syndrome, but data about this potential risk are inconclusive.[7]

Withdrawal Often known as *coitus interruptus*, **withdrawal** is an ancient contraceptive method. As the name implies, the man withdraws his penis from the woman's vagina before he ejaculates. The idea is to prevent sperm from entering the vagina by ejaculating outside the woman's body. The apparent advantage of this method is that it is available to everyone and costs nothing, but it is one of the more unreliable techniques of birth control. Not only is there a risk of impregnation from sperm in Cowper's gland fluid, it is also possible that the man will miscalculate the time for withdrawal or get carried away. Of course, there is no barrier to prevent contraction of AIDS or other STDs.

Contraceptive Methods Requiring Nonsurgical Medical Supervision

Among the available birth control methods that require some medical care and supervision are oral contraceptives, the intrauterine device, the diaphragm, and the cervical cap.

Oral Contraceptives Since 1960, when the FDA first approved **oral contraceptives** ("the pill") for use with a doctor's prescription, millions of prescriptions for them have been written in the United States alone. Except for surgical sterilization, the pill is the most widely used form of contraception among American women.[8] For the pill to be effective, the directions and schedule for taking it must be adhered to strictly; missed days make a woman susceptible to pregnancy. On average, 2 of 100 women on the pill become pregnant, but the number is even lower when the regimen is followed fastidiously.[9] Unfortunately, the pill provides no protection against AIDS or other STDs.

Most forms of the pill introduce into the body certain synthetic equivalents of the natural sex hormones in such a way that the hormonal cycle that leads the woman's body to ovulate is altered and ovulation is prevented. Research has shown that ovulation can be effectively prevented with much smaller doses of hormones than were originally used; this is fortunate, because the likelihood of developing side effects is directly related to the amount of hormone in the pill. Most brands on the market today are "combination" pills; that is, each tablet contains both progestin (a synthetic progesterone derivative) and a synthetic form of estrogen. A "minipill," which is less widely used, contains progestin in a low dose and no estrogen.

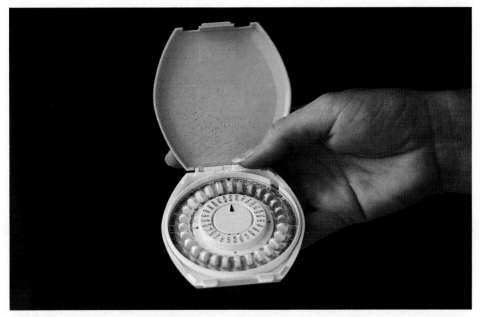

When taken regularly, birth control pills prevent pregnancy by releasing hormones that prevent ovulation. (David Young-Wolff/PhotoEdit)

For some women the pill does have troublesome side effects. The most serious are an increased risk of developing circulatory system disorders such as blood clots (usually in the legs), which can impair circulation; an increased risk of heart attacks; and a greater risk of death from a stroke. All these risks are increased if the woman smokes. The risk of pill use is greatest for women over 35 who smoke and for all women over 45.[10] Pill users also run a greater risk of developing gallbladder disease requiring surgery; benign liver tumors, which can be fatal if they rupture; and high blood pressure. If a woman takes oral contraceptives by mistake when she is pregnant, her baby may have birth defects involving the heart and the limbs.[11]

There are, however, some positive aspects of the pill. Some recent studies have suggested that pill users have a decreased risk of contracting cancer of the ovaries and uterus.[12] The pill also regulates the menstrual cycle and reduces cramps and excessive blood loss. The likelihood of developing iron deficiency anemia, acne, pelvic inflammatory disease, ectopic pregnancies, noncancerous breast tumors, and ovarian cysts has also been shown to be reduced.

Whatever the risks and benefits of oral contraceptives, they are the most effective method of birth control other than surgical sterilization, and the overall risk of death from their use is low—below that of pregnancy and childbirth itself—except among women who smoke. With all oral contraceptives, continuing medical supervision is necessary to minimize these risks and determine the appropriate pill for each woman.

The Intrauterine Device (IUD)

Intrauterine devices (IUDs) are made of soft, flexible plastic molded into various sizes and shapes; some are coated with copper. They are inserted into the uterus by a physician. Some types of IUDs must be replaced every year or so; other types can be left in place indefinitely.

Exactly how IUDs work is not completely understood, but it is thought that they interfere with the implantation of a fertilized egg in the lining of the uterus. It is also clear that they have no effect against the infectious agents of STDs and provide no protection against AIDS.

intrauterine device (IUD)— *a soft, flexible device that is inserted into the uterus to prevent pregnancy.*

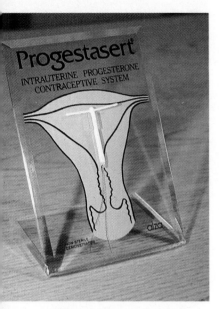

Although intrauterine devices are one of the most reliable forms of birth control, they can sometimes cause cramps and even injury. (Tony Freeman/PhotoEdit)

diaphragm—*a shallow rubber cup that is inserted into the vagina, where it completely covers the cervix, forming a mechanical barrier that prevents sperm from entering the uterus.*

Some women select the IUD as a contraceptive method because it is long-lasting, need not be put in place before intercourse, and does not alter body chemistry. IUDs are very effective, with a failure rate of 1 to 6 pregnancies per 100 women per year.[13]

IUDs do have disadvantages, however. About 15 percent have to be removed because of persistent uterine bleeding or cramps.[14] They have also been known to be expelled from the uterus without the user's noticing. This usually occurs during the first few months after insertion, but there is a continuing, although low, incidence of expulsion, particularly for a woman who has had many babies and whose uterine cavity is large. Finally, people have filed costly lawsuits charging that IUDs cause infections and infertility. These lawsuits caused the top U.S. manufacturer of IUDs to take its products off the market in early 1986.[15]

The Diaphragm   The **diaphragm** is a shallow rubber cup made of fine latex rubber stretched over a flexible, circular metal ring. The ring can be bent so that the entire device can easily be compressed and passed into the vagina. Upon release, it rests in the upper, large portion of the vagina, where it covers the cervix completely.

The diaphragm works as a mechanical barrier to prevent sperm from passing into the uterus. However, because it is not a complete barrier, it provides little protection against STDs. Spermicidal jelly or cream, which a woman must apply to the diaphragm before she inserts it, adds to its effectiveness as a contraceptive.

When a diaphragm is inserted properly, it causes no discomfort and neither partner notices it. The diaphragm does have a significant failure rate, but forgetfulness, improper insertion and use, or early removal—it should stay in place for at least 6 hours after intercourse—probably account for many of the pregnancies, as they do with many other contraceptive methods.

The Cervical Cap   The cervical cap is a soft rubber cap, smaller than a diaphragm, that fits snugly over the cervix. Variations on this device have been used by women throughout the world for centuries. The cervical cap must be fitted by a physician. Before intercourse, it is half filled with contraceptive cream or jelly and inserted. It is left in place for at least 6 hours afterward; the device remains effective for 1 to 3 days. A one-way valve lets menstrual blood and cervical mucus pass through. The cervical cap has a low failure rate, although it is sometimes accidentally dislodged during intercourse.

The cervical cap is classified by the FDA as a "significant-risk device" and should not be used by women who have diabetes mellitus, cardiovascular disease, liver or kidney disease, gonorrhea, active herpes simplex type 2 infection, an abnormal Pap smear, toxic shock syndrome, or a cervical or vaginal infection.[16] It also provides no protection against STDs.

Natural Methods of Contraception

Some people prefer not to use any methods of contraception that require medications or mechanical devices yet do not want to rely only on abstinence or withdrawal. Natural contraception requires careful planning and some initial guidance from a physician.

To use natural family planning, the couple avoids intercourse during the time when the woman may be ovulating. A number of variables are involved, including the length of time the sperm remain alive in the woman's reproductive tract and the length of time the released ovum is available for fertilization. Scientists do not know how to pinpoint these variables, and so there is about a 10 to 20 percent theoretical failure rate with natural family planning.[17] Moreover, these methods do not provide a barrier against the transmission of AIDS and other STDs.

A key variable in natural family planning is the timing of the woman's ovulation. This can be determined with fair accuracy in a number of ways, including the calendar method, the temperature method, the mucus evaluation method, and the sympto-thermal method.

The Calendar Method   This method is based on the observation that most women usually ovulate around the fourteenth day before the next menstrual period. A woman must accumulate about a 1-year record of her periods in order to be able to determine her fertile period with a reasonable degree of accuracy. Women vary considerably in the length of their menstrual cycles.

To use the calendar method effectively, the woman needs to get the advice of a doctor, at least at the beginning, to learn how to chart her menstrual periods and calculate the days when it is "safe" and "unsafe" for her to have intercourse. Unfortunately, studies have shown that this method is the least reliable natural method. The calendar method by itself is thus not currently advocated for couples who are interested in practicing periodic abstinence.[18]

The Temperature Method   With this method, a woman tries to pinpoint the time of ovulation by charting her basal body temperature every day (Figure 9.4). Ovulation will be followed by a slight rise in temperature (one-half degree Celsius) that will last until the start of the next menstrual cycle. This method is not foolproof: although the temperature change provides a fairly good indication that ovulation has occurred, a slight rise in temperature can also be caused by minor colds and infections. The temperature and calendar methods, used together, are sometimes referred to as the rhythm method.

The Mucus Evaluation Method   A third method of natural family planning is known as mucus evaluation (it is also called the ovulation method or the Billings method). It has long been known that the consistency of the mucus in the vagina changes with the menstrual cycle. At certain stages of the cycle this mucus becomes more viscous, that is, thicker and of a more gluey texture (somewhat comparable to raw egg white). It is possible to predict ovulation by examining the consistency of the cervical mucus. This technique has fairly high dependability, but it is complicated. Couples who wish to use it must obtain special training and information from a physician or other trained health care professional.

Figure 9.4 Typical changes in basal body temperature during a menstrual cycle. (The actual temperatures will vary from woman to woman.) Basal body temperature dips slightly before ovulation, indicating to the woman that ovulation is about to take place. It then increases slightly and stays slightly elevated for the rest of the woman's cycle.

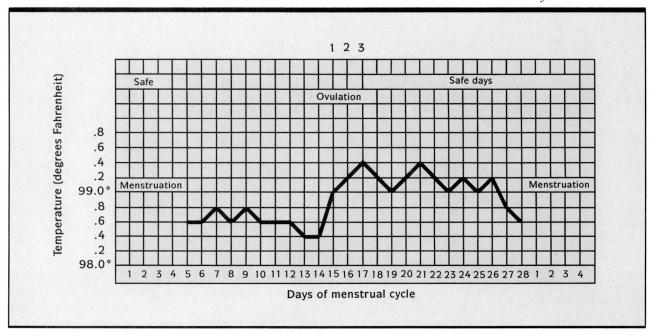

The Sympto-Thermal Method The sympto-thermal method is essentially a combination of the temperature method and the mucus evaluation method. Temperature and mucus are both observed, and intercourse must be avoided if *either* of the two appears to indicate ovulation. Intercourse should not begin again until both variables indicate that sex is safe.

Contraceptive Methods Requiring Surgery

Millions of men and women have undergone surgical sterilization as a means to prevent future pregnancy; such sterilization is virtually 100 percent effective. For individuals who are certain that they no longer wish to conceive, voluntary sterilization is the closest thing to an ideal method of contraception.

vasectomy—a surgical sterilization technique for men in which a section of each vas deferens is removed.

Every year in the United States, about 500,000 men have a **vasectomy**.[19] This simple and safe surgical procedure, which can be performed in a doctor's office, involves cutting and tying off the vas deferens, thus preventing sperm from exiting the testes (Figure 9.5). After a vasectomy the sperm are reabsorbed in the testes without harm. Many men are concerned about the effects of this operation on their masculinity, but the level of male hormones remains unchanged and there is no alteration in secondary sexual characteristics or sexual performance.

Sterilization is the most common means of fertility control. By the mid-1980s over 137 million people worldwide, male and female, had undergone voluntary sterilization.

A postoperative semen examination, normally performed about 6 weeks after the procedure, is essential to determine when the sperm count has reached zero. Another test is usually given after 4 months to make sure that the procedure was effective. Vasectomy is generally considered irreversible, although in some cases microsurgical techniques have restored fertility.

tubal ligation—a surgical sterilization technique for women in which the Fallopian tubes are severed or tied.

For women, the standard surgical technique is **tubal ligation**—dividing or tying off the Fallopian tubes—a procedure that may require hospitalization. As with a vasectomy, a tubal ligation does not affect sexual characteristics or performance. For the most part a tubal ligation should be considered permanent, although with certain techniques it is fairly reversible.

Figure 9.5 Methods of sterilization. **Top:** *vasectomy. (A) The surgeon feels the upper area of the scrotum to locate one of the two vas deferens. (B) An incision is made and the vas deferens is clamped. (C) A segment is removed. (D) The incision is sutured. The process is then repeated on the vas deferens of the other testis.* **Bottom:** *Tubal ligation (A) An incision is made and a Fallopian tube is located. (B) The tube is cut. (C) Both ends of the cut tube are tied with nonabsorbable material. The procedure is then performed on the other Fallopian tube.*

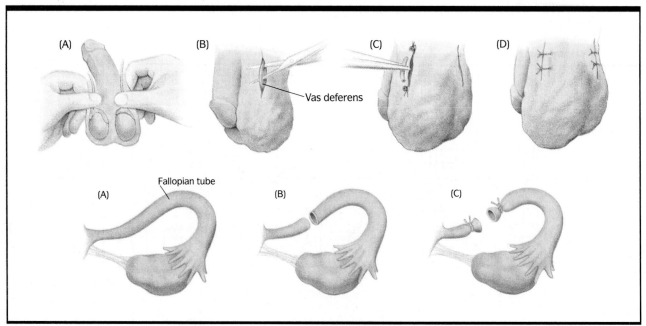

Before deciding on a vasectomy or tubal ligation, the individual should think the matter over carefully. The unforeseen death of a child may cause parents to rethink having more children. While adoption is always a possibility, it must be weighed against the desire to be the natural parents of children. The possibility of divorce and remarriage should also be considered. In general, voluntary sterilization should not be viewed as a solution to sexual or marital problems. Of course, it contributes nothing to the prevention of AIDS and other STDs.

Finally, a new surgical method that is reversible has been introduced into the United States after several years of use elsewhere in the world. This is the **contraceptive implant,** with the trade name *Norplant*, a chemical device inserted under the skin, usually on the upper arm or hip. Once implanted, it slowly releases chemicals that prevent menstruation. The effective life of Norplant is 5 years; after that it must be surgically removed and replaced. It can be removed earlier, however, if the woman wishes to become pregnant.[20]

Contraceptive Methods of the Future

Scientists continue to search for better and safer methods of contraception. In general, in addition to making contraceptives safer, the trend is toward making them easier to use so that people will be more likely to employ them. In addition, the more variety that is available, the more likely people are to find a method with which they can feel comfortable. Thus, there is a tendency to develop techniques which are effective for longer periods of time without attention.

Methods for Women Before the year 2000 additional types of contraceptive implants are expected: for example, a biodegradable rod which will not require removal and will last for 18 months and a pellet that will last for a year.[21] Other chemically based techniques are also being perfected. These include **vaginal rings,** which when placed in the vagina release chemicals that prevent ovulation or make the vaginal mucus impermeable to sperm, and **injectable contraceptives,** which release the same synthetic hormones found in most oral contraceptives and are effective for 2 or 3 months.[22]

In addition to chemical methods, a new physical barrier method is also being developed. This is the **vaginal condom,** a prelubricated latex receptacle designed to be worn by a woman instead of a man. The vaginal condom has two rings to keep it in place: an interior ring that fits into the vagina much like a diaphragm and a larger external ring to keep the condom in place during intercourse. Made of thicker and stronger latex than the male condom, it should last longer. It also provides a physical barrier against the spread of STDs.[23]

Finally, work is being done to develop an antisperm vaccine. This would work like any other vaccine in that it would produce antibodies to a foreign organism. In this case, the vaccine would sensitize a woman's immune system to sperm so that it produces antibodies to destroy the sperm as soon as they are introduced into her body.[24]

Methods for Men Chemical contraceptives are being developed that will retard the production of sperm. A substance made from cottonseed, called gossypol, was discovered a few years ago, but it causes feelings of tiredness, nausea, and lowered sex drive. However, scientists are investigating the effectiveness of similar substances with fewer side effects.[25]

The other approaches being explored are more sophisticated techniques for vasectomy. One nonsurgical technique promises no incisions or surgical stitches and almost immediate recovery. In this technique, a device much like a stapler will staple the spermatic ducts shut. Another is a "reversible" vasectomy in which a silicone plug is inserted into each vas deferens; the plugs can

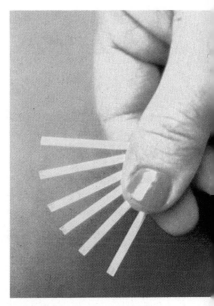

The Food and Drug Administration (FDA) finally cleared Norplant for the U.S. market in 1990. (Swersey/ Gamma Liaison)

contraceptive implant—*a device implanted under the skin that slowly releases chemicals to prevent menstruation.*

vaginal rings—*rings which, when placed in the vagina, release a chemical that prevents ovulation or makes the cervical mucus impermeable to sperm.*

injectable contraceptive—*a contraceptive that releases synthetic hormones like those found in most oral contraceptives; it is effective for 2 or 3 months.*

vaginal condoms—*a prelubricated latex receptacle designed to be worn by women during sexual intercourse.*

The Economics of Birth Control

Science and technology have made it easier for people throughout the world to decide when and whether to have children. Still, in prosperous countries as well as poor ones, unwanted pregnancies occur, and the global population continues to soar. The solution—birth control and family planning—is unevenly successful throughout the world.

One reason is that not everyone believes that birth control is desirable. To farmers in some developing nations, the advantage of creating another pair of hands to work in the fields often seems to compensate for the problem of having another mouth to feed. Resentment is also felt toward family-planning organizations from the West, which are sometimes perceived as trying to limit the growth of poorer nations.

In developed countries, too, many people believe that population growth is not necessarily going to cause economic decline. There are also many people who consider that life is an absolute value which should not be hindered by any means.

However, most nations at all levels of economic development perceive that fast-growing populations represent a real economic liability. Some, such as China, have instituted successful family-planning policies that even supporters of birth control find harsh. Many others, including Colombia in South America and Thailand in the Far East, have had surprising success in promoting family planning. Many nations in the West are getting close to zero population growth.

Ironically, one of the developed nations least successful at family planning is the United States, which has been a major advocate of birth control and is still the largest contributor to international programs. Its lack of success at home is particularly noticeable among teenagers: almost all the developed nations of Europe, even those with similar patterns of adolescent sexual activity, have lower rates of teenage pregnancy. The higher success rate in other countries compared with the United States may result from the fact that contraceptive services in Europe are more widely available, free or inexpensive, and confidential. In addition, there are fewer methods of birth control available here than in other countries: because of political and legal pressures, U.S. drug manufacturers have been reluctant to research new techniques, and the U.S. Food and Drug Administration requires particularly careful testing before a contraceptive method can be approved for sale here.

However, the failure of family planning and birth control is most severe in the developing nations, where, according to the World Health Organization, five of every six couples of reproductive age are still not using adequate methods of birth control. The problem is particularly severe in parts of Africa, Asia, and Latin America. (More than 400 million married woman do use some form of birth control today, however, up by more than 500 percent from the beginning of the 1960s.)

What are some of the reasons given for the limited success of birth control in the third world? The cost of birth control methods is one problem: although many organizations make financial and other contributions, money is a major requirement for successful programs. Recently, the United States has been less willing to support family-planning organizations, especially those which have provided abortion services in developing countries.

Religious issues also play a large role in the availability of birth control programs. Ireland has a high pregnancy rate, doubtless because of its strong Catholic tradition.

In addition to these complex issues, there are three very simple ones. In both developing and developed countries family planning is most successful if contraceptive drugs and devices are available easily and inexpensively and if information is available both about the advantages of using them and about methods for using them correctly.

Includes ideas from Peter Donaldson and Charles Keely, "Population and Family Planning: An International Perspective," *Family Planning Perspectives* (November–December 1988): 307ff; Philip J. Hilts, "Birth Control Backlash," *New York Times Magazine* (December 16, 1990): 41ff.

be removed later. A third technique involves the injection of a polymer glue into the vas deferens; it requires no incisions, takes only a few minutes, has no known side effects, and may be reversible.[26]

Pregnancy

Many people assume that having a baby is the most natural thing in the world, and in many respects it is. These people feel that when the time comes to start a family, they will be ready to make the adjustment to parenthood smoothly and effortlessly. Becoming a parent, however, involves the most profound changes the average person will ever experience. Parenthood is a lifelong responsibility, and it requires the same kind of planning as other major life decisions, such as selecting a career, getting married, and buying a house. No one can anticipate every difficulty, but there are important issues that should be considered when one is thinking about having a baby.

Planning for Pregnancy

Planning can be as useful when a couple decide to have a child as it is when they decide to avoid pregnancy. In fact, there are many more factors to consider. Some of the issues people should explore when deciding to have a child are whether genetic counseling is advisable, how to deal with problems of infertility, when they should have a child, and how having a child will affect their relationship.

Genetic Counseling   Genetic diseases, of which there are more than 2,000, affect 3 to 5 percent of all babies born in the United States.[27] Sickle-cell anemia, phenylketonuria (PKU), Tay-Sachs disease, hemophilia, a type of muscular dystrophy, cystic fibrosis, Down syndrome, and two forms of diabetes are among the conditions that may be avoided through genetic counseling.

Genetic counseling can provide prospective parents with information about whether they are likely to pass on a genetically linked disease to their child. For example, people who are carriers of Tay-Sachs disease, which condemns a

There are three genetic disorders that are related to specific ethnic groups:

- **Sickle-cell anemia** *is a blood disease that most often affects black children.*
- **Tay-Sachs disease** *is a fatal nerve disorder seen in Jewish babies with parents of Eastern European descent.*
- **Thalassemia** *is a type of anemia that occurs most often in babies born to parents of Mediterranean descent.*

Physical disorders and other health problems sometimes can be detected through ultrasound. The ultrasound machine sends thousands of harmless vibrations into the womb each second, providing an in-depth image of the growing fetus. (Alexander Tsiaras/Science Source/Photo Researchers, Inc.)

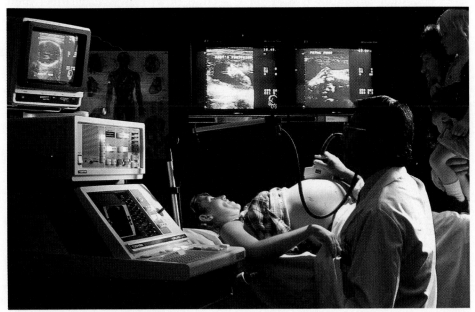

child to an early death, may decide not to risk having children in order to avoid bearing a child who may be afflicted with the disease.

A genetic counselor can explain to prospective parents how a particular disorder is transmitted from generation to generation, what the odds are that the disease will recur in their family, and what the disease is like. If the risk of passing on a disease is slight or if an effective treatment is available, the potential parents may decide to go ahead with a pregnancy despite the risks. Otherwise, adoption may be an alternative.

Some genetic disorders cannot be identified before pregnancy, but many can be identified while the fetus is still in the uterus. It is now possible to test a fetus directly for about 100 genetic disorders as early as the fourth month of pregnancy. In a procedure called **amniocentesis,** a doctor can withdraw some of the amniotic fluid that surrounds a fetus in the womb. Laboratory tests of the sloughed fetal cells in this fluid can then determine whether the fetus has a genetic disorder. A newer technique, called **chorionic villi sampling,** is sometimes preferred over amniocentesis today. It takes only 2 days to get results, compared with about 3 weeks for amniocentesis.[28]

Such tests usually are performed only if there is reason to suspect that the fetus has a particular disease, that is, if the couple have already had one diseased child or are known to be carriers of the defect. With a few of these diseases, treatments can begin before birth.

Since certain disorders are more prevalent as the age of the mother increases, doctors generally recommend that any pregnant woman over age 35—regardless of whether she has any reason to suspect the presence of a genetic disease in her family—consider amniocentesis to test for genetic disorders such as Down syndrome.

Dealing with Infertility Infertility, or the inability of a couple to achieve pregnancy, is usually impossible to predict. The many causes of infertility are more or less evenly balanced between men and women. Age—especially the mother's age—is frequently a factor to consider in family planning. A number of tests and procedures can be carried out by a physician to identify and correct many of the causes of infertility. Both the man and the woman must be involved in the process, and the procedures may take a great deal of time—often more than a year. Couples who start an infertility study should be prepared to go through the entire program.

Other Considerations Other important questions prospective parents should ask themselves concern the effect that having a child will have on their lives and their situation. If they have a child now, how will it affect their education or career, their other children and home life, perhaps even their retirement plans? A child brings new financial pressures and demands great expenditures of time, energy, and money. There are also emotional issues to consider: How will a new child affect a couple's relationship? Are the partners ready to give each other the emotional support and practical help they both need? There are still other aspects of parenthood to consider: How large a family does the couple want? How will the children be spaced in terms of age? What methods of contraception will be employed to avoid having more children than can be handled? All these questions should be considered when a couple is deciding whether to have a child. Careful planning can help ensure that pregnancy proceeds smoothly and that a couple is sufficiently prepared for the responsibilities of parenthood.

The Beginnings of Pregnancy

A pregnancy officially begins when a fertilized egg implants itself in a woman's uterine lining. Soon afterward the woman's entire body undergoes general changes that can be detected by means of pregnancy tests (see below). Meanwhile, spectacular changes occur in the uterine lining: specialized cells

amniocentesis—*a procedure in which a doctor withdraws amniotic fluid from a pregnant woman's uterus to test for certain genetic disorders in the fetus.*

chorionic villi sampling—*a new technique to test for genetic disorders in a fetus.*

More than 97 percent of women who undergo amniocentesis learn that their babies are free of the diseases they have been tested for.

The most frequent cause of female infertility is obstruction of the reproductive tract, especially blocked Fallopian tubes, and the inability to ovulate.

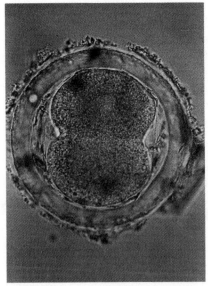
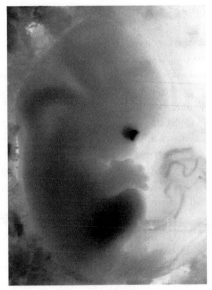
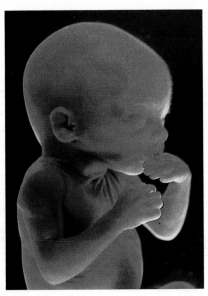

Immediately after fertilization occurs, the zygote (fertilized egg) goes through a cell division process called mitosis in which DNA from the sperm and the egg is distributed in the nuclei of the forming cells. (Petit Format/Nestle/Photo Researchers, Inc.) By the seventh week of pregnancy the head, hands, and feet of a growing embryo have taken on distinctly human form. (C. Edelmann/La Villette/Photo Researchers, Inc.) Within just 5 months a human fetus has the ability to hear; however, the other senses take more time to develop. (James Stevenson/Science Photo Library/Photo Researchers, Inc.)

from the uterus and from the now-forming embryo begin to develop into a structure known as the **placenta.** The placenta is the physical link between mother and child; it is a mass of tissue attached to the uterine lining and to what will become the child's navel. For the next 9 months the placenta will absorb life-giving nutrients and oxygen from the woman's bloodstream and transfer them to the bloodstream of the developing fetus and will also carry away fetal wastes.

The events during the rest of the pregnancy constitute one of the truly amazing phenomena of life. What starts out as a single cell—a speck barely visible to the human eye—becomes, in the space of 9 months, a fully developed baby ready to be born.

As an embryo, the organism is less than an inch long and looks a little like a curved fish. By 2 months, at which point it is called a fetus, it has developed arms and legs with fully shaped fingers and toes. By the end of the third month, although it is only about 3 inches long and weighs a mere ounce, the fetus can kick its legs, close its fingers, turn its head, and open and close its mouth. Also, by this time most of its internal organs are able to function, so that the rest of the **prenatal** period (the period before birth) can be spent in the process of growth and in putting on the finishing touches.

Throughout its prenatal life the fetus is attached to the placenta by the **umbilical cord** and is enclosed in a fluid-filled sac (the **amnion,** or **amniotic sac**) which primarily provides protection. At birth, the average full-term infant weighs anywhere from 5 to 12 pounds and may be from 17 to 22 inches long. The average length of pregnancy is 280 days, but babies born as early as 180 days or as late as 334 days after conception may be able to survive.[29]

Pregnancy: Diagnosis and Testing

Usually, the first sign of pregnancy is that an expected menstrual period does not occur. The woman may feel that menstruation is about to begin but "cannot get started." This is not, however, a definitive sign of pregnancy, since it is not unusual for women's periods to be delayed 14 to 21 days, particularly in women who are normally somewhat irregular or are under stress. A pregnant

placenta—*a mass of tissue attached to the uterine lining that during pregnancy absorbs nutrients from the mother's bloodstream and transfers them to the bloodstream of the developing baby; it also carries away fetal wastes.*

A pregnant woman and her fetus have separate blood systems. Nutrients and wastes are exchanged by diffusion between fetal and maternal capillaries in the placenta.

prenatal—*before birth.*

umbilical cord—*a ropelike tissue that links the developing fetus to the placenta nourishing its blood supply.*

amnion (amniotic sac)—*a fluid-filled sac within the uterus that encloses and protects the developing baby.*

woman may also notice breast congestion or tenderness, irritability, tenderness or a "heavy feeling" in her pelvis, and sometimes nausea.

If a woman misses her menstrual period, she may, as a preliminary to going to the doctor, use any of a number of over-the-counter home pregnancy tests. These tests should never be considered conclusive, however, since a negative reading can result from administering the test too early or improperly.

A physical exam by a qualified medical professional is necessary to confirm the diagnosis of pregnancy and begin prenatal planning and health care.[30] About 3 weeks after the missed period a physician can usually, by means of a pelvic examination, be fairly certain of the existence of a pregnancy. The pelvic tissue will be slightly softened, the vaginal opening will be slightly purplish, and the uterus will have begun to enlarge.

Medical laboratory tests may be used to confirm the pregnancy. A pregnant woman's system produces a hormone known as human chorionic gonadotropin (HCG); tests of the woman's blood or urine can show whether this hormone is present. Blood testing is available in most cities at low cost; it often requires no more than a brief visit to a clinic to leave a blood sample and a follow-up phone call to get the results. Referrals are available through local chapters of the Planned Parenthood Federation of America, local health departments, and county medical societies. There are two commonly used urine-type pregnancy tests. One takes 2½ minutes to show results and is done 42 days after the first day of the last menstrual cycle. The other test takes 1 hour to show results and can be performed right after the missed period.

Sometime during early pregnancy the woman should have a series of blood tests to check for anemia and rule out infection or other disorders. In addition, an Rh test must be done to assess the risk of Rh hemolytic disease (erythroblastosis fetalis), a genetically determined blood disorder. Most people have a substance known as the **Rh factor** in their red blood cells; if the mother lacks this substance and the baby inherits the factor from the father, the mother's blood can react against the baby's. The first pregnancy is usually not affected, but subsequent babies are at risk. Today, all mothers with the Rh condition can be immunized against this problem.

Rh factor—*a substance in the red blood cells which, if lacking in the mother and inherited by the first baby from the father, can cause the mother's blood to produce antibodies that result in a blood disorder called* **erythroblastosis fetalis** *in second and later children.*

Prenatal Health

Pregnancy is not an illness. In ordinary circumstances a pregnant woman can do almost all the things she did before she became pregnant, including working, exercising, participating in recreational activities, and having sexual intercourse. She should, however, take extra care of her health. For 9 months a fetus will be depending on her for all its body-building materials. Ideally, she should be in excellent health *before* starting the pregnancy.

A pregnant woman should think of herself as an athlete in training, building up her body to the highest level of physical fitness so that the childbirth that lies ahead will be more a natural occurrence than an ordeal. Like an athlete, she should get proper nutrition and exercise, avoid hazardous substances, guard against disease, and receive proper medical care.

Proper Nutrition and Exercise   A pregnant woman should be sure to eat adequate quantities of milk and milk products, protein foods, fruits, vegetables, and grains and to drink copious amounts of liquids. Because she is eating for two, she should expect to gain a reasonable amount of weight, ideally about 25 pounds during the course of the pregnancy. The hormonal changes that occur with pregnancy account for the woman's increased appetite; this is nature's way of providing for the developing fetus. Women who are overweight before pregnancy should cease dieting while they are pregnant because continued dieting can have an adverse effect on the health of the fetus. Pregnant women should also get regular exercise to maintain their strength and endurance.

Avoiding Hazardous Substances   It has been estimated that fully 20 percent of all birth defects are caused by environmental factors.[31] Since the mother-to-be largely controls the fetus's environment, she must protect the developing infant from as many environmental hazards as she can to ensure the health of her child.

The most common threats to fetal health come from substances which the mother ingests and which pass directly through the placenta to the fetus. Among the most hazardous substances are alcohol, tobacco, caffeine, and drugs.[32]

A woman who drinks alcohol during pregnancy is in effect giving her fetus a drink too. However, the alcohol that crosses the placenta may do far more damage to the fetus than to the mother. In the 1970s the term **fetal alcohol syndrome (FAS)** was coined in recognition of the fact that babies born to mothers who drink heavily are often born with a predictable set of abnormalities (Chapter 14).

Tobacco is also known to affect fetal development. Women who smoke have a higher than normal rate of miscarriage and stillbirth. When their babies survive, they are smaller than average and are more likely to be irritable and hyperactive. Smoking has also been associated with a higher risk of cleft palate, crossed eyes, and hernias in the newborn.

Caffeine, which is present in coffee, tea, chocolate, and cola drinks, is another potential hazard to the fetus. A high caffeine intake has been associated with an increased risk of miscarriage and birth defects.

Prescription drugs and over-the-counter medications as well as illegal drugs also pose a danger to a fetus. Since most prescription drugs have not been proved safe for pregnant women and many are known to cause birth defects, most physicians avoid prescribing any new medications for a pregnant woman. Several over-the-counter drugs often taken by pregnant women are also risky. According to current research, aspirin is dangerous to the fetus and may pose risks to the woman, particularly if she takes it near the time of labor and delivery. Aspirin decreases the blood's clotting ability and may cause either the mother or the baby to bleed excessively.

fetal alcohol syndrome (FAS)—*characteristic adverse effects (including mental retardation, slow growth before and after birth, and a wide range of physical defects) exhibited by children born to women who drink heavily during pregnancy.*

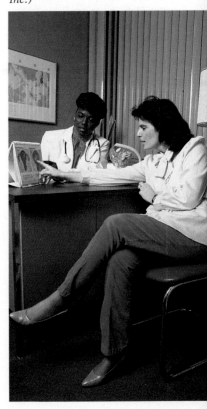

Regular medical checkups help ensure the health of the unborn baby and the mother-to-be. (Blair Seitz/Photo Researchers, Inc.)

Guarding against Infectious Diseases   Some infectious diseases can cause problems for the developing fetus as well as the mother. One such hazard is rubella (German measles), a contagious viral disease. A woman who contracts this illness early in pregnancy—even a mild case—may have a multiply handicapped baby. Other diseases, particularly STDs, may also pose hazards to the developing fetus. AIDS, for example, is transmitted from an infected pregnant woman to her fetus, condemning the future child to this fatal illness.

Receiving Proper Medical Care   Prenatal care, or medical supervision of the pregnancy, is very important for both mother and baby to help ensure that problems will be detected early and treated. Prenatal examinations routinely include a test of blood pressure. Increased blood pressure may indicate danger; a sudden rise may indicate toxemia (see below), which can result in maternal or fetal death if left untreated. Urinalysis is another vital test conducted as part of prenatal care; it can detect kidney and bladder conditions and other disorders.

Prenatal care also includes measurement of the size of the woman's abdomen to determine the baby's growth. After the fifth month the baby's heartbeat can usually be checked.

The first prenatal visit usually includes a vaginal examination, especially with a first pregnancy; the size of the birth canal is a crucial factor in safe delivery. Another examination closer to the due date helps forecast when birth will occur by observing cervical softening, thinning, and dilation.

Common Problems during Pregnancy

During pregnancy a woman may experience various problems or discomforts. While many of these problems pose little risk to the health of the mother or the fetus, a few may pose a significant threat.

Morning Sickness   Some women may experience nausea or vomiting, often called *morning sickness,* during the first 3 months of pregnancy. There are some steps a woman can take to try to reduce the discomfort of morning sickness. Arising slowly and eating a few crackers, some dry cereal, or a piece of toast first thing in the morning may help reduce its effects, as may eating four or five small meals a day instead of going for long periods without food. Avoiding greasy, fried, or highly seasoned spicy foods also helps. Drinking plenty of fluids between, rather than with, meals may lessen the effects of morning sickness.

Constipation and Hemorrhoids   Constipation is another problem frequently encountered by pregnant women. It may be caused by the position of the fetus, lying as it does near the colorectal area. Other causes may include a decrease in exercise and a lack of adequate fiber or liquids in the diet. This is another reason why proper nutrition, including lots of fruits and vegetables, is so important to a pregnant woman. Drinking plenty of liquids also helps relieve constipation. If constipation persists, the pregnant woman should consult her doctor.

Hemorrhoids—an inflammation of rectal tissue—may be brought on by persistent constipation or perhaps by the baby pressing on the veins of the rectum. Relieving constipation can help relieve hemorrhoids or reduce the possibility of their occurrence.

Heartburn and Back Pain   Some women may experience heartburn during the last months of pregnancy. It is caused by pressure placed on the stomach as the fetus grows. Eating small meals four or five times a day may help reduce heartburn, as will avoiding fatty, fried, and spicy foods.

Lower back pain caused by carrying the extra weight of a fetus as well as sharp leg pains and cramps may also be experienced during pregnancy. Varicose veins may develop because of the pressure the fetus places on the large veins of the legs. These conditions should all disappear after the birth of the baby.

Toxemia   More serious conditions can also arise during pregnancy. One such condition is **toxemia,** the presence of toxins in the bloodstream. Toxemia may occur at any time during pregnancy, and about 6 percent of pregnant women develop it. The risks are greater in first pregnancies, especially in very young or older women. In its milder form, called **preeclampsia,** the symptoms include hypertension and edema, or swelling, and protein in the urine. A more severe form of toxemia—**eclampsia**—may cause convulsions and coma.[33]

While the origin of toxemia is not fully understood, it may be related to kidney function and the utilization of salt in the body. The severity of the symptoms determines the type of treatment. For milder conditions, bed rest and sedation are prescribed and salt may be restricted to help reduce swelling. More serious symptoms require hospitalization, with sodium intake and blood pressure monitored closely. Antihypertension agents are usually prescribed as well. Marked hypertension and the onset of convulsions are an indication for terminating the pregnancy.[34]

Miscarriage   In about one of six pregnancies a woman has a **spontaneous abortion,** commonly called a *miscarriage.* A spontaneous abortion happens

toxemia—*the presence of toxins in the bloodstream during pregnancy.*

preeclampsia—*a milder form of toxemia; the symptoms include hypertension and edema, or swelling, and protein in the urine.*

eclampsia—*a severe form of toxemia; may cause convulsions and coma.*

spontaneous abortion—*the expulsion of an improperly implanted or defective embryo or fetus from the uterus; commonly called miscarriage.*

either because the fertilized ovum was not implanted correctly in the uterine lining or because the egg or sperm was defective to begin with. In a miscarriage, a woman usually starts to have vaginal bleeding and cramps, which continue until the uterus expels the defective embryo or fetus.

Spontaneous abortions are not caused by automobile trips, falls, or emotional shocks. They may be related to general glandular or body disorders; this is one reason for having a thorough medical examination before starting a pregnancy.

Terminating a Pregnancy

Spontaneous abortions are regarded with sympathy by all people regardless of their beliefs or values. They are a result of chance and may often be nature's way of preventing the birth of a baby with genetic or other serious problems. The deliberate termination of pregnancy, also called **abortion,** is a very different matter, however. Medically, abortion means ending a pregnancy before the embryo or fetus can survive on its own. This issue is at the center of one of the most heated controversies in American society today.

abortion—*the termination of a pregnancy by removal of the uterine contents before the embryo or fetus is developed enough to survive on its own.*

How a Pregnancy Is Terminated   During the first 12 weeks of pregnancy abortion is a relatively safe procedure when performed by a qualified physician. There are several techniques for terminating a pregnancy. One technique, sometimes considered a postcoital contraceptive rather than an abortion, is the use of "morning-after" pills. These pills are normally used within 72 hours of intercourse and interfere with the development of fetal tissue. One morning-after pill, called Ovral, has a low failure rate and few adverse side effects and apparently interferes with an ovarian phase of conception.[35] Another type of pill, currently unavailable in the United States, is RU 486. RU 486 contains a chemical that opposes the action of progesterone and induces menstruation, blocking a fertilized egg from attaching to the uterine lining or sloughing off an implanted ovum.[36]

A simple procedure for terminating a pregnancy, used during the first 2 weeks after a missed menstrual period, is *vacuum aspiration,* sometimes called

Though legalized in 1973 by the United States Supreme Court, abortion continues to be debated. Supporters argue that the decision to have an abortion should be a private choice, protected under the Constitution. People who are against abortion want to make it illegal, arguing that it is an immoral and criminal act. (Susan McCartney/Photo Researchers, Inc.; Bettye Lane/Photo Researchers, Inc.)

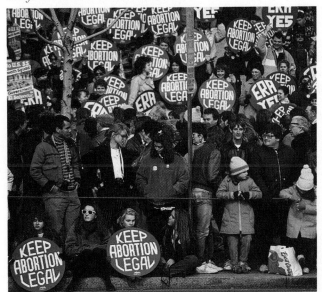

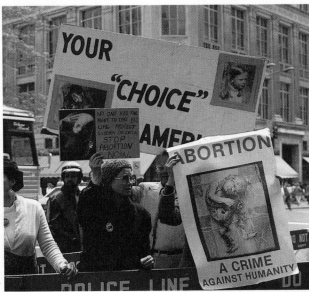

The Question of Reproductive Rights

Few issues have been as controversial over the past 20 years as whether women have the right to control their own reproduction, specifically, whether birth control and abortion should be available on demand. At the heart of this issue is a crucial question about individual rights: whether the mother has a right to individual self-determination or whether the rights of the unborn baby should be protected by the state. Two views follow, presenting both sides of this volatile question.

Self-Determination: A Basic Right   In 1973 the Supreme Court, in the landmark *Roe v. Wade* case, declared that abortion, like birth control, is included in the fundamental right to privacy that belongs to all individuals. The Court ruled that the decision to have an abortion during the first 3 months of pregnancy must be left to the pregnant woman and her doctor.

This ruling was based on the premise that our society values freedom and self-determination as a basic right. For this reason, the Court attempted to place the decision to bear a child—a decision inextricably related to the right of self-determination—beyond the reach of government. This ruling, along with earlier decisions allowing access to birth control, correctly leaves the choice to the individual most involved, the mother.

The mother is the person most closely concerned with the many issues concerning childbirth: Does she have the support a new mother needs? Will she be able to provide the child with a good home? How will an additional member affect the rest of her family? It is the mother who runs the emotional, social, spiritual, and physical risks of abortion or of not having the procedure.

Before *Roe v. Wade* millions of American women had dangerous and sometimes fatal illegal abortions, often driven to this extreme by poverty or fear. Since *Roe v. Wade* millions of women have taken advantage of their right to a safe, legal abortion. Considering the explosive growth in world population, this is a positive step contributing toward our stewardship of the planet.

There is no doubt that abortion is an emotionally charged and complex issue. However, the rights of the pregnant woman are paramount. She must have the right to choose and the fundamental right to control her own body and life.

Protecting the Rights of the Unborn Is the State's Duty   Beginning in the nineteenth century and extending through much of the twentieth, most states in the United States passed laws restricting or forbidding abortion. These laws were based on two general principles: the state's duty to protect those who cannot protect their own rights and the idea that life itself is an ultimate good.

Although various cases preceding *Roe v. Wade* established the right to birth control, there is a fundamental difference between birth control and abortion. The Supreme Court itself has declared that the decision to abort a fetus is inherently different from the decision to prevent a pregnancy, because a pregnant woman "cannot be isolated in her privacy." In other words, the pregnant woman is not just an individual but the source of a potential human life whose rights are equally important. Since the fetus cannot safeguard its own rights, it is the state's duty to intervene to ensure that they are protected.

Those who oppose abortion believe that the unborn child has a right to its own life and that this life begins at conception. No one has the right to take the life of an unborn child. To those who argue that a woman should not have to raise a child she does not want or cannot afford, they point to the thousands of childless couples who are desperate to adopt babies. The rights of the fetus, then, are of such importance that they must take precedence over the individual rights of the mother.

Do you support the first view, which emphasizes the right of the pregnant woman to individual freedom and self-determination? Or do you favor the second, in which the state intervenes to protect the rights of the unborn infant? Can you see the possibility of a viewpoint that reconciles these two opposing positions?

suction curettage or menstrual extraction. In this method, a small sterile tube is inserted into the endometrium and the menstrual tissue, fetal tissue, and placenta are extracted by suction. It is an inexpensive office procedure, requires little training, is easily performed, and poses minimal risk. However, residual tissue containing a viable embryo may remain after the procedure has been performed.

An operative procedure known as D and C—dilation of the cervix and curettage (scraping) of the uterine cavity—is also used up to about the twelfth week of pregnancy. These two techniques are frequently combined—the cervix is dilated, the uterine contents are removed with vacuum suction, and the procedure is followed by curettage to make sure that all the products of conception are removed.

After the twelfth week of pregnancy, abortion is performed in one of three ways: by *hysterotomy*, an operation which requires an abdominal incision; by introducing a salt solution into the uterus through a catheter inserted through the abdominal wall, a procedure called a *saline abortion*; or by the use of synthetic prostaglandins, either injected or administered in a vaginal suppository. Both the salt solution and the prostaglandins work by inducing contractions.

Attitudes toward Abortion   Despite its relative safety, abortion is vigorously opposed by many people in the United States, primarily on moral and religious grounds. These people wish to see abortion outlawed throughout the country. There are others who personally disapprove of abortion but believe that it should be a personal and private issue rather than a legal one decided by the government. They feel that women should have the right to make a choice about whether to have an abortion.

In 1973 the U.S. Supreme Court ruled in the case *Roe v. Wade* that a woman's right to choice should prevail and that in the first 3 months of pregnancy the decision to have an abortion should be left to the woman and her physician. The Court ruled further that in subsequent months of pregnancy, each individual state should be permitted to "regulate the abortion procedures in ways reasonably related to pregnancy" until 10 weeks before the child is due; from that point on, abortion should be prohibited except when necessary to preserve the woman's life or health.

Recent Supreme Court cases have begun to challenge *Roe v. Wade*. Although none have succeeded in overturning that decision, they have begun to limit the right to have an abortion. As Supreme Court justices age and retire, the philosophy of the Court may change, affecting the interpretation of the U.S. Constitution as it is applied to new laws regarding abortion. Whatever Court decisions are made, the issue will probably remain highly controversial in the future.

Childbirth

No one doubts that the birth of a child is one of the most amazing and awe-inspiring events in life. Witnessing the emergence of life gives a person a new perspective on what it means to be alive. In return, parents are given a tremendous responsibility as caretakers and guardians of a new human being. However, until recently the parents were given few choices about how the birth of an infant would take place.

Choices in Childbirth

Twenty years ago in most communities in the United States there were few options for childbirth. The mother and father would go to the hospital, the mother would be given a light anesthetic and would sleep through the experi-

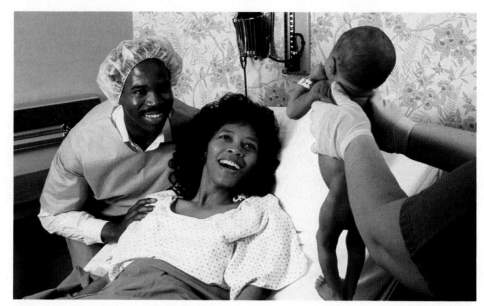

Today many hospitals provide birthing rooms where both parents can feel more at ease during labor and delivery. (Joseph Nettis/Photo Researchers, Inc.)

ence of childbirth, and the father would pace nervously in a waiting room, feeling powerless to help in any way. Today, however, there are many other alternatives to this scenario, as described in the feature on the next page.

There are also more technical medical choices which may need to be made to facilitate delivery or help ensure the health of the mother and baby. In the United States a surgical incision called an **episiotomy** is commonly made between the mother's vaginal opening and anus to prevent tearing of these tissues during childbirth. Immediately after the delivery, the incision is repaired with sutures.

Sometimes during delivery it becomes necessary to perform a **cesarean section.** Instead of being delivered through the birth canal, the baby is removed through surgical incisions in the mother's abdomen and uterus. Cesarean sections have become increasingly common in recent years. Women who have undergone this procedure can deliver through the birth canal in subsequent pregnancies as a result of improved techniques. Women's ability to have a normal delivery after a cesarean section is also enhanced if they are supervised by skilled personnel, if their contractions and vital signs are monitored closely, and if they have immediate access to compatible blood supplies and surgical facilities.[37]

How Birth Takes Place

Although birth involves hard work and often pain, people come away from the experience awed by the wonder of it. During the last month or two of pregnancy a woman may notice her uterus contracting at irregular intervals. These so-called Braxton Hicks contractions are usually not painful; they may be felt as a tightness in the back, whereas true labor contractions usually feel somewhat like menstrual cramps. Braxton Hicks contractions indicate that true labor is getting closer, but they are not a sign that it is beginning.

A day or two before labor begins the woman may notice a small amount of vaginal bleeding. Then a clear fluid will normally drain spontaneously from the vagina. This means that the amniotic sac, or "bag of waters," has broken and true labor is about to begin. At this point true contractions can usually be felt, starting at intervals of 15 to 20 minutes and gradually becoming more frequent. In some cases, however, labor sets in abruptly, with the contractions coming every 3 to 5 minutes.

episiotomy—*a surgical incision made from a mother's vaginal opening into the perineum to prevent undue tearing of tissues during the delivery of a baby.*

cesarean section—*delivery of a baby through surgical incisions made in the mother's abdomen and uterus.*

The percentage of babies born by cesarean section in the United States has been increasing dramatically:

- *1970 =   5%*
- *1980 = 18%*
- *1987 = 24%*

Considering Birthing Options

Expectant parents have many options regarding the birth of a child. They are able to select the place of birth and the type of childbirth that best suits their needs and feelings.

Over the past several decades the trend has been toward a more informal, family-centered birth experience that treats both the mother and the father as important partners in the birthing experience and encourages both to join the providers of health care in making important decisions about the birth.

A recent innovation is the birthing center, a place with a trained staff of midwives and nurses where parents can have a child without going to the hospital. Such centers offer comfortable rooms, a less technical approach, and a nurturing atmosphere as well as the capacity to use state-of-the-art equipment if necessary.

For example, they may permit family members to be present at the birth, or siblings to visit the newborn; some even offer elaborate dinners for the new parents. However, they are careful to check for any risk of medical complications resulting from the age of the mother or the position of the fetus. Patients who need it must receive hospital care.

Many hospitals now offer comfortable birthing rooms as well as the traditional delivery room with its emphasis on diagnostic and surgical techniques. Once again, instead of a physician, a nurse-midwife may be chosen to supervise the delivery. Although still controversial, home delivery with an unlicensed lay midwife has also become more popular; it offers another informal alternative to the traditional hospital environment.

As hospital costs continue to rise, home birth may be an economical choice. However, parents should be sure to consult a competent medical professional before taking this step. If there are risks of complication, a physician's skills and a hospital's elaborate equipment may be needed *within minutes.*

In addition to selecting the location and atmosphere for the birth, parents have choices about the method of delivery. Many parents today attend classes that prepare them to help as actively as possible in the birth process.

Such classes may teach ways to cope with the discomfort of labor and delivery, with the goal of reducing or eliminating the use of anesthetic and analgesic drugs. The woman's husband or other labor partner is trained to assist in the process. These courses can reduce fear and pain, overcome ignorance, and build confidence for both parents.

In the Grantly Dick-Read method of prepared childbirth, for example, parents gain a thorough understanding of labor and delivery and learn breathing techniques that will help the mother throughout the birth. The labor partner is taught to provide empathetic understanding and support.

The Lamaze method, which also uses a specific type of breathing to diminish the pains of labor, teaches a woman to replace responses of restlessness, fear, and loss of control with more useful activity. It also teaches muscular relaxation techniques and relies on the assistance of a labor partner.

The Leboyer method of delivery focuses more on the child. The emphasis is on a gentle, controlled, and subdued delivery that minimizes psychological shock and overstimulation. After delivery, the baby is placed in a warm water bath, and contact between mother and child is encouraged to increase bonding between the two.

More recently, the concepts of prepared childbirth and family-centered maternity care have been applied to cesarean births as well as vaginal deliveries. An expectant mother preparing for cesarean delivery has the option of being awake and having her husband or labor partner present.

Is there a best way to have a baby? Of course, the answer is no. The feelings of expectant parents are central to the birth experience. Choosing a method of childbirth that fits them—not their families or physicians—will bring feelings of confidence and comfort that enhance the birthing experience.

Based in part on R.W. Lubic and G.R. Hawes, *Childbearing: A Book of Alternatives* (New York: McGraw-Hill, 1987).

To understand what happens during a contraction, it helps to picture the uterus as a large muscular pouch that is upside down, with its open end leading into the vagina. Before labor, this opening is almost closed by an elastic ring, the cervix. As the walls of the pouch contract during labor, the baby's head is pressed firmly against the cervix, causing the cervix to dilate (get wider). As labor progresses, the cervix opens wide enough for the baby's head to pass through into the vagina.

When the baby's head has passed through the cervix and into the vagina, the woman feels a compulsion to bear down and push the baby out of her body. Typically, the top of the baby's head appears first; then, with succeeding contractions, the head gradually slides out, usually facedown. Once the head is out, the shoulders emerge as the body rotates, and the rest of the body usually follows easily. After the baby has left the mother's body, an attendant ties off and cuts the umbilical cord, which connects the baby's navel to the placenta. Soon the uterus contracts again and expels the placenta—the "afterbirth" (Figure 9.6).

After the birth the physician uses a suction apparatus to remove mucus from the infant's nose and mouth to make breathing easier. The newborn's breathing, muscle tone, heart rate, reflexes, irritability, and color are assessed immediately to determine whether the baby needs further medical help. If all is well, the baby is given to the mother and father, who can admire the miracle of life they have produced.

Figure 9.6 The birth process. (A) In many cases, rupture of the amniotic sac signals the onset of labor. The sac may also be ruptured purposely to stimulate labor. (B) The baby's head presses against the cervix, causing it to dilate. Reflex action causes the uterus to contract. The length and intensity of contractions increase and the interval between contractions decreases as labor continues. (C) After several hours the cervix is fully dilated to allow the baby's head to pass through the vagina. (D) Several more contractions after the delivery of the baby cause the placenta to detach from the uterine wall and be expelled.

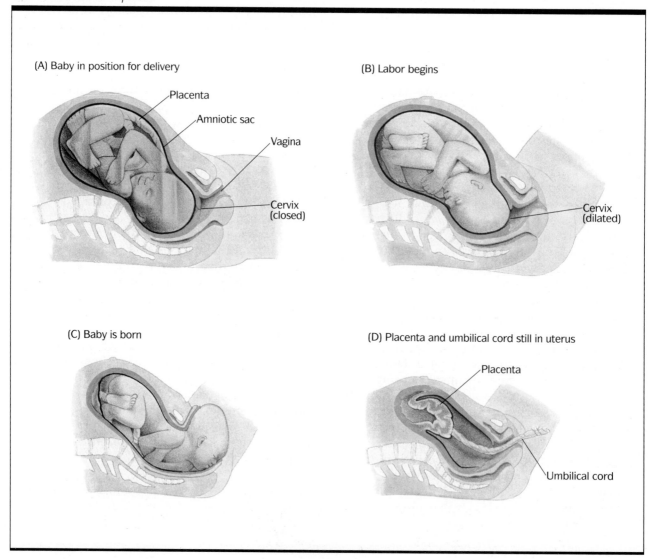

(A) Baby in position for delivery

Placenta

Amniotic sac

Vagina

Cervix (closed)

(B) Labor begins

Cervix (dilated)

(C) Baby is born

(D) Placenta and umbilical cord still in uterus

Placenta

Umbilical cord

Chapter Summary

- The female reproductive system consists of the ovaries, which contain the ova; the Fallopian tubes, which are the passages where fertilization takes place; and the uterus, which is where a fertilized ovum develops into a fetus.
- The menstrual cycle is a monthly process during which a woman's uterus prepares to receive and nourish a fertilized ovum. This cycle may cause physical discomfort, such as cramps and changes in energy level, as well as psychological changes and changes in behavior.
- The male reproductive system consists of the testes, which produce sperm; the epididymis and vas deferens, which store and nourish the sperm and transport them from the testes; and the seminal vesicles and prostate gland, which secrete fluids that combine with sperm to produce semen.
- People who approach sex responsibly and safely consider the consequences sexual activity may have on their lives, such as unplanned or unwanted children and the contraction of sexually transmitted diseases, and take precautions to avoid unplanned pregnancy and disease.
- A great variety of contraceptive methods and devices are available, including abstinence, condoms, vaginal spermicides (foams, creams, and jellies), vaginal sponges, withdrawal, oral contraceptives (the pill), intrauterine devices, the diaphragm, the cervical cap, surgical sterilization (vasectomy and tubal ligation), and the contraceptive implant. Each method and device has benefits and drawbacks.
- Natural family planning does not require medications or contraceptive devices; it makes use of the timing of a woman's ovulation to determine when sexual intercourse should be avoided. Natural contraception requires careful planning and the use of one or several techniques to determine the time of ovulation.
- Planning for pregnancy is important because of the great responsibility of parenthood. Among the issues that should be considered are whether genetic counseling is advisable and what impact a child will have on a couple's life and relationship.
- Pregnancy begins when a fertilized egg is implanted in the uterine lining. From that point on, cellular growth leads to the development of a fetus and tissues to nourish and protect the developing fetus. The fetus goes through tremendous changes from conception to birth.
- Routine testing for pregnancy includes tests to confirm pregnancy; blood tests to check for anemia, infections, and other disorders; and an Rh test to check for Rh hemolytic disease, a genetic blood disorder.
- Important factors in maximizing the health of the mother and child include getting proper nutrition and exercise; avoiding hazardous substances such as alcohol, tobacco, and drugs; guarding against infectious diseases; and receiving proper prenatal care.
- Some of the problems pregnant women may experience include morning sickness, constipation and hemorrhoids, heartburn and back pain, toxemia (a serious condition that can lead to the death of both mother and child), and miscarriage (spontaneous abortion).
- Pregnancy can be terminated by means of various techniques, including the use of morning-after pills, vacuum aspiration, an operative procedure known as D and C (dilation of the cervix and curettage of the uterine cavity), surgical hysterotomy, and saline abortion.
- There is a great controversy about the use of abortion in the United States. Some people are vigorously opposed to it on moral, ethical, or religious grounds. Others feel it is a private issue concerning a woman's control over her own body. Although a Supreme Court case in 1973 upheld a woman's right to decide, recent events and court cases are challenging that decision.
- During childbirth labor contractions force the baby's head against the cervix, causing it to dilate. As labor progresses, the baby passes through the cervix into the vagina, at which time the mother feels a compulsion to bear down and push the baby out of her body. Typically, the baby's head appears first, followed by the rest of the body.

Key Terms

Ovum (ova) (page 226)

Ovaries (page 226)

Menarche (page 226)

Ovulation (page 226)

Fallopian tubes (oviducts) (page 227)

Uterus (page 227)

Cervix (page 227)

Endometrium (page 227)

Menstrual cycle (page 227)

Menstruation (page 227)

Prostaglandins (page 228)

Premenstrual syndrome (PMS) (page 228)

Menopause (page 229)

Climacteric (page 229)

Testes (testicles) (page 230)

Sperm (page 230)

Spermatogenesis (page 230)

Epididymis (page 230)

Vas deferens (page 231)

Seminal vesicles (page 231)

Prostate gland (page 231)

Semen (seminal fluid) (page 231)

Ejaculatory ducts (page 231)

Cowper's glands (page 231)

Condom (page 232)

Withdrawal (page 234)

Oral contraceptives (page 234)

Intrauterine device (IUD) (page 235)

Diaphragm (page 236)

Vasectomy (page 238)

Tubal ligation (page 238)

Contraceptive implant (page 239)

Vaginal rings (page 239)

Injectable contraceptives (page 239)

Vaginal condom (page 239)

Amniocentesis (page 242)

Chorionic villi sampling (page 242)

Placenta (page 243)

Prenatal (page 243)

Umbilical cord (page 243)

Amnion (amniotic sac) (page 243)

Rh factor (page 244)

Fetal alcohol syndrome (FAS) (page 245)

Toxemia (page 246)

Preeclampsia (page 246)

Eclampsia (page 246)

Spontaneous abortion (page 246)

Abortion (page 247)

Episiotomy (page 250)

Cesarean section (page 250)

References

1. Robert L. Reid and S. S. C. Yen, "Premenstrual Syndrome," *American Journal of Obstetrics and Gynecology* 139, no. 1 (1981): 85–104; "Premenstrual Syndrome: An Ancient Woe Deserving Modern Scrutiny," *Journal of the American Medical Association* 245, no. 14 (April 10, 1981): 1393–1396.

2. Annete McKay Rossignol, "Caffeine-Containing Beverages and Premenstrual Syndrome in Young Women," *American Journal of Public Health* 75, no. 11 (November 1985): 1335–1337.

3. Mary Brown Parlee, "New Findings: Menstrual Cycles and Behavior," *Ms.* (September 1982): 126–128.

4. A. B. Little and R. B. Billiar, "Endocrinology," in *Obstetrics and Gynecology: The Health Care of Women,* 2d ed., S. L. Romney et al. (eds.) (New York: McGraw-Hill, 1981): 122.

5. Daniel R. Mishell, "Medical Progress: Contraception," *New England Journal of Medicine* 320, no. 12 (March 23, 1989): 777–787.

6. Ibid.

7. Denise Kafka and Rachel Benson Gold, "Food and Drug Administration Approves Vaginal Sponge," *Family Planning Perspectives* 15, no. 3 (May–June 1983): 146; Ellen Lemberg, "The Vaginal Contraceptive Sponge: A New Non-Prescription Barrier Contraceptive," *Nurse Practitioner* (October 1984): 24.

8. Jacqueline Darroch Forrest and Stanley K. Henshaw, "What U.S. Women Think and Do about Contraception," *Family Planning Perspectives* 15, no. 4 (July–August 1983): 157.

9. "Facts about Methods of Contraception," Planned Parenthood Federation of America (April 1985).

10. Rochelle G. Kanell, "Oral Contraceptives: The Risks in Perspective," *Nurse Practitioner* (September 1984): 25.

11. H. W. Ory et al., "The Pill at 20: An Assessment," *Family Planning Perspectives* 12 (1980): 278.

12. D. A. Grimes, "Birth Control Pills: A Reappraisal of the Pros and Cons," *Medical Aspects of Human Sexuality* 16, no. 8 (August 1982): 32J–32Y.

13. W. H. Masters et al., *Human Sexuality* (Boston: Little, Brown, 1982): 128–129.

14. R. A. Hatcher et al., *Contraceptive Technology 1982–1983,* 11th ed. (New York: Irvington, 1982): 84.

15. "Searle Quits IUDs," *Newsweek* (February 10, 1986): 60.

16. Mary Alice Johnson, "The Cervical Cap as a Contraceptive Alternative," *Nurse Practitioner* 10, no. 1 (January 1985).

17. Masters et al., op. cit., p. 137.

18. Mishell, op. cit.

19. "Vasectomy: Facts about Male Sterilization," (Patient Information Library, Daly City, Calif.: Krames Communication, 1987): 2.

20. Larry Wichman, "Twenty-First Century Birth Control," *Men's Fitness* 6, no. 3 (March 1990): 100–103.

21. Melanie Monier and Martha Laird, "Contraceptives: A Look at the Future," *American Journal of Nursing* 89, no. 4 (April 1989): 497–499.

22. Wichman, op. cit.

23. Ibid.

24. Ibid.

25. Monier and Laird, op. cit.

26. Wichman, op. cit.

27. H. K. Nadler and B. D. Burton, "Genetics," in *Fetal and Maternal Medicine,* E. J. Quilligan and N. Kretchmer (eds.) (New York: Wiley, 1980): 59–107.

28. W. Hogge et al., "Chorionic Villus Sampling: Experiences of the First 1,000 Cases," *American Journal of Obstetrics and Gynecology* 154 (1986): 1249–1252.

29. E. C. Sandberg, *Synopsis of Obstetrics,* 10th ed. (St. Louis: C V Mosby, 1978): 307.

30. Hatcher et al., "Pregnancy Testing and Management of Early Pregnancy," in *Contraceptive Technology 1988–1989,* 14th rev. ed. (New York: Irvington 1988): 380–387.

31. T. H. Shepard and R. J. Lemire, "Teratology," in *Fetal and Maternal Medicine,* op. cit.

32. David W. Martin, "Alcohol and Drug Abuse in Pregnancy: Information for Patients," in *Pregnancy, Childbirth, and Parenthood,* Paul Ahmed (ed.) (New York: Elsevier, 1981): 141–142; G. D. Zike, "Maternal Alcohol Use and Its Effects on the Fetus," *Physician Assistant and Health Practitioner* (February 1981): 86–94, 140–151.

33. E. Braunwald et al. (eds.), *Harrison's Principles of Internal Medicine,* 11th ed. (New York: McGraw-Hill, 1987): 1204.

34. Ibid.

35. R. A. Hatcher et al., "Postcoital Contraception," in *Contraceptive Technology 1988–1989,* op. cit., pp. 374–379.

36. Wichman, op. cit.

37. V. Rudick et al., "Epidural Analgesia for Planned Vaginal Delivery Following Previous Cesarean Section," *Obstetrics and Gynecology* 64, no. 5 (November 1984): 621–623.

PART 4

Meeting Challenges: Health and Illness

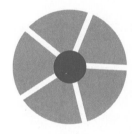

This part of the book examines the issue of disease—malfunctions of the human body due to many causes, including lifestyle. A model of disease is presented which involves not only microbial agents but also environmental and host factors: what people do to make diseases more likely to occur.

Chapter 10 explores communicable and especially sexually transmitted diseases, looking at the different types of microbes involved, how the body's natural defenses work, and precautions that can be taken to lessen the likelihood of their spread.

Chapter 11 describes the major chronic disease today: cardiovascular disease. It describes the normal functioning of the heart and circulatory system; explains major cardiovascular diseases, including heart attack and stroke; and identifies risk factors that contribute to the onset of these diseases.

Chapter 12 looks at the family of diseases called cancers: what they are, why they occur, how to detect their presence, the progress that is being made in their treatment, and steps that can minimize the risk of developing them.

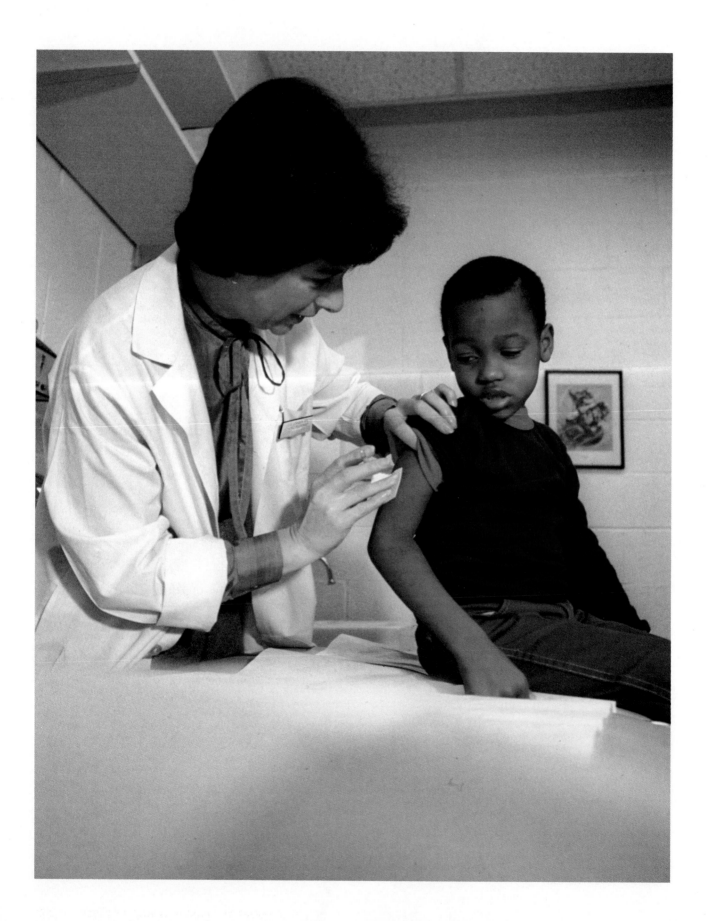

Chapter 10

Communicable Diseases

To Guide Your Reading

When you have studied this chapter, you should be able to:

- Explain the effects lifestyle, travel, and medical progress can have on patterns of diseases.

- Describe what an infection is and explain the role of agents, hosts, and environmental factors in a communicable disease.

- Identify and describe the primary agents of a communicable disease.

- Describe how the body defends itself against infection, including first-line defenses, the inflammatory response, and immunity.

- Identify major sexually transmitted diseases and describe their symptoms and potential effects.

- List the symptoms of human immunodeficiency virus (HIV) infection, AIDS-related complex, and full-blown AIDS; identify the primary modes of transmission of the HIV virus and the primary preventive measures for AIDS.

The word *disease* brings to mind a variety of ailments from the common cold to measles to appendicitis to cancer and heart disease. While these are all diseases, they are quite different from one another. Diseases can be distinguished in various ways. Some are *acute* conditions in which there is a sudden onset of illness that lasts for a relatively short period. The common cold is a familiar example. Others, such as heart disease, are *chronic* conditions that develop gradually over a relatively long period. Diseases may also be infectious or noninfectious. *Infectious* diseases are largely caused by foreign infectious agents such as bacteria and viruses, while *noninfectious* diseases are caused by other factors, such as lifestyle and genetics. Finally, diseases may also be *communicable* or *noncommunicable*; that is, they can or cannot be spread from one person to another.

Such distinctions are important, especially with regard to disease prevention. For example, prevention of acute communicable diseases such as colds and chickenpox centers on the use of vaccination to promote immunity or the avoidance of exposure to people who have these illnesses. By contrast, prevention of chronic noncommunicable diseases such as cancer and heart disease involves modifying lifestyle factors in ways that reduce the risk of developing these diseases. For example, a person may need to reduce stress to lessen the risk of developing high blood pressure, which is often linked to heart disease.

This chapter will focus on infectious, communicable diseases and will examine various agents of infection and the ways in which the body fights infection. Special attention will be given to sexually transmitted diseases because of their increasing prevalence in the United States and the dangers associated with them.

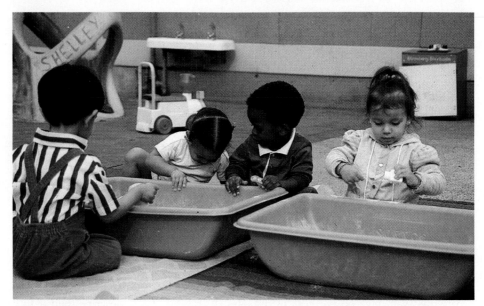

Children who spend time in child care centers are more likely to contract communicable diseases than are those who remain at home; this may give them immunities from some conditions. (Mary Kate Denny/PhotoEdit)

The Changing Face of Disease

Smallpox epidemics throughout history have killed millions of people (from 20 to 40 percent of those infected) and blinded and scarred millions more. It is the first disease to have been eradicated by medical science.

Disease has been part of the human experience since the dawn of time. Throughout their lives people are confronted with a host of diseases that can affect their health and even shorten their life span. Some diseases, such as smallpox, have been eradicated and no longer pose a threat to humanity. However, new or previously unknown diseases, such as AIDS, have appeared. Thus, the patterns of diseases change from year to year; the risk of some diseases may be reduced while the risk of others is increased. Three factors that are related to these changing patterns of disease are lifestyle, travel, and medical progress.

Lifestyle

The only constant in the lives of modern Americans seems to be the fact that their lifestyles are changing continually. Changing trends in work, diet, and activity not only influence the way people live but also affect the patterns of diseases to which people are susceptible.

As more women have entered the work force, larger numbers of young children now spend time at child care centers. At these centers, youngsters become exposed (and in turn expose others) to a greater number of diarrheal, respiratory, and other communicable diseases than they might encounter at home. Thus, the changing lifestyle of working parents has brought with it a changing pattern of disease among children.[1]

Changing diets and dietary fads also may influence the patterns of disease. For example, the increased consumption of high-fat, low-fiber foods over the past several decades may be linked to increases in cancer and heart disease among Americans. Another example is the introduction of sushi (the Japanese delicacy of raw fish) in this country. As eating raw fish has become more fashionable, cases of tapeworm *(Diphyllobothrium latum)*, normally rare in the United States, have increased.[2]

Changing activity levels among Americans also may affect the patterns of disease. For example, sedentary occupations and lifestyles seem to be linked to greater risks of developing cardiovascular disease. People who are physically active seem to be less prone to suffer heart attacks than people who live sedentary lives are. For Americans who increase their activity levels and improve their cardiovascular fitness, the risks of developing cardiovascular disease may decrease. Leisure activities also may have an effect on the patterns of disease. For example, the risks of contracting tick-borne diseases such as Lyme disease and Rocky Mountain spotted fever increase as people spend more time hiking, camping, and engaging in outdoor activities in areas where ticks are abundant.

Travel

Americans are traveling with greater frequency and to more destinations around the world than ever before. This increased travel can be a factor in the patterns of disease. Unsuspecting travelers may bring back illnesses from their trips to foreign countries. For example, throughout the 1970s and early 1980s there was a steady increase in malaria among United States citizens who acquired the disease while traveling abroad.[3] In addition to bringing back known diseases, travelers may also bring back diseases that are rare and unfamiliar to medical practitioners in their own countries, such as schistosomiasis, filariasis, and onchocerciasis. If you get sick after foreign travel, it is important to tell your doctor where you have been.

Medical Progress

Medicine has been making continuous progress in treating and preventing disease. As mentioned previously, smallpox has been eliminated throughout the world; the last case was reported in 1977. Similarly, medicine has made great progress in reducing the incidence of measles through the use of an effective vaccine, although outbreaks of the disease still occur, especially in closed populations such as college students, which may include many unvaccinated people. Medical progress and technology have also helped identify previously unknown diseases, and future developments will no doubt reveal others, along with the means for treating them.

While medical progress has resulted in improved treatment, prevention, and identification of disease, it has not been without drawbacks. The use of antibiotics has been a great help in fighting bacterial infections. However, while these antibiotics inhibit the growth of certain bacteria, they may result in mutant strains of bacteria resistant to the original antibiotic. Thus, although the use of antibiotics represents medical progress, it is also a major contributor to the problem of drug-resistant bacteria.[4]

Medical progress and technology have also contributed to **iatrogenic** (doctor-caused) and **nosocomial** (hospital-caused) problems such as adverse drug reactions, inappropriate treatments, surgical errors, and the spread of infections during hospital stays. For example, organ transplant patients face the problem of rejecting the new organ. While the use of immunosuppressant drugs has reduced the problem, these drugs also lessen the immune system's ability to fight infection.[5] Surgical procedures that implant foreign parts such as artificial heart valves and limb joints may also increase the risk of developing infection. Surgical implants have sometimes led to infection from common skin bacteria that enter the surgical wound.[6]

Perhaps the most famous epidemic was bubonic plague, or "Black Death," as it came to be called, which ravaged Asia, Europe, and the Middle East in the mid-fourteenth century. The disease was caused by a bacterium that infected rats and was transmitted to humans by fleas. The disease first appeared in Asia and spread steadily along trade routes. It is estimated that about one-third of the population of Europe died from the plague from 1347 through 1350. Population changes from plague deaths permanently altered the course of European history. Today bubonic plague is rare and can be treated with antibiotics.

iatrogenic—*referring to an illness or injury caused by a doctor's carelessness, error, or poor judgment.*

nosocomial—*referring to an illness or injury caused by contact with a hospital or other health institution, ranging from a fall from a bed to an infection to a fatal surgical error.*

The Nature of Infectious Disease

An *infection* is the invasion of the body by disease-causing organisms and the reaction of the body to their presence. Most people know what it feels like to have an infectious disease: fever, nausea or vomiting, and general malaise are a few of the symptoms that may occur.

Epidemiologists—the scientists who study human diseases as they affect populations—explain how people contract infectious diseases in terms of

*Some people never develop the symptoms of a disease but are infected nonetheless. These people are called **carriers** of the disease.*

three necessary but distinct components: host, causative agent, and environment. In the past the primary emphasis was placed on the role of the causative agent.[7] For example, if a person (the host) contracted a sore throat, most of the "blame" for the illness would be placed on streptococcus bacteria (the causative agent). However, if the bacteria did not find a susceptible host to infect or an environment (dirty hands, sneeze droplets) in which to multiply and transmit itself, the disease would not occur at all or its incidence would decrease.

Today many epidemiologists prefer to view the interactions among the causative agent, host, and environment in a more balanced way. In this view, a change in one component does not necessarily result in illness. A parent, for example, who is exposed to infectious microorganisms when caring for a child with pneumonia will not necessarily contract the disease. Perhaps the parent is in optimal health or takes precautions to prevent contracting pneumonia. In this newer model the agent, host, and environment constitute a balance of forces that determine an individual's state of health at any given time.[8]

Agent, Host, and Environmental Factors

The agent-host-environment model (Figure 10.1) makes it clear that there is no single cause of an illness. Instead, a multiplicity of factors are responsible for the onset of disease.

Figure 10.1 Communicable disease results from a complex interaction which can be visualized as a triangle consisting of a disease agent (for example, bacteria or virus), a host, and the environment. Note that the environment may have an effect on the host (making the host more susceptible to disease) and also on the agents (making them more prolific and providing a means for them to reach the host). The agents also may affect a person's environment by creating an epidemic, surrounding that individual with people who are carriers of the disease. In the case of an endogenous disease, the agents are already inside the host.

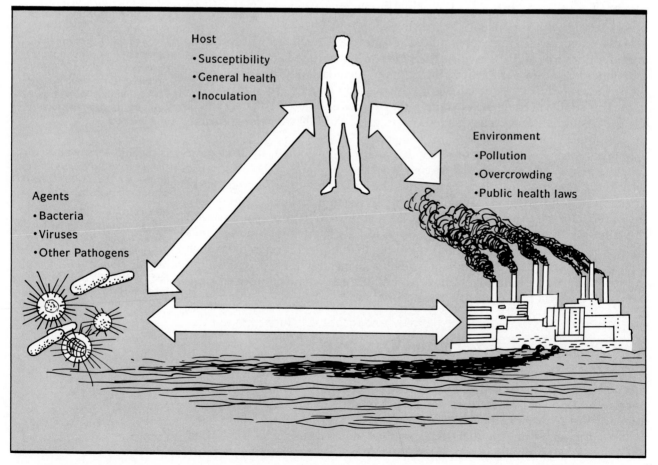

Host
• Susceptibility
• General health
• Inoculation

Environment
• Pollution
• Overcrowding
• Public health laws

Agents
• Bacteria
• Viruses
• Other Pathogens

What Is Your Attitude toward Sickness?

How do you react to disease? Are you a risk taker with your health, or do you worry too much? This activity will help you assess how reasonable you are about sickness. If a statement is one you might easily make about yourself, put a check mark in the space. If you would very rarely make the statement, leave the space blank.

_____   1. I think I am more sensitive to pain than other people.
      _____   2. I participate in activities that many people consider dangerous.
_____   3. I am afraid of getting sick.
      _____   4. I am never affected by viruses that my friends get.
_____   5. I'm afraid I will get the disease if I touch a person with AIDS.
_____   6. When I hear or read about a disease, I worry about getting it myself.
      _____   7. Good health is largely a matter of willpower.
_____   8. I worry about my health more than most people.
      _____   9. I do not think smoking is as dangerous as everybody says it is.
      _____   10. I think people who bother about diet and getting enough sleep are ridiculous.
_____   11. If I am sick and someone tells me I am looking better, it makes me mad.
      _____   12. I never give in to sickness.
_____   13. I often think I might suddenly fall ill.
_____   14. I would never touch alcohol because of the harm it can do.
      _____   15. I try to ignore physical pain.
      _____   16. When I get sick, I often feel I "deserve" the illness.
      _____   17. If I have a ride home, I usually get drunk at parties.
_____   18. I am bothered by many aches and pains.
      _____   19. I rarely finish a prescription from the doctor.
      _____   20. I do not believe in using condoms.

_____ _____   Totals

Total your check marks for each column in the spaces provided. If both scores are very low (2 or less), your attitude toward disease and risk is sensible and reasonable. A high score in the left-hand column indicates that you probably worry more about disease than you need to. A high score on the right suggests that you are more careless than you should be: no one is totally immune to disease. High scores on both sides may imply that you lack basic knowledge about disease: take the information in this chapter seriously.

Some items drawn from I. Pilowsky and N.D. Spence, *Manual for the Illness Behavior Questionnaire (IBQ).* 2nd ed. (Adelaide, Australia: University of Adelaide, 1983): appendix A. With permission.

Agent factors include the organisms that cause an infectious disease. These can be bacteria, viruses, rickettsiae, fungi, and prions. In addition to these organisms, other agent factors include the pathogenicity, or disease-causing ability, of the organism; the degree of virulence of the organism; the number of organisms necessary to cause an infection; and the ability of an organism to enter and move through living tissues.

agent factor—an organism that causes an infectious disease; includes bacteria, viruses, rickettsiae, fungi, and prions.

Host factors are attributes of individuals that may increase or decrease their susceptibility to certain diseases. They include genetic factors, immunity, health-related behaviors, and a person's general state of health. For example, a child who develops cystic fibrosis or muscular dystrophy has inherited a genetic susceptibility to these diseases. A person in poor general health is often much more susceptible to an infectious disease than is someone in ex-

host factor—an attribute of an individual that may increase or decrease his or her susceptibility to certain diseases; includes genetics, immunity, and general state of health.

cellent health. A host factor that offers special protection against disease is *immunity.*

Environmental factors are extrinsic biological, social, and physical factors that influence the probability of developing an infection. Biological factors include the source of a causative agent (for example, soil, water, or animals) and its means of transmission (for example, through the air or through insect or animal bites). Social factors include customs, behaviors, and modes of cooking and dress. The kinds of food eaten and the thoroughness of cooking, for example, may be related to illnesses such as trichinosis, which is caused by parasites in undercooked pork. Similarly, the practice of going barefoot can increase a person's risk of contracting hookworm in rural areas where these parasites are present.[9] Physical factors include the quality of air, water, and living and working environments. The hospital environment, for example, can be a significant factor in the transmission of many infectious diseases. In addition to the susceptibility of hospital patients weakened by illness, cross-infection of bacteria and viruses can be transmitted by hospital personnel as they change patients' wound dressings, adjust their intravenous equipment and catheters, and so on.[10]

The Course of Infectious Diseases

All infectious diseases depend on essentially the same mechanism: the invasion of the body by foreign organisms and the reaction of the body to them. After a person is infected, the course of the disease naturally follows a common and familiar pattern marked by five specific phases. The first is the **incubation period,** in which the organisms invade and multiply in the host. The length of this phase varies with the disease and the individual. The second phase is called the **prodrome period.** This brief phase is characterized by general symptoms such as headache, fever, runny nose, irritability, and general discomfort. A disease is highly communicable during the prodrome period. The third phase is called **clinical disease.** The illness is at its height during this phase; characteristic symptoms of the disease appear, and so a specific diagnosis can be made. During the fourth phase—the **decline stage**—symptoms begin to subside and the patient may feel well enough to become more active. The danger of relapse increases, however, if the patient becomes too active before achieving a full recovery. The final phase is **convalescence,** which is the recovery period. Although the patient is better, the disease may still be communicable. A patient who recovers but still gives off disease-causing organisms becomes a **carrier** of the disease.

Most infectious diseases can be treated to relieve the symptoms and promote healing and recovery. Bacterial infections can be treated with antibiotics, a group of drugs that help kill or disable infectious bacteria. Since some antibiotics are effective against certain kinds of bacteria but not against others, many different antibiotics have been developed to control infections. Some of the best-known antibiotics are penicillin, ampicillin, erythromycin, and tetracycline.

Agents of Infectious Disease

Vast numbers of tiny microscopic organisms too small to be seen with the naked eye share the world with humans. Billions of these microorganisms normally live on or within the human body and are called **endogenous,** or "resident," microorganisms. Billions of others are **exogenous** microorganisms; that is, they normally live outside the human body. While some microorganisms are harmless, others can be **pathogens**—agents of infectious disease.

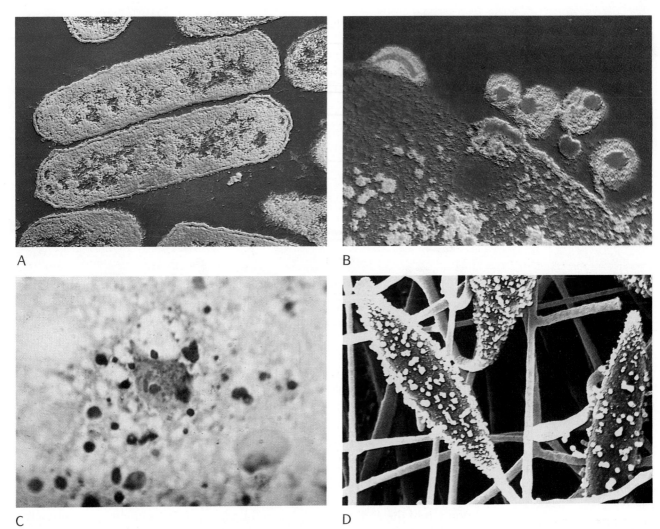

These electron micrographs show four of the main agents of infectious disease: (A) bacteria (pneumonia and meningitis); (B) virus (AIDS); (C) rickettsia (Rocky Mountain spotted fever); (D) fungus (ringworm). (A and D: CNRI/Photo Researchers, Inc.; B: Luc Montagnier, Institut Pasteur/Photo Researchers, Inc.; C: Photo Researchers, Inc.)

Bacteria

The most plentiful microorganisms endogenous to humans are the various kinds of **bacteria** (singular: *bacterium*). Each of these tiny organisms consists of just one cell with a protective cell wall and all the structures the bacterium needs to carry out its life functions.

bacteria (singular: bacterium)—*a single-celled plantlike microorganism.*

Endogenous Bacteria and Disease   Most kinds of endogenous bacteria are not harmful; some, in fact, are vital to human health. The bacterium *Escherichia coli* (often called *E. coli*) lives in the intestines and is essential in the synthesis of the B vitamins; other bacteria help kill foreign infectious organisms. However, endogenous bacteria can cause disease if they get out of hand. Skin bacteria sometimes cause acne; mouth bacteria sometimes help cause pyorrhea, a serious gum disease; and intestinal bacteria may enter the urethra, particularly in women, and cause infections of the urinary tract. Different strains of *E. coli,* perhaps introduced during travel, may cause diarrhea until the digestive system adjusts to their presence.

Streptoccocal bacteria, which usually inhabit mucous membranes, may cause diseases such as strep throat (a severe throat infection), peritonitis (a severe inflammation within the abdomen), scarlet fever (an acute fever with sore throat and rash), or rheumatic fever (an infection that primarily affects

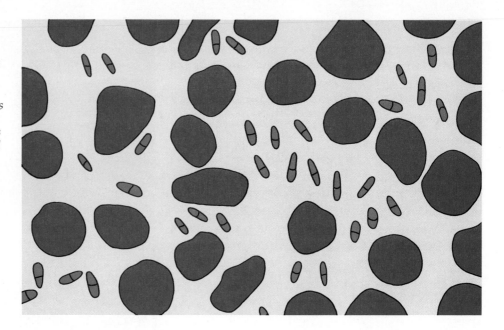

Figure 10.2 Typical staphylococcus bacteria of the type which infect boils. A single bacterium can reproduce to form a colony of 250,000 bacteria in an hour. This colony competes with body cells for food, weakening the host. The bacteria also excrete toxins that may poison body cells and result in a variety of symptoms, including skin eruptions, rashes, fever, nausea, and fatigue.

the joints and the heart). While most streptoccocal bacteria are endogenous, others may be introduced from outside the body.

Staphylococcal bacteria (Figure 10.2), which are normally present on the skin, are usually harmless. Occasionally, however, if there is a scratch or other small opening in the skin, the staphylococci will enter the wound and produce a localized infection. Staphylococci also cause boils (infections of sweat glands and hair follicles) and sties (infections on the eyelids). An exception to the typical localized infections caused by staphylococci is the condition known as toxic shock syndrome (TSS). This condition was brought to public attention in the early 1980s. Most of the victims were women who contracted an infection from the bacteria *Staphylococcus aureus* while using a particular type of tampon during menstruation. As the staph bacteria multiplied, they spread from the vagina into the bloodstream and released their toxins. The symptoms of TSS include high fever, abdominal pain, diarrhea, vomiting, and a red skin rash. Sometimes blood pressure drops suddenly, causing death. TSS can be treated with antibiotics and can be prevented by changing tampons more frequently and using sanitary napkins when the menstrual flow is light.

Attached ticks should be removed with the gentle but sustained pull of tweezers. It is not advisable to use a hot match, petroleum jelly, or a chemical irritant.

Exogenous Bacteria and Disease Stepping on a rusty nail can be a painful experience. A worse scenario will occur, however, if the nail harbors disease-causing bacteria. Tetanus, which causes a serious infection known as lockjaw—the symptoms include muscle rigidity and convulsions—is a classic example of a disease resulting from a wound infected by an exogenous bacterium, in this case *Clostridium tetani*. Exogenous bacteria are responsible for a number of major diseases, including cholera, typhus, tuberculosis, gonorrhea, and syphilis, to name just a few.

A potentially serious exogenous bacterial disease that has recently come to public attention is *Lyme disease*, which is caused by the bacterium *Borrelia burgdorferi*. In this disease the bacteria are introduced into the human body by the bite of an infected deer tick. The first stage presents as a raised red rash which develops and expands in circular fashion up to an average of 6 inches in diameter. The early symptoms may also include headache, fever, and muscle and joint pain (similar to the flu). If left untreated, Lyme disease can progress to arthritis and heart and neurological problems. In its early stages, this disease can be treated with antibiotics.[11]

Viruses

A number of diseases, including mumps, measles, rubella (German measles), smallpox, and AIDS, are caused by viruses, one of the simplest living organisms. Because viruses have a mysterious ability to exist and proliferate without carrying out the life functions of respiration and metabolism as these processes are usually thought of, some scientists question whether they should be considered living things.

A virus is nothing more than a bit of nucleic acid within a protein coat. *Nucleic acid* is the biochemical substance that carries the genetic information an organism needs to reproduce. Thus, a virus is really just a substance designed to duplicate itself. In fact, a **virus** is best defined as a microorganism that can reproduce only in living cells.

Once inside a cell, a virus takes over and directs the cell to produce many hundreds of new viruses (Figure 10.3). However, body cells can protect themselves against some viruses. When exposed to certain viruses, they may produce a protective substance called **interferon,** which helps prevent the virus from infecting other cells.

Colds and Flu Sniffling, sneezing, coughing and sore throat—the average person complains of these cold symptoms at least twice a year. The common cold is really not so common, however, as evidenced by the family of more than 100 viruses that cause it. Rhinoviruses, aptly named after the Greek word for "nose," are the major infectious agents of the common cold, especially in the fall. Among the other causal agents, over half have not been identified.[12]

Cold viruses contaminate the air and the surfaces of objects. Breathing in these viruses or touching virus-laden hands to the eyes or the inside of the mouth or nose allows them to enter the body. Once inside the host, cold viruses reproduce during a short incubation period of 1 to 3 days. For the next 4 to 7 days the immune system battles these invaders by releasing chemical substances that irritate the throat and prompt the nose and sinuses to produce fluid to soothe the irritated tissues. The results are a runny nose, watery eyes, and congestion.

Influenza, or "flu," is rarely a serious disease unless it is complicated by a secondary infection. However, if bacteria become involved or if the virus spreads to the lungs, the condition may be lethal, particularly among the very

virus—*a microorganism that can reproduce only in living cells.*

interferon—*a substance produced by the body to help protect it against disease.*

Figure 10.3 To reproduce itself, a virus must use the material in a living cell. (A) First the virus locks on to the wall of the host cell. (B) Viral DNA is injected into the cell. (C) The DNA takes over the host cell and begins to replicate. (D) New protein coats are formed around replicated viral DNA, creating new complete viruses within the host cell. Meanwhile, the attached cell may begin to release interferon. (E) The host cell bursts and releases the new viruses. (F) The new viruses attack neighboring cells. If enough interferon was created, these cells will have produced antiviral enzymes that help protect them from the virus and inhibit further viral reproduction.

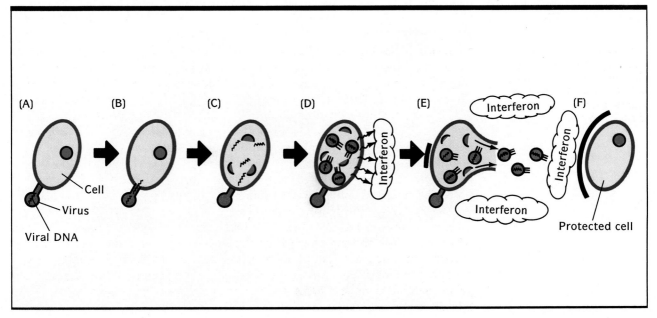

Flu shots are generally recommended only for those at risk of serious complications, for example, the elderly and people who already have respiratory or heart disease.

Some facts about the common cold:

- *The average adult has two colds a year.*
- *Colds are the cause of one-third of all work-related absences.*
- *Over $5 billion is spent annually on drugs and doctors.*

young, the elderly, and those with heart or respiratory disease. Flu complications have killed more than half a million Americans in the last 25 years.[13]

Flu viruses are "packaged" in a distinct way. In other viruses the strands of nucleic acid are strung together in one line, but with the flu virus these strands are in eight separate pieces. This makes it easier for a viral strand to become detached and change places with a strand from another virus, allowing the genetic information in the virus to change rapidly. Not surprisingly, there are not only three major varieties of flu virus—A (the most virulent), B, and C—but numerous changing strains within each major type. Immunity against one variety or strain of flu virus does not necessarily provide immunity against any other. Although there are vaccines against specific strains of flu virus, these vaccines are not effective against other strains. Also, since viral strains change, the components of vaccines are changed periodically, and individuals must be revaccinated every year.

The symptoms of flu differ from those of a cold; flu symptoms generally make a person feel more tired, achy, and weak. In general, flu develops more rapidly than does a cold, over a period of hours instead of days. A high fever usually appears within 12 hours of the first symptoms, and recuperation may last from 1 to 3 weeks.

Hepatitis Hepatitis—a viral inflammation of the liver—has increased significantly in recent years, particularly among young people. At present there are four known viral causes of hepatitis in the United States; experts suspect that there may be others as well. Of the four known types, the most prevalent are hepatitis A, B, and C. Hepatitis A, commonly called infectious hepatitis, is the most common type (and usually the least dangerous). Hepatitis B (which used to be called serum hepatitis) is far more dangerous, as is hepatitis C (once called non-A, non-B hepatitis). Hepatitis A is caused by fecal contamination of food or the environment and can be prevented with proper hygiene. Hepatitis B and C are spread primarily through the exchange of body fluids during sexual activity or through blood transfusions.[14]

The different types of hepatitis have similar symptoms: fever, headache, nausea, loss of appetite, and pain in the upper right abdomen. The urine becomes deep yellow, and the patient may become jaundiced. A primary concern with hepatitis is to prevent transmission to people in contact with those who are infected. In the case of acute type A hepatitis, all family mem-

In recent years the medical community has become aware of many new diseases that can be transmitted through blood transfusions; regardless of the donor, all blood must pass several purity tests before being accepted by a blood bank. (A. Glauberman/Photo Researchers, Inc.)

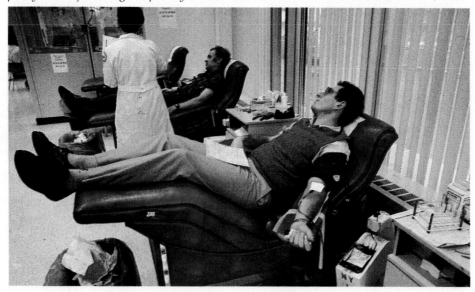

bers and close personal associates should receive immune serum globulin (ISG) as soon as possible after exposure. In acute type B hepatitis, hepatitis B immune globulin (HBIG) must be given only to the "regular" sexual contacts of the infected individual.[15] However, hepatitis B vaccine is also strongly recommended for the prevention of the disease among other high-risk individuals, including health care workers who are exposed frequently to the virus. A new blood test to detect hepatitis B and C viruses in blood used for transfusions is currently up for approval by the FDA.[16]

Antibiotics were developed to combat bacteria and fungi and are not effective in treating viral infections.

Hepatitis may be a prolonged illness and, if it causes serious damage to the liver, may be extremely dangerous. If liver failure is serious enough to cause a coma, the patient has only a 10 to 20 percent chance of surviving.[17] Up to 50 percent of hepatitis C infections cause chronic liver damage, which may lead to cirrhosis and cancer of the liver. For unknown reasons, some people are healthy carriers of the virus and escape serious liver damage.[18]

Mononucleosis Infectious mononucleosis, or "mono," is common among high school and college students. Its short-term symptoms, which can be severe, may include fever, sore throat, nausea, chills, and general weakness; the individual may sometimes have a rash, enlarged and tender lymph glands, jaundice, and/or enlargement of the spleen as well. Other symptoms may mimic those of more serious diseases such as polio, meningitis, tuberculosis (TB), diphtheria, and leukemia. Fortunately, mono can be diagnosed with a simple blood test.

The longer-term symptoms are the frustrating ones; although permanent disability is unusual, the general weakness and feeling of fatigue can last for weeks or months. Happily—for no one who has had mono ever wants to have it again—experts generally agree that the disease confers fairly long, if not permanent, immunity.[19]

Research has identified a virus known as the Epstein-Barr virus as the cause of the most common form of infectious mononucleosis.[20] Although mono is sometimes referred to as the "kissing disease," kissing is only one of several ways it is spread. Strangely, it does not spread easily by ordinary contact; in fact, it is rare to have more than one case in a household.

Rickettsiae

Rickettsiae are organisms that are considered to be intermediate between bacteria and viruses. Most rickettsiae grow as parasites in the intestinal tract of insects and insectlike creatures, with which they frequently live in peaceful coexistence. Others are disease-causing agents that are transmitted to humans and other mammals through insect and tick bites. The insect serves as a **vector,** or carrier, of the infectious agent, transferring the organism to a human host. Rocky Mountain spotted fever is transmitted to humans by ticks. Typhus fever is another major rickettsial disease that is transmitted by an insect vector—fleas, ticks, and lice. In addition to insect bites, rickettsiae may be transmitted through scratches and skin breaks and the inhalation of aerosols.[21]

rickettsiae—infectious organisms that grow in the intestinal tract of insects and insectlike creatures and can be transmitted to humans through insect bites.

vector—a carrier of an infectious disease; insects, ticks, and rats are vectors for some human diseases.

Fungi

Fungi are a type of infectious agent with which many people have had first-hand experience. Athlete's foot is caused by fungi, as are ringworm and yeast infections such as candidiasis (thrush). Fungi are many-celled organisms (mushrooms are members of this family) that lack chlorophyll and cannot manufacture their own food. As a result, they must obtain food from organic materials such as plants, animals, and, in some cases, humans. Fungi spread as bits of the organism are blown to new locations through the release of spores, or seedlike cells.

fungi—many-celled plantlike organisms that lack chlorophyll and must therefore obtain food from organic material, in some cases from humans.

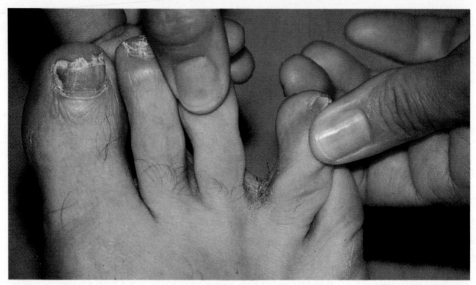

Proper hygiene can help stop the spread of all pathogens and is particularly effective against fungal infections such as athlete's foot. (Tony Freeman/PhotoEdit)

In humans, fungi tend to invade warm, moist areas such as the scalp, feet, and groin. Some generalized fungal infections may affect the lungs. Fungal infections are rarely serious and can be controlled with fungicides and proper hygiene, including regular bathing, wearing clean clothes, and avoiding the use of other people's clothing.

Prions

prion—*a small protein capable of replicating itself within the cells of mammals.*

At one time viruses were thought to be the smallest agents of disease, but today it is known that much smaller agents exist. These agents, known as **prions,** are small proteins that are capable of replicating within the cells of mammals. Prions have been implicated in certain diseases classified as slow infections with long incubation periods (months, years, or even decades) during which the host displays no symptoms. Creutzfeldt-Jakob disease—a slowly progressive illness characterized by dementia, or mental deterioration—is known to be caused by prions.[22]

Defense against Infectious Disease

Suppose a pathogenic agent does invade the body. What can the body do to fight off the pathogen and prevent it from causing disease? The body has three basic lines of defense: the skin and mucous membranes, the inflammatory response, and immunity.

First-Line Defenses

The skin and mucous membranes are the body's first line of defense. An invading microorganism must find its way through the skin or the mucosae, the mucus-coated membranes that line the respiratory, digestive, and urogenital tracts and form an "inner skin." Secretions such as tears, perspiration, skin oils, and saliva, which contain chemicals that can kill bacteria, are part of this defense system. In addition, the respiratory passages are lined with fine, short moving hairs called *cilia* that spread a carpet of sticky mucus. The mucus works like flypaper to trap inhaled microorganisms and foreign matter and carry them to the back of the throat, where they are removed by sneezing, coughing, or nose blowing or are swallowed and disposed of by digestive fluids.

Besides the cilia, other body hairs (the eyelashes, for example) may fend off invading microorganisms. Reflexes such as coughing, blinking, and vomiting are also part of the body's first line of defense, as are high acid levels in the stomach and vagina, which help destroy invaders.

The Inflammatory Response

Sometimes microorganisms get beyond the body's outer defenses—through a cut in the skin, for example. They then face a second line of defense in the blood and the tissues—**inflammation,** or the **inflammatory response.** The inflammatory response is a general one; it helps ward off any irritant or foreign matter, whether it is a relatively large physical object (such as a splinter), a chemical substance, or a microorganism.

The white blood cells in the bloodstream form a vital part of the body's defense system. Some are of a type known as **phagocytes,** a term that literally means "cells that eat." A phagocyte is made up of a semiliquid jellylike substance with a cell wall holding it together; it can actually flow around a foreign substance, take it apart chemically, and digest it (Figure 10.4).

During the inflammatory response, the supply of blood to the endangered area increases while the flow of blood through the area slows down. As a result, some *blood plasma* (the fluid that transports red and white blood cells) leaks through the walls of the blood vessels into the spaces between the cells in the endangered area, bringing with it special proteins that help destroy pathogens. Meanwhile, phagocytes rush to the area to engulf bacteria and foreign particles.

inflammation—*a general defense mechanism in the blood and tissues to ward off an irritant or foreign body. Also called the* **inflammatory response.**

phagocytes—*white blood cells that protect the body from infection by engulfing and digesting invading microorganisms, toxins, and other foreign substances.*

Figure 10.4 (A) Antibodies may help neutralize bacteria by causing them to cluster together. (B) Large cells called phagocytes detect and engulf bacteria and other foreign substances. (C) The phagocyte isolates the foreign substances within a vacuole and destroys them. The remains are then eliminated through the lymphatic system.

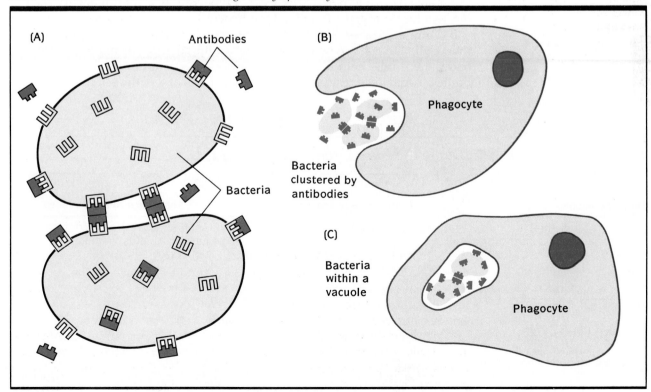

If the infection is localized in one part of the body, the patient usually shows the signs of inflammation only in that area; these signs include redness, local warmth, swelling, and pain. Such signs indicate that the invaders are being counterattacked. However, if the battle is being waged throughout the body, the patient usually will have a generalized fever, which is caused at least in part by toxins produced by the invaders or released by them while they are being destroyed. These toxins interfere with the regulatory mechanisms that control the temperature of the body. While the resulting elevated temperatures may be harmful to normal body functions, fever can be helpful as well: it stimulates the body to produce more white blood cells and may even kill the invading organism, since most pathogens cannot survive in above-normal body temperatures.

Whether the inflammatory response is sufficient to knock out the infection depends on how many invading organisms there are, how strong they are, and how well the body is able to defend itself. Sometimes the battle comes to a standstill at the local level. As more and more local tissue is destroyed, the body may form a cavity, or **abscess,** filled with sticky yellow-white pus that consists of fluid, battling cells, and white blood cells that have died in the battle. The struggle is resolved when enough invading organisms have been killed or inactivated to halt the infection. In more severe cases, this line of defense fails and the invading organisms begin to spread through the tissues and even into the bloodstream. The infection then becomes generalized and highly dangerous.

abscess—a pus-filled cavity formed as a result of destruction of local tissue in the inflammatory response.

Immunity

immunity—a group of mechanisms that help protect the body against specific diseases.

The body's third line of defense against disease is **immunity,** a group of mechanisms that help protect the body against specific diseases (Table 10.1). Immunity is the body's most efficient disease-preventing weapon; it can help fight either a viral infection or a bacterial one.

lymphocytes—protective white blood cells in the immune system that fight infection.

antibodies—chemical substances produced in response to an invading microorganism (the antigen) that can inactivate that microorganism.

The Role of Lymphocytes In the immune mechanism, as in the inflammatory response, white blood cells become involved in fighting infection. Here the protective white blood cells are of a type known as **lymphocytes,** including two key subtypes: B and T lymphocytes.

B lymphocytes, or B cells, are believed to originate in the bone marrow (hence the letter B). When foreign or invading pathogens are present in the body, these cells help produce substances called immunoglobulins, or **antibodies.** Antibodies react specifically to the parts of a pathogen that link up to

Table 10.1   Types of Immunity: Active and Passive, Natural and Acquired

Type of Immunity	Active Antibodies Are Manufactured	Passive Antibodies Are Introduced
Natural (Without Medical Intervention)	Antibodies are manufactured following natural exposure to a foreign agent; immunity is long-term and specific or Interferon is produced following exposure to viruses; immunity is temporary and specific	Antibodies are transferred from mother to fetus; immunity is temporary and specific
Acquired (With Medical Intervention)	Immunization with vaccine triggers manufacture of antibodies; immunity is long-term and specific	Antibodies are administered in immune serums or antitoxins; immunity is temporary and specific

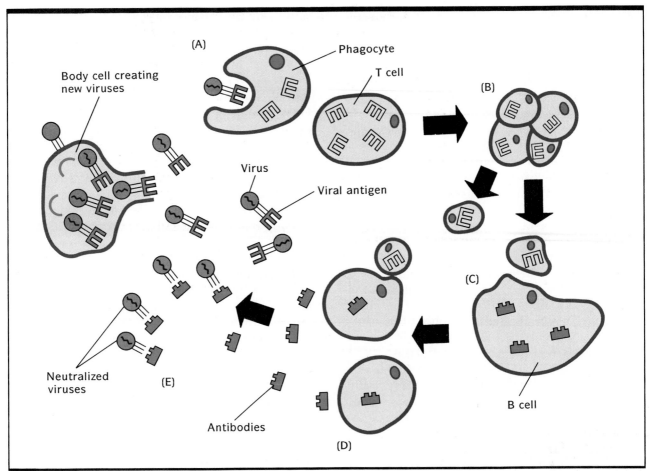

(A) Phagocyte

Body cell creating new viruses

T cell

(B)

Virus

Viral antigen

(C)

Neutralized viruses

(E)

Antibodies

B cell

(D)

human cells and cause damage. These parts, which are called **antigens,** are thus neutralized (Figure 10.5). If the invaders are viruses, the antibodies lock on to their antigens and prevent them from entering the target cells. If the invaders are bacteria, the antibodies lock on to them and cause them to clump together, making it easier for phagocytes to engulf and digest them. These bacterial-antibody clumps also activate certain *bactericidal* (bacteria-killing) substances in the blood. Antibodies can also lock on to bacterial toxins to make them less harmful to the body.

T lymphocytes, or T cells, named for their origin in the thymus gland, fight infection in three major ways. First, some T lymphocytes spur the phagocytes to eat foreign substances faster. Second, some help stimulate the production of antibodies by B lymphocytes. Third, some can attack foreign cells (such as cells in tissues that have been transplanted), cells that have been killed by viruses, and possibly cancer cells.

Natural Immunity As discussed earlier, when a virus attacks the body, it helps bring about its own destruction by triggering the production of interferon. Natural immunity works in somewhat the same way. When an invading antigen enters the body, it stimulates the body to produce certain antibodies that can inactivate it. When antigens lock on to specific receptor sites on a body cell's plasma membrane, the immune response is set in motion and antibodies are produced. As was mentioned above, antibodies work only on the specific antigens that trigger them: measles antibodies work only on the measles virus, mumps antibodies on the mumps virus, and so on. There are over a million different specific antibodies, each capable of fighting one antigen. That means that over a million different foreign antigens can stimulate the immune system to take action.

Figure 10.5 The immune system mobilizes against a virus. (A) A phagocyte engulfs a virus and transfers information about its antigen to a T cell. (B) The T cell multiplies and contacts B cells. (C) The B cells develop specific antibodies against the viral antigen. (D) The B cells multiply and release their antibodies. (E) The antibodies lock on to the viruses, preventing them from attacking other body cells. Antibodies and some of the activated T cells remain in the bloodstream, providing acquired immunity to the virus for long periods.

antigen—*part of an invading microorganism that stimulates the body to produce a chemical substance (antibodies) that can inactivate a microorganism.*

A Broader View

Eradicating a Killer Disease

Thanks to medical research and knowledge about disease transmission, communicable diseases no longer cause widespread sickness and death. Outbreaks still occur and cause great fear—especially outbreaks of newly discovered diseases such as AIDS—but the horror of communicable diseases in the Middle Ages is almost unthinkable now. Smallpox, cholera, tuberculosis, typhoid, and bubonic plague were all great killers until medical science began to develop and test techniques for their cure and prevention. Now they have been largely eliminated in the developed nations, and smallpox is thought to have been eradicated throughout the world.

Smallpox was the most feared disease— very contagious and deadly. Up to 40 percent of its many victims did not survive, especially the very old and the very young. Those who lived through severe cases suffered fever and pain for several weeks, were sometimes blinded, and were often left badly disfigured, with deep pockmarks all over the skin. Edward Jenner, who developed the technique of vaccination in England, called smallpox "the most dreadful scourge of the human species." However, less than two centuries after vaccination was first used, it is no longer

needed: smallpox appears to be extinct.

The tale of the end of smallpox begins, as many medical stories do, in folk medicine: it ends with modern technology and painstaking detective work. The crowded cities of eighteenth-century Europe and North America made smallpox dangerous among the wealthy and influential as well as the poor. Finding methods to combat it became a high priority. Fortunately, exploration and trade brought stories from all over the world about different folk methods for providing protection against this disease. One method, used in different forms in Africa, China, and Turkey, involved a preparation from the scabs of smallpox itself: the scabs were either blown into the patient's nose or applied to a scratch on the skin. It sounds very dangerous, but it met with some success both in London and in Boston.

The Royal Society of London, one of the most prestigious groups of scientists at that time, kept track of some of these successes and found that statistically the technique seemed to work. Then, in 1788, Jenner found that the same effect could be produced with the harmless scabs of a related disease known as cowpox. He called the technique

---

vaccine—*killed or weakened viruses that are taken orally or by injection to stimulate the body to produce antibodies that give immunity to the specific disease caused by a virus.*

active immunity—*long-lasting resistance to an infectious disease acquired through the production of antibodies as a result of having the disease or being vaccinated against it (compare with* passive immunity*).*

passive immunity—*short-term resistance to infectious disease acquired through the administration of antibodies formed by another person or an animal (compare with* active immunity*).*

Acquired Immunity   In the past, having a disease was the only way to develop immunity to it (natural immunity through the development of antibodies to fight the current infection and subsequent ones). Today, however, immunity may be induced artificially by means of **vaccines,** which consist of killed or weakened viruses, taken orally or by injection. Several days or weeks after an individual receives a vaccination, the body starts to produce specific antibodies, which circulate in the bloodstream, ready to attack the initiating antigen.

People who contract a disease or receive a vaccine for it usually develop **active immunity.** But what happens if a person is exposed to a serious disease and it is too dangerous to wait for the person's body to produce its own antibodies? In this instance a physician may confer **passive immunity** by giving the person antibodies from another person or an animal. These antibodies are found in certain proteins in the donor's blood that are collectively called **gamma globulin.** Gamma globulin is used to confer passive immunization against infectious hepatitis and other diseases for which an effective vaccine has not been devised.

In general, active immunity is long-term and in some cases lifelong, whereas passive immunity generally lasts only a few weeks or months. Babies have passive immunity at birth because antibodies that pass through the placental membrane become part of the fetus's immune system. Within 6 weeks

vaccination: it was the first form of immunization invented.

The technique underwent several improvements over the next century and a half: methods were developed for producing the vaccine in large quantities and preserving it effectively under refrigeration. By 1940 compulsory vaccination programs had all but eliminated smallpox from many countries in Europe. In the United States the last case officially recorded occurred in 1949. Efforts to use mass vaccination in other nations met with only partial success, however. A 1950 drive to defeat smallpox in the Americas was successful in the Caribbean and Central America but failed in some South American countries. A 1959 resolution to achieve global vaccination proved too expensive and hard to enforce.

In 1967 another approach was tried. Instead of relying only on mass vaccination, health workers would seek out reports of all cases of smallpox. Each would be investigated, and every contact would be tracked down, treated if necessary, and kept in quarantine until safe.

The last person to be diagnosed with smallpox was a Somalian named Ali Maalin in 1977. When Maalin came down with a high fever and a headache, he was admitted to a hospital and treated for malaria. A few days later other symptoms appeared, and it was realized that Maalin was suffering from smallpox; he had recently been exposed to two other cases of smallpox, the only two known cases in Somalia at that time.

Maalin's illness ignited what has turned out to be the last campaign to find people with smallpox. Maalin was a cook in a hospital. He had exposed 161 people to the disease, 41 of whom had never been vaccinated against it. Medical workers found all 41, vaccinated them, and monitored their health; none came down with smallpox.

Over the next 6 months medical teams scoured the villages near Maalin's hometown in search of others who might have been exposed. They investigated thousands of rash and fever cases, and the World Health Organization Smallpox Reference Center in Atlanta, Georgia, examined more than 500 specimens. No new cases of smallpox were found.

Based on Donald A. Henderson, "The History of Smallpox Eradication," in *Times, Places, and Persons: Aspects of the History of Epidemiology,* A. M. Lilienfeld (ed.) (Baltimore: Johns Hopkins University Press, 1980): 99–107. With permission.

---

after birth, however, passive immunity begins to weaken, and the baby will need to receive vaccinations to start the development of active immunity against certain diseases.

gamma globulin—certain blood proteins that contain antibodies.

Types of Vaccines Some vaccines, such as those used against yellow fever and measles and the Sabin oral polio vaccine, contain living infectious agents. Although these agents have been weakened in the laboratory, they still provoke the formation of antibodies. Other vaccines contain killed infectious agents; included among these are the whooping cough and Salk polio vaccines. The killed infectious agents do not produce the disease but stimulate the production of antibodies to protect the body from future infection.

Along similar lines, acquired immunity can be induced against certain microbial toxins that produce disease. Diphtheria and tetanus, for example, produce disease through their toxins. Modified toxins called **toxoids,** which are no longer poisonous, are used in vaccines to stimulate the production of antibodies that will inactivate the toxins if the invading organism strikes.

toxoids—modified toxins which are no longer poisonous; used to induce the production of antibodies that will inactivate specific microbial disease-producing toxins.

Maintaining Immunity Vaccines have greatly limited the number of people who may be carrying certain infectious diseases and thus have reduced the risk of contracting these diseases in the United States and elsewhere. Effective and safe vaccines are now available for many infectious diseases.

Table 10.2 Recommended Schedule for Active Immunization

Age	Vaccines
2 months	Diphtheria-tetanus-pertussis (DTP), oral polio vaccine
4 months	DTP, oral polio vaccine
6 months	Oral polio vaccine (recommended for infants in areas where polio is endemic)
15 months	Measles, rubella, mumps
18 months	DTP, oral polio booster
4 to 6 years (school entry)	DTP booster, oral polio booster
14 to 16 years	Combined tetanus and diphtheria toxoid, adult type (repeat every 10 years)

Source: American Academy of Pediatrics.

Tuberculosis has recently been seen more often in the United States, particularly as an opportunistic infection associated with AIDS.

Some vaccines have to be administered only once; others require periodic boosters to keep the level of antibodies high enough to confer immunity. Because of vaccinations, American children today are avoiding many of the diseases their parents experienced during childhood. Rubella (German measles), varicella (chickenpox), and pertussis (whooping cough) are much less common today than ever before. More serious diseases, such as polio, tuberculosis, diphtheria, and tetanus, have also decreased to almost insignificant levels.

Widespread regular immunizations (Table 10.2) not only defend individuals against disease, they lessen the presence of the disease organism itself. This benefits the whole population, including those who have not been vaccinated. In fact, some Americans have been lulled into complacency about infectious diseases. They are not as well informed as they should be, nor are they as careful as they should be to keep up with the necessary immunizations. This may lead to trouble. Although it is not necessary for everyone in the population to be immune in order to prevent a disease from spreading, scientists do not know how far below 100 percent immunity the population can go without having new outbreaks of these diseases. That is one reason why school systems and colleges often require proof of immunizations before registration or for giving out grades. It is important for everyone to keep vaccinations up to date and urge others to do the same.

Malfunction of the Immune System Experts suspect that disorders of the immune system may be involved in many puzzling medical problems. At times the body's defenses seem to act against the body's best interests. This can be seen in allergies and connective tissue diseases.[23]

In response to dust, pollen, bee or wasp venom, and certain other substances, some people produce antibodies in such large quantities that they cause harm. The overabundant antibodies attach themselves to *mast cells* in certain body tissues. The mast cells then release toxins that cause the individual to cough, produce large amounts of mucus, and suffer other allergic symptoms.

A number of mysterious diseases afflict the various kinds of connective tissue in the body, such as the cartilage that holds the joints together. In the disease known as lupus, the immune system somehow attacks the body's connective tissue. In rheumatoid arthritis, certain antibodies actually behave like antigens: they cause the body to put out other antibodies, which lock on to them and cause inflammation in the joints.

In addition to allergies and diseases of connective tissues, malfunction of the immune system can be seen most devastatingly in acquired immune deficiency syndrome. This disease, which presents a major challenge to the immune system, will be discussed in detail later in this chapter.

Sexually Transmitted Diseases

Although AIDS has received a great deal of publicity recently, it is just one of a great number of **sexually transmitted diseases (STDs),** which include herpes genitalis, syphilis, gonorrhea, condyloma, and chlamydia (Table 10.3). In general, STDs are on the increase in the United States, with individuals under age 25 accounting for the majority of cases. In addition to young people, other groups at high risk for contracting STDs are minorities, the medically under-

sexually transmitted disease (STD)—*an infectious disease that is almost always transmitted during sexual intercourse, homosexual relations, or other sexual activity.*

Table 10.3 Common STDs: Risks, Symptoms, and Treatments

STD	Risks	Symptoms	Treatments
Acquired immune deficiency syndrome (AIDS)	Opportunistic infections, cancers, death	Vary with the afflicting diseases: common symptoms include fatigue, loss of appetite or weight, skin rashes, chronic cough, diarrhea and/or bloody stools, and a whitish coating on the tongue or in the throat	No drugs yet shown to have antiviral impact on AIDS virus; AZT and other experimental drugs may slow disease; treatment often focuses on opportunistic infections and cancers
Chlamydia	*Women:* pelvic inflammatory disease (PID); infertility *Men:* nongonococcal urethritis *Newborns:* infection, death	*Women:* vaginal itching, discharge; but often asymptomatic *Men:* burning, itching in genital area; discharge	Tetracycline, erythromycin
Condyloma	Obstruction of birth canal	Warty growths around anus or genitals	Chemical ointments or surgery
Gonorrhea	PID; arthritis; endocarditis; infertility; blindness in newborns	*Women:* painful urination; vaginal inflammation; usually asymptomatic *Men:* discharge; painful urination	Tetracycline, ampicillin, penicillin
Herpes genitalis	Eye infection; neurological damage; miscarriage, infection of newborn, infant blindness, neurological damage and death; recurrent infection; cancer of the cervix and prostate	Sores and blisters around genitals; possible fever, chills, headache; painful urination	No cure yet; symptoms respond well to acyclovir
Hepatitis	In severe cases: liver damage; death	Mild flulike symptoms to high fever with vomiting and severe abdominal pain	Gamma globulin; bed rest; adequate fluid intake
Pubic lice (crabs)	Secondary infections	Persistent itching; lice are visible in pubic and other body hair	Topical treatments such as γ-benzene hexachloride
Syphilis	If untreated: paralysis, blindness, insanity, death; birth defects, transmittal to fetus	In early stage: chancre sores; second stage: flulike symptoms, rash, hair loss; late stage: brain, heart, liver damage	Penicillin and other antibiotics
Trichomoniasis	*Women:* Form of vaginitis that can lead to cystitis; abnormal Pap smear *Men:* urethritis	*Women:* yellowish-green discharge; inflammation of vagina; often asymptomatic *Men:* usually asymptomatic	Oral metronidazole given to both partners
Yeast infections (candidiasis, moniliasis)	Rarely, systemic infection	Itching, yeasty white discharge	Prescription suppositories

Source: Marilynn Larkin, ''Not the End of Sex,'' *Health* (December 1985): 51.

served, and people who partake in risky sexual behaviors.[24] These diseases pose a real problem to people's health and well-being. Some have serious consequences, including chronic pain, sterility, abnormal pregnancy, cancer, and, in the case of AIDS, death.

Many STDs are bacterial and can be conquered or controlled with antibiotics. Some cannot always be cured, however. For example, resistant strains of the bacteria that cause gonorrhea have developed, making this disease less easily cured than it was in the past.[25] Other STDs are caused by viruses. Because there is no cure for viral infections, treatment of these diseases is aimed at controlling symptoms and reducing spread to others. With all STDs, the most important step in prevention is to avoid infection. One of the keys to this is knowledge about these diseases coupled with safer sexual practices.

Herpes Genitalis

In recent years genital herpes *(herpes genitalis),* which is caused by the herpes simplex virus (HSV), has become one of the most prevalent STDs in the United States. An estimated 200,000 persons are infected by herpes simplex viruses each year. There are two types of HSV: type 1 and type 2. Formerly, HSV type 1 (HSV-1) was associated with fever blisters and cold sores while HSV type 2 (HSV-2) was blamed for herpes genitalis. Today, however, it is known that genital herpes can be caused by either HSV-1 or HSV-2, although HSV-2 infections are much more likely to recur than are infections caused by HSV-1.[26]

Symptoms of Genital Herpes The symptoms of herpes genitalis include blisterlike sores that appear anywhere on the genitalia about 6 days after sexual contact or other direct physical contact with herpes blisters. These sores rupture spontaneously to form shallow ulcers that may be very painful. The first occurrence of these lesions lasts about 12 days; this is followed by a latency period during which the symptoms disappear. Subsequent, usually milder recurrences last about 4 days. Other symptoms of herpes genitalis include difficult urination, swelling of the legs, watery eyes, fatigue, and a general feeling of illness. The symptoms usually respond well to treatment; the antiviral drug *acyclovir* has been helpful in reducing or suppressing symptoms.[27] Unfortunately, no cure has been found for the herpes simplex virus, which remains in the body indefinitely.

Herpes is a cyclical disease in which the virus retreats periodically to the base of the spine. During these periods the risk of transmitting the disease to a partner is low. Sometimes herpes lies dormant for years. When the symptoms recur, they are often activated by sexual intercourse. Exposure to the sun, lack of sleep, infections, and physical or emotional stress can also bring them on. In some women the symptoms tend to reappear just before the menstrual period. The disease can be spread any time during the recurrence of symptoms. Occasionally the symptoms are too mild to be noticeable, and a sexual partner may be infected without knowing it.

While the physical symptoms of herpes can be painful, many victims find the emotional impact even more distressing. Herpes sufferers often feel isolated, angry, and ashamed. The disease can ruin relationships and make one's social life difficult. In fact, sufferers' feelings of frustration and unhappiness are so characteristic that some psychologists refer to a "herpes syndrome." Since emotional stress can trigger an outbreak, it is important for herpes sufferers to learn how to live with the disease.

Dangers of Herpes Genital herpes can pose a significant problem for pregnant women, whose miscarriage rate is more than three times that of the general population.[28] When miscarriage does not occur, the birth process may expose the infant to the virus, causing death or irreversible brain damage. As a preventive measure, the baby may be delivered by cesarean section; if the child is delivered vaginally, there is about a 50 percent chance that it will contract the disease. Herpes is fatal for more than half of the infants who contract it.[29]

Research has also indicated a strong relationship between HSV-2 and cancer of the cervix and prostate. Women with HSV-2 are more likely to develop cancer of the cervix than are other women.[30] Presumably, the virus penetrates the cervical cells, disrupting their normal metabolism and setting off the typical uncontrolled growth of cancer. As a result, women with genital herpes should have Pap smears annually or more often to check for the early signs of cervical cancer.

Syphilis

Syphilis, which is caused by a spiral bacterium (a spirochete) known as *Treponema pallidum,* is an extremely dangerous STD. Without treatment, the disease remains in the body for years, moving through a number of stages. Fortunately, it can be cured with antibiotics during the first two stages. If left untreated, however, it can have serious consequences. Therefore, it is important for people who even suspect they may have syphilis to seek medical treatment as quickly as possible.

First Stage   In the first stage of syphilis a spirochete enters a person's body through a small break in the skin. Syphilis usually enters through the warm, moist mucous membrane of the genital tract, rectum, or mouth. After 10 to 28 days a dime-sized moist lump appears where the spirochete entered the body. This painless *chancre* is sometimes invisible but always extremely contagious. With or without treatment, the chancre disappears in a few weeks, deceiving many people into thinking they are cured. However, the disease is still very much present.

Second Stage   In the second stage the spirochetes travel through the bloodstream to all parts of the body. During this stage the symptoms appear any time from a few weeks to a year after the disappearance of the chancre. These symptoms may include a skin rash, small flat sores on moist areas of the skin, whitish patches in the mouth and throat, patches of temporary baldness, general discomfort, a low fever, headache, and swollen glands. Syphilis is more contagious during this stage than it is at any other time. The secondary stage lasts 3 to 6 months.

One of the most notorious victims of syphilis was the Chicago gangster Al Capone, who died at the age of 48 after succumbing to the tertiary symptoms during his 9-year jail sentence. (UPI/Bettmann Newsphotos)

Latency Phase   After the second stage of syphilis, all signs and symptoms of the disease disappear and the infected individual appears to be disease-free. The disease has entered the latency phase, but it is not gone: spirochetes are invading various organs, including the heart and brain. This phase sometimes lasts only a few months, but it can last for 20 years or longer. Although there are no symptoms during this phase, a blood test will reveal the presence of the disease.

During the latency phase the individual is usually not infectious, with one important exception: a pregnant woman can pass the infection to her unborn child, causing congenital syphilis. Early in pregnancy the infection may kill the fetus, produce various malformations, or result in an obviously diseased baby. A fetus infected late in pregnancy may seem healthy at birth, only to develop syphilis later. Treatment of an infected pregnant woman within the first 4 months of pregnancy halts the spread of the disease in her unborn child.

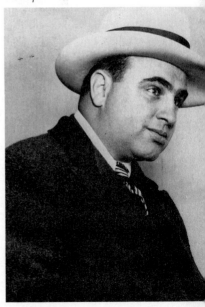

Tertiary Stage   The tertiary stage generally begins 10 to 20 years after the beginning of the latency phase, but it sometimes occurs much earlier. With

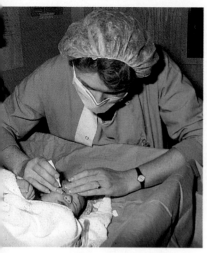

Application of a 1% silver nitrate solution to a newborn's eyes is a simple and effective precaution against gonococcal conjunctivitis, a form of blindness caused by the gonorrhea bacterium. (Susan Leavines/Photo Researchers, Inc.)

tertiary syphilis about one-fourth of all untreated patients become incapacitated.[31] Many develop serious cardiovascular disease. Some die of severe heart damage or rupture of the aorta. Others have slowly progressive brain or spinal cord damage which eventually leads to crippling, blindness, or insanity.

Gonorrhea

More than 850,000 cases of gonorrhea were reported in the United States in 1984, making it the most commonly reported communicable disease in the nation. It is estimated that if unreported cases were included, the number would reach 2 million cases annually.[32]

Gonorrhea is caused by gonococcal bacteria and is transmitted through sexual contact. It usually starts in the lower urinary and genital areas in both men and women. If left untreated, it can spread upward in the genital tract and cause sterility. It can also enter the bloodstream and cause severe arthritis and *endocarditis* (an inflammation of the heart). Thus, gonorrhea can be very serious. Fortunately, it is easily treated with antibiotics such as penicillin if caught early.

Women may not even suspect that they have the disease at first. The early symptoms are frequently not pronounced, and most women never develop early symptoms. A few days after exposure they may notice a mild burning sensation in the genital region and perhaps a vaginal discharge. (Occasionally the individual develops severe pain in just one joint.) Later, after the disease has spread from the vagina up through the uterus and into the Fallopian tubes and ovaries, they may have pain and fever. These symptoms may be severe or may be so mild that they are attributed to stomach upset. Sometimes a woman does not suspect she has gonorrhea until informed of the fact by a sexual partner.

Women who suspect that they have been exposed to gonorrhea or have a vaginal discharge of any sort should see a physician promptly for diagnosis and treatment. If left untreated, the symptoms of gonorrhea may diminish, but the disease will continue unabated. The whole pelvis may eventually become inflamed by **pelvic inflammatory disease (PID),** a painful condition that can damage the reproductive organs and cause infertility. If gonorrhea organisms are present in a woman's birth canal, they may infect her baby's eyes during childbirth. To prevent blindness, most states require that silver nitrate solution be put in every baby's eyes shortly after birth.

The early symptoms of gonorrhea are more evident in men, although some men do not experience these symptoms. About 3 to 8 days after exposure men may notice a sharp, burning pain during urination. At about the same time pus begins oozing from the penis; this causes many men to seek treatment.

If a man does not receive prompt treatment, the infection spreads to his prostate gland and testicles, where it can cause sterility. In time, the infection can cause the urethra to become narrowed, making it difficult to urinate. If the infection is severe, men can suffer arthritis as well as heart damage.

Condyloma

Condyloma acuminata, or genital warts, are caused by the human papillomavirus (HPV). Genital warts account for more than 1 million visits to physicians annually, making condyloma the most commonly diagnosed viral STD in the United States.[33] The symptoms are warty growths around the anus, vulvovaginal area, penis, urethra, or perineum. In women, the warts may develop inside the vagina and on the cervix. These growths can be painful; if they enlarge, they may destroy healthy tissue. In women, genital warts may enlarge and obstruct the birth canal during pregnancy, necessitating a cesarean section. Early treatment of genital warts can prevent their spread. The warts may be removed surgically or with the use of chemical ointments.

pelvic inflammatory disease (PID)—*inflammation of the pelvis; a painful condition that can damage the reproductive organs and cause infertility.*

HPV has also been associated with an increased incidence of cervical cancer. Among the strains of this virus which appear to be most closely connected with cervical cancer, the most virulent does not cause warts but is still easily spread through unprotected sexual contact.

Chlamydia

While condyloma is the most commonly diagnosed STD, chlamydia (caused by the bacterium *Chlamydia trachomatis*) is the most commonly occurring one, striking over 3 million American men, women, and children every year.[34] In men chlamydia causes infections of the urethra, epididymis, and prostate; in women it causes inflammation of the cervix and Fallopian tubes. Most women experience no symptoms from chlamydial infections, but if left untreated, these infections may spread throughout the pelvic area, causing PID, which, as mentioned earlier, may damage the reproductive organs and cause infertility.[35] Untreated chlamydia also causes infections in pregnant women and in infants before and after birth; it is associated with higher rates of infant deaths and with eye, ear, and respiratory infections in newborns.

The symptoms of chlamydia include pain in the lower abdomen, vaginal discharge, and difficulty in urinating. A pelvic examination may show that a woman's cervix is swollen and inflamed and is discharging pus. Pain during this examination suggests inflammation of the Fallopian tubes.[36] Chlamydia is found most often among young, sexually active men and women. The more sexual partners a person has, the greater is the likelihood of contracting the disease.[37] In many cases, sexually active individuals suffer from chlamydia and other STDs simultaneously. For example, many men with urethritis are found to have chlamydia plus another infection at the same time. Up to half of all women with gonorrhea also have a chlamydial infection of the cervix.

Chlamydia in college males (also called nongonococcal urethritis or NGU) is the number one STD reported to university health services.

Because of the damage untreated chlamydia can cause, it is important that people with symptoms of the disease seek diagnosis and treatment promptly. Doctors usually prescribe a 7- to 10-day course of tetracycline or another antibiotic for both the patient and the patient's sexual partners, even those without symptoms. When one sexual partner is not treated—even if nothing seems to be wrong—the infection is likely to be passed back. Fortunately, chlamydia responds well to antibiotic treatment, and people can protect themselves against contracting the disease (as well as other STDs) by using barrier methods of contraception such as condoms and diaphragms with spermicides.

AIDS

Acquired immune deficiency syndrome has increased rapidly throughout the world since it was first diagnosed in 1981. In the United States the Centers for Disease Control estimate that between 246,000 and 298,000 Americans will develop the disease by the end of 1993.[38] In this country about 93 percent of AIDS cases so far have occurred in men, mainly between ages 25 and 44 years. Although these cases have occurred primarily among homosexual men, the number of cases among heterosexuals is now increasing at a rate twice that for homosexual and bisexual men. Moreover, the disease is occurring more frequently among the young, the poor, women, and members of minority groups. In some areas and in some age groups, AIDS is now the leading cause of death for women.[39]

Before any causes are understood or tests devised, diseases may be recognized by sets of symptoms which commonly occur together. These groups of symptoms are called syndromes.

AIDS is a collection of diseases caused by the human immunodeficiency virus (HIV). This virus invades and destroys the T cells (T lymphocytes), resulting in a defective immune system. Instead of recognizing and launching an immune response against foreign substances, the T cells actually begin producing HIV themselves. Without opposition from the T cells, HIV and other viruses multiply rapidly. The longer a person is infected with HIV, the more likely it is that his or her immune system will be impaired.

Initially, the majority of people infected with HIV exhibit no symptoms. Two to 5 weeks after infection, however, many suffer a viral syndrome similar to infectious mononucleosis, with fever, fatigue, or a variety of neurological signs such as meningitis, a red rash on the face or trunk of the body, mild

Congenital AIDS, passed from mother to child, has become one of the fastest-growing types of the disease.

hepatitis, and swollen lymph glands. These symptoms pass, and a latency period of 5 to 10 years may occur. With the passage of time, people infected with HIV normally progress to a number of syndromes that indicate advancing immunodeficiency. These syndromes include generalized chronic swelling of the lymph glands, night sweats, fever, diarrhea, weight loss, fatigue, and rare infections such as oral candidiasis (a fungal infection) and herpes zoster (a viral disease characterized by skin eruptions and pain along the course of sensory nerves).[40]

AIDS is the most severe form of HIV infection. Twenty to 30 percent of HIV-infected persons develop AIDS within 5 years.[41] In the later stages of full-blown AIDS, the severely weakened immune system leaves the infected person vulnerable to a variety of opportunistic diseases, including *Pneumocystis carinii*, an unusual form of pneumonia; tuberculosis; and a rare form of skin cancer known as Kaposi's sarcoma. (Such opportunistic diseases are not normally seen in people whose immune systems are functioning properly.) Among those whose infection progresses to AIDS, 50 percent die within 18 months and 80 percent die within 3 years.[42]

AIDS has been projected to become the second leading cause of death by disease for people under age 65 by 1992.

Modes of Transmission

The human immunodeficiency virus is transmitted through the exchange of body fluids—principally blood and semen—during sexual contact and blood transfusions or by exchanging needles during intravenous (IV) drug use. During sexual contact, permeable membranes in the vagina, cervix, mouth, rectum, and urethra can allow the virus to enter the body. Although HIV once was thought to be transmitted by saliva, urine, feces, and tears as well, the Centers for Disease Control no longer regard these as high-risk fluids unless they are contaminated with infected blood.[43] The virus can also pass from mother to child during the perinatal period, leading to an increasing number of newborns with HIV.[44] HIV is *not* spread through casual contact such as hugging and kissing. In addition, there is no evidence to suggest that the virus is spread by insects or in food or water.[45]

The tragedy of AIDS was personified in the middle 1980s by Ryan White, a hemophiliac who contracted the disease from blood transfusions. Fearing for their children, the parents of some of his schoolmates tried to keep him out of classes even though the HIV virus does not spread by casual contact. (UPI/ Bettmann)

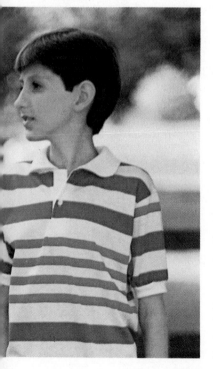

Preventive Measures for AIDS

At the present time prevention is the *only* way to control the spread of AIDS. People can take steps to protect themselves from contracting HIV. The primary step is knowing how HIV is transmitted and what precautions individuals can and should take to avoid infection.

Because one of the primary modes of HIV transmission is sexual activity, knowledge about the safety of sexual behavior and activities is essential. The safest sexual behavior is abstinence, since refraining from sexual activity ensures that a person will not be exposed to HIV sexually. The practice of mutual monogamy also helps control the spread of AIDS; a completely monogamous noninfected couple cannot contract the virus sexually. The fewer the number of individuals a person engages in sexual activity with, the lower is the likelihood of being exposed to an infected person.[46]

No sexual activity involving direct contact with sexual secretions should be considered safe unless the people involved are known to be free of infection. Unfortunately, many people infected with HIV show no signs of the disease but can still transmit the infection to others. As a result, people need to be aware of and use self-protective measures, or safe sex practices.

Such practices include the use of chemical and physical barriers during sexual activity. These barriers include latex condoms used during vaginal intercourse and oral sex performed on a man, latex dental dams or plastic wrap used as a barrier to vaginal secretions during oral sex on a woman, and the use of more than one latex condom or an extra strong condom during anal intercourse (the form of intercourse which carries the highest risk of HIV

Comfort Level

Fear of the Unknown

Regardless of the type of disease a person has, fear of the unknown can have a powerful effect. For example, in a story in *The Healing Heart* the writer describes a golfer who had a heart attack on the golf course. The writer saw the man being attended to by paramedics and noticed his ashen color and trembling body. He also noticed that while everyone was tending to the man's physical needs—giving him oxygen, placing him on a stretcher, and starting an intravenous—no one was attending to his panic.

The writer put his hand on the man's shoulder and said, "You are going to be all right. You are in very good hands, and you will be going to the best hospital in a few minutes." Less than a minute after those few comforting words, the man's cardiogram showed that his heartbeat had slowed. Color returned to his face. He began to look around and take an interest in what was going on.

Fear of the unknown can increase stress and make symptoms worse. It can also cause people to be so afraid that they deny their symptoms and fail to seek medical treatment. Some people would rather ignore symptoms than take the chance of finding out they have a "dreaded" disease.

Fear of the unknown can also affect how people treat those who are ill. Years ago people shunned victims of Hansen's disease (leprosy). Because sufficient scientific knowledge did not exist and because adequate thought was not given to the consequences, those patients were placed in quarantine. This probably furthered the spread of the illness by distancing the sick from centers of medical research.

Fear of the unknown continues to affect how people deal with the victims of certain diseases. The irrational fear that accompanied leprosy is similar to the fear that is associated with AIDS today. Just as many people viewed leprosy victims as "unclean," today's AIDS victims are viewed as having "fallen from grace."

People who understand AIDS know that it is just another disease—no more, no less. When Dr. C. Everett Koop was surgeon general, he spent much of his term disseminating knowledge about AIDS. He knew that many people were worried about getting the AIDS virus, and so he wanted everyone to know how the disease is transmitted. He also encouraged the public to practice responsible behavior based on understanding and on strong personal values in order to stop the spread of the AIDS virus.

Through knowledge and accurate information, fear of the unknown can be overcome. This knowledge cannot be the kind that pushes the public toward hypochondria. Rather, what is needed is the comfort that knowledge brings. For instance, when people have adequate knowledge, they are not afraid to see a doctor if they have pain. They also experience less stress because they are not afraid of every disease.

People need to have confidence in their bodies so that not every pain is considered a harbinger of disaster. They need to understand how to promote good health and a personal lifestyle that reduces negative stress to the fullest possible extent.

Materials drawn from Norman Cousins, *The Healing Heart* (New York: W W Norton, 1983); Douglas Shenson, "When Fear Conquers," *New York Times Magazine* (February 28, 1988): 34–48; C. Everett Koop, "Understanding AIDS: A Message from the Surgeon General" (HHS Publication [CDC] HHS-88-8404, 1988).

infection). In all cases, the use of a lubricant containing the spermicide nonoxynol-9 is recommended to help reduce the risk further.

Besides sexual activity, HIV is transmitted by the sharing of needles used for the IV injection of drugs. Sharing needles when injecting cocaine or other drugs may be responsible for the increase in HIV infection among teenage addicts and their sexual partners. If an individual does inject drugs, needles, syringes, cookers, and other paraphernalia should never be shared. The use of nonintravenous drugs may also increase the risk of infection by making users irresponsible about their sexual behavior.[47]

The use of self-donated blood is referred to as autologous donation. *If it is not used immediately, such blood can be frozen and stored up to 2 years.*

Transfusion of blood and blood products is another known route of transmission of HIV infection. Although blood used for transfusions is routinely tested for HIV, about 1 in every 100,000 pints may be contaminated with the virus.[48] The safest type of transfusion involves the use of self-donated blood, which can eliminate even this risk. With surgery, for example, if the timing and conditions allow it, patients can donate a pint of their own blood every week up to 6 weeks before the operation, ensuring that the blood used is free from infection.[49]

Because HIV infection is transmitted from mother to fetus, all women who may have been exposed to the virus should be tested before becoming pregnant. An HIV-infected woman should be counseled about the risk of transmitting the virus to her fetus if she becomes pregnant.

Current Treatment Options

Treatment of AIDS has involved attempts to treat complications such as infections and tumors, reestablish immune defenses, and control or destroy the virus.[50] Research to date has not been successful in developing a cure.

In 1987 zidovudine (azathioprine [AZT] or Retrovir) was the only anti-HIV drug available commercially for the treatment of AIDS. Since then, eight other drugs have been approved for the treatment of AIDS-related conditions, and as of 1989, 55 companies were testing other medicines and vaccines in human clinical trials (Figure 10.6).[51]

At present, AZT remains the cornerstone of HIV therapy and continues to improve the prognosis of HIV-infected persons. While AZT does not cure

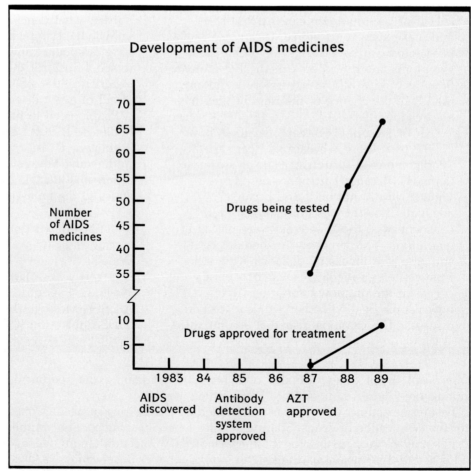

Figure 10.6 Since AIDS was discovered, pharmaceutical researchers have rushed to contain the epidemic and treat its victims. An HIV antibody detection system was developed and approved in less than 2 years. (Medicines are approved only after successful clinical testing.) AZT began clinical testing and was approved for use against the HIV virus in 1987. By 1989 a total of nine medicines had been approved for use against various AIDS-related conditions. The number of medicines being tested rose from 35 to 67.

Sources: John C. Petricciani, "The Pharmaceutical Industry's Perspective on Clinical Trials for AIDS Drugs and Vaccines," *AIDS Patient Care* (October 1989): 2; Gerald J. Mossinghoff, "AIDS Medicines in Development," *AIDS Patient Care* (October 1989): 4.

AIDS, it has been found to prolong survival and reduce mortality in AIDS patients. The earlier the patient starts AZT therapy after the initial diagnosis of the disease, the better are the chances of long-term survival.[52]

In the future, AZT most likely will be used in combination with other drugs. Such combinations could lead to more complete suppression of the virus than can be achieved with any single drug. Since HIV mutates rapidly and may become drug-resistant, the use of combinations of drugs may help reduce the emergence of viral strains that are resistant to any particular drug. Also, since many of the drugs used in treating AIDS have toxic side effects, the use of several drugs will allow less toxic, lower doses of each drug to be used.

Finally, the Centers for Disease Control advise HIV-infected individuals to remain as healthy as possible through proper nutrition, adequate exercise, stress reduction, and avoidance of nonprescribed drugs, alcohol, and tobacco.

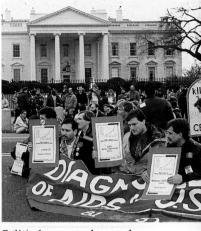

Political pressure by people with AIDS and their friends has had positive results. For example, some promising drugs have been made available on accelerated schedules. (Cynthia Johnson/Gamma-Liaison)

The Politics of AIDS

AIDS is not only a serious health threat but a political issue as well. One of the basic concerns has been the need to balance the rights and needs of AIDS-infected persons with those of the community. The U.S. Supreme Court, for example, has classified AIDS as a handicap protected under federal law in order to protect persons with AIDS from discrimination. The courts continue to debate whether an employer has the right to fire a person with AIDS if other employees are unduly afraid or if the place of employment will suffer as a result of the AIDS-infected person's employment.[53]

Another important politically related issue concerns where the money will come from to treat AIDS victims. Increasingly, AIDS is a disease of the poor and disenfranchised. Even in the best of times the groups now hardest hit by the disease—drug abusers, blacks, and Hispanics—are the most difficult to reach with disease-prevention messages. These groups also have less access to health insurance and medical care. Because of budgetary constraints, government health care programs will not be able to absorb the rising cost of AIDS treatment easily, and help may come too late for many victims. Controversies surrounding such issues are sure to intensify as the number of AIDS cases increase in the years to come.[54]

The Future of AIDS

Despite estimates by the Centers for Disease Control and other groups, no one knows for sure how many people are infected with HIV. What is certain, however, is that without a cure, the HIV epidemic and the AIDS problem will continue to expand, increasing the need for adequate care and treatment of AIDS patients.

Although unprecedented efforts have been made to find drugs that will decrease the transmission of the virus and halt the progression of the disease, the key issue is time: time to evaluate and test new drugs, time to continue research on the disease in hopes of finding a vaccine and/or a cure, and time to teach people how to prevent HIV infection as well as infection from other STDs. With education and time, not only AIDS but other STDs as well may eventually be conquered.

Chapter Summary

- Changing trends in work, diet, and activities may affect people's susceptibility to disease as they become exposed to infection or their bodies become less resistant to disease. Travel to other cultures may also expose people to dis-

eases. Medical progress has resulted in improved identification, prevention, and treatment of disease, but it also may contribute to other medical problems.

- An infection is the invasion of the body by disease-causing organisms and the reaction of the body to their presence. A multiciplicity of factors—agent, host, and environmental factors—are responsible for the onset of disease. Agent factors include the organisms that cause disease. Host factors include attributes of individuals that may affect their susceptibility to disease. Environmental factors are biological, social, and physical factors that may influence the probability of developing an infection.
- An infectious disease normally follows a common pattern marked by five phases: the incubation period, the prodrome period, clinical disease, the decline stage, and convalescence.
- The primary agents of infectious disease include bacteria, viruses, rickettsiae, fungi, and prions. Bacteria are tiny one-celled organisms; some are helpful to the human body, while others are harmful pathogens. Viruses are biochemical microorganisms that reproduce within living cells. Rickettsiae can be either parasitic organisms that coexist peacefully within insects or disease-causing agents transmitted to humans by insect bites. Fungi are many-celled organisms (such as mushrooms) that must obtain food from other organic materials, including humans. Prions are small proteins capable of replicating within the cells of mammals.
- Strep throat, scarlet fever, rheumatic fever, tetanus, cholera, tuberculosis, and gonorrhea and syphilis are bacterial diseases. Mumps, measles, smallpox, AIDS, colds and flu, hepatitis, and mononucleosis are viral diseases. Rocky Mountain spotted fever and typhus are rickettsial diseases. Athlete's foot is a fungal disease. Creutzfeldt-Jakob disease is caused by prions.
- The skin and mucous membranes are the body's first line of defense against infection. Cilia in the respiratory passages also fend off invading microorganisms. If microorganisms get through the body's first-line defenses, the inflammatory response wards off and defeats them. White blood cells rush to infected areas to engulf and consume foreign organisms. Redness, local warmth, swelling, and pain are signs that the body is counterattacking invading organisms.
- In the immune system, B and T lymphocytes play a role in producing antibodies that help eliminate foreign antigens from the body. People may develop natural immunity when the body manufactures antibodies in response to disease, or acquired immunity through the use of vaccines that stimulate immunity before disease can strike.
- Some of the major sexually transmitted diseases include herpes genitalis, syphilis, gonorrhea, condyloma, and chlamydia. The symptoms of these diseases vary, but they all hold potential danger for people suffering from them.
- The symptoms of HIV infection include fever, fatigue, and a variety of neurological signs. The disease may then progress through a number of syndromes including generalized chronic swelling of the lymph glands, night sweats, fever, diarrhea, weight loss, fatigue, and the occurrence of rare infections such as oral candidiasis and herpes zoster. With full-blown AIDS, the patient's immune system is seriously impaired and the patient is susceptible to a variety of opportunistic and life-threatening diseases.
- The human immunodeficiency virus is transmitted through the exchange of body fluids—principally blood and semen—during sexual contact, blood transfusions, and the exchange of needles during intravenous drug use.
- At present AIDS cannot be cured; prevention is the only way to control its spread. Preventive measures include safer sex practices, such as the use of condoms, abstinence, and monogamous relationships with noninfected partners, along with the avoidance of shared intravenous drug paraphernalia. Current treatment options for persons with AIDS include the use of AZT and other experimental drugs, established medical procedures to stem infections and tumors, and the maintenance of a healthy lifestyle.
- Two of the political issues surrounding AIDS are the rights of AIDS-infected persons and the availability of money to treat AIDS victims and conduct research on the disease.

Key Terms

Iatrogenic (page 259)

Nosocomial (page 259)

Agent factor (page 261)

Host factor (page 261)

Environmental factor (page 262)

Incubation period (page 262)

Prodrome period (page 262)

Clinical disease (page 262)

Decline stage (page 262)

Convalescence (page 262)

Carrier (page 262)

Endogenous (page 262)

Exogenous (page 262)

Pathogen (page 262)

Bacterium (bacteria) (page 263)

Virus (page 265)

Interferon (page 265)

Rickettsiae (page 267)

Vector (page 267)

Fungi (page 267)

Prion (page 268)

Inflammation (page 269)

Inflammatory response (page 269)

References

1. Bennett Lorber, "Changing Patterns of Infectious Diseases," *American Journal of Medicine* 84, no. 3 (March 1988): 569–578.

2. Ibid.

3. Ibid.

4. Ibid.

5. Ibid.

6. Ibid.

7. Judith S. Mausner and Shira Kramer, *Epidemiology: An Introductory Text* (Philadelphia: W B Saunders, 1985).

8. Ibid.

9. Ibid.

10. F. D. Daschner, "The Transmission of Infections in Hospitals by Staff Carriers, Methods of Prevention and Control," *Infection Control* 6, no. 3 (1985): 97–99.

11. Peter A. Schlesinger, "Lyme Disease: Prevention and Intervention," *Hospital Medicine* (October 1989): 92–119.

12. Joanne Silberner, "Best Ways to Fight That Cold," *U.S. News and World Report* (January 29, 1990): 54–60.

13. Lawrence K. Altman, "Infections Still a Big Threat," *New York Times* (July 20, 1982): C2.

14. Abram S. Benenson (ed.), *Control of Communicable Diseases in Man,* 13th ed. (Washington, D.C.: American Public Health Association, 1981): 161–169.

15. J. H. Hoofnagle, "Acute Hepatitis," in *Principles and Practice of Infectious Diseases,* 2d ed., G. L. Mandell et al. (eds.) (New York: Wiley, 1985).

16. Gary P. Barnas and Linda J. Hanacik, "Hepatitis B Vaccine: Persistence of Antibody Following Immunization," *Infection Control & Hospital Epidemiology* 9, no. 4 (1988): 147–150.

17. C. C. Boyd and H. Sheldon, *An Introduction to the Study of Disease,* 7th ed. (Philadelphia: Lea & Febiger, 1977): 304.

18. Lawrence K. Altman, "Quandary for Patients: Have Surgery, or Await Test for Hepatitis C?" *New York Times* (February 13, 1990): C3.

19. A. S. Evans et al., "Seroepidemiologic Studies of Infectious Mononucleosis with EB Virus," *New England Journal of Medicine* 297 (1968): 1121.

20. Ibid.

21. Benenson, op. cit.; John M. Last, *Maxcy-Resenau Public Health and Preventive Medicine,* 14th ed. (E. Norwalk, Conn.: Appleton & Lange, 1985): 384–388.

22. Lorber, op. cit.

23. B. H. Park and R. H. Good, *Principles of Modern Immunology: Basic and Clinical* (Philadelphia: Lea & Febiger, 1974).

24. Hatcher et al., *Contraceptive Technology 1988–89,* 14th ed. (New York: Irvington, 1988): 14–45.

25. Ibid.

26. Ibid.

27. Ibid.

28. C. E. Campbell and R. J. Herten, "VD to STD: Redefining Venereal Disease," *American Journal of Nursing* 81, no. 9 (September 1981): 1629–1635.

29. L. B. Meeks and P. Heit, *Human Sexuality: Making Responsible Decisions* (Philadelphia: W B Saunders, 1982).

30. A. J. Nahmias et al., "Epidemiology of Cervical Cancer," in *Viral Infections of Man: Epidemiological Control,* A. S. Evans (ed.) (New York: Plenum, 1975).

31. Boyd and Sheldon, op. cit.

32. Hatcher et al., op. cit.

33. Ibid.

34. Mark Bricklin (ed.), "Making Chlamydia Detection Easier," *Medical Care Yearbook 1990* (Emmaus, Pa.: Rodale Press, 1990).

35. C. I. Fogel and N. F. Woods, *Health Care of Women: A Nursing Perspective* (St. Louis: C V Mosby, 1981).

36. Neville Golden, "Treating the Adolescent with *Chlamydia trachomatis* Infection," *Medical Aspects of Human Sexuality* 19, no. 7 (July 1985): 80.

37. Centers for Disease Control, "*Chlamydia Trachomatis* Infections, "*Morbidity and Mortality Weekly Report* (January 29, 1990): 28.

38. Steven Findlay with Joanne Silberner, "The Worsening Spread of the AIDS Crisis," *U.S. News and World Report* 34, no. 3 (August 23, 1985): 53ff.

39. Lauren Poole, "HIV Infection in Women," in *The AIDS Knowledge Base,* P. T. Cohen et al. (eds.) (Waltham, Mass.: Medical Publishing Group, 1990): 4.2.9, p 1.

40. P. Samuel Pegram, "Human Immunodeficiency Virus Infection," *North Carolina Medical Journal* 50, no. 3 (March 1989): 151–154.

41. Hatcher et al., op. cit., pp. 1–13.

42. Ibid.

43. Joseph E. Smith et al., "Everyday Ethics in AIDS Care," *AIDS Patient Care* (October 1989): 27–31.

44. Samuel Pegram, op. cit.

45. Hatcher et al., op. cit., pp. 1–13.

46. Edward A. Kezer and Steven A. Weinstein, "Risk Reduction Guidelines for Your Patients," *AIDS Patient Care* (October 1989): 23–26.

47. Michael S. Gottlieb and Mark Katz, "A Clinician's Report from the AIDS Conference," *AIDS Patient Care* (October 1989): 9–12.

48. Lawrence K. Altman, "Quandary," op. cit.

49. Ibid.

50. Pegram, op. cit.

51. Gerald J. Mossinghoff, "AIDS Medicines in Development," *AIDS Patient Care* (October 1989): 4–8.

52. Gottlieb and Katz, op. cit.

53. Smith et al., op. cit.

54. Findlay with Silberner, op. cit., p. 28.

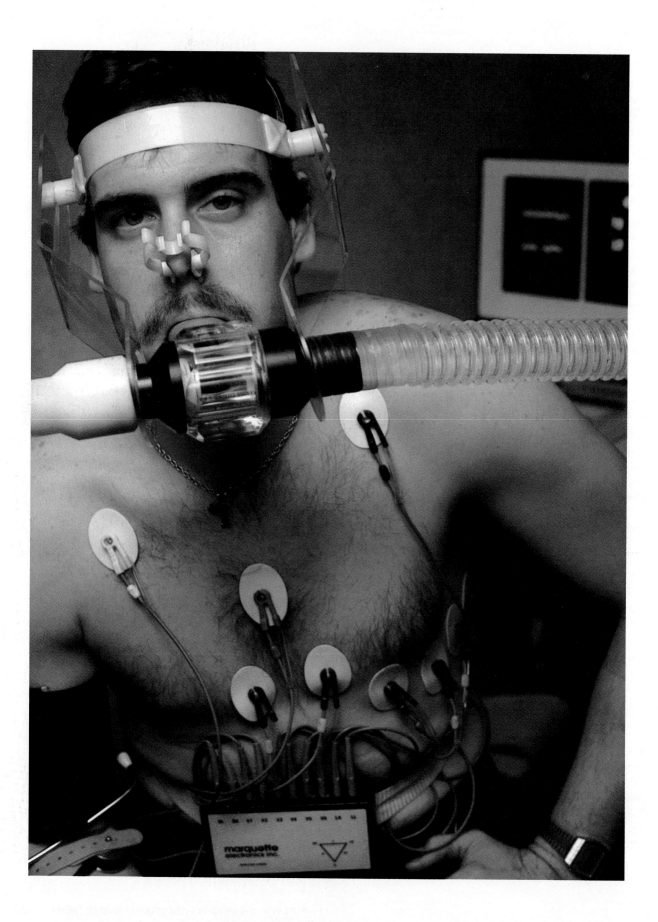

Chapter 11

Cardiovascular Health and Disease

To Guide Your Reading

When you have studied this chapter, you should be able to:

- Identify the components and structures of the heart and circulatory system and explain how they work.

- Define hypertension and atherosclerosis and discuss their cause and treatment.

- Explain how heart attacks and strokes occur and describe several treatments for them.

- Describe cardiovascular diseases other than heart attack and stroke.

- Identify several of the controllable risk factors for contracting a cardiovascular disease and discuss how they can be reduced.

It is one of the ironies of life that people who rarely forget to fasten their seat belts, scrupulously eliminate all known carcinogens from their diet, and install sophisticated burglar alarm systems take few precautions against cardiovascular disease (CVD), a class of highly preventable disorders of the heart and blood vessels that pose a severe threat to health, well-being, and even life.

According to the 1990 edition of *Heart and Stroke Facts,* a booklet published by the American Heart Association, cardiovascular diseases claim more American lives—nearly 1 million people a year—than do all other causes of death combined. A stealthy killer that develops slowly and without noticeable symptoms over a number of years, CVD takes many forms, including high blood pressure, coronary artery disease (disease of the arteries that supply the heart muscle), stroke, abnormal heart rhythms, and rheumatic heart disease. A staggering total of nearly 66 million Americans—more than one in four—have some form of CVD.[1]

Although CVD usually manifests itself during middle age, the seeds of the disorder are sown decades earlier. In one famous study, army pathologists examined the hearts of 300 American soldiers killed in combat in Korea. These young men (their average age was 22) were apparently in good health when they were killed, and none were known to be suffering from CVD. However, in more than 75 percent of these men the coronary atherosclerotic process (a process in which the coronary arteries are narrowed) had already begun.[2] The study showed that CVD can begin "silently" while people are still in their late teens and twenties.

However, people can protect themselves against CVD. Individuals who make an effort to control major risk factors—such as stress, smoking, high blood pressure, lack of exercise, obesity, and a high-fat diet—can reduce their chances of developing CVD. In fact, death rates from heart attack, stroke, and other CVDs are declining. Contributing to this improvement are advances in medical treatment and the fact that many people have adopted healthier lifestyles in recent years.[3]

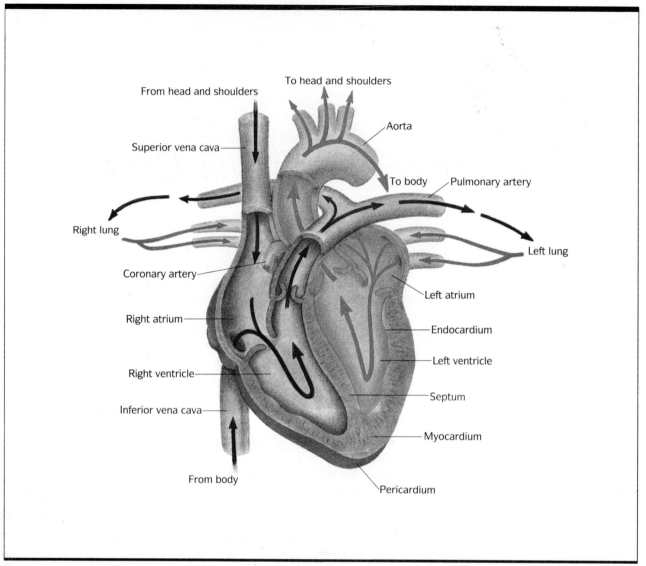

From head and shoulders

To head and shoulders

Superior vena cava

Aorta

To body

Pulmonary artery

Right lung

Left lung

Coronary artery

Left atrium

Right atrium

Endocardium

Left ventricle

Right ventricle

Septum

Inferior vena cava

Myocardium

From body

Pericardium

Figure 11.1 The heart is a four-chambered pump that moves blood first through the lungs and then throughout the body. The right half of the heart pumps deoxygenated blood from the vena cava through the pulmonary arteries to the lungs. Reoxygenated blood returns to the heart through the left atrium. The left half of the heart pumps this blood through the aorta to the body.

The removal of carbon dioxide from the blood is almost as important as oxygen supply. A by-product of metabolism, this gas can cause the blood vessels to constrict if it is not eliminated by the lungs as one breathes out.

Although the situation is improving, people should not relax their guard against CVD, because a sizable percentage of the population is still at risk. As a result, it is important to know what causes CVD and what steps can be taken to help prevent it. First, however, it is necessary to know a few basic facts about the heart and circulatory system.

The Heart and Circulatory System

The major function of the heart is to pump blood into the lungs to pick up oxygen and then to pump that blood throughout the body to supply the tissues with fresh, oxygen-rich blood (Figure 11.1). This pumping process is carried out through a continuous series of contractions and relaxations of the heart. Blood is pushed out with each contraction and pulled in with each relaxation, over and over again.

Unlike organ systems such as the kidneys, which can shut down for a short time without causing permanent harm to the body, the heart must work nonstop. The only time it rests is during the split second between beats. The reason for this is that the cells of the body need a constant supply of oxygen—the fuel that keeps them alive. As oxygen is used up, it must be replenished constantly to prevent *oxygen starvation,* which causes destruction of body tissue, including the brain, the body's master control. Brain death, which results if the brain is deprived of oxygen, causes irreversible loss of consciousness and, sooner or later, death.[4]

A Look at the Heart

The heart is a four-chambered muscular organ the size of an adult's fist that weighs less than 1 pound. It beats about 100,000 times a day, pumping about half a cup of blood with each beat. Its thick muscular wall (the *myocardium*) is surrounded by a tough protective sac (the *pericardium*) and is lined on the inside by a thin membrane (the *endocardium*).

Divided down the center by a solid sheet of muscle (the *septum*), the heart consists of four distinct chambers. The top chambers, one on each side of the septum, are called the *atria* (singular: *atrium*). The lower chambers, which also are located on each side of the septum, are called the *ventricles.* As the heart beats, the left atrium and ventricle work together to form one pump, while the right atrium and ventricle form another.

Deoxygenated blood enters the right atrium through the central veins of the body, known as the *inferior* and *superior venae cavae;* it then passes through the right ventricle and into the *pulmonary artery,* which leads to the lung. In the lung there are millions of tiny air sacs *(alveoli)* at the ends of the branches of the respiratory tract. There the blood is cleaned of waste gas (carbon dioxide) and saturated with a fresh supply of oxygen. Thus revitalized, the blood moves from the lungs back to the heart, passing first into the left atrium, then through the left ventricle, and finally out of the heart through the **aorta,** the main artery of the circulatory system. Branching off from the aorta are the many smaller arteries that carry blood bearing oxygen and other nutrients to all the organs and tissues of the body.[5]

This constant process of oxygenation is made possible by the heart's natural **pacemaker,** an electrical impulse center in the upper wall of the right atrium. This center regulates the heartbeat by stimulating the heart muscles to pump in a coordinated fashion. Valves separating the heart's chambers open and close to regulate the flow of blood through the heart and out into the body. These valves ensure that the blood always passes through the heart in the proper direction. Damage to any of the heart valves can result in backward movement of blood within the heart, causing reduced efficiency and even failure of the whole system.

In a lifetime, a person's heart beats about 2.5 billion times, pumping a total of over 100 million gallons of blood through the body. While the average heart rate at rest of an adult is 70 beats per minute, the heart of a baby beats more rapidly. At birth, a baby's heart rate is about 150 beats a minute, settling down to about 100 beats a minute by the first birthday.

aorta—*the main artery of the circulatory system; carries blood from the heart to the arteries.*

pacemaker—*an electrical impulse center in the upper wall of the right atrium that regulates heartbeat by stimulating the heart muscles to pump in a coordinated fashion.*

The Circulatory System

The circulatory system consists of the heart and blood vessels (Figure 11.2). It takes approximately 10 to 15 seconds for blood to make a complete circuit of this system. Oxygenated blood leaving the heart through the aorta travels through a complex network of **arteries** to the head, the shoulders and arms, the digestive system, the legs, and the heart muscle itself. These arteries divide and subdivide into smaller and smaller branches until they finally become tiny **capillaries.** Capillaries have very thin walls through which nutrients and oxygen can pass directly from the blood into the tissues and waste matter and carbon dioxide can pass from the tissues into the blood. This deoxygenated blood then travels from the capillaries through a network of **veins** leading back to the heart, which then returns the blood to the lungs to receive a fresh supply of oxygen.

In contrast with the capillary walls and the walls of the veins, arterial walls are thick and muscular. When the powerful left ventricle contracts to pump blood throughout the body, the arteries receive more blood than can be moved instantly through the capillaries. Thus, the walls must stretch and

arteries—*blood vessels that carry blood from the heart to the various parts of the body.*

capillaries—*very small blood vessels that serve as a link between the smallest arteries and veins.*

veins—*blood vessels that carry blood from the body back to the heart.*

Figure 11.2 The heart beats about 100,000 times a day, circulating the average person's 9 pints of blood 1,900 times. This stylized picture shows how blood is replenished in the lungs and the digestive organs, and driven to nourish the brain and the rest of the body, all in less than half a minute.

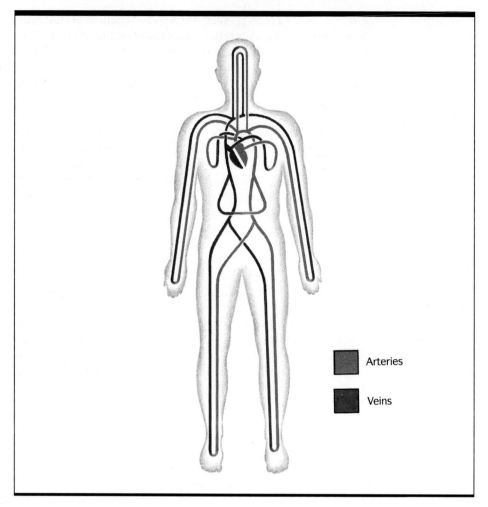

Arteries

Veins

then, using their own muscles, contract to squeeze the extra blood through the system.

Of vital importance among the arteries are the *coronary* arteries, which supply blood to the heart muscle, and the *carotid* and *vertebral* arteries, which bring blood to the brain. Sometimes branches of these arteries become blocked, cutting off the flow of blood from vital tissues. This is when heart attack and stroke, the major CVDs, occur.

The Causes of Cardiovascular Disease

Two important causes of blockage in the circulatory system are hypertension (high blood pressure) and atherosclerosis. In fact, because of the problems they lead to, these two conditions are usually considered dangerous types of CVD themselves.

Blood Pressure and Hypertension

blood pressure—*the force exerted by the blood on the walls of the arteries. It is measured by two separate figures taken when the heart is pumping and when it is at rest.*

Blood pressure is the force exerted by the blood on the walls of the arteries. It varies greatly during each heartbeat: when blood is being pumped out and the arteries are expanding, blood pressure is considerably higher than it is when the heart is refilling for the next beat. For this reason, a person's blood pressure is measured in two figures: the *systolic pressure*, when blood is being forced into the arteries from the heart, and the *diastolic pressure*, when the arteries are waiting for the next beat.

Both of these figures can vary considerably in an individual, depending on activity and emotional state as well as many other factors, for example, infections, the use of nicotine and other drugs, and even the time of day. However, a person who is rested and relaxed yet has a systolic pressure above 140 or a diastolic above 90 is considered to have high blood pressure, or **hypertension.**

Hypertension is thought to be the root cause of many of the problems that plague the heart and blood vessels. The dangers of untreated high blood pressure cannot be overstated. In Framingham, Massachusetts, the adult population was studied for more than 25 years. An analysis of the Framingham data showed that a persistent 5 milligram increase in diastolic blood pressure over the usual measurement for the individual was associated with a 34 percent increase in the risk of stroke and a 21 percent increase in the risk of coronary heart disease.[6]

hypertension—an elevation of blood pressure from the normal range; increases the risk of developing a cardiovascular disease.

Who Gets High Blood Pressure?
Called the silent killer because it rarely produces noticeable symptoms, high blood pressure affects some 60 million American adults—roughly one in four—and accounts for about 30,000 deaths annually.[7] It is rarely found in persons under 20 years of age, but by age 50 approximately one-half of the population has hypertension in some form. Until about age 50 to 55 men are far more likely than women to have high blood pressure. Some women, however, become hypertensive during pregnancy, and women who take oral contraceptives are more likely to develop high blood pressure than are those who do not. Nonwhites are two to five times as likely to be affected as are whites. Also at risk are people who have a family history of high blood pressure, those who are overweight, smokers, and individuals with chronic conditions such as diabetes.[8]

In 90 percent of cases the cause of high blood pressure is not known. In these cases it is called essential hypertension.

How Can You Tell If You Have High Blood Pressure?
Advanced cases of hypertension may be accompanied by headaches (frequently at the back of the head), feelings of tension and irritability, dizziness, and fatigue. Generally, the only way to tell if you have high blood pressure is to have your blood pressure checked regularly. A single elevated reading does not necessarily mean that a person has hypertension. It is normal for blood pressure readings to vary from time to time, decreasing during periods of rest and increasing during periods of anxiety, excitement, anger, strenuous physical activity, and other stressful situations that make the heart pump more vigorously.

If your blood pressure is repeatedly above the normal range for your age, you should see a physician without delay and follow his or her instructions. Blood pressure that is below normal should probably not be of great concern. Low blood pressure is generally a problem only in certain medical emergencies, such as hemorrhage and shock, and among the elderly.

The technique for measuring blood pressure is described in Chapter 19.

People under age 40 rarely have occasion to find out their normal blood pressure, because they rarely have physicals. As a student, however, you may be able to receive a series of tests free at your college health service. This is useful as it establishes your baseline blood pressure. (Tony Freeman/ PhotoEdit)

Treatment of High Blood Pressure
Most cases of hypertension, from the mildest to the most severe, can be treated effectively provided that the disorder is recognized. Treatment is often remarkably easy, is usually inexpensive, and reaps huge dividends: protection against early disability or death from heart attack or stroke. While many medications act as antihypertensives, helping to lower high blood pressure, dietary change and improved exercise habits may control hypertension by themselves.

People can often reduce high blood pressure by decreasing the amount of salt in the diet, losing weight if they are obese, and restricting their intake of alcohol. Before prescribing drugs, doctors often recommend these methods, especially for people who have only mildly elevated blood pressure.[9]

If medications are indicated, there are several types to choose from. One group—the diuretics—rid the body of excess fluids and sodium. Others, known as beta blockers, reduce the heart rate and the heart's output of blood. Another type—the sympathetic nerve inhibitors—can inhibit the ability of

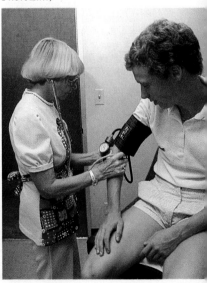

Estimate Your RISKO Score for Heart Disease Risk

Find the column for your sex and age group. Everyone starts with a score of 10 points. Work down the page selecting the letter that fits you for each item, then add or subtract the number of points indicated in your column opposite that letter.

		MEN		WOMEN	
		54 OR YOUNGER	55 OR OLDER	54 OR YOUNGER	55 OR OLDER
STARTING SCORE		10	10	10	10

1. Weight

Locate your weight category in the table on the opposite page. If you are in . . .

		MEN 54 or younger	MEN 55 or older	WOMEN 54 or younger	WOMEN 55 or older
a. _____	weight category A	−2	−2	−2	−2
b. ✓ _____	weight category B	−1	−0	−1	−1
c. _____	weight category C	+1	+1	+1	+1
d. _____	weight category D	+2	+3	+2	+1
	EQUALS	___	___	−1	___

2. Systolic Blood Pressure

Use the "first" or "higher" number from your most recent blood pressure measurement. If you do not know your blood pressure, estimate it by using the letter for your weight category. If your blood pressure is . . .

		MEN 54 or younger	MEN 55 or older	WOMEN 54 or younger	WOMEN 55 or older
a. _____	119 or less	−1	−5	−2	+3
b. _____	between 120 and 139	−0	−2	−1	−0
c. _____	between 140 and 159	+0	+1	+0	+3
d. _____	160 or greater	+1	+4	+1	+6
	EQUALS	___	___	−1	___

3. Blood Cholesterol Level

Use the number from your most recent blood cholesterol test. If you do not know your blood cholesterol, estimate it by using the letter for your weight category. If your blood cholesterol is . . .

		MEN 54 or younger	MEN 55 or older	WOMEN 54 or younger	WOMEN 55 or older
a. _____	199 or less	−2	−1	−1	−3
b. _____	between 200 and 224	−1	−1	−0	−1
c. _____	between 225 and 249	+0	+0	+0	+1
d. _____	250 or higher	+1	+0	+1	+3
	EQUALS	___	___	−0	___

4. Cigarette Smoking

If you . . .

(If you smoke a pipe, but not cigarettes, use the same score adjustment as those cigarette smokers who smoke less than a pack a day.)

		MEN 54 or younger	MEN 55 or older	WOMEN 54 or younger	WOMEN 55 or older
a. _____	do not smoke	−1	−2	−1	−2
b. _____	smoke less than a pack a day	−0	−1	−0	−1
c. _____	smoke a pack a day	+1	+0	+1	+1
d. _____	smoke more than a pack a day	+2	+3	+2	+4
	FINAL SCORE EQUALS	___	___	−1	___

What Your Score Means

0–4 You have one of the lowest risks of heart disease for your age and sex.

5–9 You have a low to moderate risk of heart disease for your age and sex but there is some room for improvement.

10–14 You have a moderate to high risk of heart disease for your age and sex, with considerable room for improvement on some factors.

15–19 You have a high risk of developing heart disease for your age and sex with a great deal of room for improvement on all factors.

20 & over You have a very high risk of developing heart disease for your age and sex and should take immediate action on all risk factors.

Look for your height (without shoes) in the far left column and then read across to find the category into which your weight (in indoor clothing) would fall. Because both blood pressure and blood cholesterol are related to weight, an estimate of these risk factors for each weight category is given in items 2 and 3 opposite.

	MEN Weight Category (Lbs.)					WOMEN Weight Category (Lbs.)			
Your Height	**A**	**B**	**C**	**D**	**Your Height**	**A**	**B**	**C**	**D**
5′1″	up to 123	124–148	149–173	174 +	4′8″	up to 101	102–122	123–143	144 +
5′2″	up to 126	127–152	153–178	179 +	4′9″	up to 103	104–125	126–146	147 +
5′3″	up to 129	130–156	157–182	183 +	4′10″	up to 106	107–128	129–150	151 +
5′4″	up to 132	133–160	161–186	187 +	4′11″	up to 109	110–132	133–154	155 +
5′5″	up to 135	136–163	164–190	191 +	5′0″	up to 112	113–136	137–158	159 +
5′6″	up to 139	140–168	169–196	197 +	5′1″	up to 115	116–139	140–162	163 +
5′7″	up to 144	145–174	175–203	204 +	5′2″	up to 119	120–144	145–168	169 +
5′8″	up to 148	149–179	180–209	210 +	5′3″	up to 122	123–148	149–172	173 +
5′9″	up to 152	153–184	185–214	215 +	5′4″	up to 127	128–154	155–179	180 +
5′10″	up to 157	158–190	191–221	222 +	5′5″	up to 131	132–158	159–185	186 +
5′11″	up to 161	162–194	195–227	228 +	5′6″	up to 135	136–163	164–190	191 +
6′0″	up to 165	166–199	200–232	233 +	5′7″	up to 139	140–168	169–196	197 +
6′1″	up to 170	171–205	206–239	240 +	5′8″	up to 143	144–173	174–202	203 +
6′2″	up to 175	176–211	212–246	247 +	5′9″	up to 147	148–178	179–207	208 +
6′3″	up to 180	181–217	218–253	254 +	5′10″	up to 151	152–182	183–213	214 +
6′4″	up to 185	186–223	224–260	261 +	5′11″	up to 155	156–187	188–218	219 +
6′5″	up to 190	191–229	230–267	268 +	6′0″	up to 159	160–191	192–224	225 +
6′6″	up to 195	196–235	236–274	275 +	6′1″	up to 163	164–196	197–229	230 +

Warning

* If you have diabetes, gout, or a family history of heart disease, your actual risk will be greater than indicated by this appraisal.
* If you do not know your current blood pressure or blood cholesterol level, you should visit your physician or health center to have them measured. Then figure your score again for a more accurate determination of your risk.
* If you are overweight, have high blood pressure or high blood cholesterol, or smoke cigarettes, your long-term risk of heart disease is increased even if your risk in the next several years is low.

How to Reduce Your Risk

* Try to quit smoking permanently. There are many programs available.
* Have your blood pressure checked regularly, preferably every twelve months after age 40. If your blood pressure is high, see your physician. Remember blood pressure medicine is only effective if taken regularly.
* Consider your daily exercise (or lack of it). A half hour of brisk walking, swimming, or other enjoyable activity should not be difficult to fit into your day.
* Give some serious thought to your diet. If you are overweight, or eat a lot of foods high in saturated fat or cholesterol (whole milk, cheese, eggs, butter, fatty foods, fried foods) then changes should be made in your diet. Look for the *American Heart Association Cookbook* at your local bookstore.
* Visit or write your local Heart Association for further information and copies of free pamphlets on many related subjects including:
  • Reducing your risk of heart attack.
  • Controlling high blood pressure.
  • Eating to keep your heart healthy.
  • How to stop smoking.
  • Exercising for good health.

Some Words of Caution

* If you have diabetes, gout, or a family history of heart disease, your real risk of developing heart disease will be greater than indicated by your RISKO score. If your score is high and you have one or more of these additional problems, you should give particular attention to reducing your risk.
* If you are a woman under 45 years or a man under 35 years of age, your RISKO score represents an upper limit on your real risk of developing heart disease. In this case, your real risk is probably lower than indicated by your score.
* Using your weight category to estimate your systolic blood pressure or your blood cholesterol level makes your RISKO score less accurate.
  • Your score will tend to overestimate your risk if your actual values on these two important factors are average for someone of your height and weight.
  • Your score will underestimate your risk if your actual blood pressure or cholesterol level is above average for someone of your height or weight.

*Nitroglycerin, available in tablets, skin patches, and a spray, is also used to relieve the symptom called **angina pectoris**, which is described later in this chapter.*

sympathetic nerves in the brain to narrow blood vessels and cause blood pressure to rise. Still another type—the vasodilators—cause the muscles in arterial walls to relax, allowing the arteries to widen. Nitroglycerin is a vasodilator that is commonly prescribed for recovering heart attack patients.

In most cases, such drugs can help lower blood pressure. It is usually necessary, however, for patients to go through a trial period with a drug to determine its effectiveness for the individual and to monitor any undesirable side effects.

Dangers of High Blood Pressure In a person with hypertension, the muscles of the arterial walls are constricted, causing the blood vessels to become narrower and less flexible. If the condition remains untreated, the heart must pump unnaturally hard to force blood through the network of constricted arteries. In severe cases, the heart may fail from the added strain.

Unrelieved high blood pressure also may cause arteries to become damaged as a result of blood pressing against their walls with added force. Fatty substances and other debris collect on the inner walls of the damaged arteries. This contributes to the other major cause of serious cardiovascular disease: atherosclerosis.

Atherosclerosis

atherosclerosis—narrowing of the arteries caused by fatty deposits on the inner arterial walls.

In **atherosclerosis,** the arteries grow narrower as a result of fatty deposits on the *endothelium*—the inner lining of arterial walls (Figure 11.3). These deposits

*Atherosclerosis is the most important type of **arteriosclerosis,** a more general term used to describe hardening of the arteries— thickening and loss of elasticity in the arterial walls.*

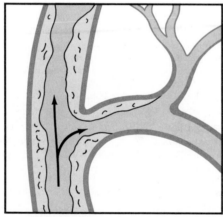

(A) Narrowed artery

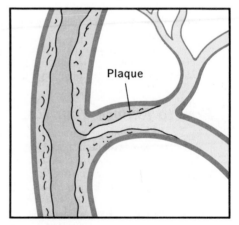

(B) Ischemia

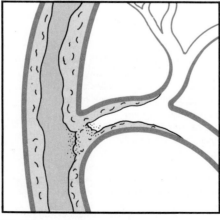

(C) Thrombus

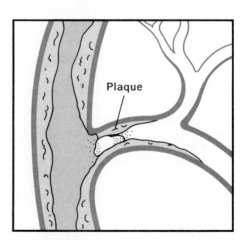

(D) Embolism

Figure 11.3 Atherosclerosis is a disease that develops over many years. (A) The effects of the narrowing arteries can go unnoticed even when the artery is more than half occluded. (B) As atherosclerosis progresses, it can cause ischemia, in which pain is caused by lack of blood flow. (C) If the narrowed artery is damaged, a blood clot (thrombus) may form, causing sudden ischemia or even total blockage. (D) The blood vessel may also be blocked by material carried in the bloodstream (an embolus). Blocked arteries result in the death of cells deprived of their blood supply.

are called **plaque** and are composed of fatty substances, cholesterol, cellular waste products, calcium, and fibrin (a clotting material in the blood).

The Cause of Atherosclerosis   Atherosclerosis is not completely understood, but it is thought to begin as a result of damage to the endothelium. In addition to hypertension, scientists point to other factors that are associated with damage to the arterial walls, including high levels of fat and cholesterol in the blood, and cigarette smoking.[10]

Damage to an arterial wall triggers the body's usual healing mechanism. The blood thickens around the damaged area and forms a **thrombus,** or blood clot. Blood clots are a normal part of the healing process and usually dissolve harmlessly. In patients with atherosclerosis, however, the damaged arterial walls heal only partially. A jagged lesion remains, and as blood flows past the affected area, this rough surface attracts fatty debris and causes a buildup of plaque. In a final effort to heal the wound, the body covers the area with scar tissue, creating a permanent deposit of plaque and a permanently narrowed artery.

The Role of Fats and Cholesterol   A large body of scientific evidence has linked high levels of saturated fats and cholesterol in the blood to the development of atherosclerosis.[11]

The fatty molecules in the blood that increase the tendency toward developing atherosclerosis are called *lipoproteins*. These molecules are produced primarily by the liver and consist of fats (triglycerides and cholesterol) and a blood protein that makes the fats soluble in the watery portion of the blood (Chapter 5). Two types of lipoproteins are of concern here. Low-density lipoproteins (LDLs) carry triglycerides and cholesterol to the capillaries, where they can be used by the body cells. However, LDLs appear to carry an excessive amount of cholesterol. Some of this cholesterol is returned to the liver, but the rest continues circulating in the bloodstream. High levels of LDLs in the bloodstream are associated with the formation of cholesterol deposits on arterial walls, adding to any plaque buildup there. (This is why LDLs are sometimes called "bad" cholesterol.) High-density lipoproteins (HDLs), by contrast, carry excess cholesterol away from the cells and back to the liver, where it is metabolized and excreted. (Hence, HDLs are known as "good" cholesterol.) Actually, it seems to be the balance or *ratio* of lipoproteins in the bloodstream which can be good or bad—relatively low levels of HDL appear to predispose a person to atherosclerosis (Table 11.1).

Because of evidence linking saturated fat and cholesterol with atherosclerosis, federal health officials recommend that all Americans (not just those with high cholesterol levels) reduce the fat content of their diets to lower their risk

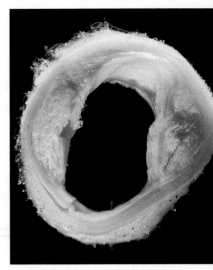

This cross section of a human aorta reveals atherosclerosis, a partial obstruction created by fat deposits; when this occurs in smaller arteries, such as those in the heart and brain, it can lead to thrombosis, or total blockage. Part of the deposit may also break away and be carried by the blood to block a smaller artery, causing an embolism. (Richard Kirby, David Spears, Ltd./Science Photo Library/Photo Researchers, Inc.)

plaque—*fatty deposits made up largely of cholesterol that can build up on the inner walls of blood vessels, narrowing them and eventually closing them completely.*

thrombus—*a blood clot.*

Table 11.1   Cholesterol Ratios and the Average American

Risk Level	Ratio of Total Cholesterol to HDL Cholesterol[a]	
	Men	Women
Average American	5.0	4.4
Average victim of heart disease	5.4–6.1	4.6–6.4
Twice the average risk	9.6	7.1
Triple the average risk	23.4	11.0

[a]*Total cholesterol divided by HDL cholesterol is a good indicator of risk for heart disease. Relatively more HDL reduces this ratio and thus reduces the risk. Note that the average American's cholesterol ratio is too high—close to that of the average heart disease victim. Vegetarians and marathon runners have lower ratios (2.8 and 3.4, respectively).*
Source: National Heart, Lung and Blood Institute, Bethesda, Md.: 1987.

Lipoproteins are substances containing both fat and protein that transport fat molecules through the body. Low-density lipoproteins (LDLs) contain little protein and are the major medium of cholesterol transport. High-density lipoproteins (HDLs) are heavier, and higher concentrations of them in the body seem to provide some protection from heart disease.

of developing CVD.[12] The verdict on fats and cholesterol is not yet final, however, and many fundamental questions remain. Future research will no doubt provide other insights into fats and cholesterol and their role in atherosclerosis and CVD.

Dangers of Atherosclerosis Generally, the heart can continue pumping effectively even through arteries that have been reduced 60 percent in size. The narrowing of an artery in a person with atherosclerosis may first become noticeable when it is severe enough to cause **ischemia**—inadequate blood circulation to the body cells that it supplies. This can take many years to develop because of the extremely slow buildup of plaque.

However, after a certain time ischemia can occur more suddenly: if the blood vessel sustains further damage, a blood clot may develop in addition to the plaque. This type of clot is called a **thrombosis**, and it may block the vessel totally. Blockage can also occur if a blood clot or piece of plaque breaks off from an arterial wall somewhere else and becomes wedged in the narrowed vessel; such as a wedge is called an **embolus** (a Greek word meaning "stopper"), and the condition is known as an **embolism**.

These complications of atherosclerosis can occur anywhere in the body. In a condition called *peripheral vascular disease,* which is most common among the aged, loss of the blood supply to a leg or arm muscle may lead to weakness, pain, or even atrophy (shrinking). However, the most severe results of atherosclerosis occur when the damage is sustained in the blood vessels that supply the heart or the brain.

Major Cardiovascular Diseases

As was mentioned earlier, CVD takes many forms. The most catastrophic of these are heart attack and stroke. Together, these two diseases claim close to 700,000 lives a year, somewhat more than two-thirds of the total number of deaths due to all forms of CVD.[13]

Heart Attack

Essentially, a **heart attack** is a loss of function in the heart. Most commonly, there is a total interruption in the supply of blood to a portion of the heart muscle, and that portion dies from lack of oxygen. This is known technically as a **myocardial infarction.** In 1987 heart attacks claimed the lives of more than 514,000 Americans.[14] Heart attacks result from blood vessel disease in the heart, usually referred to as coronary artery disease or coronary heart disease; this disease often results from atherosclerosis.

Prior to causing a full-fledged heart attack, coronary heart disease may lead to a condition called **myocardial ischemia,** or ischemic heart disease, in which a portion of the heart gets too little blood and oxygen. Ischemic heart disease is often accompanied by a chest pain called **angina pectoris,** which is felt during exertion but goes away if one rests. While angina can be a warning sign that a person is at risk for a heart attack, it does not always lead to a heart attack. Heart muscle can and often does recover from minor ischemic episodes, even those which result in pain. Some people have ischemia without experiencing any pain, although there may be undetected damage to the heart. This so-called *silent ischemia* may lead to a sudden heart attack without any warning.

How a Heart Attack Happens A heart attack occurs when a blockage forms in a branch of one of the coronary arteries, cutting off the blood supply to a portion of the heart. Thus deprived of oxygen and nourishment, the heart

ischemia—*narrowing of the arteries sufficient to cause inadequate blood supply to the body cells they serve.*

thrombosis—*the development of a blood clot within an artery that severely constricts or blocks the flow of blood.*

embolus—*a blood clot that breaks off an arterial wall, flows through the circulatory system, and becomes lodged in a smaller artery, where it blocks the flow of blood.*

embolism—*a sudden blockage of a blood vessel by a blood clot* (embolus).

heart attack—*the death of a portion of the heart muscle from lack of oxygen.*

myocardial infarction—*the death of a section of the heart muscle caused by a reduction in the supply of blood to that area.*

myocardial ischemia—*insufficient blood flow through partially blocked coronary arteries; starves a portion of the heart of oxygen.*

angina pectoris—*tightness, pressure, and intense pain in the chest caused by insufficient blood flow through partially blocked coronary arteries.*

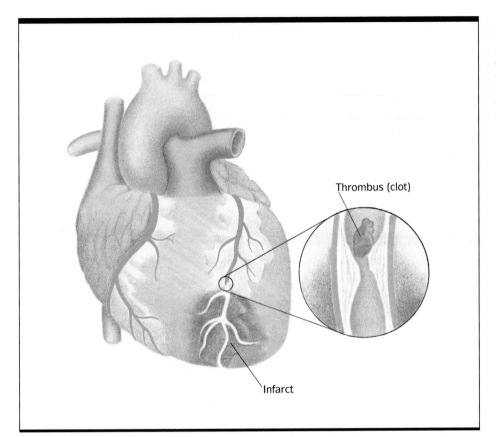

Figure 11.4 Coronary thrombosis. When a clot suddenly forms or migrates to a part of the heart muscle, the central area deprived of blood may die. The dead tissue is called a myocardial infarction or infarct.

Thrombus (clot)

Infarct

muscle that is fed by the affected artery dies. This may occur as a result of a **coronary thrombosis**—a blood clot that forms in a coronary artery (Figure 11.4). It can also occur as a result of a **coronary embolism,** in which a piece of clotted material breaks away from an arterial wall elsewhere in the body and travels with the bloodstream until it lodges in—and blocks—a coronary artery.

Whether the victim of a heart attack lives or dies depends in part on where the arterial blockage occurs. If the flow of blood through one of the main arteries is blocked, large portions of the heart muscle may die, irreparably damaging the heart's pumping mechanism. A total stoppage of the heart—called **cardiac arrest**—may result. When cardiac arrest occurs, immediate action is necessary or the patient will die; the brain can survive without damage for only about 4 minutes after the heart stops circulating blood. If, however, the main coronary arteries are unaffected and only a small arterial branch is blocked, other areas of the heart may be able to compensate for the loss and the attack will not be life-threatening.

What It Feels Like to Have a Heart Attack Occasionally, heart attacks occur quietly and painlessly and are not discovered until months or even years later, during the course of a routine electrocardiogram or perhaps during an autopsy. Such "silent" heart attacks can be just as damaging to the heart muscle as overtly painful ones and are extremely dangerous because the victim rarely seeks medical attention or takes steps to ward off further episodes.

In most heart attacks, however, the victim knows something is wrong, although he or she may initially think the sensations have been caused by indigestion or "heartburn." The typical symptoms of a heart attack may vary from an uncomfortable feeling of pressure, fullness, and squeezing to a crushing pain in the center of the chest lasting 2 minutes or longer. The pain may

coronary thrombosis—*a blood clot in a coronary artery.*

coronary embolism—*blockage of a coronary artery that occurs when a piece of clotted material breaks away from the arterial wall and dams a narrowed coronary artery.*

cardiac arrest—*any stoppage of the heartbeat.*

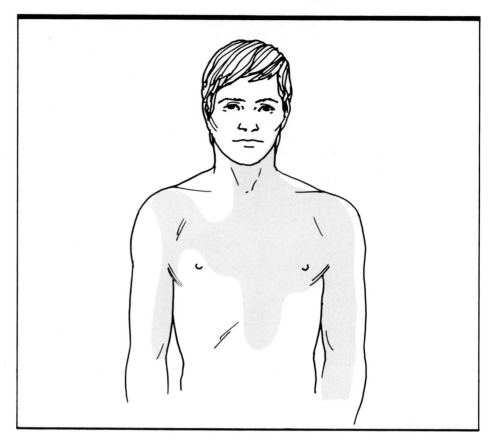

Figure 11.5 The pain of a heart attack and the pain of angina may not be felt as heart pain—it may be felt in the upper arms, shoulders, or neck. It may also radiate from the chest to these areas. Scientists suggest that internal organs such as the heart, which have few pain receptors and very rarely experience pain, may confuse the nervous system: the pain is "felt" as if it were in nearby areas that are served by closely related nerves. Sharp "referral" pains in the areas shaded here should be considered a danger signal, especially if they are spreading and last more than 2 minutes. Do not deny the problem—get help.

then spread to the shoulders, neck, or arms (Figure 11.5). The victim may experience severe pain, dizziness, fainting, sweating, nausea, or shortness of breath. It is not uncommon to experience feelings of terror or a sense of impending doom. While these are some of the common signs of a heart attack, it is important to note than they may not be felt at all and may not be continuously present—they may subside and then return.[15]

About 60 percent of the more than 500,000 deaths from heart attack each year occur within the first hour.

Dealing with a Heart Attack   Heart attack can strike anyone at any time. When it occurs, there is no time for delay. Most victims survive if they recognize what is happening and get help quickly. During a heart attack, the cardiac muscle does not die all at once. Prompt intervention—within 1 to 3 hours—can restore the flow of blood to the heart with a minimum of damage.

It is therefore critical that a person who experiences the warning signs of a heart attack take action promptly. Heart attack victims commonly deny the presence of symptoms and delay getting help. Such delays should be avoided—help should be sought by calling a rescue squad, the police, the fire department, or whatever group handles medical emergencies in the community. People at risk and their families should know who to call and should post emergency telephone numbers in a conspicuous place.

If it is faster to get to a hospital than to call for help, the victim should be taken there immediately. Someone in cardiac arrest from a heart attack (or from drowning, electrocution, or strangulation) can be saved if cardiopulmonary resuscitation (CPR) is performed. When administered properly by a trained individual, CPR can help sustain the victim until medical help arrives. (A local American Heart Association or Red Cross chapter can provide information on CPR training.)

Recovery from a Heart Attack   After a heart attack, the patient must rest for a while to reduce the work load on the heart and allow it to heal. During the healing process, scar tissue forms around the area where the heart muscle

A Second Chance at Life

Heart disease runs in my family. And even though I had high cholesterol, I ate poorly and did not exercise. No one ever saw me without a cigarette. In addition, I had an aggressive personality and a stressful job that I spent too much time at. After 7 years of battling angina and ignoring other warning signs, I suffered a heart attack.

I'll never forget it. I felt as if an elephant were sitting on me. The pain hit me like a thunderbolt—it went down my left arm and into my elbow. It made me sweat. My skin was clammy and gray. If I hadn't made it to the emergency room, I don't know what would have happened. I kept repeating to myself, "Am I going to die?"

Even after I pulled through, the fear of death remained. I was afraid to be alone and kept the lights on all night. Little by little the fear subsided. Time and reality were effective antidotes. I felt as if I had a second chance at life.

One thing having a heart attack made clear to me was that I had to make some changes in the way I was living. First, there was the matter of smoking. Cigarettes were almost part of me. I had smoked since I was 17, and I smoked while I did most things—two to three packs a day for more than 30 years. But as I lay in the hospital emergency room with medical personnel rushing around trying to save my life, I vowed to do everything possible to prevent this from happening again. I knew I had to quit smoking, so I did.

Changing my diet was harder. I used to eat foods that "tasted good" and were "easy." For breakfast I had toast with cream cheese and jelly and coffee with cream and sugar. Lunch consisted of a cheeseburger and French fries. I had pizza for dinner. I never ate vegetables or concerned myself with fiber. After my heart attack I learned to make healthy choices. If the guys at work ordered food from the deli, I would order turkey without mayo and would pass on the coffee. I found out that the pizza I enjoyed could be healthful when made with low fat cheese, and I now eat red meat only once a week. To lose weight and have a substitute for a cigarette, I eat carrot sticks. They're low in sodium and calories and kill hunger.

Walking helped me lose weight. I found that I actually enjoyed exercise. When the weather got too cold, I had to switch to a treadmill. It wasn't as much fun, but at least I was still exercising.

For the first few months I really tried to stay calm in stressful situations. Then, sure enough, I found myself getting angry over little things, just as I had in the past. It's been really hard for me to modify the way I react. After all, I'm still the same person. I've always been that intense. That intensity probably helped me make all the other changes in my life—my smoking, diet, and exercise.

My doctor says that people who have had a heart attack often make these changes in lifestyle. In the beginning they're motivated to stop smoking, eat right, and get exercise. But it's the day-to-day, year-to-year living that's harder. He said that if you want to live badly enough, you simply do what you have to do.

died. This scar tissue cannot contract, but if the scar is small, the heart may continue to function well and the patient may recover. Eighty percent of people who survive heart attacks can return to work and their usual activities within 3 months.[16] In fact, physicians today are advising a shorter period of bed rest than they did in the past. They encourage patients to begin a planned program of exercise under medical supervision as soon as they are well enough.

After a heart attack, emotional recovery is as important as physical recovery. People who suffer the trauma of a heart attack become more aware of their mortality. A vital organ—the heart—has failed. As a result, most victims experience depression and fear. They may have the idea that it will be dangerous to put any strain whatsoever on the heart. Thus, they may be afraid to exercise at all, even to get out of a chair and walk across the room.

Their families are also affected by the experience. Spouses may try to encourage recovering heart patients to avoid exercise, including sexual activity, and thus may reinforce the doubts the victim already has about his or her heart. The patient's fear of a recurrence of heart attack symptoms or even of sudden death may interfere with rehabilitation. Patients who continue to experience fear and depression after several months should probably seek professional counseling.

The first step toward emotional recovery is for heart attack patients to recognize that lifestyle changes can have a positive effect on their cardiovascular health and that they can help themselves return to a normal life. Patients must be reassured that an exercise program will not hurt them. In fact, moderate exercise not only will help improve overall health, it also can aid the process by which the heart develops **collateral circulation**—a system of smaller blood vessels that provide alternative routes for blood when a main artery is blocked.

The affection of a loving relationship also aids a patient's recovery. While couples can expect the emotional ups and downs that often follow a crisis such as a heart attack, their relationship should gradually return to normal. Heart attack patients and their spouses often fear that by increasing heart rate and blood pressure, sexual activity will cause undue strain and lead to further crises. This fear is unfounded. Most people can return to their usual sexual activities after a brief recovery period.[17] As heart attack patients modify some aspects of their lifestyle and ease back into others, their confidence will grow and their lives will return to normal.

Stroke: When CVD Affects the Brain

A **stroke**—also known as a *cerebrovascular accident* or *cerebrovascular occlusion*—is a sudden loss of brain function resulting from interference with the blood supply to part of the brain (Figure 11.6). After heart attacks and cancer, stroke is the leading cause of death in the United States.[18]

The word *stroke* is particularly apt: victims compare the experience to being struck on the head with a blunt instrument. There are three types of stroke: cerebral thrombosis, cerebral embolism, and cerebral hemorrhage. A **cerebral thrombosis** is caused by a blood clot forming in a cerebral blood vessel. A **cerebral embolism** occurs when material from outside clogs a cerebral blood vessel. In a **cerebral hemorrhage,** blood flow to the brain is impaired by the rupture of a cerebral blood vessel. In all three cases, the flow of oxygen to parts of the brain is impaired, resulting in the death of some brain tissue.

Some strokes are so severe that they kill within minutes by destroying the part of the brain that regulates heart and lung functions. Others may be very mild, causing only temporary dizziness or slight weakness or numbness; such strokes are called **transient ischemic attacks (TIAs)** and are often ignored.

However, when a stroke, even a transient one, has occurred, the chances of having a second stroke are increased. This is one reason why it is a good idea to be alert to a possible TIA. The symptoms of a TIA may include brief unexplained numbness, tingling, unusual weakness, or paralysis of any part of the body; difficulty in swallowing, speaking, phrasing sentences, or thinking clearly; and sudden dizziness, fainting, altered vision, or severe headaches. Such an attack may last anywhere from a few minutes to a few hours. A person who has clearly experienced the symptoms of a TIA should seek immediate medical attention.

In a stroke, the nearby brain cells, no longer fed by the blocked or ruptured artery, are deprived of oxygen and begin to die. Depending on what part of

collateral circulation—*a system of smaller blood vessels which develop to provide alternative routes for blood when a main artery is blocked.*

stroke—*also called a cerebrovascular accident or cerebrovascular occlusion; a sudden loss of brain function resulting from interference with the blood supply to a part of the brain.*

cerebral thrombosis—*impaired blood flow to the brain caused by a clot blocking a cerebral blood vessel.*

cerebral embolism—*impaired blood flow to the brain caused by a mass of abnormal material clogging a cerebral blood vessel.*

cerebral hemorrhage—*impaired blood flow to the brain caused by rupture of a cerebral blood vessel.*

transient ischemic attack (TIA)—*a mild stroke that causes only temporary dizziness or slight weakness or numbness; such a stroke is often ignored.*

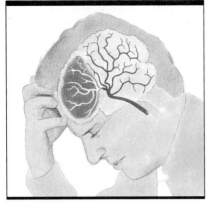 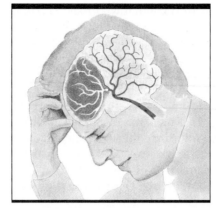 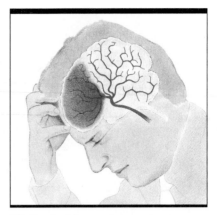

(A) Cerebral thrombosis   (B) Cerebral embolism   (C) Cerebral hemorrhage

Figure 11.6 Strokes usually occur as a result of localized blood loss in the brain. (A) In cerebral thrombosis, a blood clot forms within a cerebral blood vessel or in one of the arteries that supplies the brain. (B) A cerebral embolism occurs when a solid particle from elsewhere lodges in a cerebral artery. (C) Cerebral hemorrhage is a third cause of stroke. In this case, a diseased blood vessel ruptures and floods the brain tissue with blood that does not circulate.

the body or mind was controlled by these cells, the victim may suffer partial paralysis and other crippling afflictions.

Hypertension has been identified as the single most important risk factor for stroke.

Recovery from Stroke The patient's condition soon after a stroke can be very discouraging. The key factor determining the outcome is the part of the brain affected by the stroke. Many stroke victims suffer from loss of memory—especially short-term memory—and many exhibit general confusion. They become tired easily, and their ability to concentrate may be impaired. Sudden and extreme mood fluctuations and inappropriate emotional reactions are fairly common.

Many stroke victims are left with permanent physical impairment, yet in many cases there is hope for at least a partial recovery. Although brain cells do not regenerate (unlike most other body tissues), one area of the brain can learn to take over the functions of another area after brain damage has occurred. With appropriate physical therapy, it is often possible for a stroke victim to relearn basic self-care skills and sometimes other skills as well. Often the degree of recovery is remarkable, as in the case of the actress Patricia Neal, who went on to win an Academy Award; a slight limp was the only evidence of the stroke that almost killed her.

Recovery from a severe stroke is a slow, painstaking process. It requires enormous effort, patience, and strength on the part of the victim and those around him or her. The most dramatic improvements occur in the first weeks and months after the incident. Subsequent progress may be extremely slow. Physical therapists and others who help in the rehabilitation of stroke victims stress the importance of encouraging patients to do as much as possible for themselves, helping them regain confidence in their abilities, and preventing them from becoming too dependent on well-meaning friends and relatives.[19]

Early Diagnosis of Major Cardiovascular Disease

Since CVD sometimes is not accompanied by overt symptoms, it is important for people, especially those over age 40, to get regular checkups and periodic blood and blood pressure tests to detect potential problems. Of course, anyone who experiences severe chest pains or the symptoms of stroke should immediately consult a physician.

Tests for CVD fall into three categories: imaging, measuring electrical activity, and charting blood flow. The tests are painless and can be done on an outpatient basis.[20]

Imaging tests include computerized axial tomographic scanning (CAT scan), magnetic resonance imaging (MRI), and radionuclide angiography (nuclear scan). Each of these tests can be used to create pictures of the heart and brain to identify areas of damage or potential blockage.

Physicians measure electrical activity with electroencephalograms (EEGs)—tests that chart the electrical activity of the brain so as to assess the damage caused by a stroke—and electrocardiograms (ECGs)—tests that chart the electrical activity of the heart to reveal cardiovascular abnormalities. ECGs may be done while the patient is at rest or on a treadmill to explore how the heart functions under stress.

A variety of tests are available to chart blood flow. One of the most common is cardiac catheterization, or *angiography*, a procedure in which x-ray pictures are taken of different areas in the cardiovascular system. A catheter, or small tube, is inserted into an artery in the leg or elsewhere and guided to the area to be studied. A dye is injected through the catheter, and x-ray pictures are then taken to detect the dye. With this process, doctors can get detailed pictures of narrowed arteries and potentially dangerous blood clots. Generally, catheterization is a safe procedure, but there are some risks, including an allergic reaction to the dye, disturbances of heart rhythm, arterial damage, blood clots, and bleeding.[21] Another procedure—the thallium radioactive isotope x-ray—is used today as a safer method.

Treatment of Major Cardiovascular Disease

In many instances lifestyle changes and "healthier living" alone can prevent or reduce the risk of a recurrence of major cardiovascular episodes. Sometimes, however, other steps must be taken to control the conditions that lead to CVD or to treat the victims.

Using Drugs to Control CVD Drugs offer doctors and patients a means of combating many of the conditions that lead to cardiovascular episodes. Several drugs are available for lowering the high cholesterol levels associated with atherosclerosis. Bile acid sequestrants, one commonly used type of medication, act by causing the body to produce extra bile acids for the digestive system. Body cholesterol is used up to produce these bile acids. Another type of medication, lovastatin, an enzyme inhibitor, limits production of an enzyme that controls the synthesis of body cholesterol and thus stimulates the removal of low-density lipoproteins. Another drug, gemfibrizol, has also shown positive results in lowering cholesterol. In a 1987 study, this drug reduced LDL cholesterol and triglycerides and raised HDL levels in the blood. Mortality from heart disease was reduced 26 percent in one group that received the drug, and the total incidence of coronary heart disease was reduced 34 percent among all those participating in the study.[22]

Aspirin, long known as a painkiller and anti-inflammatory agent, has also proved useful in the treatment of CVD. It acts to slow the clotting of blood—a capability that suggests its use as a therapy for the prevention of heart attacks and strokes in which blood clotting is a factor. The results of a study which tested 22,000 male physicians between the ages of 40 and 84 suggested that aspirin may be an appropriate therapy for some people who already have a CVD. In that study, doctors with evidence of CVD who received aspirin had fewer heart attacks than did those in a control group who received a placebo. However, while the study seemed to suggest a reduction in the risk of developing a heart attack, the evidence concerning stroke and total cardiovascular deaths was inconclusive. For this reason, people should not begin a regular therapeutic course of aspirin without consulting a physician.[23]

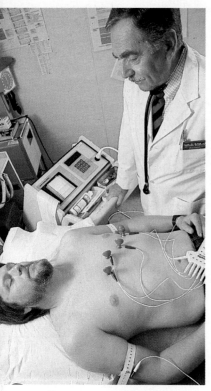

Doctors can gather a large amount of cardiovascular data with an electrocardiogram (ECG). This is done using electrodes to record electrical activity from the heart at several locations in the body. The electroencephalogram (EEG) measures similar impulses from the brain. (Doug Plummer/Photo Researchers, Inc.)

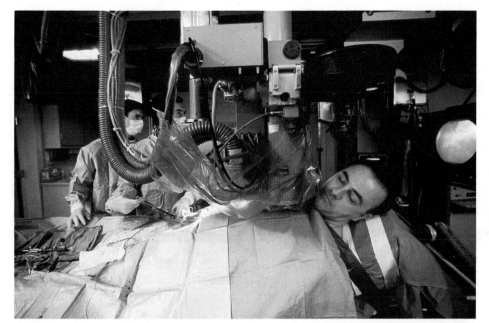

Now a standard procedure for treating constricted arteries, angioplasty is about a 2-hour procedure that is carefully monitored on a fluoroscope, or moving x-ray picture. (Alexander Tsiaras/Science Source/Photo Researchers, Inc.)

Other Types of Treatment Certain other types of treatment are also available for dealing with CVD. Among these are angioplasty, bypass surgery, and the use of transplants and artificial hearts.

Angioplasty is the process of squeezing the plaque within a coronary artery to increase the flow of blood. The procedure is initiated by inserting a catheter into an artery in the leg or arm and guiding it to the site to be treated in the coronary artery. A second catheter with a balloon tip is then inserted inside the first. At the site of blockage, the balloon is inflated, causing the plaque to be flattened against the arterial wall. When the balloon is deflated, the blood can flow more freely through the widened passage created within the artery. In about 25 percent of cases the artery renarrows after the angioplasty has been performed, usually within 6 months. At that point, the doctor will consider whether to repeat the procedure or suggest open-heart surgery.[24]

angioplasty—*the process of increasing the diameter of the opening in a narrowed artery by expanding a balloonlike device.*

If a coronary artery is damaged beyond repair, a doctor may consider **bypass surgery.** A portion of a healthy blood vessel, usually from the patient's leg, is removed and then used to replace (or bypass) the section of the coronary artery that is blocked. One end of the vessel is attached to the artery above the blockage, and the other end is attached below it, restoring blood supply to that area of the heart. Of the approximately 332,000 bypass operations performed in 1987, 74 percent were performed on men.[25]

bypass surgery—*surgery during which a portion of a healthy blood vessel, usually from the patient's leg, is removed and used to replace (bypass) the section of the coronary artery that is blocked.*

When a patient's heart is irreversibly damaged by heart disease and the patient is at risk of dying, sometimes the only feasible treatment is heart, or cardiac, transplantation. Cardiac transplantation is now an accepted procedure for patients who have been adequately screened and for whom it represents the only hope for survival. Over 164,000 heart transplants were performed in 1988.[26]

Other Cardiovascular Diseases

Although the greatest cardiovascular dangers are heart attack and stroke, a number of other cardiovascular conditions threaten the health of thousands of Americans. These include arrhythmias, rheumatic heart disease, congenital heart defects, and congestive heart failure.

Arrhythmias

As was mentioned earlier, the beating of the heart is timed by electrical impulses that originate in the specialized group of cells known as the pacemaker in the right atrium. Sometimes there is an irregularity, or **arrhythmia,** in the rhythm of the heartbeat. In one type of abnormal rhythm known as **ventricular fibrillation,** the ventricles beat irregularly at an extremely fast rate—hundreds of times a minute—and in an uncoordinated manner. When this happens, the heart is incapable of pumping blood; unless the fibrillation can be stopped and normal circulation can be restored, the patient will die.

Arrythmias can develop when the pacemaker develops an abnormal rate or rhythm, the normal pathways of the pacemaker's electrical impulses are interrupted, or another part of the heart takes over for a failed pacemaker. Irregularities in heartbeat can be precursors to heart attacks or may result from heart attacks.

Arrhythmias can usually be treated with drugs, but if the drugs fail, an artificial pacemaker can be implanted in the chest. An artificial pacemaker is a small battery-operated device that produces electrical impulses and transmits them through tiny wires to the heart. These impulses prompt the heart to beat with a more normal rhythm.[27]

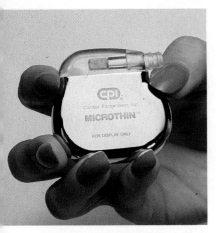

If the heart's natural pacemaker fails, this artificial device can be implanted in the heart muscle to take its place. (SIU School of Medicine/Peter Arnold, Inc.)

arrhythmia—*an irregularity in the rhythm of the heartbeat.*

ventricular fibrillation—*an arrhythmia in which the ventricles beat irregularly at an extremely fast rate.*

rheumatic fever—*an inflammatory disease that affects the connective tissues of the body, especially in the brain, the joints, and the heart.*

Rheumatic Heart Disease

Rheumatic fever is an inflammatory disease that affects the connective tissues of the body, especially those of the brain, the joints, and the heart. When rheumatic fever permanently damages the heart, the damage is called *rheumatic heart disease.*

Rheumatic fever often begins with a streptococcal infection, usually of the throat (strep throat). It usually strikes children between ages 5 and 15, although it occurs in older people as well. While prompt treatment with antibiotics can prevent serious heart complications, approximately one-third of all victims of rheumatic fever are left with heart damage, particularly damage to the valves.[28]

The damage to the heart from the scarring of the heart muscle and valves is the greatest danger with this disease. Depending on the extent of scarring, rheumatic heart disease can interfere with the normal functioning of the heart and make it work much harder than normal. An attack of rheumatic fever does not necessarily leave a person with a damaged heart. The disease tends to recur, however, and with each episode the chance of permanent damage increases.

Congenital Heart Defects

Every year about 25,000 infants—about 1 in every 100—are born with congenital heart defects—inborn defects or abnormalities of the heart.[29] (This sometimes is referred to as congenital heart disease.) Congenital heart defects vary in severity and can affect any part of the circulatory system, including the pumping chambers of the heart, the valves that separate these chambers, and the blood vessels leading from the heart to the lungs and other parts of the body. Most heart defects obstruct the flow of blood in the heart or in the blood vessels near it or cause blood to flow through the heart in an abnormal manner.

For the most part, scientists do not know why congenital heart defects occur. Some think that viral infections such as rubella (German measles) contracted during pregnancy may cause abnormal development of the baby's heart. Other viral diseases may also produce congenital defects. Drinking too much alcohol or taking drugs during pregnancy may lead to a higher number of congenital defects.

Some congenital defects can be corrected surgically after the baby is born; in some cases, more than one surgical procedure is needed. Sometimes medications are used to prevent complications caused by the defect or to relieve symptoms. More recently, physicians have been trying to develop ways to detect and correct some congenital defects before birth, while the baby is still in the womb.

Congestive Heart Failure

Congestive heart failure is a condition sometimes caused by damage to the heart muscle. In a patient with congestive heart failure, the heart cannot keep the blood circulating normally throughout the body. The result is a congestion, or backing up, of blood in the body's tissues. As this fluid collects, it causes **edema,** or swelling, in various parts of the body, especially the legs and ankles. Fluid sometimes collects in the lungs as well, causing shortness of breath.

Almost every known type of CVD can produce congestive heart failure. Sometimes this condition can be aggravated by high blood pressure, which forces the heart to work harder to deliver an adequate supply of blood to the organs and tissues. It can also be caused by heart attack, defective heart valves, and weakening of the entire heart by disease or toxins. Finally, it can be caused by problems elsewhere in the circulatory system, for example, chronic lung disease.

Most cases of congestive heart failure are treatable. The treatment generally combines rest, proper diet, modified daily activities, and the use of certain drugs such as digitalis (to increase the heart's pumping action), diuretics (to help eliminate excess salt and water), and vasodilators (to expand blood vessels and allow blood to flow more easily). With proper medical supervision, people with congestive heart failure can live normal lives.[30]

congestive heart failure—a condition in which the heart cannot pump enough blood, resulting in congestion, or backing up, of blood in the lungs and other body tissues.

edema—swelling caused by fluid collecting in the tissues.

Preventing Cardiovascular Disease

While there are many medical treatments for the different types of cardiovascular disease, the most important approach remains prevention. Many deaths from CVD could be prevented if people had a better understanding of the associated risk factors and took steps to modify their behaviors and lifestyles accordingly.

Of course, some of the risk factors associated with CVD—age, gender, race, and heredity—are beyond the individual's control. For example, the risk of heart attack increases with advancing age; 55 percent of all heart attack victims are age 65 or older, and about 80 percent of fatal heart attacks strike people of that age. Before age 60, heart attack is more common among men than among women, although the difference decreases after menopause. Whites suffer heart attacks with greater frequency than do blacks and Asians. People with blood relatives who have had CVD are at greater risk of developing CVD than are people with no familial history of cardiovascular problems.[31]

While there is nothing a person can do to reduce such risk factors, being aware of them can help an individual compensate for them in terms of lifestyle and medical treatment.

When the left side of the heart fails first, fluid is likely to back up into the lungs, causing breathing problems, especially at night. (SIU School of Medicine/Peter Arnold, Inc.)

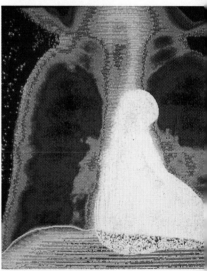

Controllable Risk Factors

Although some risk factors are uncontrollable, many can be controlled. Included among these are tobacco smoking, diet, lack of exercise, weight and obesity, hypertension, stress, and combinations of these and other factors.

A great deal of evidence has been amassed about the behaviors and habits associated with CVD.[32] Based on this evidence, the medical community has

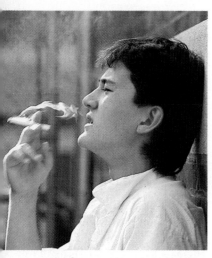

The damage that cigarette smoke can do to the lungs is rivaled by the damage it can do to the heart and the circulatory system. The likelihood of having a fatal heart attack can be lessened considerably by quitting smoking. (Richard Hutchings/InfoEdit)

been able to make certain recommendations about lifestyles and ways of healthier living that can help prevent CVD. Real gains in preventing CVD could be made if people would modify the aspects of behavior and lifestyle that are within their control.

Tobacco Smoking   Tobacco smoking is very hard on the heart and circulatory system. It speeds the heart rate, raises blood pressure, and constricts blood vessels. It raises the fatty acid level in the blood and deprives red blood cells of oxygen.[33] It also contributes to atherosclerosis and therefore increases the risk of developing both stroke and heart disease. As a result, smokers have twice the risk of heart attack that nonsmokers have. In fact, tobacco smoking is the most important factor in sudden fatal heart attacks: smokers face two to four times the risk that nonsmokers face. A smoker who has a heart attack is more likely to die and to die suddenly (within an hour) than is a nonsmoker.[34]

In recent years these effects of tobacco smoking have been shown to be increased by oral contraceptive use. Women who smoke and use the pill have a higher risk of heart attack than do nonsmoking pill users and smoking nonpill users.[35] Smoking is also the greatest risk factor for *peripheral vascular disease*—the narrowing of the blood vessels that nourish the leg and arm muscles. In fact, this condition is confined almost exclusively to smokers.

The preventive value of *not* smoking has been clearly demonstrated. When people stop smoking, their risk of contracting heart disease decreases rapidly regardless of how long or how much they have smoked. Ten years after stopping smoking, a formerly moderate smoker's risk of death from heart disease is almost the same as that of a nonsmoker.[36]

Diet   People have become accustomed to the irony that the foods they like best—chocolate, hot dogs, French fries—are not good for them. Indeed, many specialists regard diet as the single most important factor in atherosclerosis, especially a diet high in fats and cholesterol (as was discussed earlier in this chapter).

As a result, experts recommend limiting the intake of saturated fats in one's diet and increasing the intake of complex carbohydrates. Eating a high-quality diet full of nutritious, natural foods is one of the best ways to reduce the risk of contracting a CVD (Chapter 5).

Lack of Exercise   Although the value of exercise in preventing CVD has not been proved conclusively, recent studies have shown an association between regular moderate exercise and a reduced risk of contracting CVD.[37] People who are physically active seem to be less prone to heart attacks and to tolerate them better than are those who lead sedentary lives.

The *type* of physical activity undertaken is important. Certain forms of aerobic exercise (Chapter 4), such as running, cycling, and swimming, enhance the development of an extensive collateral circulation. Thus, if a coronary artery is blocked, it can be immediately bypassed and circulation can be continued through these collateral arteries. This helps avert death and disability from heart attack.

Exercising regularly is also an excellent way of balancing the HDL/LDL ratio, that is, of raising the level of artery-protecting HDLs and reducing the level of artery-damaging LDLs in the blood. One study demonstrated that people considered to be at high risk for heart disease were able to improve their HDL ratios significantly by running regularly.[38]

If a person is already suffering from atherosclerosis, exercise may provide a warning signal that something is wrong. The reduced blood flow to the heart produced by narrowed coronary arteries may not be noticeable when the heart is beating routinely and is under little stress. However, when extra demands are made on the heart muscle—for example, when a person sprints or shovels snow—blood flow to the heart becomes insufficient and the individual may experience angina, an important indicator of coronary heart disease.

Regular aerobic exercise also tends to lower blood pressure, reduce stress, and help control obesity, all of which are potential risk factors for CVD. Before undertaking strenuous exercise, however, individuals over 35 years old should consult a physician to determine whether there are any cardiovascular irregularities that may suggest avoiding severe physical exertion.

Weight and Obesity   While the evidence linking obesity to coronary heart disease is unclear, excess weight does make the heart work harder. The link between weight and coronary heart disease is also based on the relationship between obesity and high blood pressure, high blood cholesterol levels, and possibly diabetes.[39]

Recent evidence has shown that the location of excess fat on the body can affect the risk of contracting heart disease; studies have suggested that the waist-hip ratio is a possible factor in increased risk. In men, the waist measurement should not exceed the hip measurement. In women, the waist measurement should be no more than 80 percent of the hip measurement. (For instance, a woman with 36-inch hips should ideally have a waist measuring 29 inches or less.) Ratios greater than these may put a person at greater risk for CVD.[40]

Hypertension   As you learned earlier in this chapter, high blood pressure is an underlying condition in many heart attacks and strokes. Unfortunately, although hypertension is one of the most treatable disorders, only a minority of people with high blood pressure bring it under control.[41] Through regular blood pressure checks, the condition can usually be identified and irreparable damage can be avoided. People with high blood pressure can work with their doctors to control the condition through a program of diet, weight reduction, regular exercise, low salt intake, and medication. (See the section on treatment of high blood pressure earlier in this chapter.)

Stress   While there is no proof that stress in itself helps cause CVD, some scientists have noted a relationship between the risk of developing CVD and certain types of stress. For example, it has been suggested that people with Type A personalities, with their competitive, aggressive, impatient, fast-paced, and highly pressured lifestyle, may be more prone to heart attacks, although not all researchers agree with this conclusion. In any case, it is highly unlikely that stress will prove to be as important a direct factor in heart disease as smoking, diet, and hypertension, all of which can, of course, be affected by stress.

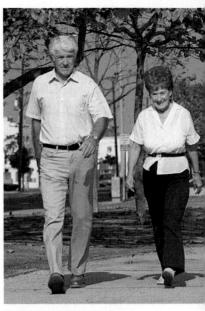

Regular aerobic exercise, walking as well as running, helps maintain the body's stamina and reduces the threat of contracting cardiovascular disease. (David Young-Wolff/ PhotoEdit)

The Danger of Multiple Risks

One of the most troublesome aspects of CVD risk factors is the way they tend to reinforce one another. People often eat or smoke more when they are under stress; overweight people tend to shun exercise. Separately, the risk factors represent a considerable threat; in combination, they are even more deadly. For example, a person with normal blood pressure and blood fat levels who neither smokes nor has diabetes has a 5 percent chance of having a heart attack before age 65. If one of these risk factors is present, the chance doubles to 10 percent; with two risk factors, it becomes 50 percent.[42]

Consider a fairly common combination of risk factors—obesity plus smoking. Obesity puts a strain on the cardiovascular system as a whole; for every pound gained, the body must circulate more blood to provide nourishment. Obese persons thus put much more stress on their hearts than leaner people

Recovering from a Heart Attack

In times not long past, a heart attack survivor often had to choose between living as an invalid and dying an early death. Today, thanks to medical technology and a better understanding of how diet and exercise contribute to coronary health, the outlook for heart attack victims is much brighter.

Some 10 million Americans who have survived heart attacks are living full, active lives today. While heart attack survivors need not restrict their activities completely, they generally need to make major changes in the way they live. Coronary patients face the challenge of learning new, healthier habits without taking the pleasure out of their lives or making themselves miserable. They must face up to the fact that life now requires a new compromise.

Heart attacks illustrate an important fact about comfort level compromises: hard facts should not be ignored. While it may seem more comforting to try to forget one's problems, this cannot lead to true comfort levels in one's lifestyle. Although there are modern medications, pacemakers, and other products of technology to help the heart mend, the most important factor in recovery is patients' willingness to change their lives in ways that strengthen their heart muscles and circulatory systems.

Risk factors that were present before are now more immediate; consequently, they require people to make a new arrangement. Smokers, for example, are at higher risk of suffering heart attacks than other people are. However, those who stop smoking after a heart attack are only half as likely to suffer another attack as are those who continue to smoke. In fact, giving up smoking is the most important step a patient can take toward establishing coronary health. People with high cholesterol levels or high blood pressure are also at high risk for having heart attacks and repeat attacks.

People can control their blood pressure and cholesterol levels with diet, exercise, and medication. Other risk factors that can be controlled include psychological stress, diabetes, obesity, and lack of exercise.

Although it is easy to identify the lifestyle changes that can improve a patient's chances of recovery, it is not easy to make them. For many people, exercising is not enjoyable or a priority. Others feel that smoking cigarettes, eating whatever they want, or succeeding in a stressful job makes life worth living. However, if coronary patients wish to maximize their chances of recovery, such behaviors need to be changed.

One's comfort level is an important element in making such changes. Recovering patients are often advised to alter their lifestyles bit by bit. Coronary patients who are willing to adopt healthier habits should make the changes gradually. Their new behavior is more likely to last if they make only one or two changes at a time. Suppose an overweight smoker with high blood pressure has just suffered a heart attack and knows she should make changes in her lifestyle. She begins by making the following compromises: she will give up smoking cigarettes and adopt a mild exercise program right away. Both changes will help reduce her blood pressure. For the time being she will not worry about losing weight.

While coronary patients need to exercise, they also may need to overcome their fear of exercise and activity after a heart attack. Medical professionals can help by working with them to develop exercise plans that are appropriate for their medical conditions. For instance, the best exercises are generally those that build endurance, such as hiking and ballroom dancing. Exercises that can be dangerous, such as weight lifting, usually involve sustained contraction of muscles.

Recovery from a heart attack requires effort, but many survivors are healthier and happier than they were before their illnesses. New exercise routines may give them more stamina for the activities they enjoy. Diet and exercise may help them feel better about their looks. By learning new ways to handle stress, they may find that they can do their jobs more effectively and get along better with other people. Even though they have put aside some old pleasures, they may have found new activities that they enjoy at least as much. At the very least, by developing new habits, they may live longer.

do. If the obese person also smokes cigarettes, the risk is compounded: smoking lessens the adaptability of the cardiovascular system as a whole. Consequently, a system that is already stressed by obesity is additionally stressed by smoking much more than it would be by nicotine alone. When uncontrollable risk factors such as age and heredity are added to the equation, the chance of an overweight smoker having a heart attack skyrockets.[43]

The Challenge of Changing Behavior

Although there are uncontrollable risk factors for CVD, the fact remains that more than any other major disease, CVD has its roots in lifestyle—the behaviors in which people choose to indulge and which they can choose to limit. The good news is that behaviors *can* be changed.

The bad news is that in the case of many risk factors for heart disease, such change is difficult. Smoking, for example, is a notoriously hard habit to break, and if one succeeds, other problems may become more severe—for example, weight gain.

However, with CVD the stakes are high—it is a matter of life or death. Of course, avoiding heart disease and stroke is not the only reward: quitting smoking provides many other benefits, such as added stamina, a whole new world of smells and tastes, and protection from diseases such as cancer. A healthful diet and exercise can bring similar benefits, together with vibrant confidence born of new physical fitness and a new appearance.

The challenge of behavior change is not a matter of a sudden revolution. Habits are best changed little by little, with a carefully calculated plan. Reconsider the discussion of behavior change in Chapter 1. Then concentrate on the change you think is most necessary for you and perhaps also the change with which you think you will be most comfortable—these are the changes you will find most rewarding.

Above all, do not be discouraged and give up. There is no life without risk, so if you are aware of some of them, no great harm will result. You may even choose to accept a few, believing that the gains of living hard, for example, are worth the possible price. However, if you can lessen some of the other risks and thus lessen the possibility of having a heart attack or stroke, that is certainly worth some aggravation.

The cost of cardiovascular disease in 1990 was estimated at $94.5 billion. This includes the cost of physicians, hospitals, nursing home services, medicines, and loss of productivity as a result of disability.

Chapter Summary

- The heart is a four-chambered muscular organ that pumps blood through the circulatory system, providing the cells of the body with oxygen and other nourishment. Along with the heart, the circulatory system consists of networks of arteries and veins which branch out to carry blood to all parts of the body.

- Hypertension is a condition in which blood pressure is sustained at a highly elevated level. High blood pressure can be reduced by reducing sodium intake, losing weight if one is obese, and restricting the intake of alcohol. It can also be treated with antihypertensive drugs, including diuretics, beta blockers, sympathetic nerve inhibitors, and vasodilators. Because it puts a strain on the blood vessels, chronic high blood pressure may cause arteries to become damaged and can lead to or accelerate atherosclerosis.

- Atherosclerosis is a condition characterized by a narrowing of the blood vessels. It is caused by the accumulation and hardening of fatty deposits on the inner walls of the arteries, possibly as a result of damage to the arterial wall. Evidence suggests that excess fats and cholesterol in the blood contribute to the development of atherosclerosis.

- Heart attacks occur when a blockage forms in one of the coronary arteries, cutting off the supply of blood to a portion of the heart. This blockage may result from a coronary thrombosis or coronary embolism. The symptoms of heart attack include pain in the center of the chest, which then radiates to the shoulders, neck, or arms. The victim also experiences dizziness, fainting, sweating, nausea, or shortness of breath.

- A stroke is a sudden loss of brain function resulting from the blockage of blood to a portion of the brain. Strokes may be caused by a cerebral hemorrhage, cerebral thrombosis, or cerebral embolism, usually as a result of degenerative cardiovascular disease.
- Early diagnosis of cardiovascular disease may be determined by imaging tests (including a CAT scan), tests to measure electrical activity (including EEGs, and ECGs), and tests to chart blood flow (including cardiac catheterization, or angiography).
- Cardiovascular disease can sometimes be controlled with drugs, which can lower cholesterol levels or slow the clotting of blood. CVD can also be treated with angioplasty, bypass surgery, and heart transplants and artificial hearts.
- Other types of cardiovascular disease include arrhythmias, or irregular heartbeats; rheumatic heart disease, caused by rheumatic fever; congenital heart defects, inborn defects or abnormalities of the heart; and congestive heart failure, a backing up of blood in the tissues.
- Controllable risk factors for cardiovascular disease include tobacco smoking, diet, lack of exercise, obesity, hypertension, and stress. These risk factors can be reduced by modifying one's behavior and adopting a healthier lifestyle based on many of the principles discussed in this book.
- The presence of multiple risk factors increases the danger of developing a cardiovascular disease because risk factors tend to reinforce one another in a synergistic manner.

Key Terms

Aorta (page 289)

Pacemaker (page 289)

Arteries (page 289)

Capillaries (page 289)

Veins (page 289)

Blood pressure (page 290)

Hypertension (page 291)

Atherosclerosis (page 294)

Plaque (page 295)

Thrombus (page 295)

Ischemia (page 296)

Thrombosis (page 296)

Embolus (page 296)

Embolism (page 296)

Heart attack (page 296)

Myocardial infarction (page 296)

Myocardial ischemia (page 296)

Angina pectoris (page 296)

Coronary thrombosis (page 297)

Coronary embolism (page 297)

Cardiac arrest (page 297)

Collateral circulation (page 300)

Stroke (page 300)

Cerebral thrombosis (page 300)

Cerebral embolism (page 300)

Cerebral hemorrhage (page 300)

Transient ischemic attack (TIA) (page 300)

Angioplasty (page 303)

Bypass surgery (page 303)

Arrhythmia (page 304)

Ventricular fibrillation (page 304)

Rheumatic fever (page 304)

Congestive heart failure (page 305)

Edema (page 305)

References

1. American Heart Association, *1990 Heart and Stroke Facts* (Dallas: American Heart Association, 1989).

2. W. F. Enos et al., "Coronary Disease among United States Soldiers Killed in Action in Korea," *Journal of the American Medical Association* 152, no. 12 (1953): 1090.

3. American Heart Association, op. cit., p. 1.

4. Ibid.

5. L. M. Elston, *It's Your Body: An Explanatory Text in Basic Regional Anatomy with Functional and Clinical Considerations* (New York: McGraw-Hill, 1975): 485–486; Robert C. Schlandt et al., "Anatomy of the Heart," in *The Heart*, 7th ed., J. Willis Hurst et al. (eds.) (New York: McGraw-Hill, 1989).

6. Norman M. Kaplan, *Clinical Hypertension*, 5th ed. (Baltimore: Williams and Wilkens, 1990): 2.

7. American Heart Association, op. cit., p. 9.

8. Ibid., pp. 11–12; W. Boyd and H. Sheldon, *An Introduction to the Study of Disease*, 7th ed. (Philadelphia: Lea & Febiger, 1977); William C. Roberts, "The Hypertensive Disease," in *Topics in Hypertension*, J. H. Laragh (ed.) (New York: Dun Donelly, 1980).

9. American Heart Association, op. cit., p. 11.

10. Ibid., p. 6.

11. Ibid.

12. Gina Kolata, "Report Urges Low-Fat Diet for Everyone," *New York Times* (February 28, 1990): A-1, A-22.

13. Ibid., pp. 17–21.

14. Ibid., p. 12.

15. Ibid., p. 17.

16. Ibid., p. 15.

17. American Heart Association, *Sex and Heart Disease* (Dallas: American Heart Association, 1983).

18. American Heart Association, *1990 Facts*, p. 2.

19. R. S. Fowler and W. E. Fordyce, *Stroke: Why Do They Behave That Way?* (Dallas: American Heart Association, n.d.); *Self-Care for the Hemiplegic* (Minneapolis: Sister Kenny Institute, 1977).

20. American Heart Association, *1990 Facts*, p. 150.

21. Frederic R. Kahl et al., *A Patient's Guide to Cardiac Catheterization* (Raleigh, N.C.: Bowman Gray School of Medicine, North Carolina Baptist Hospital, 1986).

22. William H. Wiist, "A Cholesterol Primer for Health Educators," *Health Education* (April–May 1989): 24–32.

23. Steering Committee of the Physicians' Health Study Research Group, "Final Report on the Aspirin Component of the Ongoing Physicians' Health Study," *New England Journal of Medicine* 321, no. 3 (July 20, 1989): 129–135; Valentin Fuster et al., "Aspirin in the Prevention of Coronary Disease," *New England Journal of Medicine* 321, no. 3 (July 20, 1989): 183–185.

24. American Heart Association, *1990 Facts,* pp. 14–15.

25. Ibid., p. 4.

26. Ibid., p. 34.

27. Ibid., p. 16.

28. Boyd and Sheldon, op. cit., pp. 228–234.

29. American Heart Association, *1990 Facts,* p. 29.

30. Ibid., pp. 33–34.

31. Ibid., p. 18.

32. S. P. Fortmann et al., "Effect of Long Term Community Health Education on Blood Pressure and Hypertension Control," *American Journal of Epidemiology* 132, no. 4 (1990): 629–646; J. A. Berlin and G. A. Colditz, "A Meta-Analysis of Physical Activity in the Prevention of Coronary Heart Disease," *American Journal of Epidemiology* 132, no. 4 (1990): 612–627.

33. *You and Your Heart* (South Deerfield, Mass.: Channing L. Bete, 1986): 12.

34. American Heart Association, *1990 Facts,* p. 18.

35. L. Rosenberg et al., "Oral Contraceptive Use in Relation to Non-Fatal Myocardial Infarction," *American Journal of Epidemiology* 111, no. 1 (1980): 59; D. E. Krueger et al., "Fatal Myocardial Infarction and the Role of Oral Contraceptives," *American Journal of Epidemiology* 111, no. 6 (1980): 655.

36. American Heart Association, *1990 Facts,* pp. 18–19.

37. R. S. Paffenbarger et al., "A Natural History of Athleticism and Cardiovascular Health," *Journal of the American Medical Association* 252 (1984): 491–495; J. N. Morris et al., "Incidence and Prediction of Ischaemic Heart Disease in London Busmen," *Lancet* ii (1966): 553–559; H. Blackburn, "Physical Activity and Coronary Heart Disease: A Brief Update and Population View," *Journal of Cardiac Rehabilitation* 3 (1983): 101–111, 171–174; K. E. Powell et al., "Physical Activity and the Incidence of Coronary Heart Disease," *Annual Review of Public Health* 8 (1987): 253–287.

38. M. W. Buckalew, "Type A People and the Type B Solution," *Running Times* (March 1985): 9.

39. American Heart Association, *1990 Facts,* p. 20.

40. Ibid.

41. Ibid., p. 3.

42. T. Gordon et al., "High Density Lipoprotein as a Protective Factor against Coronary Heart Disease," *American Journal of Medicine* 62 (1977): 707; U. S. Public Health Service, *Cardiovascular Primer for the Workplace.*

43. W. Windelstein and M. Maimot, "Primary Prevention of Ischemic Heart Disease: Evaluation of Community Intervention," *Annual Review of Public Health* 2 (1981): 253–273.

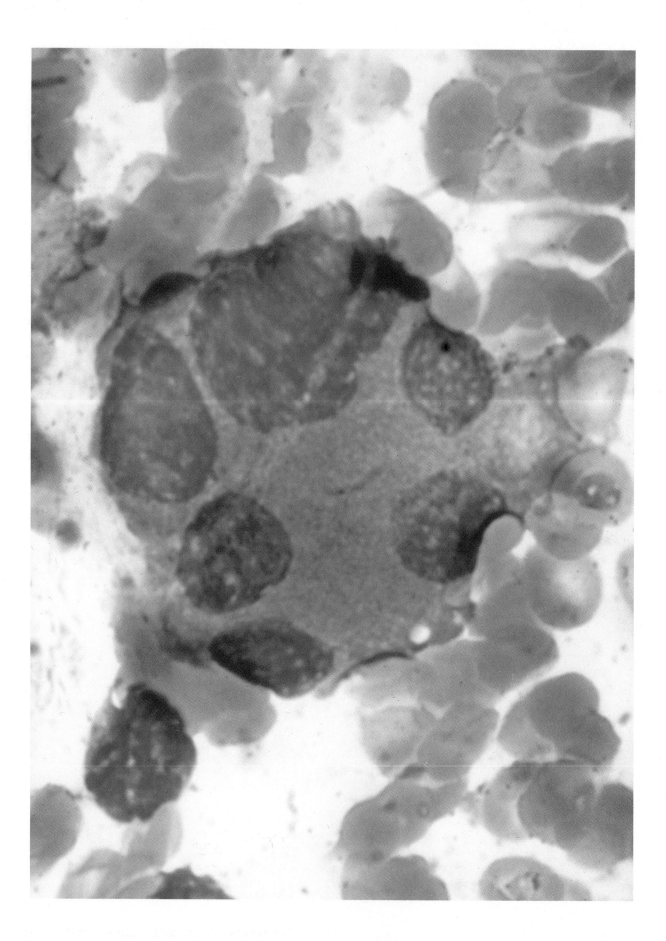

Chapter 12

Cancer: Some Cause for Hope

To Guide Your Reading

When you have studied this chapter, you should be able to:

- Explain what cancer is, describe the process of metastasis, and identify various types of cancer.

- Discuss some of the emotional, psychological, and social effects of cancer.

- Identify and discuss several risk factors associated with cancer.

- Explain the importance of early detection of cancer and describe procedures and recommendations for self-examination and early diagnosis.

- Define the procedure known as staging and explain its importance in determining an appropriate treatment.

- Identify and discuss the primary treatments available for dealing with cancer and the dangerous appeal of quack remedies for the disease.

- Describe some new developments in treatment and diagnosis that offer hope for cancer patients.

- Discuss some of the ways in which people attempt to cope with cancer and explain how cancer patients can be helped to deal with the disease.

Although it once was talked about in hushed, fearful tones, cancer has become a much more openly acknowledged disease. Thanks to medical research, greater public knowledge, more open communication, and greater understanding, people today are better able to cope with this disease and their fear of it. However, while the fear of cancer has abated in recent years, the disease still constitutes a major health problem in the United States. One of every five deaths in this country is caused by cancer. With over 500,000 deaths per year, cancer is second only to heart disease as a cause of death.[1]

The death rate from cancer has increased from less than 6 percent of all deaths in 1900 to about 20 percent today. There are several reasons for this increase. First, today's technology and medical techniques permit earlier, more accurate diagnosis than was possible in the past, when many patients who had other disorders died without knowing that they also had cancer. Second, since the risk of getting cancer increases with age, the increasing life span of Americans has automatically increased the prevalence of the disease. Third, the mortality rate from certain other diseases has decreased, resulting in a larger proportion of total mortality attributable to cancer. Fourth, changing lifestyles have increased people's exposure to certain causative factors, such as tobacco and other cancer-producing agents.

Although the statistics on the incidence of cancer and cancer deaths are troubling, the statistics on the long-term survival of cancer patients offer hope. In the early 1900s few cancer patients survived; today, however, about 405,000 Americans—4 of 10 cancer patients—will be alive 5 years after diagnosis.[2] More and more, cancer is seen less as a death sentence than a challenge along the road to optimal health and well-being (Figure 12.1).

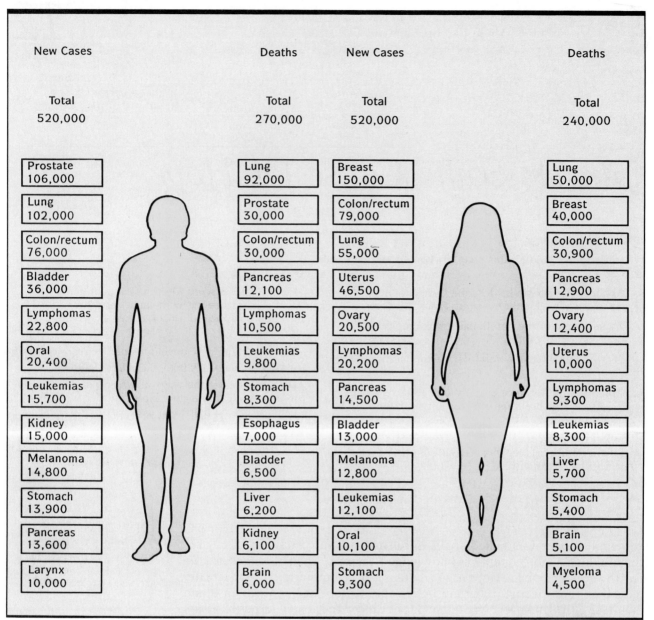

New Cases	Deaths	New Cases	Deaths
Total 520,000	Total 270,000	Total 520,000	Total 240,000
Prostate 106,000	Lung 92,000	Breast 150,000	Lung 50,000
Lung 102,000	Prostate 30,000	Colon/rectum 79,000	Breast 40,000
Colon/rectum 76,000	Colon/rectum 30,000	Lung 55,000	Colon/rectum 30,900
Bladder 36,000	Pancreas 12,100	Uterus 46,500	Pancreas 12,900
Lymphomas 22,800	Lymphomas 10,500	Ovary 20,500	Ovary 12,400
Oral 20,400	Leukemias 9,800	Lymphomas 20,200	Uterus 10,000
Leukemias 15,700	Stomach 8,300	Pancreas 14,500	Lymphomas 9,300
Kidney 15,000	Esophagus 7,000	Bladder 13,000	Leukemias 8,300
Melanoma 14,800	Bladder 6,500	Melanoma 12,800	Liver 5,700
Stomach 13,900	Liver 6,200	Leukemias 12,100	Stomach 5,400
Pancreas 13,600	Kidney 6,100	Oral 10,100	Brain 5,100
Larynx 10,000	Brain 6,000	Stomach 9,300	Myeloma 4,500

Figure 12.1 1990 estimates: new cases of cancer and deaths. This graph gives estimates for each sex of the top 10 types of cancer identified in 1990 and the top 10 types that caused deaths in that year. Note that the lists do not correspond; for example, bladder cancer in men was diagnosed far more often than was stomach cancer but caused fewer deaths.

Source: Adapted from American Cancer Society, *1990 Cancer Facts and Figures,* p. 12.

What Is Cancer?

Cancer is considered a modern disease, although it was not unknown in ancient times. (The condition is named from the Latin word for "crab," presumably because the ancients saw its clawing, crablike growth.) Rather than a single disease, **cancer**—also known as **malignant neoplasm**—is a group of more than 100 diseases characterized by the uncontrolled growth and spread of abnormal cells.

cancer—*a condition of abnormal cell growth; also known as* **malignant neoplasm.**

Cell Division, Growth, and Tumors

Cancer starts when one or a few cells undergo changes that leave them unable to perform their intended functions. These altered, or *mutant,* cells then begin to reproduce very rapidly; if reproduction continues unchecked, the affected organs or body systems will be impaired and the victim will die.

To understand the nature of cancer, it is necessary to know how cancerous tissues are distinguished from other kinds. The term **tissue** refers to a collection of specialized cells that are united to perform a specific function. Muscle tissue is composed of cells that are specialized to fulfill the function of muscles, nerve tissue is made up of cells specialized to fulfill the function of nerves, and so on. The tissues of the body undergo constant change as cells die and new ones replace them.

Most cells in the body are continually reproducing. Normally, an individual cell divides to produce two new cells through an orderly process known as **mitosis.** This process is controlled through a complex mechanism that directs the body to replace worn cells when necessary or to produce additional cells for growth and the repair of damage.

Sometimes the controls that govern cell reproduction break down, and the reproductive process goes out of control. Cells within a tissue that normally cooperate with one another in performing a useful function cease to do so. They begin to multiply independently, often rapidly, sometimes forming an abnormal swelling or mass known as a **tumor** or **neoplasm** (a term that means "new growth"). Such growths have no physiological use.

When this type of uncontrolled growth occurs, it does not necessarily mean that the individual has cancer. The person may have a **benign tumor**—a tumor that grows relatively slowly with a growth pattern that keeps it localized. Benign tumors usually do not recur once they have been removed. The fact that they are called benign, however, does not mean that they do no damage. They can cause pressure and subsequent harm to surrounding structures and can rob normal tissues of their blood supply. A benign tumor can have serious consequences if it occurs in a vital organ such as the brain, but such tumors can be treated successfully with radiation and/or surgery.

tissue—a collection of cells in the body that are specialized to perform certain functions.

mitosis—the orderly division of a cell into two new cells.

tumor—a swelling or mass formed by a group of cells within a tissue that grow to an abnormal size and shape and multiply in an uncontrolled fashion.

neoplasm—a group of cells growing in an uncontrolled fashion to form a tumor.

benign tumor—a tumor that grows relatively slowly and remains localized.

Cancer and Metastatic Growth

Uncontrolled cell growth can also lead to the development of a **malignant tumor,** or cancerous growth (*malignant* means "growing worse"). The cells that form a malignant tumor, or *malignant neoplasm,* are of a special type: they grow in abnormal ways and may invade healthy tissues. Cancerous cells may break away and enter the lymphatic channels and blood vessels. The lymphatic and circulatory systems can then carry the cancerous cells to other parts of the body, where they may settle and form new cancerous tumors.

malignant tumor—a tumor whose cells grow in abnormal ways and may break away and spread to other parts of the body.

The new, or secondary, tumors that form when cancerous cells break away from the original malignant tumor are called **metastases,** and the process by which they spread is called **metastatic growth.** These new growths may develop a considerable distance from the original tumor, and each metastasis may be capable of seeding more new tumors. In this way, cancer can spread widely throughout the body (Figure 12.2).

As cancer cells invade an organ or organ system and begin to spread, they act as disruptive elements in that organ or organ system. As the cancer spreads, the disruption becomes more severe and the functioning of the organ is progressively reduced. For example, if the cancer is in the stomach, digestion will be impeded and the patient will lose weight and progress toward starvation. If the cancer involves the blood or the blood-forming organs (for example, the bone marrow), the patient may become more susceptible to infection, tire easily, or suffer internal hemorrhage (profuse bleeding). If the cancer is in the liver or kidneys, toxins and other harmful substances that normally would be removed circulate through the blood to most body tissues. When such disruptions become severe, death results because the affected organs cannot function properly.

metastases—secondary tumors that form when cancerous cells break away from the original malignant tumor and are transferred to a new location in the body.

metastatic growth—the process by which cancerous cells break away from the original malignant tumor and are transferred to a new location in the body.

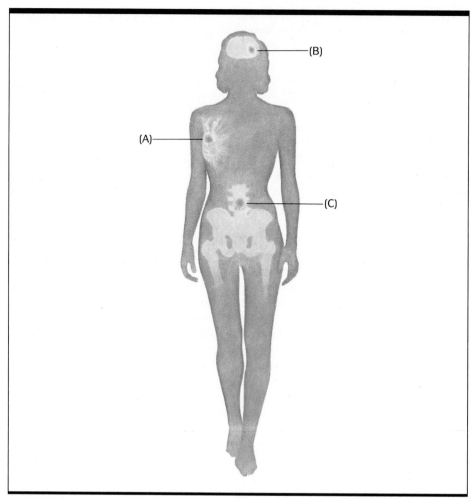

Figure 12.2 Cancer cells can spread throughout the body by traveling through the blood or lymphatic system in a process called metastasis. Here cancer cells from a tumor in the breast (A) have traveled through the lymphatic system and triggered cancerous growths in the brain (B) and spine (C). These new tumors are known as metastases.

carcinomas—*cancers that arise from the epithelium.*

epithelium—*the cells forming the skin, the glands, and the membranes that line the respiratory, urinary, and gastrointestinal tracts.*

sarcomas—*cancers that arise from supporting or connective tissues, such as bone, cartilage, and the membranes covering muscles and fat.*

adenocarcinomas—*cancers arising from glandular epithelial cells, such as the cells lining the milk ducts in the breast.*

lymphomas—*cancers arising from lymphatic cells.*

leukemias—*cancers of blood-forming cells.*

melanomas—*cancers of the pigment-carrying cells of the skin.*

anaplastic—*refers to cancers whose cellular structure is so abnormal that they no longer resemble the cells of the tissue from which they originated.*

Types of Cancer

There are more than 100 different forms of cancer, most of them classified according to the tissues or organs from which they arise. About 30 types of malignant neoplasms are fairly common.[3]

Carcinomas are cancers that arise from **epithelium**—the cells forming the skin, the glands, and the membranes that line the respiratory, urinary, and gastrointestinal tracts. Carcinomas tend to spread to other parts of the body through the lymphatic system. **Sarcomas** are cancers that arise from supporting or connective tissues, such as bone, cartilage, and the membranes that cover muscles and fat. Sarcomas tend to spread to other parts of the body through the bloodstream. The terms *carcinoma* and *sarcoma* are often modified to indicate more specifically the type or location of the disease. In cancer of the breast, for example, cancers derived from the cells that line the milk ducts are called **adenocarcinomas,** meaning that they are composed of glandular (*adeno-*) epithelial cells.

Other major forms of cancer include **lymphomas,** cancers of lymphatic cells; **leukemias,** cancers of blood-forming cells; and **melanomas,** cancers of the pigment-carrying cells of the skin. There are also cancers whose cellular structure is so abnormal that they no longer resemble the cells of the tissues in which they originated; such cancers are termed **anaplastic.**

Psychological and Social Aspects of Cancer

Cancer profoundly affects not only a person's body but also his or her psychological state and relationships with other people. Besides the physical changes that occur with cancer, the disease brings patients face to face with their own mortality. The way in which they and the people around them deal with the disease can mean the difference between confronting it with courage and hope and accepting it with depression, isolation, and despair.

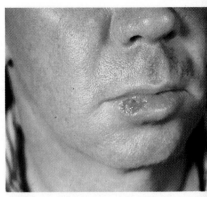

Most often caused by overexposure to the sun, skin cancer can take the form of unsightly sores like this one; these sores should be removed promptly to prevent further damage to the skin. (AFIP/ Science Source/Photo Researchers, Inc.)

The Psychic Pain of Cancer Since cancer is not a single disease but a collection of illnesses that differ in terms of onset, prognosis, treatability, and other features, it is difficult to generalize about the kind of emotional turmoil and psychic pain each cancer patient feels.[4] However, most people would agree that a diagnosis of cancer is a powerful stressor.

Almost all cancer patients are initially concerned about dying as a result of the disease. While this concern is understandable, for some people it is unrealistic thanks to new methods of treating cancer and prolonging life or perhaps even curing the disease. A realistic appraisal of the disease and its prognosis can often alleviate some of the fear.

Most cancer patients are also concerned about the treatment of the disease. Many fear the effects of chemotherapy, radiation therapy, and surgery and the possibility of being bedridden and unable to carry on normal activities. Medical personnel and people who have undergone treatment can be supportive and can reassure patients that although some unpleasant side effects may result from certain treatments, many of these effects can be alleviated.

Such concerns can cause a great deal of emotional stress. Cancer patients must come to terms with a disabling illness that may result in the loss of a body part or death. Their usual methods of coping with the world and striving for fulfillment no longer work, and their emotional needs and defenses are knocked off balance. Anxious about whether they can continue meeting the ordinary demands of life, they often lose self-esteem, becoming more vulnerable to their own feelings and fears and to the feelings and actions of others around them. Psychological problems may be particularly severe if the disease seems likely to interrupt valued life activities and disturb the patient's body image. Such expectations may be psychologically painful, and the patient may feel under attack on all fronts.[5]

Feelings of Depression, Anxiety, and Anger When they are confronted with cancer, many patients have to deal with depression, anxiety, or anger. Those accustomed to leading very active lives may feel depressed, especially on days when they do not feel well. Some develop excessive anxieties about their bodies, feeling that they have become very fragile and unreliable. Others believe that they have somehow brought the disease on themselves, and this makes them feel guilt-ridden and angry. Such feelings can be very harmful to a cancer patient's emotional health.[6]

Disruptions in Personal and Social Life Being ill with cancer can sometimes disrupt a patient's personal and social life and lead to feelings of loneliness. Treatments are often time-consuming and exhausting, leaving little energy for interactions with family members and friends or for various activities. In addition, friends and some family members may avoid interactions with a cancer patient because they do not know what to say or do. For their part, patients often do not want to burden people with their concerns and feelings and thus limit their communication with others. Moreover, friends and family members, in an effort to maintain a positive attitude around the patient, often fail to share their true emotions. Faulty communication can lead to feelings of isolation and exclusion that can hamper a person's ability to cope with the disease. By contrast, simple, direct, and supportive communication frequently provides much of what a patient genuinely hopes for and needs.[7]

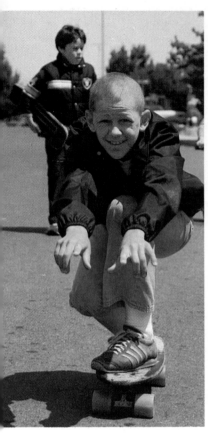

The more a person with cancer can join in normal social activities, the less likely it is that emotional stress will create additional problems related to the disease. (Tom Tracy/ MediChrome)

About 90 percent of the 600,000 cases of skin cancer diagnosed in 1990 could have been prevented through protection from the sun.

Cancer can also alter family dynamics as a result of changing roles. For example, the burden of certain responsibilities may shift to a healthy spouse or to children, who may resent the added responsibilities. This shift of responsibilities can cause feelings of guilt on the part of the patient, leading to a reluctance to ask for help and contributing to feelings of isolation and stress.

Work-related problems can also disrupt the lives of cancer patients. Attitudes such as the idea that cancer is contagious or that cancer patients are unproductive, although false, can lead to a person's dismissal or demotion or to a reduction of work-related benefits. Some cancer patients also face problems maintaining adequate health insurance, especially if they are not covered by group policies.[8]

Fortunately, many of the psychological stresses associated with cancer are not inevitable. Accurate knowledge about cancer coupled with open communication, patience, and understanding on the part of the patient and others can help reduce the stress and anxiety associated with the disease; this sometimes contributes to a patient's recovery.

Understanding Risk Factors for Cancer

Over the years health professionals and researchers have identified a number of risk factors implicated in the development of cancer. Some of these factors are hereditary and some are environmental, but several—for example, use of tobacco and alcohol and an inadequate diet—are directly related to individual lifestyles and behaviors. This means that, for many people, behavior changes may actually reduce the risk of developing cancer by eliminating many of the factors associated with the disease. Experts estimate that 75 percent of all cancer deaths in this nation could be avoided by eliminating or minimizing risk factors that can be controlled.[9]

Hereditary and Genetic Risk Factors

As with any disease, the chances of developing cancer depend in part on the individual's genetic constitution. Many skin cancers, for example, are triggered by exposure to the ultraviolet rays of the sun. However, genetic "host" factors also appear to be involved—persons with fair complexions are more likely to develop skin cancer than are persons with heavy pigmentation.[10]

In a slowly developing disease such as cancer, it is often difficult to pinpoint genetic factors. For example, there is a high rate of stomach cancer among the Japanese. Does this mean that as an ethnic group the Japanese are at high risk, or could there be a typical element in the Japanese diet which adds to the likelihood of developing this type of cancer? Such questions can be answered only by means of carefully designed studies which investigate the histories of particular families and groups of individuals.

A few rare types of cancer, such as cancer of the retina, have been identified as definitely being hereditary. With other types of cancer, however, there is evidence that families tend to inherit an increased risk of contracting a particular form of the disease. It is this predisposition to certain cancers, rather than a direct genetic link to a particular form of the disease, that is the most common type of hereditary risk factor. For example, women with several close female family members who have had breast cancer are at higher risk of developing the disease. A family history of cancer of the colon or rectum is thought to be associated with a greater risk for developing these forms of the disease. There also seems to be a hereditary association in regard to prostate cancer, although it is unclear whether this disease is due primarily to genetic or environmental factors.[11]

Knowing one's family medical history is thus important when one is taking preventive measures against cancer. When a woman knows that there is a

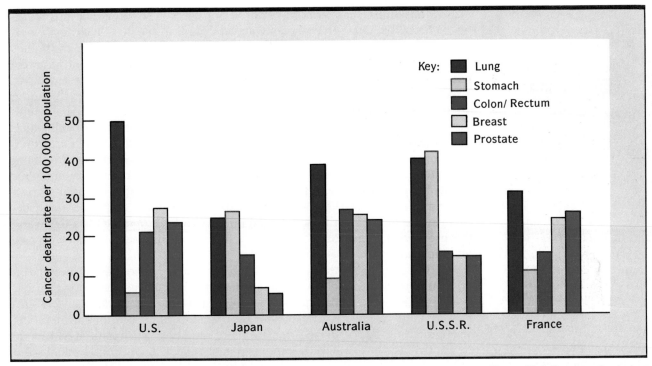

Source: American Cancer Society, *1990 Cancer Facts and Figures*, p. 30.

Figure 12.3 Cancer rates in different nations can tell investigators many things. Note the similarities between the United States, Australia, and France on the one hand and Japan and the Soviet Union on the other. However, this pattern does not appear in the lung cancer figures, suggesting that a different environmental factor may be operating.

history of breast cancer in her family, for example, she can take special precautions: monthly breast self-examinations, annual physicals, and regular mammograms after age 39 can help ensure early detection of breast cancer or its precursers and can reduce the mortality rate by as much as 35 percent.[12]

Environmental Risk Factors

Although experts disagree about certain points, research strongly suggests a connection between environmental factors—such as chemicals and pollutants—and cancer (Figure 12.3). Animal studies have suggested that many chemicals have carcinogenic properties: animals given high doses of these chemicals tend to develop cancer. It is not clear, however, how closely these carcinogenic chemicals are connected with cancer in humans, because the conditions under which humans are exposed to them vary so widely. Among the chemicals suspected of being contributors to human cancer are nitrites (used in curing ham, bacon, frankfurters, salami, and other processed meats), saccharin, hair dyes, and certain pesticides.

The evidence is sometimes confusing, however: cancer of the stomach, which might be thought to be closely related to chemical additives or preservatives in food, has actually been *decreasing* in the United States over the past 25 years. Furthermore, countries such as Poland and Czechoslovakia, which do not use American methods of food production or preservation, have overall cancer rates similar to or higher than those of the United States. Thus, connections between cancer and food additives and preservatives remain doubtful.[13]

What about the connection between cancer and environmental pollutants and chemicals in the workplace? It has been well established that lung cancer rates are higher in urban areas, even after smoking has been taken into account.[14] The role of water contaminants has also been debated extensively. However, studies aimed at resolving this issue have generally been inconclusive. Such is not the case, however, with hazardous chemicals found in the workplace.

A **mammogram** *is an x-ray examination of the breast using a low level of radiation. It can reveal cancers too small to be felt by even an experienced physician, well before signs and symptoms appear.*

Cigarette smoke is the number one air contaminant associated with an increased risk of developing cancer.

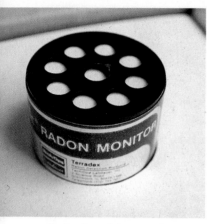

A simple and inexpensive radon test kit can lessen a naturally occurring risk of cancer that has only recently been identified. (Todd Jacobs/Custom Medical Stock Photo, Inc.)

The sun's ultraviolet rays are strongest between the hours of 10 A.M. and 3 P.M. People should take extra care with exposure during these hours. Protective clothing and sunscreen are advisable for all prolonged exposures to the sun.

Evidence linking cancer to high-dose, long-term exposure to various workplace chemicals has been more conclusive. Chemicals such as asbestos (found in insulating and fireproofing), vinyl chloride (found in plastics), chromates (found in paint), benzene (found in rubber), and benzidine (found in dyes) have been shown to increase the risk of developing certain forms of cancer. Asbestos has been linked to *mesothelioma*, a rare cancer that attacks the lining of the chest or abdominal cavity; vinyl chloride has been associated with cancers of the liver, lungs, and brain; benzene has been associated with leukemia (a blood cancer); and benzidine has been linked to bladder cancer.[15]

Unfortunately, it is not always easy to avoid chemicals in the environment and the workplace. People who are exposed to potentially carcinogenic agents have little choice but to change jobs or move. Perhaps a more appropriate alternative would be to reduce exposure as much as possible and become aware of, and perhaps involved in, efforts to change the laws regarding the use and disposal of hazardous chemicals and the reduction of air and water pollutants.

Another environmental risk associated with cancer—one that is more natural in origin—is ultraviolet radiation from sunlight. As was mentioned earlier, excessive exposure to the sun's ultraviolet rays can lead to skin cancer; sunbathing is therefore a risky behavior that most experts recommend reducing or eliminating. Exposure to other forms of radiation, such as x-rays, can increase the risk of developing other types of cancer, including leukemia and cancers of the thyroid gland, skin, and bone. This does not mean that x-rays should never be used diagnostically, but they should be used with discretion, and exposure should be kept to a minimum.

Another environmental cancer risk is associated with radon, a naturally occurring radioactive gas found in many homes throughout the nation; radon has been linked to lung cancer. Therefore, if people have their homes tested and discover high levels of radon, they should take steps to see that those levels are reduced.[16]

Lifestyle and Behavioral Risk Factors

A high proportion of cancer in the United States is associated with people's personal habits and lifestyles. Smoking tobacco, drinking alcohol, and dietary factors are of major importance, and other factors are also related to lifestyle.

carcinogenic—cancer-producing.

Smoking and Drinking Each year in the United States, many people die needlessly as a result of cigarette smoking. In 1990, an estimated 142,000 Americans died from lung cancer. The incidence of this particular form of the disease has been rising among both men and women. Among women, it has now surpassed breast cancer as the number one cancer killer.[17]

How is smoking related to lung cancer? Both the tar and the smoke from tobacco contain specific **carcinogenic,** or cancer-producing, chemicals. Evidence indicates that inhaling these chemicals over a period of time triggers the cancerous potential in susceptible lung tissue cells. When tobacco smoke is inhaled, it paralyzes the bronchial cilia, interfering with their natural cleansing mechanism. Carcinogenic agents can thus enter the lungs and linger there, irritating the lungs and causing damage that can eventually trigger cancerous growth.

Lung cancer is not the only type of cancer associated with tobacco. Cigarette, cigar, and pipe smoking and the use of smokeless tobacco are also risk factors in oral cancer, which can affect any part of the oral cavity, from the lips to the tongue to the mouth, throat, and jaws. Smoking is also one of the greatest risk factors in bladder and pancreatic cancers, with smokers having twice the risk of nonsmokers.[18] In the case of the bladder, the body apparently attempts to excrete tobacco carcinogens through the urinary tract, irritating the bladder in the process.

Chronic excessive consumption of alcohol also seems to be associated with a higher risk of developing certain cancers. For example, oral cancer and cancers of the larynx, throat, esophagus, and liver occur more frequently among heavy drinkers of alcohol, especially when accompanied by cigarette smoking or the use of smokeless tobacco.[19]

Avoiding tobacco and alcohol can reduce the risk of getting cancer, but quitting is often a problem. Tobacco contains nicotine, an addictive drug, and people can become physically and psychologically dependent on alcohol as well (Chapters 14 and 15).

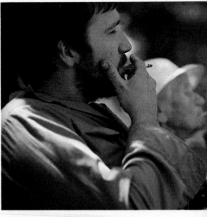

Many people still choose to smoke even though the link between smoking and cancer has been publicized extensively. (Jan Halaska/Photo Researchers, Inc.)

Dietary Factors It has been suggested that diet accounts for approximately 35 percent of avoidable cancer deaths.[20] Evidence seems to link certain dietary factors with specific types of cancer. For example, individuals who are 40 percent or more overweight seem to have an increased risk of developing colon, breast, prostate, gallbladder, ovarian, and uterine cancers.[21] Some studies have linked breast, prostate, and colon cancers to a high dietary intake of fat, while others have found that foods high in fiber seem to have a protective effect against colon cancer.[22]

Extensive research is under way to evaluate and clarify the role diet and nutrition play in the development of cancer, but no direct cause-and-effect relationship has been proved. Nevertheless, most experts recommend that all Americans reduce fat intake, increase fiber consumption, increase their intake of fruits and vegetables rich in vitamins A and C, and increase their consumption of cruciferous vegetables such as broccoli and cauliflower. Such recommendations coincide with the principles of good nutrition that were discussed in Chapter 5.

Other Lifestyle Risk Factors While smoking, drinking, and diet may be the most pervasive risk factors, other behaviors and lifestyle occurrences have been associated with cancer as well. A study by the American Cancer Society has suggested a correlation between exercise and cancer. The study, although far from conclusive, found that the degree of exercise a person engages in is negatively correlated with cancer death rates. In other words, the more exercise a person gets, the lower is the incidence of death from cancer.[23]

Cancer of the cervix has been associated with factors such as sexual intercourse at an early age and sex with multiple partners. Women who have been infected with the herpes simplex 2 virus or human papillomavirus are also at increased risk for developing cervical cancer. This does not mean that a woman with these viral infections will develop cancer of the cervix. It does mean, however, that the risk is higher, and women with these viruses would be wise to have more frequent medical examinations.[24]

The use of certain drugs may also increase a person's risk of getting cancer. Estrogen, birth control pills, and some drugs used in conjunction with organ transplants have come under scientific scrutiny as being potentially carcinogenic. Estrogen, which sometimes is used in high doses to control menopausal symptoms, is associated with an increased risk of developing uterine cancer; short-term, low-dosage use does not appear to present as great a risk.[25]

Researchers are unsure about the relationship between oral contraceptives and cancer of the cervix and have found no clear-cut evidence of an increased or decreased risk of breast cancer among women who use oral contraceptives. Research among women using the pill is ongoing. To date, cancer of the endometrium (the lining of the uterus) is the only form of the disease that has been linked to oral contraceptive use, and this may be limited to only one type—perhaps even a single brand—of oral contraceptive, Oracon.

In 1971 a very small but still unusual series of cases of a rare form of vaginal cancer were reported among women age 14 to 22 whose mothers had taken the drug DES (diethylstilbestrol) to prevent miscarriage. Recent research has shown that DES is associated with many kinds of cancer. Women who were exposed to DES before birth are now entering the age range when cancers of the cervix and breast begin to appear, and it will be a number of years before they reach the usual age for cancers of the endometrium and ovary. Men whose mothers took DES also may be at risk. It is estimated that between 4 million and 6 million Americans, including mothers, daughters, and sons, were exposed to DES.

Certain drugs used during organ transplants to suppress the immune response and thus lessen the chances of the body's rejecting a new organ have been implicated as increasing the risk of developing cancer. The results of one study of over 16,000 kidney transplant patients showed that one type of lymphatic cancer developed at 35 times the normal rate.[26] Presumably, this increased risk is due to suppression of the immune system rather than to any carcinogenic properties of the drugs.

Early Detection of Cancer

Early detection of cancer can save a person's life. The American Cancer Society continually emphasizes this message in the hope that people will take appropriate precautionary steps to reduce the risks of contracting the disease. The more people take action to ensure early detection, the greater the chances of finding cancer early enough to treat it effectively and facilitate a complete recovery.

The Importance of Early Detection

The American Cancer Society estimates that 42,500 of the cancer deaths that occurred in 1989 could have been prevented through early detection and treatment.

Case histories of cancer survivors indicate that early detection often saves lives. The more time that elapses between the beginning of the disease and its detection and treatment, the greater the chances of the cancer spreading locally or metastasizing to other sites, where it can damage or destroy vital organs.

Early detection is helping to make breast cancer survivable. Mammogram X-rays clearly show when a breast is normal (left); performed regularly, they will locate a tumor well before it reaches the size of that shown at right. (Breast Screening Unit, Kings College Hospital, London/Science Photo Library)

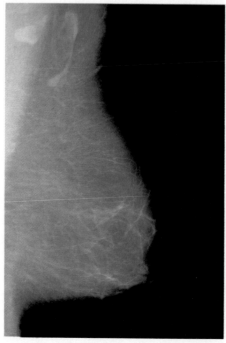
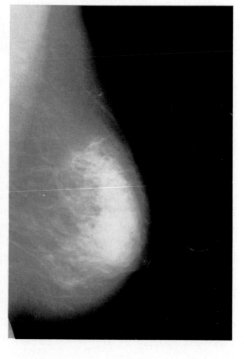

A look at the statistics provides proof that time is of the utmost importance. For example, when the disease is detected early and treated promptly, over 75 percent of people with cancer of the colon and rectum can be cured.[27] When breast cancer is caught in the earliest stage—that is, when there is just a small localized tumor—the survival rate approaches 100 percent. However, as the size of the tumor increases and the cancer spreads, survival rates drop dramatically to about 60 percent.[28] A woman's options for treatment of breast cancer also depend on how far the disease has progressed. With surgical treatment, for example, it may mean the difference between a *lumpectomy*—removal of just the tumor and the surrounding tissue—and a *mastectomy*—removal of the entire breast.[29]

Further evidence of the value of early detection can be seen by looking at the cure rates for cancers which are more easily detectable versus the rates for those which are not. Skin cancers are easily visible to the trained eye; as a result, they frequently receive early attention and are readily accessible for treatment. Except for *melanoma*, a form of skin cancer particularly resistant to treatment, the cure rate for other skin cancers is 95 percent.[30] Lung cancer, by contrast, is difficult to detect early; it often does not produce obvious symptoms until it has gotten out of control. As a result, only 13 percent of lung cancer patients (considering all stages of the disease) live 5 or more years after diagnosis. The survival rate is 36 percent for cases detected while the cancer is in a localized stage, but only 21 percent of lung cancers are discovered that early.[31]

Self-Examination and Seeking Further Advice

Paramount in the early detection of cancer is a thorough familiarity with the warning signs of the disease (Figure 12.4). Some of these signs can be detected by means of a simple, painless self-examination; others are often found during routine medical checkups. While the presence of these symptoms does not necessarily indicate that a person has cancer, they should not be ignored.

The most curable cancers are those which are detected early, and most tumors are first discovered by the patients themselves. For that reason, women are advised to examine their breasts for lumps every month from

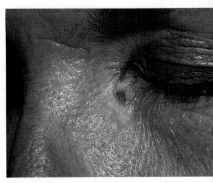

Like many curable cancers, this basal cell carcinoma can be identified because of its distinctive appearance. (J. F. Wilson/Photo Researchers, Inc.)

The American Cancer Society outlines the ABCD warning signals for melanoma:

- *A—asymmetry: one-half of the growth does not match the other half.*
- *B—border irregularity: ragged-type edges.*
- *C—color: pigmentation is not uniform.*
- *D—diameter: greater than 6 millimeters.*

Source: American Cancer Society, 1990 Cancer Facts and Figures, p. 18.

CANCER'S SEVEN WARNING SIGNALS

1. Change in bowel or bladder habits

2. A sore that does not heal

3. Unusual bleeding or discharge

4. Thickening or lump in breast or elsewhere

5. Indigestion or difficulty swallowing

6. Obvious change in wart or mole

7. Nagging cough or hoarseness

Figure 12.4 Cancer's seven warning signals. If you have any of these signals, do not panic: they may occur for many other reasons. However, be sure to see your doctor, especially if the symptom lasts longer than 2 weeks.

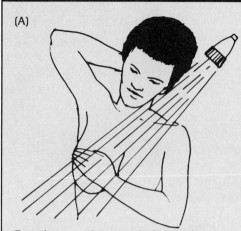

(A)

Examine your breasts during bath or shower; hands glide easier over wet skin. Fingers flat, move gently over every part of each breast. Use right hand to examine left breast, left hand for right breast. Check for any lump, hard knot, or thickening.

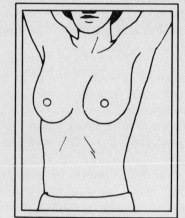

(B)

Stand before a mirror and inspect your breasts, first with arms at your sides, then with arms raised high overhead. Look for any changes in the shape of each breast, swelling, dimpling of the skin, or changes in the nipple. Then rest your palms on your hips and press down firmly to flex your chest muscles. Left and right breasts will not exactly match; few women's breasts do.

(C)

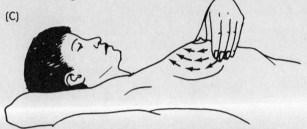

Lie down on a bed and put a pillow or folded towel under your right shoulder. Place your right hand behind your head; this distributes breast tissue more evenly on the chest. With left hand, fingers flat, press gently in small circular motions around an imaginary clock face. Begin at outermost top of your right breast for 12 o'clock, then move to 1 o'clock, and so on around the circle back to 12. A ridge of firm tissue in the lower curve of each breast is normal. Then move in an inch toward the nipple and keep circling to examine every part of your breast, including the nipple. This requires at least three more circles. Repeat this procedure on your left breast with a pillow under your left shoulder and your left hand behind your head.

(D)

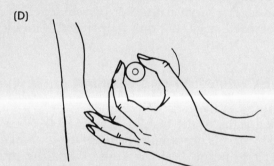

Finally, squeeze the nipple of each breast gently between thumb and index finger. Any discharge, clear or bloody, should be reported to a doctor immediately.

Figure 12.5 How to examine your breasts. Breast cancers were diagnosed in 150,000 women in 1990. Many were first discovered through monthly self-examinations for unusual lumps and other changes. Even though the large majority of these changes are due to other causes, it is vital to see a doctor as soon as possible. The best time to perform the examination is about a week after menstruation, when the breast is unlikely to be swollen or tender.

The best time for a woman to give herself a breast self-examination is just after her menstrual period.

Testicular cancer is the most common cancer in the United States among men age 15 to 34.

puberty through old age to detect breast cancer (Figure 12.5). In addition to breast self-examination, regular pelvic examinations and Pap smears (microscopic examination of cells scraped from the cervix and uterus) are also recommended for detecting cervical and uterine cancers. Men are urged to spend 3 minutes once a month on a testicular self-examination; testicular lumps or abnormalities warrant prompt medical attention (Figure 12.6).

Recommended for both men and women are monthly self-exams of the skin to detect growths, unusual discolorations, sores or lumps, and changes in the appearance of warts or moles—signs that skin cancer may be developing. Malignant melanomas, for example, often start as small molelike growths that increase in size, change color, become ulcerated, and bleed easily from a slight injury. A skin self-examination should include a survey of all the surfaces of the skin, using a mirror for hard-to-see areas.

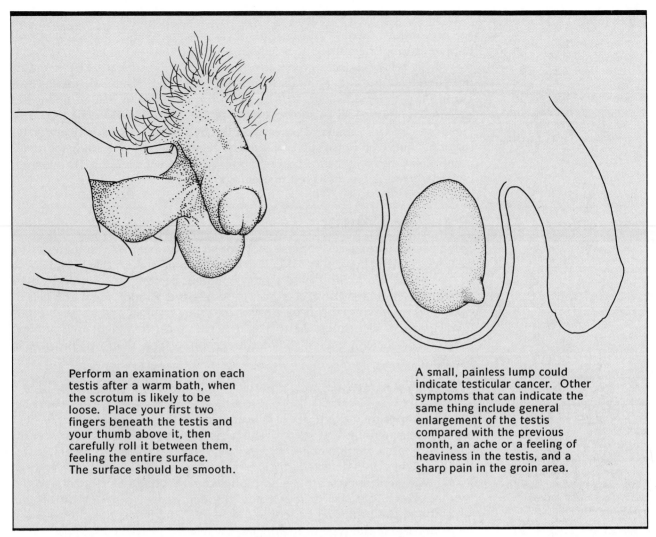

Perform an examination on each testis after a warm bath, when the scrotum is likely to be loose. Place your first two fingers beneath the testis and your thumb above it, then carefully roll it between them, feeling the entire surface. The surface should be smooth.

A small, painless lump could indicate testicular cancer. Other symptoms that can indicate the same thing include general enlargement of the testis compared with the previous month, an ache or a feeling of heaviness in the testis, and a sharp pain in the groin area.

Figure 12.6 How to examine your testes. Men are encouraged to do monthly self-examinations for cancer of the testes. Although this is a much less common cancer than female breast cancer, it can still cause fatalities: if it metastasizes, it can spread to the lung tissues. Although lumps may be found in the epididymis—the soft tissue behind the testis—lumps on the testis itself are the main danger signal.

Source: Dept. of Biomedical Communications, Bowman Gray School of Medicine of Wake Forest University, Winston-Salem, N.C.

To detect colon and rectal cancers, it is recommended that as part of a regular physical exam individuals obtain a stool sample at home and return it to the physician or clinic to be tested for hidden blood. New self-tests allow people to get instant test results themselves. A positive result from this type of screening, however, does not necessarily indicate cancer; further testing is needed to make that determination. A rectal exam and proctoscopic exam are also recommended as part of regular periodic checkups.

Dangers Associated with Delay and Denial

It was discussed earlier how cancer can affect a person's psychological and emotional state. Among the most common initial reactions is fear. This fear may cause a person to deny that there is a problem and thus delay doing anything about it. One study found that delay in seeking medical help seems to be a conscious, deliberate act rather than a failure to notice the symptoms of a potential problem or understand the consequences.[32]

Self-help tips:

- *Watch for the seven warning signals.*
- *Learn your own risk factors.*
- *See your doctor for a cancer-related checkup appropriate to your age, gender, and risk factors.*

When people let fear take over their lives, the latest knowledge about cancer prevention, causes, and cures is of little value. What people *think* will happen during the course of the disease can produce so much anxiety that they delay seeing a doctor. Such fear, of course, is normal; it takes time during periods of stress to adjust and adapt to new, frightening circumstances. During this time, however, it is essential for a person to realign his or her defenses for coping. If this takes too long, the self-defense mechanism may cross over into self-destructiveness and the individual can actually endanger his or her survival. Since survival often depends on early detection and treatment, delay can result in a progression of the disease to the point where it becomes irreversible and life-threatening.

Treating Cancer

Some people fear cancer because they are afraid of what will happen during treatment. Will it be painful? Will it disable them or make it hard for them to live a normal life? Will it help them or merely prolong and intensify their suffering? These are all valid concerns. While the outlook for many cancer patients is improving, the disease *can* be disabling or fatal, and treatment may involve pain or discomfort. However, modern cancer treatments can prolong survival and make a patient's life far more comfortable than was possible in the past.

Types of Cancer Treatment

The study of cancer is known as oncology. *An* oncologist *is a physician who specializes in the treatment of malignancies. Both words are derived from the Greek word* onkos, *which means "mass."*

The number of treatable types of cancer is increasing, and treatment has become increasingly individualized. The basic goals of treatment for cancer include cure, prolongation of life, and *palliation* (the control of symptoms). After the disease has been detected, physicians use a procedure known as *staging* to assess treatment options. In staging, physicians evaluate factors such as the type of cancer, the size of the tumor, the degree to which the cancer has spread, and the health and condition of the patient. This type of evaluation helps determine the type of treatment that will be most effective and appropriate for the needs of the individual patient.[33]

Physicians often elect to use a combination of treatments, which may include surgery, radiation therapy, and/or chemotherapy together with psychological, nursing, and nutritional support services. In many cases it is possible actually to cure cancer with some of these treatment approaches. If a total cure is not realistic, treatment can often extend the life of the patient and make the symptoms less severe.

Surgery Medical science has come a long way since antiquity, when the only known way of treating cancer was to cut out the diseased tissue. Since then, medical thinking about the use of surgery has evolved, and some specialists are now challenging the use of radical surgical operations for treating cancer. Nevertheless, for many forms of cancer, surgical removal of cancerous tissue remains the most effective method of treatment.[34]

Because of improved diagnostic equipment and laser instruments, cancer surgery has become more precise. It has proved very successful against various malignancies, especially tumors involving the lung, colon, stomach, bowel, liver, and skin. However, when surgery involves removing or disrupting entire organs, it can mean more physical problems for the patient, sometimes with profound psychological effects. Some specialists question whether it is necessary to perform a radical mastectomy (surgical removal of the entire breast and the neighboring lymph nodes) in patients with breast cancer. If superior results can be achieved without resorting to such radical surgery, some of the emotional and physical trauma associated with losing a breast can be eliminated.

By helping doctors make more accurate diagnoses of cancers, medical imaging technologies such as the CAT scan have played an important role in increasing the survival rate of cancer patients. (Larry Mulvehill/Photo Researchers, Inc.)

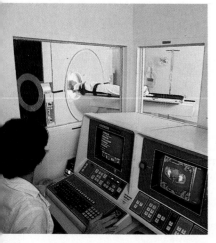

Communicating About

Communicating with Your Doctor about Fears

When you have concerns about health, whether you feel the problem is minor or are fearful about a serious problem such as cancer, you need to communicate those concerns to your doctor. Good communication is the key to getting your fears addressed and getting good medical care.

Often people are reluctant to go to the doctor. Some hesitate because of the cost, some because they fear they will seem stupid or worried about nothing. Some are fearful of what they may learn that is bad, and some worry that they will not understand the doctor. However, with a serious illness such as cancer, early detection can mean the difference between life and death.

Doctors and patients use different languages to refer to the same symptoms; this can be a barrier to good communication. Many patients are reluctant to speak about intimate topics even to the doctor. Sometimes people are so fearful of what they may learn that they omit or distort information because they are afraid of what it may mean.

When you have fears about your health, remember that no matter how alarming something seems to you, you do not have the medical knowledge to make a diagnosis. For example, a lump that seems like cancer to you may be no more than a cyst. Only a doctor can diagnose such a problem. That is why it is so important that you do not withhold facts from the doctor. A doctor must have all the facts about your condition to deal with and relieve your fears.

To communicate well with the doctor, be prepared by having the kind of information the doctor needs from you. Either get it clear in your mind or write it down ahead of time. First, be ready to tell the doctor what is wrong using simple, clear language. Give your symptoms, not a diagnosis. Do not say, "I've had this virus for a few days." Instead, say, "I've had diarrhea and a high fever for 2 days." Let the doctor interpret the cause and importance of each symptom. Do not fail to mention symptoms that seem intimate—doctors deal with them all the time.

Then, for each symptom—pain, nausea, itching, bleeding, faintness, vision problems, coughing, and so on—try to pinpoint when it started. For instance, if the symptom is pain, what kind of pain is it? Where is it located? Is there a pattern to the symptom (time of day when it occurs, activities that bring it on, positions that make it worse, its relation to meals or sleeping)? When did it come on? Has the symptom gotten worse? Have you had it before? If so, how was it treated? In addition, provide a list of any drugs you are taking for this condition or any other conditions. You should also describe any other medical conditions you have.

Once you have told the doctor about your symptoms and answered any questions, the doctor will respond to you. At this point you should be ready to ask questions of the doctor. For instance, if the doctor asks you to have certain medical tests, by all means ask about the costs, what the doctor is looking for in the tests, whether they are dangerous or painful, and when you will get the results.

When the doctor makes a diagnosis and recommends treatment, you can ask how you got the condition and what the usual course of the disease is. Be sure to request a definition of any terms you do not understand. You should also ask questions about the treatment the doctor has recommended. For example, what results can you expect and what kinds of things should you call the doctor about? You should ask about the reason for treatment and the risks, if any. If the doctor recommends surgery, ask about the chances of complete recovery and the length of your stay in the hospital and of your recovery at home afterward.

After a doctor has recommended treatment, you may want to get a second opinion. This is especially important if you question the doctor's judgment or have been diagnosed as having a serious disease such as cancer. Seeking advice from another doctor may help calm your fears or help you find alternative forms of treatment.

Based on J. Alfred Jones and Gerald M. Phillips, *Communicating with Your Doctor* (Carbondale and Edwardsville: Southern Illinois University Press, 1988).

Radiation Radiation therapy uses energy in very high, concentrated doses to destroy cancer cells. Once the location and extent of cancerous growths are determined, highly trained health professionals deliver radiation treatments in an attempt to cure patients or make them more comfortable. The decision to use radiation treatment depends on the type of tumor, evaluations by physicians about whether radiation therapy is appropriate, and the wishes of the patient. When detected early, skin cancers and some stages of cancers of the oral cavity and throat, uterus, cervix, and prostate are often treated solely with radiation.[35]

The rate of success with some cancers can be improved by combining radiation therapy and surgery. For example, radiation is sometimes given before surgery to shrink a tumor before it is removed. Postoperative radiation—given after a surgical wound has healed—is used to destroy the microscopic cancerous growths that may remain. This treatment is often used as a curative adjunct with a variety of cancers, including cancers of the kidney, bladder, pancreas, and breast.[36]

Many patients with noncurable cancer receive radiation therapy to shrink tumors and reduce their level of pain. Although such use of radiation treatment sometimes increases the duration of survival, the main object is to improve the quality of life by relieving symptoms without adding the more drastic side effects of chemotherapy.

With any radiation treatment, of course, it is impossible to avoid exposing some normal tissue to radiation. As a result, side effects such as skin redness, hair loss, loss of appetite, and fatigue can and do occur, depending on the site treated and the dose of radiation. Some of these side effects become apparent within weeks of treatment; others may not become noticeable for months or even years. A few of these late side effects, such as damage to arteries, can result in major complications. Most of the early side effects usually clear up shortly after treatment has been stopped.

Although such problems do exist, radiation therapy today is more effective, less dangerous, and far more predictable and results in fewer ill effects and long-term complications than was the case in the past. The crucial thing to remember is that radiation must be handled by a specialist who tailors the therapy to the individual patient. No two cancers are alike, and no two people respond to radiation therapy in the same way.

Chemotherapy The use of chemicals to treat cancer is called *chemotherapy*. In recent years chemotherapy has become the major weapon against cancers that have metastasized; it is also used as an adjunct to surgery or radiation when it is likely that the cancer has not been cured by surgery or radiation alone.[37]

While chemotherapeutic drugs may be taken orally or injected, depending on the drug and the type of cancer, intravenous injection is the most common method of administration. Sometimes the drugs are used in combinations to achieve a greater effect. Basically, chemotherapeutic drugs kill cancer cells because they are toxic to cells that spend a great deal of time growing and dividing (as cancer cells do). Unfortunately, other fast-growing normal cells—such as those in the bone marrow, skin, hair, and stomach lining—also are affected by chemotherapeutic drugs. For this reason, chemotherapy often results in temporary side effects, including total hair loss, nausea, diarrhea, and suppression of the ability of bone marrow to produce blood cells, thus increasing susceptibility to infection. Ways to decrease chemotherapy-induced side effects are being studied.

While traditional chemotherapy uses drugs that are toxic to cells, other chemicals are also used in the treatment of cancer. Among these are antihormones and hormones, which are used for the treatment of cancers of hormone-responsive organs such as the breast and prostate. Tamoxifen is an antihormone which slows down the production of estrogen and is therefore

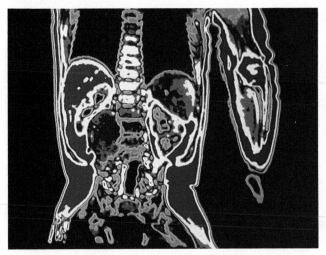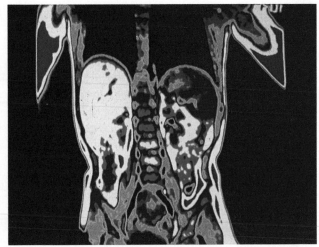

The effects of chemotherapy on cancers can be quite dramatic. Here are two MRI scans of a 7-month-old girl's kidneys. In the later picture (right), the cancerous pressure on the child's spine has totally disappeared. (Howard Sochurek/Medical Images Inc.)

useful for treating breast cancer. Megesterol acetate, a synthetic progesterone, is sometimes used in the treatment of breast, uterine, and prostate cancers. Another group of chemicals used in chemotherapy are immune modifiers such as interferon, a chemical that the body normally produces in response to viral infections. When injected in large amounts, interferon may have some antitumor effects either through direct action or through its effect on the immune system. Many cancer researchers believe that proper understanding and use of the immune system will ultimately provide the key to curing many forms of cancer.

Positive Developments in Treatment

Progress in cancer treatment is being made every day. An important example is the improvement in the survival rate of persons with acute lymphocytic leukemia, a cancer of the blood-forming tissues. Chemotherapy has proved to be quite effective in killing the abnormal cells produced by this disease. In addition, continuing research is yielding new and better drugs for treating leukemia patients. As a result, the 5-year survival rate for patients with acute lymphocytic leukemia has increased from only 4 percent in the early 1960s to 48 percent in the early 1980s. In children, the improvement has been even more dramatic—from 4 percent to 71 percent.[38]

Another sign of improvement has been seen in the management of testicular cancer in young men. The use of more precise diagnostic tools has allowed a better selection of treatment, and this has resulted in improved survival. Over the course of 20 years, the 5-year survival rate for men with testicular cancer rose from 63 to 87 percent.[39]

Meanwhile, scientists continue researching new and better treatments for cancer. Some are working on the theory that genetics can be used to enhance the tumor-fighting capacity of the immune system.[40] Another area of research involves cancer vaccines. Clinical trials performed with vaccines derived from tumor cells have indicated that they are safe and may be effective in some circumstances. They appear to be able to help cancer patients fight off metastases by stimulating immune responses to the growth of tumors.[41]

New approaches to drug therapy use combinations of chemotherapeutic drugs as well as chemotherapy combined with radiation and surgery. New substances are also being tested for their effectiveness in treating patients who are resistant to the drug therapies now in use.

*A person should go to reputable sources for information on cancer. The National Cancer Institute, an agency of the U.S. government, sponsors a toll-free Cancer Information Service, with a computerized data base known as **Physician Date Query (PDQ).** The phone number is 1–800–4–CANCER. The American Cancer Society's Response system can be reached at 1–800–ACS–2345. **Anyone** wanting information on cancer, not just health professionals, can call either of these numbers.*

Progress in the Fight

It seems that almost every day one hears about new cancer risks associated with lifestyle or the environment. However, one also learns about medical breakthroughs and sophisticated new treatments. Are people making progress in fighting cancer? Two opinions follow. The first says people are still fairly helpless in combating cancer; the second concludes that people can do a great deal to prevent—and cure—this disease.

Our Knowledge and Technology Are Not Yet Effective in Combating Cancer I am pretty discouraged by the incidence and risks of cancer today. Every time you pick up a newspaper or turn on the news, there's yet another study that's identified more possible cancer causes: our morning coffee, "secondhand" cigarette smoke, even sunshine—the list seems endless. Sometimes I feel overwhelmed trying to keep track of the things I should do to reduce my risk of getting cancer.

We have very little control over most cancer-causing factors, especially heredity, viruses, and radiation. In addition, the list of environmental carcinogens continues to grow. Some, like asbestos, have been identified and are slowly being eradicated, while others, including radon gas, are imperceptible dangers. I've read that there's no compelling reason to believe that all carcinogens will eventually be identified.

When someone is diagnosed as having cancer, that is the result of a very long process. It may, for example, have taken 40 years for that person to develop cancer after being exposed to asbestos. At Hiroshima and Nagasaki the high incidence of lung cancer among those exposed to the atomic explosion was not apparent until after 30 years or more. Who knows what cancer seeds we are planting in this age of ozone depletion, extensive air and water pollution, and growing reliance on nuclear energy.

I've tried to become knowledgeable about cancer, but the data are pretty discouraging. Sometimes I think that instead of spending time worrying, I should just enjoy myself and take my chances.

Our Knowledge Is Helping Us Prevent and Cure Cancer I think that each of us has an important tool to decrease cancer occurrence and deaths—and that tool is knowledge. Knowing the risk factors in your own lifestyle and understanding the value of early diagnosis and treatment may very well save your life.

We've made a lot of progress both in identifying the causes and in cures through early treatment. Today there are over 5 million Americans who have survived cancer.

About 90 percent of all types of cancer are caused by environmental factors and lifestyle—all things that we can control. The guidelines are simple: eat plenty of high-fiber foods, foods rich in vitamins A and C, and vegetables of the cabbage family. Eat limited amounts of high-fat foods and salt- and nitrite-cured foods. Avoid tobacco, alcohol, excessive weight gain, exposure to work-related carcinogens, and too much sun.

You can educate yourself about cancer's warning signals—ask your doctor or call the local office of the American Cancer Society for the list. Learn the risk factors that affect you personally (perhaps a family history of a certain type of cancer) and see your doctor for cancer-related checkups according to your age, gender, and risk factors.

The major methods for treating cancer—surgery, radiation therapy, and chemotherapy—are growing increasingly sophisticated. Physicians keep informed about the latest proven treatment methods through a computer network sponsored by the National Cancer Institute. With factual information, cancer *is* preventable and curable. Knowledge and initiative give you the best advantage over cancer.

What is your opinion? Would you agree that people are still helpless in fighting cancer? Are attempts to reduce the risk of getting cancer futile because it will take decades to know what cancer seeds have been planted? Or do you think this society is well on its way to controlling cancer?

Includes ideas from Lorenzo Tomatis, *Environmental Cancer Risk Factors* (Paris, France: International Agency for Research); *Knowledge Is Power* (Winston-Salem, N.C.: Southeast Cancer Control Consortium).

New technologies are also proving helpful in fighting cancer. For example, high-technology diagnostic techniques have replaced exploratory surgery for some cancer patients, and advances in technology have also enabled physicians to locate tumors more precisely, making more accurate treatment possible. New technologies have also enabled doctors to use bone marrow transplantation as a treatment option in some cancer patients with leukemia; the use of this technique for other cancers is under study.[42]

With medical progress having led to some optimism about the physical well-being of cancer patients, psychosocial needs and support of patients are now emerging as important areas of research as well. The concern is no longer a matter only of treating and dealing with the physical aspects of cancer but one of helping people learn to live with the disease as well.

The Dangers of Quackery

Unfortunately, in addition to or instead of going to qualified health professionals for cancer treatment, some people fall prey to medical quackery. *Quackery* (Chapter 18) refers to incompetence in a licensed health professional or, more commonly, an unlicensed and unorthodox practitioner. Cancer quacks prosper because of patient ignorance and because patients are afraid and desperate for some type of cure. Quack treatments for cancer include the use of ineffective drugs, special diets, and other controversial methods. Among the publicized treatments that lack scientific support are laetrile, krebiozen, nucleic acid diets, vegetarian diets, and a variety of mechanical devices.

Laetrile, also known as vitamin B_{17} or aprikern, is one of the most notorious quack cancer treatments. There is no such vitamin as B_{17}; the substance is an extract of apricot pits that costs about 2 cents a pill to produce and sells for $1.25 or more. Studies at reputable cancer and medical research institutes have failed to disclose any evidence that laetrile can cure or prevent any form of cancer. Nevertheless, advocates of laetrile as well as other quack treatments often claim success and offer testimonials by "cured" patients. What they do not say is that the cure they attribute to their treatment may well result from a naturally occurring improvement (*remission*) or a standard medical treatment such as chemotherapy.

The greatest tragedy of any type of cancer quackery is that a patient who might be cured often delays making a trip to the doctor and instead relies on useless drugs and treatments. When he or she does finally seek appropriate treatment, it may be too late to curb the disease.

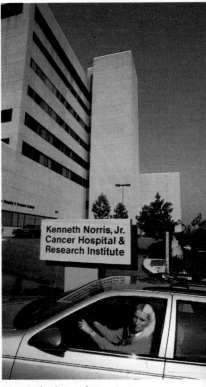

Hospitals devoted to cancer research have led the fight against cancer in the United States. (Tom Tracy/ MediChrome)

Living with Cancer

There are over 6 million Americans living who have a history of cancer; nearly 3 million of these people are considered cured of the disease. ("Cured" means that a person is free of evidence of the disease 5 years or more after the initial diagnosis and treatment.[43]) Thanks to earlier detection and new methods of treatment, many of these cancer survivors will have the same life expectancy as people who never had the disease; others will live a longer time while continuing to battle the disease from day to day (Figure 12.7).

Making Each Day Count

For many long-term survivors, cancer can be thought of as a chronic disease that must be dealt with over a long period. Just like people with chronic conditions such as hypertension and diabetes, cancer survivors need to take special care of themselves on a daily basis. They may or may not have to adhere to medication regimens or follow special diets, but they will need routine periodic health exams throughout their lives.

Figure 12.7 Early detection of cancers in their localized stages results in much higher survival rates. For instance, 90 percent of female breast cancer patients survive at least 5 years when the disease is diagnosed in its local stage. When breast cancer has already spread regionally, about 68 percent of patients survive. Only 18 percent survive when the cancer has metastasized to distant sites before diagnosis.

Over the years, improved cancer treatment has increased the overall 5-year survival rate, from about 20% in 1930 to 50% in 1990.

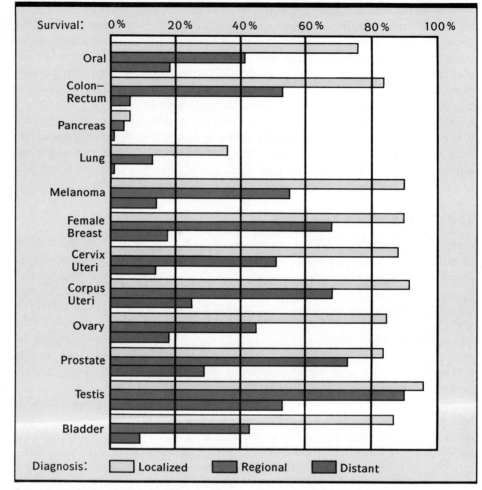

Source: American Cancer Society, *1990 Cancer Facts and Figures*, p. 17 citing "Cancer Statistics Branch, National Cancer Institute."

Living with cancer from day to day means trying to focus on living rather than dying, but it also means working through one's feelings about death, fear, and isolation. When former cancer patient Orville Kelly realized this, he wrote a newspaper article that prompted the American Cancer Society to sponsor a program called Make Today Count. With over 700 local chapters, this self-help organization helps cancer patients and their families learn to live each day as fully and completely as possible. Groups such as this, along with other efforts to keep cancer patients active and involved, help improve a patient's outlook; this in turn promotes a patient's overall health and well-being. "Making today count" is a good motto not only for cancer patients but for all people concerned with the quality of their life and health.

Coping with Cancer

Cancer patients and survivors have to cope with a great deal. Many must deal with fears of disease recurrence and possible death. Disabilities resulting from the disease or its treatment may remain a source of ongoing psychosocial distress. Anxiety, fear, and panic attacks can develop after cancer treatments have been completed. The experience of having had cancer produces clear, long-lasting memories characterized by an easy recall of the initial feelings and emotions associated with the illness and its recovery period, a continuing concern about one's mortality, and a lasting sense of vulnerability.[44]

People with cancer use various types of coping behavior to help them deal with the disease. They may use denial as a temporary protection against being overwhelmed by the experience. They may intellectualize the problem by detailing the medical aspects of their illness in a manner completely devoid of personal involvement. They may suppress their feelings, project them onto others, or displace feelings such as anger to less threatening targets (such as a spouse rather than a physician) or more socially acceptable ones (such as an adult rather than a child). They may also search for a meaning for the illness and for their lives; for some people, faith in God may offer consolation.[45]

With the number of cancer survivors increasing and with those survivors living longer, it is important for cancer patients as well as their families and friends to learn how to define and live with their feelings about the disease. Since people's sense of mastery and control over their lives can be affected by cancer, attempts to increase personal control are significantly beneficial in helping them cope with the disease.

Some people are able to cope with cancer by themselves or with the help of their families and friends. For others, support programs such as those offered by the American Cancer Society can provide information and counseling services—including group education programs, pamphlets, and visitor programs—to help them deal with the medical, social, and psychological aspects of living with cancer. Through their own efforts and with the help of others, most cancer patients are able to lead normal, active lives filled with hope and optimism for the future.

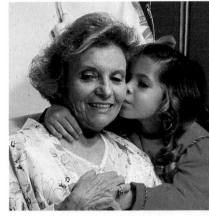

The love of friends and family members can be very important to cancer patients, who need the warmth of human contact and communication to help them get through difficult times. (Werner Bertsch/Medical Images, Inc.)

Chapter Summary

- Cancer is a group of more than 100 diseases characterized by the uncontrolled growth and spread of abnormal cells. Sometimes these cells form an abnormal mass of tissue known as a tumor. Sometimes new, or secondary, tumors form when cancerous cells break away and spread to other parts of the body; this process is known as metastatic growth.

- There are more than 100 forms of cancer; some of the more common types are carcinomas, sarcomas, lymphomas, leukemias, and melanomas.

- Cancer brings people face to face with their own mortality and often causes a great deal of psychological pain and emotional distress. Cancer patients often fear dying, the possible pain and side effects associated with treatment, and not being able to lead a normal life. They may also face disruptions in personal and social life that can lead to loneliness and depression. Family dynamics may change as roles and responsibilities shift as a result of dealing with the disease.

- A number of risk factors—including some that are genetic, some that have to do with the environment, and some, such as smoking and drinking, that have to do with individual lifestyle—have been associated with the development of cancer. Certain cancers seem to be more strongly associated with some of these risk factors than with others.

- To help reduce the possibility of developing cancer, it is often suggested that people change their lifestyles and behaviors so as to avoid the risk factors associated with the disease. This includes avoiding tobacco smoking and excessive alcohol consumption, eating a nutritious diet, exercising, avoiding hazardous chemicals and other environmental pollutants, and avoiding excessive exposure to the sun's ultraviolet rays.

- Early detection of cancer can save a person's life. The earlier the disease is detected, the better the prognosis for treatment, longer survival, and even complete recovery.

- Regular self-examinations should be performed to ensure early diagnosis of breast cancer and testicular cancer. Such self-examinations are easy to perform and can save a person's life.

- In staging, physicians evaluate a number of factors, including the type of cancer, the size of the tumor, the degree of metastasis, and the health and condition of the patient. This procedure helps determine the most appropriate and effective form of treatment.

- The primary treatments for cancer are surgery, radiation therapy, and chemotherapy. The choice of treatment depends on the nature of the cancer, its spread, the health of the patient, and other factors similar to the ones evaluated during staging.

- Since early detection of cancer is crucial to a patient's survival, medical quackery is particularly dangerous in regard to this disease. Not only is quackery ineffective, by delaying treatment it allows the cancer to spread to a point where proper medical treatment is less effective.

- New developments in the treatment and diagnosis of cancer include the use of more precise diagnostic tools, combined drug therapies, and the potential for developing vaccines for some forms of the disease.

- Cancer patients must cope with the fears associated with the disease. To do this, they use many of the normal coping mechanisms, such as denial, intellectualizing the problem, suppressing feelings, projecting feelings onto others, and searching for meaning in their lives. While some cancer patients cope well with the disease by themselves, family members and friends can be crucial; organized support groups can help provide information and counseling.

Key Terms

Cancer (page 314)

Malignant neoplasm (page 314)

Tissue (page 315)

Mitosis (page 315)

Tumor (page 315)

Neoplasm (page 315)

Benign tumor (page 315)

Malignant tumor (page 315)

Metastases (page 315)

Metastatic growth (page 315)

Carcinomas (page 316)

Epithelium (page 316)

Sarcomas (page 316)

Adenocarcinomas (page 316)

Lymphomas (page 316)

Leukemias (page 316)

Melanomas (page 316)

Anaplastic (page 316)

Carcinogenic (page 320)

References

1. American Cancer Society, *Cancer Facts and Figures—1990* (Atlanta, Ga.: American Cancer Society, 1990): 3.

2. Ibid.

3. G. R. Newell et al., "Epidemiology of Cancer," in *Cancer Principles and Practices of Oncology*, V. T. DeVita et al. (eds.) (Philadelphia: Lippincott, 1982): 3–32.

4. Bobbie M. Atwell, "Psychosocial Aspects of Cancer," in *Understanding Cancer*, Bobbie M. Atwell and Robert Michiellutte (eds.) (Winston-Salem, N.C.: Oncology Research Center, Bowman Gray School of Medicine, 1986): 196–206.

5. Arthur M. Sutherland, "Psychological Impact of Cancer and Its Therapy," *Ca* 31, no. 30 (May–June 1981): 159–171.

6. Ibid.

7. Rob Buckman, "Communicating with Cancer Patients," *The Practitioner* 233 (October 22, 1989): 1393–1396.

8. Deborah Welch-McCaffrey et al., "Surviving Adult Cancers: Psychosocial Implications," *Annals of Internal Medicine* 111, no. 6 (September 15, 1989): 517–524.

9. Caryn Lerman et al., "Reducing Avoidable Cancer Mortality through Prevention and Early Detection Regimens," *Cancer Research* 49 (September 15, 1989): 4955–4962.

10. American Cancer Society, op. cit., p. 13.

11. American Cancer Society, op. cit., p. 12.

12. Lerman et al., op. cit.

13. D. Schottenfield, "The Epidemiology of Cancer," *Cancer* 47 (1981): 1095–1108.

14. Norton Nelson, "Cancer Prevention: Environmental, Industrial, and Occupational Factors," *Cancer* 47 (1981): 1065–1070.

15. G. Marie Swanson, "Cancer Prevention in the Workplace and Natural Environment," *Cancer* 62 (October 15, 1988): 1725–1745; L. Tomatis, "Environmental Cancer Risk Factors," *Acta Oncologica* 27 (1988, Fasc. 5): 465–472.

16. American Cancer Society, op. cit., p. 18.

17. Ibid., p. 9.

18. Ibid., p. 13.

19. Ibid., p. 18.

20. Lerman et al., op. cit.

21. American Cancer Society, op. cit., p. 22.

22. Lerman et al., op. cit.

23. American Cancer Society, op. cit., p. 27.

24. Judy Bahnson, "What You Must Know about the Pap Smear and Cancer Prevention" (Winston-Salem, N.C.: Cervical Cancer Prevention Project at Bowman Gray School of Medicine).

25. American Cancer Society, op. cit., p. 10.

26. R. Hoover, "Effects of Drugs—Immunosuppression," in *Origins of Human Cancer*, H. H. Hyatt et al. (eds.) (Cold Spring Harbor, N.Y.: Cold Spring Harbor Laboratory, 1977): 369–379.

27. American Cancer Society, "Colorectal Cancer: Go for Early Detection" (Atlanta, Ga.: American Cancer Society).

28. American Cancer Society, op. cit., p. 10.

29. "Getting Good Care Means Knowing All the Choices," *U.S. News & World Report* (July 11, 1988): 56.

30. American Cancer Society, op. cit., p. 13.

31. Ibid., p. 9.

32. Thomas P. Hackett et al., "Patient Delay in Cancer," *New England Journal of Medicine* 28, no. 1 (July 5, 1983): 14–20.

33. J. Michael Sterchi, "Surgical Management of the Cancer Patient," Atwell and Michiellutte (eds.), op. cit., pp. 11–21.

34. Ibid.

35. Damon D. Blake, "Radiation Therapy," Atwell and Michiellutte (eds.), op. cit., pp. 22–34.

36. Ibid.

37. Douglas R. White, "Chemotherapy," Atwell and Michiellutte (eds.), op. cit., pp. 35–51.

38. American Cancer Society, op. cit., p. 14.

39. Ibid., p. 4.

40. Barbara J. Culliton, "Fighting Cancer with Designer Cells," *Science* 244 (June 23, 1989): 1430–1433.

41. Jean L. Marx, "Cancer Vaccines Show Promise at Last," *Science* 245 (August 25, 1989): 813–815.

42. American Cancer Society, op. cit., pp. 4–5.

43. Ibid., p. 3.

44. Welch-McCaffrey et al., op. cit.

45. Atwell, op. cit.

PART 5

Avoiding Danger: Health and Common Sense

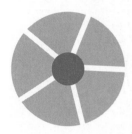

This part of the book studies types of damage other than disease that can affect one's health: from the deterioration that can be caused by drugs, including alcohol and tobacco, to the injuries that afflict many people. The causes of such damage are compared with the causes of disease itself; prevention is emphasized.

Chapter 13 surveys the field of medicinal and illegal drugs. It explores how a drug's beneficial or harmful effects on the body and brain are a function of time and dose and emphasizes the damage that can be caused by the use of harmful drugs or of other drugs in excessive doses or damaging combinations.

Chapter 14 describes the effects of alcohol on the body, including pleasurable and harmful short-term effects, as well as long-term, life-threatening implications. It discusses treatment programs for those who have problems controlling its use.

Chapter 15 covers the toxic effects of tobacco, including smokeless tobacco; the many types of chronic disease it can cause to both users and bystanders; and techniques one can employ to counter the dependence it causes.

Chapter 16 studies different types of accidental and violent injuries and explores approaches to injury prevention and control. It also stresses the value of knowing first-aid procedures if one is confronted with an emergency.

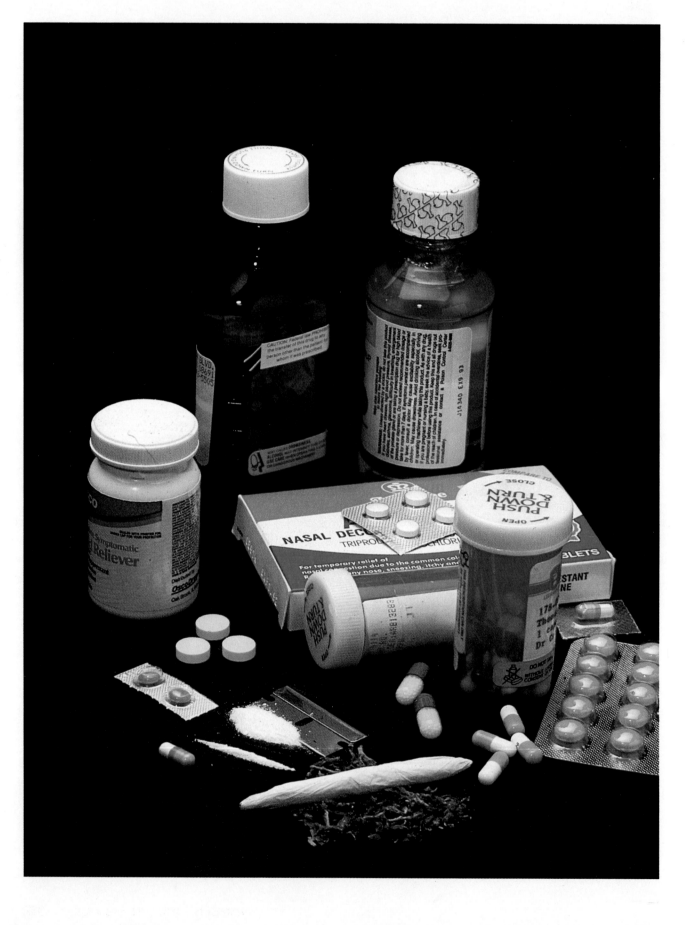

Chapter 13

Drug Use and Abuse

To Guide Your Reading

When you have studied this chapter, you should be able to:

- Explain what drugs are, why people use them, and how drug addiction can develop.

- Describe patterns of drug use and explain the relevance of the agent-host-environment model to drug dependence.

- Summarize the main effects of drugs, describe the different ways in which drugs are administered, and discuss the relationship between methods of administration and effects.

- List, describe, and give examples of the main types of drugs, including sedatives/hypnotics, stimulants (including cocaine), marijuana, volatile solvents, opiate narcotics, and psychedelics/hallucinogens.

- Discuss programs that help drug abusers and efforts at the societal level to combat the drug problem.

Many Americans begin the day with a drug, although most people would probably not think of the caffeine in a cup of coffee, tea, or cocoa as a drug. As the day goes on, other drugs may be added: the nicotine in a cigarette, caffeine in a cola drink, alcohol in a beer, perhaps an over-the-counter drug such as aspirin for a headache, or a prescription drug such as a diuretic for a more serious condition. Some people use illicit drugs such as marijuana and cocaine.

An enormous variety of chemical substances—available both legally and illegally—play a significant role in the lives of millions of Americans. Drugs are used as a part of most medical regimens; the way in which medical care has benefited from the application of drugs is one of the miracles of the twentieth century. Americans also use drugs to ease uncomfortable social occasions, give themselves a lift, and help themselves relax or feel better or simply out of habit. People seem to believe that drugs can provide easy solutions to many of their physical, emotional, intellectual, social, and spiritual problems. However, drugs have been implicated in a host of problems, including accidents, crime, illness, violence, and family and community disintegration.

The question for most people is not whether to use drugs; almost everyone does that if caffeine, nicotine, and alcohol are included. The issues people should be concerned about include the purposes for which drugs are used and the benefits, risks, and consequences of drug use for themselves and for society. The challenge for individuals as well as for society is to maximize the benefits of drugs while reducing the associated risks. This is the basis for responsible drug use.

Drugs and Why People Use Them

Drugs include an enormous number of substances. Since the dawn of recorded history people have used and abused these substances for a variety of reasons: to escape boredom, relieve pain and discomfort, reduce frustration,

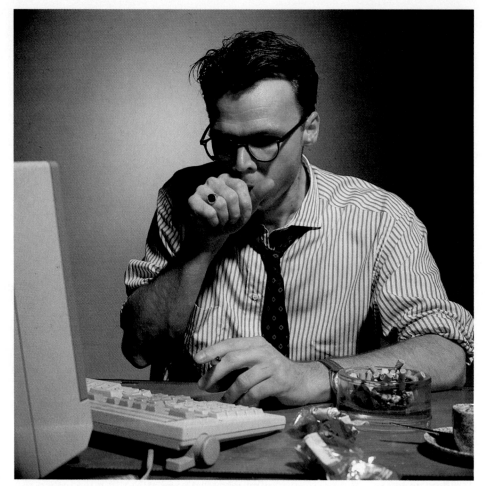

The nicotine in tobacco is one of many drugs that can induce dependence in users so that they feel they cannot function without their drug. (Johannes Hofman/Okapia/Photo Researchers, Inc.)

overcome feelings of alienation, escape problems, achieve togetherness, experience pleasure, relieve stress or tension, improve performance, and enhance mystical or religious experiences and rites of passage.

Sometimes people experience little difficulty with the use of a drug; the vast majority of people, for example, can moderate their use of alcoholic beverages. At other times, however, drugs may cause problems. These problems may be minor compared with the benefits a drug brings—think of the slight drowsiness that may accompany the use of an allergy medicine and the relief that medicine brings from sneezes, a runny nose, and watery eyes. However, drug use can create serious problems both for users and for society.

What Are Drugs?

drug—*any nonnutritional substance that is* **deliberately** *introduced into the body to produce a physiological and/or psychological effect.*

psychoactive drug—*a drug that acts primarily on the brain, producing altered states of mood, perception, consciousness, and central nervous system activity.*

The term **drug,** as defined in this book, refers to any nonnutritional substance that is *deliberately* introduced into the body to produce a physiological and/or psychological effect. Drugs that act primarily on the brain, producing altered states of mood, perception, consciousness, and central nervous system activity, are called **psychoactive drugs.** Drugs that do not act in this way are referred to as *nonpsychoactive drugs.*

Psychoactive drugs, such as marijuana or cocaine, have the potential for abuse, while nonpsychoactive drugs, such as penicillin and other antibiotics, do not. Two psychoactive drugs that affect the health of millions of people are alcohol and tobacco. Because they are so widely used and cause such pervasive problems, they will be considered separately in the next two chapters.

The Use of Drugs

Most people who take drugs do so legally, using them to prevent or treat health disorders, not to get high or feed an addiction. Nearly everyone takes aspirin, cold remedies, and other over-the-counter (OTC) drugs now and then to treat common ailments. There is a wide range of medical problems for which people can purchase such drugs. In addition, most people occasionally use drugs that require a doctor's prescription. For many people with chronic diseases such as heart disease, daily life includes taking a broad assortment of prescription drugs to treat their illnesses.[1]

When prescribing a drug, a doctor must prescribe the right medicine for a particular problem *and* for a particular patient, given that some people have allergic reactions to certain drugs. Doctors can choose from a huge assortment of drugs, each with its own specific effects on the body. Prescription drugs are available to

- *Relieve symptoms*, for example, analgesics to control pain such as a headache
- *Prevent illness*, for example, vaccines to prevent diseases such as polio
- *Control chronic conditions*, for example, diuretics to control chronic conditions such as hypertension
- *Treat diseases*, for example, antibiotics to treat infectious diseases such as syphilis and gonorrhea

Any drug can be harmful if a person ingests enough of it, but some drugs have much more potential for harm than others do. In addition, certain combinations of drugs can be lethal even when taken in small quantities. For example, even a small amount of certain sedatives can cause death if taken in combination with alcohol or other depressant drugs.

The drugs with the greatest potential for harm—including many that are medically useful but potentially addictive—are regulated by federal and state laws. This is why certain drugs can be obtained legally only with a prescription. Some drugs offer so little medical benefit compared with the harm they can cause that they are rarely or never prescribed and can be obtained only illegally; examples are heroin, crack, LSD, and marijuana.

Drug Tolerance, Dependence, and Addiction

Among the factors that must be considered when one is making decisions about using drugs is the risk of becoming too accustomed to a drug—of becoming tolerant of, dependent on, or addicted to it.

Tolerance In many cases it is possible to develop a dangerous tolerance to a drug. **Tolerance** means that the body becomes adapted to the drug so that increasingly larger dosages are needed to produce the desired effect; this increases the hazard of any undesired effects the drug may have as well.

People have been known to develop a tolerance to nonpsychoactive drugs. In this book, however, *tolerance* is used in reference to both legal and illegal psychoactive drugs that some people use nonmedically to alter their mental state.

Dependence There is often a very fine line between tolerance and **dependence**—a condition in which individuals become so accustomed to a drug that they cannot, or feel they cannot, function without it. Dependence may refer to psychic dependence or physical dependence; both conditions can exist at the same time.

Psychic dependence, sometimes referred to as habituation, involves the idea of compulsive drug use for the sense of well-being it gives the user. With psychic dependence, a user deprived of the drug may feel restless, irritable, or anxious but does not usually become physically ill.

Labels on OTC medications should be read carefully. Certain medicines should not be taken by people with high blood pressure or diabetes except on the advice of a physician. Other medicines are not advised for pregnant or nursing women. Labels also provide information on maximum doses for a 24-hour period as well as the names of other drugs that may not interact well. A great deal of information is given in the fine print.

tolerance—*a situation in which the body becomes adapted to a drug so that increasingly larger doses are needed to produce the desired effect.*

dependence—*a condition in which users become so accustomed to a drug that they cannot, or feel they cannot, function without it; may be physical, psychic, or both.*

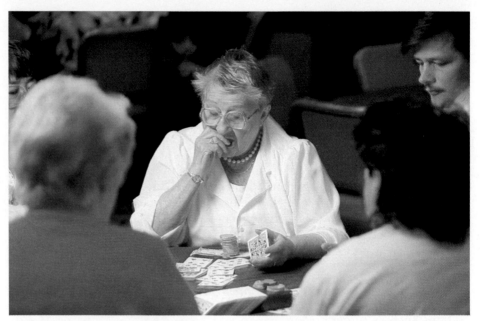

Gambling is a type of compulsive behavior that can be explained by the theory of psychic addiction; gamblers often have the sense that the hopeless aspects of their lives can be eliminated by success in gambling. (PhotoEdit)

With *physical dependence,* the body's systems have been altered: an abnormal situation—the continuous presence of the drug—has become the norm. If a physically dependent person is deprived of the drug, he or she experiences the **withdrawal syndrome** (sometimes known as abstinence syndrome—an unpleasant and possibly painful experience and sometimes even a life-threatening one). The well-known delirium tremens (DTs) of the alcoholic is an example of a withdrawal syndrome (Chapter 14). Withdrawal from heroin may bring symptoms such as nausea and vomiting, runny nose, sweating, fever, increased pulse and blood pressure, tremors, and joint and muscle pains.

withdrawal syndrome—*an unpleasant and possibly painful condition that an individual who is physically dependent on a drug experiences when deprived of that drug.*

Addiction The term **addiction** has received mixed usage by experts, in part because it has come to imply criminality and other socially value-laden ideas. Some experts use the term to emphasize a compulsive quality in a person's drug use. This pattern is marked both by tolerance and by psychic and physical dependence.[2]

addiction—*a compulsive pattern of drug use marked by both tolerance and psychic and physical dependence.*

How People Become Dependent on Drugs

Dependence can develop both with drugs used medically and with those, such as alcohol and marijuana, used for recreational or social purposes. In either case, a person can fall into a pattern of dependence in essentially the same way.

Relief of Discomfort People sometimes take drugs, with or without a prescription, to relieve discomfort such as physical pain or anxiety. If a person follows the instructions of a physician or those indicated on the drug label, there should be no problem. However, a person may deviate from these instructions in two ways, each of which can lead to drug dependence.

- If the drug acts quickly to ease pain, the person may unconsciously begin to lower the level of "tolerable" pain and start taking the medication to achieve lower and lower pain levels (in other words, more and more often). Such a pattern is less likely to develop with a drug that acts slowly.
- Since the drug eliminates pain, a person may reason that it is better to *anticipate* the recurrence of pain and take the drug ahead of time, thus

avoiding discomfort entirely. Now the person is on an "avoidance sched-ule," which can lead quickly to regular but unnecessary use of the drug and can greatly increase the chance of developing psychic and/or physical dependence.

Replace the word *pain* in the description above with *anxiety, depression,* or even *nervousness,* and it is clear how dependence can develop with the use of any substance that promises relief from unpleasant feelings.

Levels of Drug Use   Not everyone who uses a drug a few times is destined for destructive dependence. There are actually several levels of nonmedical drug use. Whether a person is likely to develop a drug dependence depends in part on which level of use that person follows. The following are the major levels of drug use in roughly chronological order.

1. *Experimental use.* At this level the individual "samples" a drug, typically in social situations, but uses it very infrequently. The risk of dependence is usually low, though it *may* occur. The first-time use of some drugs can occasionally cause death.
2. *Recreational use.* The individual uses modest amounts of a drug in social settings where such use is accepted or even expected. The individual's level of use reflects that of his or her social group. The widespread use of alcohol and marijuana and the use of cocaine in some social circles typify recreational use. Risk of dependence, though a little higher than at the experimental level, is still relatively low.
3. *Situational use.* The individual uses a drug in order to experience effects that he or she considers beneficial in a particular situation or in certain circumstances. An example of a situational user is a salesperson who typically takes a stiff drink before visiting a customer. In contrast to recreational use, no one else need be present. At this level, the risk of dependence may be considerable, depending on the situation, frequency, and particular drug used.
4. *Intensified use.* The individual uses a drug regularly to reduce perceived physical, psychological, or social discomfort. The frequency of use generally increases and becomes self-reinforcing, and—depending on whether tolerance occurs—the amount of the drug the individual uses may increase. The risk of developing dependence is usually high at this level of use.

People who use pain relievers or sleeping pills on a regular basis run the risk of becoming addicted to these drugs. (Arthur Sirdofsky/The Stock Shop)

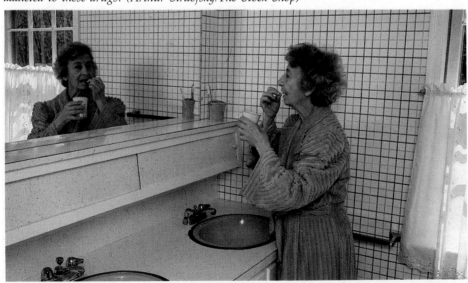

5. *Compulsive use.* The individual is preoccupied with obtaining and using a drug. Tolerance has often developed, and the drug has become less able to produce the anticipated effect. Normal functioning is markedly impaired; the individual's social relationships are superficial; he or she usually develops some degree of physical debilitation; and vocational or academic pursuits are imperiled or abandoned. The individual's physical and emotional health are at risk of being seriously compromised.

The Agent-Host-Environment Model   The levels of drug use just described are primarily from the perspective of the individual, but it is important to view drug dependence as more than an individual problem. Since many of the pressures to take drugs and the availability of drugs come from outside the individual, the role of society and other factors must also be considered (Figure 13.1).

The agent-host-environment model (the public health paradigm for the epidemiology of disease discussed in Chapter 10) can be helpful in explaining the epidemiology of drug dependence. In terms of drug use, agent factors include the pharmacological characteristics of a drug—dose, purity, toxicity, interaction with other drugs, and method of administration. Clearly, these factors can influence the potential for drug dependence. Host factors involve the physical, emotional, intellectual, social, and spiritual characteristics of the individual drug user. Emotional problems and physical illness, for example, can be factors in increased drug use and thus may play a role in drug dependence. Environmental factors include peer pressure, family patterns and behaviors, cultural mores, religious practices and beliefs, and laws. Pressures from family members, friends, and society may act to inhibit or encourage drug use and thus can be a factor in drug dependence as well.

Figure 13.1 The agent-host-environment model. Three complex sets of factors interact to determine drug use and abuse. Potential hosts bring their individual needs to social interactions. The social environment influences individual decisions by encouraging or discouraging drug use. As agents, drugs can change the characteristics of a host, and hosts select agents with different characteristics.

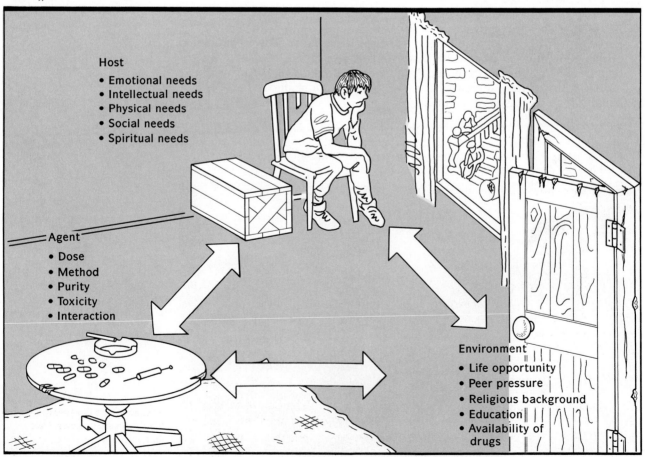

Host
• Emotional needs
• Intellectual needs
• Physical needs
• Social needs
• Spiritual needs

Agent
• Dose
• Method
• Purity
• Toxicity
• Interaction

Environment
• Life opportunity
• Peer pressure
• Religious background
• Education
• Availability of drugs

There is no such thing as a "safe" or "unsafe" drug. What determines a drug's safety is the interaction of these three factors—agent, host, and environment. Drug dependence should not be seen as just a function of the individual drug user but as a result of the interplay between the individual (the host), a particular drug (the agent), and the setting in which the drug is taken (the environment).

Trends in Drug Use

The most frequently used illegal drug in the United States today is marijuana, although its popularity is nowhere near that of alcohol, even among people too young to obtain alcohol legally. A 1989 survey of 1,200 college students found that 16.3 percent had used marijuana in the past month, 2.8 percent had used cocaine, and 76 percent had drunk alcohol. Compared with previous studies, the survey showed a decline in the use of all three drugs through the 1980s, although the use of alcohol declined much less rapidly during that time than did the use of marijuana and cocaine.[3]

According to a recent survey by the National Parents Resource Institute for Drug Education (PRIDE), drug use is declining among younger students as well. This survey of students in junior and senior high schools found that 4.6 percent had tried cocaine—down from 6.4 percent in a similar survey done two years earlier.[4]

Despite the decline in drug use among students, drug abuse has become a pervasive and critical national problem among other segments of the population. According to the National Institute on Drug Abuse, the number of people addicted to cocaine increased at least 33 percent between 1985 and 1989.[5] The term *cocaine* as used in this book also includes cocaine derivatives such as crack. These derivatives are less expensive than cocaine and have quicker, more intense, and more dangerous effects. Their lower price has been a factor in their increased use.

The American Council for Drug Education has reported that women between ages 18 and 34 constitute one of the groups in which cocaine addiction is spreading most rapidly. This situation is especially lamentable because pregnant women can pass the addiction on to their babies. One-tenth of all babies born in 1988 had illegal drugs—usually cocaine—in their bodies and faced the prospect of severe health problems.[6] In New York City alone, an estimated 10,000 mothers were addicted to crack at the beginning of 1990—a threefold increase over 1988.[7] In Philadelphia, doctors at Temple University Hospital reported in 1989 that 16 percent of the women delivering babies had used cocaine—four times more than in 1987—and the University of Pennsylvania Hospital reported that one-fifth of the women giving birth had used cocaine or cocaine derivatives just before going into labor.[8]

The Effects of Drugs

Drugs can produce a wide range of effects, desirable and undesirable, on the body as well as the mind. People take drugs to relieve pain, calm upset stomachs, cure bacterial infections, or fight cancerous tumors. They also take drugs to feel calmer, more energetic, less anxious, or more cheerful. Whether a drug affects a person physically, mentally, or both, it produces its effects by interacting with specific parts of the body.

How Drugs Interact with Body Cells

How does a particular drug act on a specific problem? Why does one drug act on the blood vessels and another on nerves? One explanation is the "receptor theory"—the idea that a drug affects only specific **receptor sites** on cells where the drug molecules "fit." (A *molecule* is the smallest functional unit of a

receptor sites—*specific spots on cells where the molecules of a specific drug "fit."*

Talking about Drug Use with Your Children

Finding out that a child is using drugs is every parent's nightmare. How do you prevent your children from using drugs? How do you deal with suspicions that your child is becoming addicted? Because drug use is so prevalent in American society and because so many teenagers and even children experiment with drugs, parents have to be prepared to deal with these issues.

If you have established good, open communication with your children, talking about drugs should not be very difficult or require special techniques. However, because this is an emotion-laden topic for most parents and because many teenagers are sensitive about their independence, many parents have great difficulty handling it. As a result, communication breaks down and parents do not accomplish anything.

Parents need to begin communicating about drugs when their children are very young. They should present information to children simply and in a matter-of-fact way. They should not dramatize the problem or make drug use seem exciting. Instead, they need to give clear messages that are appropriate to the child's age. For example, when you give your 3-year-old an antibiotic from the pediatrician, you might say, "We have to take care with medicines. The doctor says this is good for your earache, but we have to follow his directions carefully." You can follow this up by talking about good medicines that the doctor prescribes and bad drugs that can hurt people.

As your child grows, be sure he or she understands your views on drugs, but do not put the child's friends down for using drugs. Suppose an 8-year-old reports that a friend has said that marijuana is cool. You should not say, "Jamie is a bad kid, and I don't want you to play with him anymore." Instead you should say something like, "I know that some people think that it's okay to use drugs sometimes, but I feel that any kind of drug is dangerous. Drugs can hurt your mind and your body."

Some of the messages you give your child about drugs are nonverbal. For example, if your child sees you using drugs, you will be sending the message that drugs are okay. Do not expect more of your child than you do of yourself.

If you suspect that your teenager is using drugs or alcohol, it is vital to keep the channels of communication open in order to help. Do not yell or lecture; instead, encourage him or her to talk to you. Listen for clues to the feelings that underlie drug use. Then reflect those feelings back to your child to see whether you are right. Suppose your child says, "Oh, everyone else was smoking this stuff and I didn't want to look like a geek." You might say, "I know it's important to be part of your group, but this really might hurt you." If the child replies, "This stuff isn't going to hurt me," you might say, "It's good to feel confident about things, but it has hurt a lot of people; what did it seem to do to you?"

Whenever you talk about drugs, make it clear that you accept and like your teenager even though you may not accept his or her behavior. Try to focus on how bad drugs are and what their negative effects are instead of on how foolish or bad your teenager is for trying them. Talk about your feelings honestly. You might say, "I worry that if you use drugs even once, you could damage your health" or "I'm afraid that when your good judgment is impaired by drugs you might drive a car and be hurt or killed."

Listen to what your child says and try to decide whether this was a one-time thing, perhaps caused by peer pressure, or a chronic problem. Once you have an idea what caused the drug use and how serious the problem is, you can plan your next steps, such as working on the problem with your child, getting counseling, going to a rehabilitation clinic, and so on. Whatever steps you decide to take, remember that your communication should be focused on resolving the problem rather than on criticizing your child. Your ultimate goal is to help the child make good choices about drug use.

Based on Marlene Brusko, *Living with Your Teenager* (New York: McGraw-Hill, 1986).

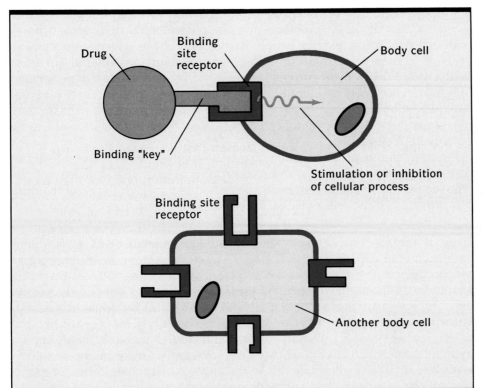

Figure 13.2 Cells in the body have receptors in their membranes that can affect their functioning. Drugs stimulate these receptors when their chemical "keys" fit into, or bind with, the receptor "locks." Since receptors in different cells may be similar, drugs can affect several types of tissues. However, the effects on these tissues can be very different, depending on the number of receptors and their function in a particular cell. Opiates, for instance, inhibit muscle contractions in the intestine and create euphoria when they bind with receptors in the brain.

chemical substance.) Drug molecules do not act on the whole cell—only on the receptor sites. A drug acts only on cells that have receptor sites compatible with its molecules (Figure 13.2).

This compatibility between drug molecules and receptor sites is similar to the mechanism of a key placed in a lock. If the teeth of the key match the tumblers in the lock, the lock responds by opening (the interaction produces the desired effect). To determine whether a drug will act on a given type of cell, it is necessary to find out *how much* compatibility there is between the drug molecules and the receptor sites in the cell, in other words, to find out the "degree of fit."

Side Effects of Drugs

If a drug acted on only one site in the body—the place where there is a problem—the physician's task would be relatively simple. Unfortunately, drugs cannot be counted on to act this way in all circumstances. All drugs have **side effects**—effects that are unwanted and unrelated to the essential purpose of a drug. Some side effects may occur immediately, and some over a period of time; some are transient, and some permanent; some are mildly annoying, and some much worse—perhaps even life-threatening. A side effect of crack is paranoia that may inspire violence.[9] Even aspirin can have the side effect of upsetting one's stomach.

What causes the side effects of drugs? Basically, some drugs are much less selective than others about the receptor sites with which they interact. Certain drugs used to treat bacterial infections, for example, go on a search and destroy mission that requires them to interlock with invading bacteria and combat those harmful organisms. Unfortunately, these drugs may interlock with and destroy healthy blood cells or glandular cells housing the bacteria, resulting in damage to the blood, glands, or vital organs.[10] Medical descriptions of drugs sometimes include terms that denote hazards to specific organs, such as *ototoxity* (harm to the ears), *nephrotoxicity* (harm to the kidneys), and *hepatotoxicity* (harm to the liver).

Drug use can pose greater risks for some people than it does for others because of variations in host factors or characteristics such as a compromised

side effects—*effects of a drug that are unwanted and unrelated to its essential purpose.*

Some drugs may have side effects that increase the chance of having accidents. Be sure to find out if the drug you are taking will affect your motor coordination, balance, or vision. Pharmacists are a valuable source of this type of information. Do not be afraid to ask questions.

immune system, damaged organs, and pregnancy. A recent study found that a combination of health problems and the physiological decline that comes with age may make elderly people more apt to have adverse reactions to drugs.[11] Certain OTC antacids contain large amounts of sodium. For most people these drugs pose virtually no risk, but for people with hypertension they can cause medical complications. Other drugs pose little risk except when taken by a pregnant woman; while unlikely to injure the woman, they can cause birth defects. (Drugs that can cause birth defects are said to be potentially **teratogenic.**)

When giving or prescribing *any* drug, especially if there is a possibility of critical or permanent injury, a physician must always take into account the risk-versus-benefit ratio. That is, the physician must weigh the good the drug can provide against any potential threat to the patient.

teratogenic—*pertaining to a drug which, if taken by a pregnant woman, can interfere with the crucial stages of a baby's prenatal development and is thus associated with birth defects.*

allergy—*an acquired overreaction to a specific substance by the immune system. Also called hypersensitivity.*

anaphylactic shock—*a life-threatening allergic reaction in which blood pressure can drop so low that a person dies.*

cross-sensitivity—*a situation in which an allergy to one drug warns the user of possible similar reactions to other, chemically related ones.*

Drug Allergies An **allergy**—also called *hypersensitivity*—is an acquired overreaction to a specific substance by the immune system. Allergies to drugs can produce many reactions, ranging from mild rashes to life-threatening **anaphylactic shock,** in which blood pressure can drop so low that the person dies. Allergy to drugs is not as widespread a problem as is popularly believed, but with some drugs it can represent a major difficulty. This is especially true when a patient has an infection and is allergic to the antibiotic that is known to fight it most effectively. Fortunately, alternative medications are often available. A person who is allergic to the antibiotic drug penicillin, for example, can be given another antibiotic known as erythromycin. In some instances, an allergy to one drug will warn a person of possible similar reactions to other, chemically related drugs; this situation is known as **cross-sensitivity.**

How Drugs Are Administered

There are two fundamental principles of responsible drug use: take the right drug for the specific effect needed or desired and be aware of the other effects the drug can have. Another important principle is that the way a drug is administered can make a big difference in terms of whether it will have the desired effect.

route of administration—*the way a drug is introduced into the body.*

The way a drug enters the body is known as the **route of administration.** Drugs may be swallowed, injected, inhaled, implanted, applied to the skin, or administered through body orifices (as with rectal suppositories). The route of administration can be a crucial factor in a drug's effect. The most common routes of administration are by mouth, by injection, and by inhalation.

Oral Administration Most medicinal drugs are administered orally, or taken by mouth. Drugs designed to be taken orally dissolve in the stomach and mix with the contents of the stomach and small intestine. Thus, they can pass through the walls of the gastrointestinal (GI) tract into the bloodstream, where they are circulated to the rest of the body.

A drug administered orally is absorbed more rapidly if the stomach is empty. Therefore, if rapid absorption is desired, a doctor may direct that the drug be taken before meals. Some drugs, however, tend to irritate the stomach and are best taken when it is cushioned with food. In this case, the drug should be taken *after meals.*

Sometimes drugs cannot be taken orally. Some drugs—such as insulin, the hormone taken regularly by diabetics—are destroyed by digestive juices in the stomach. A person may be so nauseated that he or she cannot keep down anything taken orally. Some people—a small child or an unconscious person, for example—have difficulty swallowing a pill.

Injections A drug that is administered **parenterally** goes into the body in a manner other than through the digestive tract. The most common means of parenteral administration is injection—either **subcutaneously** (under the skin), **intramuscularly** (into a muscle), or **intravenously** (into a vein). Intravenous injection, which places drugs directly into the blood, is the quickest way of getting a drug into the bloodstream; in life-threatening situations this time advantage can be crucial. Another advantage is that the walls of blood vessels are relatively insensitive and can tolerate certain irritating substances better than the stomach can. A disadvantage of intravenous injection is that it requires special equipment and skill and thus should be attempted only by trained medical personnel.

Inhalation Breathing a drug into the lungs allows the drug to be absorbed rapidly into the bloodstream without the paraphernalia required for injections. A drug that is inhaled comes into direct contact with the rich supply of capillaries (tiny blood vessels) in the nose, throat, bronchi, and lungs and is absorbed into the bloodstream through the capillary walls.

Inhalation has disadvantages: dose levels are more difficult to regulate, and certain drugs do not diffuse through the lung tissues to reach the bloodstream. Moreover, the inhalation of some drugs can injure the body and irritate the delicate tissues that line the respiratory system.

parenteral—*pertaining to the introduction of a drug in a manner other than through the digestive tract.*

subcutaneous—*pertaining to the administration of a drug under the skin.*

intramuscular—*pertaining to the injection of a drug into a muscle.*

intravenous—*pertaining to the injection of a drug into a vein.*

The Time-Response Relationship

Another important factor in the effect of a drug is the time-response relationship—how much time it takes for the drug to produce the desired effect and how long that effect will last (Figure 13.3). If there is a possibility of side effects, it is important to know how long it will take for the body to "fend off" the drug by transforming it chemically, excreting it, or both.

Figure 13.3 Routes of administration and time response. The time it takes the body to begin responding to a drug and the time the drug's effect lasts vary with the size of the dose and the route by which the drug is administered. For example, a drug administered intravenously (by injection into a vein) reaches a high level in the bloodstream quite rapidly, and its effects wear off relatively soon; the same drug administered orally takes longer to reach the bloodstream and begin having an effect, and its action lasts longer. A drug is effective when its concentration in the blood is above the threshold level.

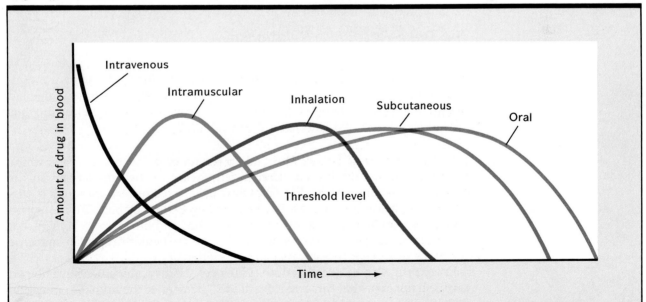

Distribution and Speed of Effect

The movement of drugs through the body is called **pharmacokinetics.** Different drugs have different ways of spreading through the body. Most drugs affect the parts of the body that are the most richly supplied with blood vessels (the brain, heart, liver, and kidneys) before moving on to other internal organs and to the muscles, fat tissue, and skin. Some drugs, however, gravitate toward specific places in the body. Iodine, for example, usually winds up in the thyroid gland.

The speed with which drugs take effect can vary, depending in part on the way a drug is distributed. Some drugs react with the body almost immediately (alcohol moves quickly through the bloodstream to the brain), whereas others act more slowly. The duration of a drug's effect also depends in part on the way in which it is stored in the body. Drugs stored in fat tissues, for example, remain in the body longer than do drugs stored in muscle tissues.

Biotransformation and Duration of Effect

Certain reactions inside the body may chemically alter a drug, or **biotransform** (metabolize) it, so that it is a very different compound by the time it leaves the bloodstream. Some drugs combine with body proteins in the bloodstream; others are broken into smaller chemical components by the liver, kidneys, and GI tract.

A drug that is biotransformed is less likely to linger in the body in active form after it is needed or wanted. Research has shown, for example, that biotransformation leaves heroin, alcohol, amphetamines, and nicotine only a relatively short time to work their effects on the body. Drugs that are not biotransformed are excreted more slowly and can continue to be active in the body for days. For example, small amounts of diazepam (Valium) may remain in the body as long as 8 days. Certain substances, such as marijuana, are actually stored by body tissues and are retained long after absorption.

Excreting Drugs from the Body

Drugs may be eliminated from the body either unchanged or as **metabolites**—the substances they become through biotransformation. The kidneys do most of the work in eliminating drugs and metabolites by excreting them in the urine, but there are other means of excretion, including feces, respiration, tears, sweat, and saliva.

An often overlooked route of excretion is mother's milk. When drugs are taken by a nursing mother, they are often excreted in breast milk, sometimes in concentrated form. Since this can pose a danger to an infant, nursing mothers should take drugs only under medical supervision.

The Dose-Response Relationship

The least amount of a drug needed to produce a particular effect—known as the *threshold dose*—varies from person to person (Figure 13.4). Some tranquilizers, for example, are used in doses of 2 to 50 milligrams; an amount needed to calm a seriously disturbed person would probably make a mildly anxious person feel dazed and extremely drowsy.

Effective Dose and Lethal Dose

As a reference point, doctors refer to the dose that causes the desired effect in 50 percent of the population. This is called the effective dose 50 (ED 50). Obviously, the effective dose for a particular individual is not necessarily the same as ED 50. Depending on factors such as weight, sex, health, overall metabolism, and other drugs being used, one person may need to take more or less of a particular drug than someone else does to receive the same therapeutic effect.

Every drug also has a lethal dose (LD) level. Statistical studies have helped establish the dose that can cause death in 50 percent of the human population (LD 50). This is crucial because doctors need a reasonable margin of safety between the effective dose and the lethal dose. They refer to this safety mar-

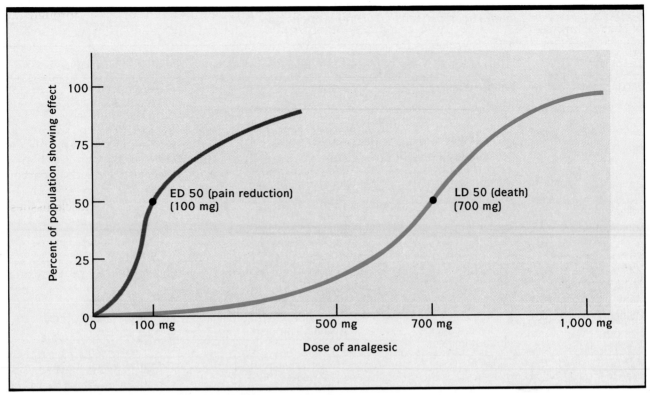

Figure 13.4 The dose-response relationship. The drug in question—for example, an analgesic or pain reliever—has an effective dose 50 of 100 milligrams (that is, a 100-milligram dose effectively reduces pain in 50 percent of the population). Its lethal dose 50 is 700 milligrams. Thus, its therapeutic index, or the margin of safety between the effective dose and the lethal dose, is 700 ÷ 100, or 7.

gin as the **therapeutic index.** Obviously, a drug with a high therapeutic index (a large difference between the effective dose and the lethal dose) is safer than one with a low index.

With many drugs, the potential to cause harm is specifically related to the amount taken; moreover, overdose is less likely to occur with some drugs than it is with others. No one has ever been known to take a lethal overdose of an antibiotic, but many deaths have occurred, accidentally and otherwise, from overdoses of sleeping pills, alcohol, and powerful stimulants such as amphetamines.

Drug Interactions A serious and often unpredictable risk of drug use is interaction between two or more drugs (Table 13.1). An interaction problem occurs when one drug blocks or counteracts the effects of another. For example, an antacid may prevent an antibiotic from effectively battling an infection by decreasing its absorbability.[12]

A second interaction problem concerns increasing side effects: one drug may, by means of its side effects, provide a setting that heightens the side effects of another drug. One effect of aspirin is that it interferes with blood clotting, resulting in an increased tendency to bleed.[13] If alcohol is taken at the same time as aspirin, the effect may be additive; that is, the anticoagulant effect of aspirin may be increased.

A third drug interaction problem is **synergism** (potentiation). When two drugs, both with similar effects, are taken together or in rapid sequence, the end result may be not simply additive but much more extreme: the desired effect of one drug may be made much too powerful by the addition of another. A classic and potentially lethal synergistic combination is that of alcohol with any of a number of sedatives, ranging from mild anxiety-reducing

therapeutic index—*the safety margin between the effective dose of a drug and a lethal dose.*

synergism—*a type of drug interaction in which two drugs taken at the same time or in rapid sequence have more powerful effects than the two drugs would have if taken alone.*

Table 13.1 Possible Interactions between OTC Preparations and Other Drugs

Use of OTC	Ingredient that Causes Interaction	Interacts with	Result
Decongestants	Antihistamines	MAO inhibitors Phenothiazines Alcohol	Hypertensive crisis Increased drowsiness Increased drowsiness
Pain and fever	Asprin Aspirin Acetaminaphen Acetaminaphen Acetaminaphen Acetaminaphen	Anticoagulants Oral antidiabetics Alcohol Anticoagulants Phenobarbital Tetracyclines	Increased effect Increased effect Drowsiness Hidden bleeding Decreased effect Slowed absorption
Indigestion	Magnesium hydroxide	Iron tetracycline	Reduced effect
Constipation	Gut irritants	Oral anticoagulant, by reducing vitamin K absorption	Increased effect
Cough (mixture); sore throat (lozenges)	Iodine	Diagnostic test for thyroid function	Falsely high test results
Many preparations	Sugar	Diabetic therapy	Decreased effect
Multicontent products	Paracetamol, aspirin, codeine, caffeine, antihistamines	Other medications containing the same ingredients	Increased danger of toxic effect

Sources: Jill David, "Do-It-Yourself Medicine, Part 2," *Nursing Times* (February 19, 1981): 329; Griffith, H. Winter, *Complete Guide to Prescription and Non-Prescription Drugs* (Tucson, Ariz.: HP Books, 1985).

drugs such as Valium to barbiturates. All these drugs are in a broad sense depressants, meaning that they relax a person, slow things down, and decrease excitability and anxiety. When combined, such drugs can increase those effects to the point where they do not merely calm but can kill. Many people have died as a result of combining alcohol with sedatives. Even OTC preparations and foods can interact synergistically with other drugs to cause undesirable effects.

The Use of Psychoactive Drugs

Although all drugs can cause problems, the psychoactive drugs have the greatest potential for abuse. These substances affect different structures in the brain that are thought to control mood, consciousness, and behavior (Figure 13.5). As was mentioned earlier in this chapter, two important psychoactive drugs—alcohol and nicotine—are associated with such pervasive problems that separate chapters have been devoted to them. Among the remaining types of psychoactive drugs, some are prescription medications subject to abuse by patients or others who obtain them legally, and some are illegally marketed versions of those drugs. Others are strictly "street drugs" that are not used medically; their sale and use are wholly outside the law (Table 13.2 on page 352).

Two groups of psychoactive prescription drugs will not be examined in this chapter simply because they have not posed a problem in terms of abuse. One group consists of clinical antipsychotics, which are powerful drugs used primarily to treat acute emotional and mental problems. The other group consists of clinical antidepressants; these drugs have also proved useful in treating psychoses and acute emotional difficulties but do not produce the type of stimulation that invites recreational use.

The groups of psychoactive drugs to be discussed in this chapter are sedatives/hypnotics, stimulants including cocaine, marijuana, volatile solvents, opiate narcotics, and psychedelics/hallucinogens (Table 13.3 on pages 354–5).

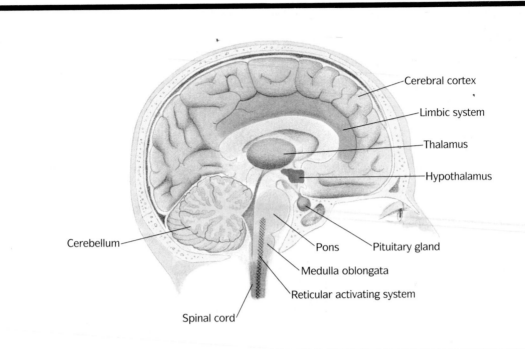

Cerebral cortex

Limbic system

Thalamus

Hypothalamus

Pituitary gland

Pons

Medulla oblongata

Reticular activating system

Cerebellum

Spinal cord

Brain Structure	Function	Drug Effects
1. Medulla oblongata	Monitors respiration and cardiac activity	Alcohol, analgesics, and sedatives/hypnotics can cause cardiovascular or respiratory failure
2. Reticular activating system (RAS)	Alerts brain to stimuli or blocks out certain stimuli; activates other parts of the brain	Sedatives/hypnotics dampen RAS activity, and stimulants overcome RAS underactivity; psychedelics distort perception and stimuli interpretation; PCP may prevent stimuli from different parts of the body from being correctly processed by the brain
3. Cerebellum	Controls the senses, motor coordination, balance, and agility	Alcohol and sedatives/hypnotics can produce uncoordinated movements and impair sensory perception, hearing, smell, taste, and touch; psychedelics can evoke vision distortion and alter time and space perception; marijuana can cause disoriented behavior
4. Thalamus	Communication center; directs messages to and from brain	Alcohol and sedatives/hypnotics can cause slurred speech and distortion of communication patterns; psychedelics can disrupt the transmission of impulses controlling cognitive, sensory, and motor functions
5. Hypothalamus	Control center for autonomic nervous system; regulates hormone production, temperature, fluid balance, feelings of hunger and fullness, thirst, pleasure, pain	Analgesics and sedatives/hypnotics can alter the pleasure-pain response; marijuana may affect testosterone production and feelings of hunger and fullness
6. Cerebral cortex	Controls learning, memory, thinking, integration of sensory impressions, inhibitions and emotions, time and space orientation, vision and hearing, speech and motor skills	Volatile solvents alter thought processes and behaviors; alcohol dulls discrimination, memory, concentration, and insight and disrupts motor processes while causing quick mood shifts; long-term marijuana use has been linked to apathy, disturbed self-awareness, and confusion; LSD may cause perceptual alterations and in large doses can produce paranoia and other psychotic reactions; PCP often induces psychosis, coma, or a comatose state
7. Limbic system	Connects cerebral cortex, thalamus and hypothalamus; involved with emotions and short-term memory	Antianxiety drugs alter physiological responses to emotions; opiates affect memory, spatial orientation, and emotions

Figure 13.5 Different structures of the brain are affected by different drugs. This view through the middle of the brain shows the major structures which drugs may affect.

Table 13.2 Schedules of Psychoactive Drugs under the Federal Controlled Substances Act

Schedule[a]	Types of Drugs and Examples	Comments
I	Certain opium derivatives and opiates (heroin) Some psychedelics/hallucinogens (LSD, mescaline, psilocybin, PCP, STP) Marijuana, THC	High potential for abuse; no currently accepted medical use; psychedelics/hallucinogens included in Schedule I purely for regulatory purposes
II	Opium Coca leaf derivatives (cocaine) Class A narcotics (methadone, morphine) Amphetamines	High potential for abuse and severe physical and psychological dependence; have currently accepted medical uses; must be dispensed only on written prescription (except in emergencies) and may not be refilled without new written prescription
III	Short-acting barbiturates (Nembutal, Seconal) Class B narcotics (Empirin, codeine preparations) Paregoric	Less potential for abuse than drugs in Schedules I and II but may lead to moderate physical and psychological dependence; may be dispensed on either oral or written prescription but may not be refilled more than five times or more than 6 months after date
IV	Certain major tranquilizers, antianxiety drugs, and long-lasting barbiturates (barbital, phenobarbital, chloral hydrate, meprobamate)	Lower potential for abuse and more limited physical and psychological dependence than drugs in Schedule III; may be dispensed on either oral or written prescription but may not be refilled more than five times or more than 6 months after date
V	Exempt OTC narcotic preparations, usually for treatment of coughs and diarrhea	Lower potential for abuse and more limited physical and psychological dependence than drugs in Schedule IV

[a] The federal government places drugs in schedules, or classes, on the basis of their degree of abuse potential and risk for psychological or physical dependence. In general, the lower a drug's schedule number, the more severe the penalties for possession or sale. No drug listed in Schedule I has a currently accepted medical use in the United States, although marijuana is currently being used on an experimental basis in 16 states; the drugs in all the other schedules do have accepted medical uses, so the criteria for classifying drugs into the other schedules are relative to one another.

Source: Adapted from Brent Q. Hafen and Brenda Peterson, *Medicines and Drugs: Problems and Risks, Use and Abuse*, 2d ed. (Philadelphia: Lea & Febiger, 1978): 206–207.

Sedatives/Hypnotics

sedatives/hypnotics—*drugs that have both sedative (calming) and hypnotic (sleep-inducing) effects.*

The **sedatives/hypnotics** are drugs that have either sedative (calming) or hypnotic (sleep-inducing) effects; the difference between these effects is just a matter of dosage. Technically, these drugs, more commonly known as "downers," are depressants—they slow the activity of the central nervous system. This group of drugs includes barbiturates and anxiolytics (antianxiety drugs).

barbiturates—*sedative/ hypnotic drugs that are used primarily to treat insomnia and, less often, for daytime sedation; some also have anticonvulsant properties.*

Barbiturates The **barbiturates** range from short-acting drugs with effects lasting less than 6 hours—such as amobarbital (Amytal), pentobarbital (Nembutal), secobarbital (Seconal), and Tuinal (a combination of amobarbital and secobarbital)—to longer-acting ones such as butabarbital (Butisol) and even longer-acting ones such as phenobarbital (Luminal) whose effects may persist up to 24 hours. The barbiturates are used primarily to treat insomnia or, less often, for daytime sedation; certain barbiturates also have anticonvulsant properties.

anxiolytics—*sedative/ hypnotic drugs used to reduce anxiety; some are also used as muscle relaxants and to control certain types of convulsive seizures.*

Antianxiety Drugs The **anxiolytics,** or relaxants, include meprobamate (Equanil and Miltown), hydroxyzine (Atarax), and many others. A number of the anxiolytics—chlordiazepoxide (Librium), diazepam (Valium), chlorazepane (Tranzene), oxazepam (Serax), alprazolan (Xanax), and triazolam (Halcion)—are in a chemical group called the benzodiazepines. Anxiolytics are widely used to reduce anxiety. Some have muscle-relaxant

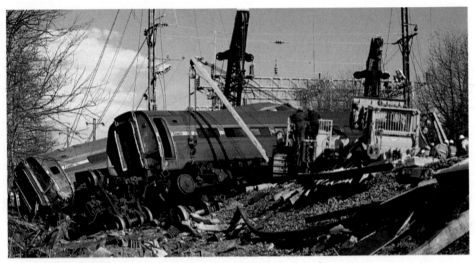

Drug abuse has led to major transportation accidents even though there are strict laws intended to prevent such occurrences. (Marty Katz/Gamma-Liaison)

properties as well, and a few have proved useful in controlling specific types of convulsive seizures.

Potential Risks A variety of side effects may occur with sedatives/hypnotics, including hangovers, nausea, headaches, dizziness, and drowsiness; users may be at risk for accidents at home, at work, and while driving. Furthermore, these drugs are all potential killers through overdose. According to the National Institute on Drug Abuse, sedatives/hypnotics are involved in 18 percent of all drug-related visits to hospital emergency rooms and 30 percent of all drug-related deaths.[14]

A special danger exists with the synergistic interaction of these drugs—the concurrent use of one sedative/hypnotic with another or with a different type of depressant. In fact, aside from the problem of dependence, the most serious danger with sedatives/hypnotics is combining the drug with another depressant—especially alcohol. Young people have been known to combine sedatives/hypnotics with alcohol to achieve heightened intoxication. The depressant effects of both drugs on the central nervous system can act synergistically to cause critical conditions, including coma and death. People taking these drugs should be aware of the lethal potential for synergistic action and should heed warnings about not drinking while taking them.

Another risk with sedatives/hypnotics is the potential for dependence. The daily use of 500 milligrams or more of barbiturates or equivalent doses of other sedatives/hypnotics usually produces classic physical dependence. Users can rapidly develop a tolerance for up to 15 times the normal dose.[15]

The withdrawal symptoms experienced by people dependent on these drugs are very severe. These symptoms begin with nervousness, trembling, and weakness. If they are not treated, the users of these drugs can suffer epileptic-like seizures or a toxic psychosis with delusions and hallucinations and can lose consciousness. The most severe symptoms of untreated withdrawal last about 4 days *and can be fatal.* If a pregnant woman is dependent on sedatives/hypnotics, her baby will have to suffer through the withdrawal syndrome shortly after birth.

Stimulants

The most widely used stimulant in the United States is caffeine. Drinking large amounts of beverages that contain caffeine, such as coffee and cola, *can* cause harm. Two other kinds of stimulants—amphetamines and cocaine—can be extremely dangerous.

Table 13.3 Comparison Chart of the Major Psychoactive Drugs

Name of Drug or Chemical	Schedule	Trade or Other Name	Medical Uses	Physical Dependence
Opiate Narcotics				
Opium	II, III, V	Dover's Powder, paregoric, parepectolin	Analgesic, antidiarrheal	High
Morphine	II, III	Morphine, pectoral syrup	Analgesic, antitussive	
Codeine	II, III, V	Codeine, Empirin Compound with Codeine, Robitussin A-C	Analgesic, antitussive	Moderate
Heroin	I	Diacetylmorphine, horse, smack	Terminal cancer and analgesic (Canada)	
Hydromorphone	II	Dialudid	Analgesic	High
Meperidine		Demerol, Pathadol	Analgesic	
Methadone		Dolophine, methadose	Analgesic, heroin substitute	
Other narcotics	I, II, III, IV, V	LAAM, Leritine, Levo-Dromoran, Percodan, Tussionex fentanyl, Darvon, Talwin, Lomotil	Analgesic, antidiarrheal, antitussive	High-low
Sedatives/hypnotics				
Chloral hydrate	IV	Noctec, Somnos	Hypnotic	Moderate
Barbiturates	II, III, IV	Amobarbital, phenobarbital, Butisol, Luminal, secobarbital, Tuinal, Nembutal	Anesthetic, anticonvulsant, sedative, hypnotic	High-moderate
Glutethimide	III	Doriden	Sedative, hypnotic	High
Methaqualone (no longer manufactured in U.S.A.)	II	Optimil, Parest, Quaalude, Somnafac, Sopor		
Benzodiazepines	IV	Ativan, triazotam, diazepam, Librium, Serax, Tranxene, Valium, chlorazepane	Antianxiety, anticonvulsant, sedative, hypnotic	Low
Other sedatives/hypnotics	III, IV	Equanil, Miltown, Noludar, Placidyl, Valmid	Antianxiety, sedative, hypnotic	Moderate
Stimulants				
Cocaine	II	Coke, flake, snow, crack	Local anesthetic	Possible
Amphetamines	II, III	Benzedrine, Dexedrine, methamphetamine, Desoxyn, Mediatric, ice	Hyperkinesis in children, narcolepsy, short-term weight control	
Phenmetrazine	II	Preludin		
Methylphenidate		Ritalin		
Other stimulants	III, IV	Adipex, caffeine, Didrex, Ionamin, Plegine, Prolamine, Dexatrim Tenuate, Tepanil, Voranil, Theophylline		
Psychedelics/hallucinogens				
LSD	I	Acid, microdot	None	None
Mescaline		Mesc, buttons, peyote, mushroom	None	
Psilocybin				
Amphetamine variants		2,5-DMA, PMA, STP, DMT, MDA, TMA, DOM, DOB, MMDA, MDMA		Unknown
Phencyclidine		PCP, angel dust, hog	Veterinary anesthetic	Degree unknown
Phencyclidine analogs		PCE, PCPy, TCP	None	
Other psychedelics/hallucinogens		Bufotenine, ibogaine, DET, psilocyn		None
Cannabis				
Marijuana	II	Pot, Acapulco gold, grass, reefer, weed, sinsemilla, Thai Sticks	Nausea of cancer chemotherapy, glaucoma treatment (under investigation)	Degree uncertain
Tetrahydrocannabinol		THC		
Hashish		Hash	None	
Hashish oil		Hash oil		
Volatile solvents				
Glue, gasoline, paint thinner, cleaning and lighter fluids, aerosols	None	Plastic model cement, hydrocarbons, Toluene, acetone, naphtha	None	Unknown
Nitrous oxide		"Laughing gas"	General anesthetic	
Amyl nitrite		Locker room, Rush	Angina pectoris	
Butyl nitrite			None	

Table 13.3 Comparison Chart of the Major Psychoactive Drugs (continued)

Psychological Dependence	Tolerance	Duration of Effects (hours)	Usual Methods of Administration	Possible Effects	Effects of Overdose or Long-Term Use	Withdrawal Syndrome
High			Oral, smoked	Euphoria, drowsiness, respiratory depression, constricted pupils, nausea	Slow and shallow breathing, clammy skin, convulsions, coma, possible death	Watery eyes, runny nose, yawning, loss of appetite, irritability, tremors, panic, chills and sweating, cramps, nausea
Moderate			Oral, injected			
High	Yes	3–6	Injected, sniffed, smoked			
		12–24				
High-low		Variable	Oral, injected			
Moderate	Possible	5–8	Oral	Hangovers, headaches, nausea, slurred speech, disorientation, drunken behavior without odor of alcohol, subject to accidents	Shallow respiration, cold and clammy skin, dilated pupils, weak and rapid pulse, coma, possible death; suppressed immune system could worsen AIDS-related diseases	Anxiety, insomnia, tremors, delirium, convulsions, possible death
High-moderate		1–16	Oral, injected			
High	Yes	4–8				
Low						
Moderate						
	Yes	1–2	Sniffed, injected	Increased alertness, excitation, euphoria, increased pulse rate and blood pressure, insomnia, loss of appetite	Agitation, increase in body temperature, hallucinations, convulsions, psychosis, sexual dysfunction, possible death	Apathy, long periods of sleep, irritability, depression, disorientation
High			Oral, injected			
	Yes	2–4	Oral			
Degree unknown	Yes	8–12	Oral	Illusions and hallucinations, poor perception of time and distance, severe panic, synesthesia	Longer, more intense "trip" episodes, psychosis, possible death	Withdrawal syndrome not reported
			Oral, injected			
		Up to days	Oral, injected,			
High			Oral, injected, smoked			
Degree unknown	Possible	Variable	Oral, injected, smoked, sniffed			
Moderate	Yes	2–4	Smoked, oral	Euphoria, relaxed inhibitions, increased appetite, distorted time perception, muscular weakness	Fatigue, paranoia, possible psychosis, sensory distortion, negative effect on reproductive system, respiratory damage, reduction in antibacterial defenses	Insomnia, hyperactivity, and decreased appetite occasionally reported
	Possible	1–2		Loss of muscle coordination, euphoria, confusion, disorientation	Organic brain syndrome, nerve damage, liver and kidney disease, possible death	Withdrawal syndrome not reported
Minimal to moderate	Not known		Sniffed	Euphoria, shortness of breath, nausea	Bone marrow and nerve damage, hearing loss, severe anemia	
	Yes	1		Euphoria, headache, dizziness, perspiration, nausea, fainting, vasodilation	Cardiac arrhythmias, organic brain syndrome	

Source: National Institute on Drug Abuse, adapted from *Health Management: Promotion and Self-Care* (Englewood, Colo.: Morton, 1982): 162–163; (inhalants) Annabel Hecht, "Inhalants: Quick Route to Danger," *FDA Consumer* (May 1980): 19–22.

Basically, **stimulants** rev up the neural network known as the sympathetic nervous system, the part of the autonomic nervous system that prepares the body to cope with stress in what is known as the fight-or-flight response (Chapter 2). Stimulants mobilize this mechanism inappropriately, when it may not be needed. While caffeine does this on a relatively low level, more powerful stimulants do so on a larger scale which may endanger rather than protect the body.

Caffeine Few people realize how potent caffeine is or how fast it can act. In less than 5 minutes after one drinks a cup of coffee, caffeine has raced to every part of the body: it increases the flow of urine and stomach acid, relaxes involuntary muscles, steps up the intake of oxygen, and speeds the basal metabolic rate. It also increases the pumping strength of the heart, but too much caffeine can lead to an irregular heartbeat. Although caffeine sometimes improves a user's physical coordination, it can also hinder a person's efforts by making it far more difficult to perform a painstaking task that requires a steady hand and accurate timing.

Amphetamines The **amphetamines,** sometimes known as pep pills or uppers, are synthetic drugs that include amphetamine (Benzedrine, or "bennies"), dextroamphetamine (Dexedrine, or "dexies"), and methamphetamine (Methedrine, or "meth" or "speed"). The word *speed* is often used to refer to this group of drugs.

People have been using and misusing amphetamines since they were introduced 50 years ago. Amphetamines have some legimate medical uses: to treat an extremely rare condition called *narcolepsy* (an uncontrollable need for short periods of deep sleep) and to treat *hyperkinetic* (uncontrollably overactive) children. Interestingly, the effects of amphetamines are paradoxical in hyperkinetic children: they seem to calm these children rather than stimulate them.

In addition to those uses, some amphetamines have been combined with others or with barbiturates or tranquilizers in a variety of products aimed at achieving weight control. (Prominent OTC brands include Anorexin, Appedrine, Dex-A-Diet II, Dexatrim, Pro-Dax, and Prolamine.) It is unwise to use amphetamines as an appetite suppressant. After 2 to 4 weeks they are no longer effective, and the risks are hardly worth it—many people dependent on amphetamines started out by using them as weight-loss aids.

Recently a new form of methamphetamine has become available on the illegal drug market. Called "ice," "glass," "freeze," or "quartz," it looks like rock candy and is inhaled after being heated in a glass pipe. The immediate result is a lengthy high with euphoria and feelings of alertness and confidence, but the withdrawal causes an intense depression, and irritability and insomnia are also frequent effects. More serious psychotic effects have also occurred.

Potential Risks People can become physically dependent on both caffeine and amphetamines, and these drugs pose other risks as well. For most people, 400 milligrams of caffeine (about three to four cups of coffee) can cause irritability, headaches, tremors, and nervousness. Double that amount can cause hallucinations and perhaps even convulsions. The fatal dose of caffeine is about 10 grams, but to ingest that much would require drinking 67 to 100 cups of coffee in a brief sitting.[16] People who drink at least five cups of coffee a day can suffer several days of withdrawal symptoms—including nausea, headaches, irritability, and lassitude—when they kick the habit. People who drink a lot of coffee regularly can experience "caffeinism," a syndrome characterized by rapid breathing, heart palpitations, agitation, and mood changes.

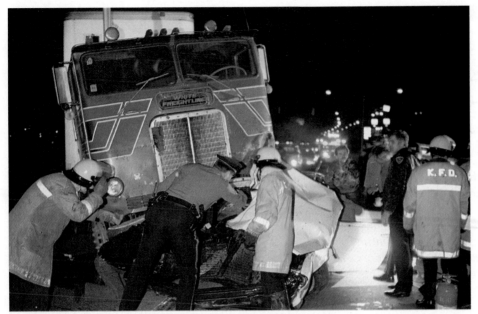

There is a limit to how long amphetamines can keep a person awake; abusing that limit can result in injury or death. (Kenneth Murray/Photo Researchers, Inc.)

Caffeine may pose other dangers as well. Studies have linked it to heart disease, benign and malignant tumors, pancreatic cancer, and birth defects; other studies, however, have refuted these links.[17] Nevertheless, it is a good idea for pregnant women to avoid caffeine as they would avoid any other drug. Recently, there has been increased concern about children who get too much caffeine. Even one cola drink gives an 8-year-old a hefty jolt of the drug, and many children consume much more than that every day.

Amphetamines often bring on unwanted side effects such as nervousness, elevated blood pressure, and headache with just one small dose. If the drug is used on a single occasion (to help a student study for an exam, for example), there may be no further detrimental effects. (It should be noted that amphetamines do *not* improve intellectual functioning, and knowledge gained while using the drug may well be lost after the drug wears off.) However, if the drug is taken in a situation that is inherently risky, such as by a trucker traveling a superhighway, there is an additional peril. The effects of amphetamine often cease abruptly and unpredictably, and sleep or even death can be the result in such circumstances.[18]

In large doses or over prolonged periods, amphetamines have unpredictable effects, including insomnia, dizziness, agitation, confusion, delirium, and malnutrition. A user may develop wildly exaggerated feelings of confidence and power which can lead to errors of judgment such as crossing a busy intersection without taking proper precautions. For some people, prolonged use of amphetamines can lead to psychosis. For example, ice has caused hallucinations, paranoia, and violent behavior. In other instances the elevated blood pressure caused by continued amphetamine use can put a strain on blood vessels. Intravenous use of amphetamines can lead to death from ruptured blood vessels such as in a stroke.

As a rule, amphetamines are not used recreationally. They tend to be taken by individuals who want them or think they need them rather than shared in social situations. Thus, the first two levels of drug dependence—experimental use and recreational use—are often omitted. Individuals may proceed fairly quickly to situational, intensified, and compulsive use. Once they are into this pattern, users may find that they need increased amounts of the drug. Tolerance does develop, and psychic dependence is strong.[19] Al-

Other than caffeine and nicotine, amphetamines are the most widely used stimulants in the United States.

Should Drugs Be Legalized?

One of the most intractable problems in the United States in the late twentieth century is the widespread use of illegal drugs. Drug use is largely responsible for the epidemic of violent crime that has swept through the cities and for the spread of AIDS and other serious diseases. By the early 1990s the problem had become so serious that for the first time, serious discussion of legalizing drugs began to enter the public debate, not only among extreme liberals and members of the counterculture but also among conservatives and mainstream politicians. Following are the arguments often propounded on both sides of the legalization debate.

Pro-Legalization: Weighing the Costs of Drug Use For over 100 years this society has made the use of certain drugs illegal and has penalized illegal drug use. But during that time the use of marijuana, heroin and other opiates, and cocaine has become an epidemic into which Americans have poured countless dollars in law enforcement resources. Most recently, Americans have spent billions on arresting and imprisoning sellers and importers of crack cocaine, with almost no effect on the supply or street price of the drug.

The societal costs of illegal drugs are immense. They include the costs of law enforcement, criminal proceedings against those arrested, and jails and prisons. They also include the spread of deadly diseases such as AIDS and hepatitis through the use of shared needles; the cost to society of raising "crack babies," children poisoned by drugs even before birth; and the cost of raising a generation of young people who see illegal drug selling and violence as their only escape from poverty and desperation. Finally, the societal costs include the emotional cost of the violence that no one in this society can now escape.

Legalizing drug use in this country would eliminate many of these costs. Billions of dollars would be saved on interdiction, law enforcement, trials, and prisons. This money could be spent on treatment of addicts, job training, and education programs to help disadvantaged young people assume valuable roles in society. Using the model already in place for alcohol and cigarettes, the government could make drug use legal for adults but impose severe penalties on anyone who sells drugs to young people. Drug sales could be heavily taxed, thus deterring drug purchases and giving society as a whole the

though the potential for physical dependence is not as great as with sedatives/hypnotics and opiate narcotics, there is often *some* degree of physical dependence as evidenced by depression, an increased appetite, and an increased need for sleep when the drug is stopped.

Cocaine

cocaine—a stimulant drug extracted from the leaves of the South American coca bush.

Among the most popular illicit drugs in use today, **cocaine** may also be the most dangerous.[20] Extracted from the leaves of the South American coca plant, cocaine is a stimulant closely related to caffeine, although it is much more potent. Cocaine initially decreases appetite and produces feelings of well-being, confidence, and alertness that last 20 to 90 minutes, depending on the form in which the drug is taken.[21] As these effects wear off, users experience feelings of anxiety which can last several hours.

The National Institute on Drug Abuse estimates that there are 2 million cocaine addicts in the United States, about four times the number of heroin addicts.

Uses of Cocaine Medically, cocaine is used as a local anesthetic in certain types of surgery; it numbs tissues and constricts blood vessels, helping to reduce bleeding. Recreationally, cocaine is inhaled ("snorted") through the nostrils, injected, or smoked. Cocaine users inhale a powdery form of the drug, cocaine hydrochloride, commonly known as coke, blow, toot, or flake. This powder can also be mixed with water and injected; this causes a faster

additional benefit of tax revenues that could be used for drug treatment and education. Instead of throwing away billions of dollars on ineffective law enforcement efforts, money could be spent on the real cause of the drug problem—the social conditions that give rise to the drug culture.

Anti-Legalization: Providing a Positive Role Model Drugs are illegal because they are dangerous and deadly and provide no societal value. To make their possession or use legal would send a message to young people that using drugs is acceptable and that drugs are not treacherous or life-destroying. It would tell 8-year-olds in the ghetto who are being recruited to work for drug sellers that dealing drugs is okay and that society condones it.

Making drugs illegal has not increased the number of drug users or sellers, just as making alcohol legal after Prohibition did not reduce the number of people who drink. Recent law enforcement efforts have indeed made a difference. Over the past few years, as law enforcement efforts have sent more and more people to jail, the number of young people who use illegal drugs has steadily

declined. Furthermore, education about the ill effects of drug use has begun to deter people from buying and using illegal drugs.

Recently, the incidence of drug-related deaths and violence has begun to level off even in the areas of the most hard-core drug use. This is proof that strict law enforcement is working. This country has begun to turn the corner on this drug epidemic, and Americans will soon see real fruits for the money they have been spending on the war on drugs.

Which position do you favor? Do you think that legalizing drug use in this country would eliminate the societal costs of illegal drugs? Are recent law enforcement efforts ineffective, or are they making a difference so that the number of young people using illegal drugs is declining? Would legalizing drugs simply send a message to young people that using drugs is acceptable?

Based on information from *Atlantic Monthly* (November 1990); Richard Schlaad and Peter Shannon, *Drugs of Choice: Current Perspectives on Drug Use,* 2d ed. (Englewood Cliffs, N.J.: Prentice-Hall, 1982).

high. Some users seek more intense highs by injecting cocaine with heroin, an extremely dangerous combination known as a speedball.

Cocaine users also smoke a form of cocaine known as freebase or a form known as crack. Smoking the drug produces a quicker high than does snorting or injecting it, although the high is shorter-lived.[22] While cocaine hydrochloride is only 20 to 50 percent pure, freebase cocaine is nearly 100 percent pure, and so the smoker gets an extremely concentrated dose of the drug. Crack, a "rock" form of the drug, is 25 to 90 percent pure freebase cocaine. The introduction of prepackaged crack pellets has increased the availability of cocaine to lower-income people and adolescents because of the lower cost.[23]

Once inhaled, crack reaches the brain in as little as 8 seconds and provides about 10 minutes of euphoria. The drug is highly addictive because this short high is followed by an intense depression, making multiple doses seem necessary.

Potential Risks According to the National Institute on Drug Abuse, cocaine is the illicit drug that currently poses the greatest threat to public health in the United States. It has been estimated that 2 million people are addicted to cocaine—about four times as many as are addicted to heroin.[24]

Although it was once thought that cocaine use does not lead to dependence, animal experiments have demonstrated its addictiveness. In these experiments, monkeys that were allowed unlimited access to cocaine continued ingesting the drug until they died from exhaustion and malnutrition. This type of behavior is reflected in human users, who often pursue the drug without regard for their own health, safety, or welfare.[25] Although reliable

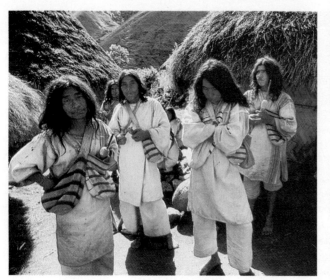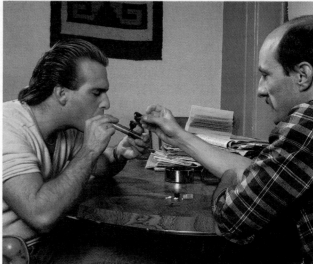

Coca leaves produce a numbing effect when they are chewed, but when the leaves are refined into cocaine powder and then inhaled, the effect is dangerously enhanced. (Jose Azel/Contact Stock; James Prince/Photo Researchers, Inc.)

data have not been accumulated, most experts believe that crack is very addicting and that addiction may occur after relatively few experiences with the drug.[26]

Cocaine has been implicated in cardiovascular problems, including heart attacks and abnormal heart beat *(arrhythmia),* and in pulmonary problems and strokes.[27] Regular use of cocaine can lead to tolerance and dependence and is often accompanied by increased anxiety and depression, paranoid delusions, and malnutrition.[28] While cocaine may produce heightened sexual performance at first, long-term use can cause sexual dysfunction in both men and women.[29] Heavy, prolonged use of cocaine can also produce tremors and convulsions as a result of loss of motor coordination. Repeated inhalation of cocaine can cause the mucous membranes in the nostrils to atrophy and in rare instances can lead to perforation of the nasal septum (the membrane between the nostrils).[30] Yet another danger associated with cocaine and other illicit drugs is related to the purity of the drug. Users can never be sure about what they are buying and what additives have been used.

Pregnant women who use cocaine are at higher risk for having miscarriages and premature deliveries than are women who do not use the drug. Moreover, babies born to users are likely to show signs of underdevelopment, including short bodies, lower birth weights, and small heads, along with neurological impairment. Cocaine use by pregnant women has been linked with other birth defects, including malformations of the heart, skull, and genitourinary tract. The babies of users may also be at greater risk for developing sudden infant death syndrome (SIDS).[31]

Marijuana

marijuana—*material from* **Cannabis sativa** *(the hemp plant); it is dried and prepared for smoking and has a variety of mind-altering and physiological effects.*

hashish—*a concentrated and potent resin of* **Cannabis sativa** *(the hemp plant).*

Marijuana—also called pot or grass—is the third most popular recreational drug in the United States (after alcohol and nicotine) and is possibly the most widely used of all controlled substances. *Cannabis sativa* (the botanical name for the hemp plant) is the source of **marijuana** and **hashish,** a concentrated and more potent resin from the plant. The chief psychoactive ingredient in *Cannabis sativa* is *delta-9 tetrahydrocannabinol (THC);* the amount of this chemical in a given quantity of marijuana determines its potency.

Cannabis has a 5,000-year history of medical use, mostly as an analgesic, or pain reliever. Largely superseded by aspirin and other pain-relieving drugs for that purpose, cannabis nevertheless appears to have a therapeutic potential for treating glaucoma and the GI side effects of cancer chemotherapy.

Short-Term and Long-Term Effects

When it is taken in average doses, the effects of marijuana are not much different from those of moderate quantities of alcohol, with the addition of distortion of time perception, an increase in heart rate, dilation of blood vessels in the eyes, increased appetite and thirst, and some muscular weakness. These effects can last as long as 8 hours.[32]

Other effects vary with the individual and the setting and may sometimes be like those of a mild sedative or, conversely, a mild stimulant. Marijuana may also intensify the effects of alcohol, caffeine, and barbiturates.[33] A marijuana user who is emotionally unstable may react in an exaggerated manner in almost any direction, including severe panic or paranoia, as may a user who is anxious or under stress.[34] Higher doses may bring on significant sensory distortion. The ability to think clearly and learn is usually reduced by marijuana, as are short-term memory and psychomotor performance.

While long-term marijuana users can develop a tolerance to the drug, the reverse also occurs: an experienced user may require less of the drug to experience its effects. Although the risk of physical dependence is probably insignificant, psychic dependence is entirely possible.

Potential Risks

Short-term marijuana use can endanger individuals in situations that require fully functioning perceptual ability and motor coordination, such as driving. In one study subjects who had used marijuana were unable to make the swift decisions that are sometimes necessary in driving,[35] and another study found that drivers' perceptions and motor coordination were hindered if they were under the influence of this drug.[36] The combination of marijuana and alcohol can be especially hazardous when one is driving.

With long-term use, the major risk of marijuana is respiratory damage. Like tobacco, marijuana may decrease the efficiency of the lungs. There is also evidence that marijuana smoke impairs antibacterial defense systems within the lungs, posing an increased risk of developing an infection.[37] Although there is no direct proof that marijuana smoking is correlated with lung cancer, cannabis smoke residuals (like the "tar" in tobacco smoke) have been found to produce tumors in experimental animals. Benzopyrene, a known cancer-causing chemical in tobacco smoke, is found at higher levels in marijuana smoke.

Another serious concern with long-term marijuana use is its effect on the reproductive system, notably because of its proven impact on the secretion of certain hormones. A number of studies have found lowered testosterone levels in men who are heavy marijuana smokers, along with two abnormalities in the structure, count, and motility of sperm. It is believed that these effects are reversible when the drug is discontinued.[38] In women, marijuana use has been associated with disruption of the menstrual cycle and possibly with miscarriage.[39] Since harmful effects on fetal development are known to occur with alcohol and are suspected with other drugs, the use of marijuana during pregnancy probably poses additional risks. One study reported a significant reduction in the birth weight of babies whose mothers used marijuana.[40] Some experts also question the potential impact on the development of various systems, such as the reproductive system, in a developing fetus.

A third concern with marijuana use is its impact on a person's mind. Although a wide variety of psychotic phenomena—delusional thinking, paranoia, and visual and auditory hallucinations—have been attributed to the use of cannabis, it is unclear whether the drug causes these problems or precipitates an underlying predisposition to them.[41] It has also been suggested that long-term marijuana use leads to decreased drive and ambition, loss of motivation, apathy, inactivity, self-neglect, and lack of concern about the future.

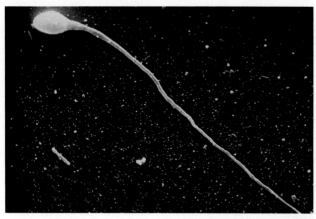 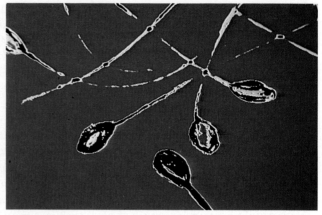

Normal sperm have a vibrant, healthy appearance, whereas the sperm of marijuana users (on right) appear stunted and lack vitality. (Dr. G. Schatten/SPL/Photo Researchers, Inc.; Howard Sochurek/Medical Images, Inc.)

Studies have failed to prove such a connection; instead, it has been suggested that such personality features are due to preexisting traits or to sociocultural factors.[42]

Volatile Solvents

inhalants—*a group of substances containing volatile chemical solvents that have psychoactive and other effects when breathed into the lungs.*

Substances containing volatile chemical solvents that have psychoactive and other effects when breathed into the lungs are called **inhalants**. Substances that have been inhaled for a quick high include gasoline, furniture polish, insecticides, transmission fluid, paint thinners, aerosols, cleaning and lighter fluids, and model airplane glue. All these substances can damage vital organs such as the lungs, kidneys, liver, and brain and can cause death.

Nitrous Oxide Used by dentists as an anesthetic since the 1840s, nitrous oxide (laughing gas) is among the least toxic inhalants. Death can occur, however, if it is inhaled with insufficient oxygen. Furthermore, repeated long-term use can result in nerve damage, muscle weakness, hearing loss, changes in heart rate, impotence, and life-threatening anemia. A study of 60,000 dental workers found that their exposure to nitrous oxide increased the rates of miscarriage, birth defects in the children of both male and female workers, and the incidence of certain types of cancers.[43]

amyl nitrite—*a prescription drug used to treat angina; it sometimes is used recreationally as a euphoriant and sexual stimulant.*

butyl nitrite—*an analogue of amyl nitrite that is used recreationally as a euphoriant and presumed sexual stimulant.*

Amyl Nitrite and Butyl Nitrite **Amyl nitrite** is a prescription drug used to treat angina (severe chest pain due to insufficient blood and oxygen supply to the heart). Its analogue **butyl nitrite** has never been used medically to any significant extent. Both drugs have been used recreationally as euphoriants and sexual stimulants. A related substance, isobutyl alcohol, produces similar but less powerful effects than those of butyl nitrite.

The immediate effects of nitrite inhalation include headache, dizziness, flushing, muscle relaxation, heightened heart rate, and lowered blood pressure, with possible nausea, vomiting, and fainting. These effects may be especially dangerous for people with low blood pressure or glaucoma. Users can develop tolerance to nitrites, although physical dependence has not been reported. Inhaling substantial amounts over time can lead to a condition called methemoglobinemia, in which normal hemoglobin has been chemically converted and can no longer carry oxygen. There is also a long-term risk of developing heart and blood vessel damage.[44]

Nitrite use may also be related to the development of opportunistic infections associated with AIDS, such as *pneumocystis carinii* (Chapter 12). A study of homosexual men with Kaposi's sarcoma—a rare cancer of the connective tissues associated with AIDS—found that almost every patient had a prior history of nitrite use. It is generally thought that the drug contributes to suppression of the immune system, increasing the risk of contracting an opportunistic disease.[45]

Opiate Narcotics

The word *narcotic* comes from the Greek word *narkoun*, meaning "to make numb." The opiate narcotics do indeed make the user numb in both mind and body (Figure 13.6). They act as an analgesic on the central nervous system, relieving pain without causing a loss of consciousness. They also have a strong potential to create physical and psychological dependence.

The **opiate narcotics** include the **opiates**—opium, morphine, and heroin—and the **opioids**—a group of synthetic drugs, such as methadone and meperidine, that are chemically similar to the opiates. **Opium,** the parent substance, comes from the opium poppy, which is native to Asia Minor; its active ingredient is **morphine. Heroin,** a derivative of morphine, is more than twice as potent as morphine.

A recent variant of heroin is "tango and cash," which combines heroin with a tranquilizer. A dangerous synergistic effect results, which caused several deaths during the first months that the drug was out on the street.

Medical Uses The opiate narcotics are useful medically to relieve pain, control diarrhea, and suppress coughs. While most people who take these

opiate narcotics—*group of narcotics made from the opium poppy; includes the opiates and opioids.*

opiates—*a group of narcotic analgesics that includes opium, morphine, and heroin.*

opioids—*a group of synthetic drugs, such as methadone and meperidine, that are chemically similar to the opiates.*

opium—*a narcotic analgesic substance made from the opium poppy; it is the parent substance of the opiate narcotics.*

morphine—*a narcotic analgesic that is the active ingredient in opium.*

heroin—*a narcotic analgesic derived from morphine and more than twice as powerful.*

Figure 13.6 Pain relief from opiates. (A) Normal nerve transmission involves electrical transmission within a nerve cell, and chemical (neurotransmitter) transmission from one cell to the next. (B) Opiates mimic the effect of natural endorphins by attaching to endorphin receptors and thus blocking the action of neurotransmitters between the nerve cells. While endorphins are rapidly dispersed, however, opiates linger at the receptor sites, causing tolerance and addiction.

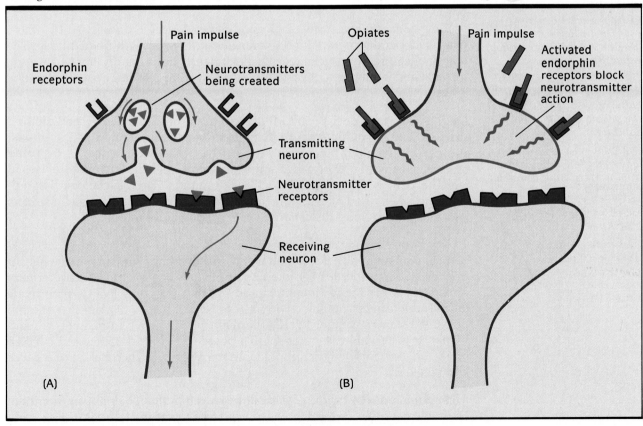

drugs under a prescription do not become dependent on them, a few do. If morphine is prescribed to relieve the severe pain of an injury, the individual taking it may develop a dependence by the time the injury has healed and the drug is no longer needed.

Potential Risks   Until the increase in cocaine use in the 1980s, heroin represented the nation's most prevalent illicit drug problem. Heroin is typically injected intravenously, although it is also sometimes injected subcutaneously (a practice known as skin popping) or sniffed (snorted). A person who uses heroin by any method is at great risk of becoming physically dependent on the drug.

Typically, a heroin user seeks the drug's mind-numbing effect, its blurring of thought and feeling, which can include the "rush"—feelings of ecstasy similar to sexual orgasm. When a user has become dependent, the drug is also needed to avoid the distress of withdrawal. As the user becomes dependent, he or she is also likely to develop a tolerance: the usual initial dose of heroin, about 3 milligrams, can escalate to 1,000 milligrams within a matter of months, with large sums of money required to support the user's habit.

Psychedelics/Hallucinogens

The **psychedelics/hallucinogens** are drugs that create illusions, distorting the user's mind by creating moods, thoughts, and perceptions that would otherwise take place only in a dream state. The earliest forms of these substances were derived from plants and have been employed in folk medicine and as part of religious rituals. Other forms have been developed in recent years.

The well-known hallucinogen **LSD** ("acid") was developed in the late 1940s. In addition to LSD, this group of drugs includes a variety of substances, some natural plant derivatives and other concocted in chemistry labs. Among them are **PCP** (an animal tranquilizer), **mescaline** (derived from the peyote cactus), **psilocybin** (a mushroom derivative), and other substances known by abbreviations of their chemical names (DMT, DET, DOM, and so on).

None of these drugs causes physical dependence, and there is little if any psychic dependence, although tolerance can develop with frequent use. The real dangers of the psychedelics/hallucinogens lie primarily in their unpredictable and sometimes devastating effects during use and occasionally long afterward.

LSD   An average dose of 50 to 100 micrograms of LSD (lysergic acid diethylamide, "acid") produces slight dizziness, weakness, dilation of the pupils, and perceptual alterations such as intensive visual experiences, a distorted time sense, sharpened hearing, and **synesthesia**—a blending of the senses in which a person "hears" colors or "sees" sounds. The psychological symptoms include a flood of thoughts in new combinations, rapid mood changes, and a feeling of body distortion.[46]

PCP   Phencyclidine, also known as PCP, "angel dust," and other nicknames, was originally developed as an anesthetic for humans, but when its unpredictable properties became known, its use was restricted to veterinary applications. No longer manufactured for that purpose, PCP is now made illegally and can be combined with or represented as any of a number of other illegal substances (notably THC, the main psychoactive ingredient in marijuana). It is available as water-soluble powder, liquid, or tablet and is taken orally, sniffed, injected, or sprinkled on marijuana, kitchen herbs, or tobacco and smoked.[47]

Mescaline and Psilocybin   Mescaline is used in the religious ceremonies of Native Americans. Psilocybin has also played a part in Native American religious lore since the days of the ancient Aztecs. When taken in connection with traditional rituals and under the supervision of experienced users, these substances probably do no lasting harm. Outside such highly controlled settings, however, the effects of these drugs can be unpredictable and hazardous.[48]

Potential Risks Both PCP and LSD can cause strong adverse reactions, including death. LSD users sometimes experience "bad trips," complete with monstrous perceptions, extreme delusions, and severe panic. Such reactions are common with high doses and impure drugs, although they can occur for no apparent reason. In some people LSD can trigger serious depression, paranoia, and chronic psychoses. Even occasional users of LSD can experience **flashbacks**—brief, sudden perceptual distortions and bizarre thoughts that can occur as long as 5 years after the user's last experience with the drug.

PCP is a perplexing and alarming drug with conflicting and paradoxical properties. It can act not only as a deliriant but also as a stimulant, a depressant, and an analgesic. Its effects can vary from person to person and from one time to another in the same person. Low doses may produce a feeling of intoxication, euphoria, overall numbness, thought disorganization, slurring of speech, hostile and bizarre behavior, or any combination of these effects.[49] Somewhat larger doses may cause nausea and vomiting, fever, loss of muscle control, or coma. Still larger doses may lead to any of these conditions plus large increases in blood pressure and heart rate, psychotic behavior (including violence), convulsions, and coma. PCP has been known to cause a psychosis similar to schizophrenia and occasionally catatonia (an inability to move).[50]

Designer Drugs

In an attempt to circumvent laws against particular drugs, a new class of drugs began to appear during the 1980s. Called *designer drugs,* these substances were created in underground labs with slight molecular variations from controlled drugs, so that they mimicked the effects of those drugs. However, mistakes were sometimes made with serious consequences, such as the development of a Parkinson's-like condition. These drugs are now also illegal, due to a law passed by the U.S. Congress in 1986.

Dealing with Drug Use and Abuse

Some drugs can and do save lives and improve human health. Many people, however, use drugs as agents they feel they need to solve life's problems, and in this way, drugs often become a problem. Substances, both legal and illegal, that can ease pain, reduce tension, or make life seem more pleasant may quickly turn a person's life into a nightmare of physical illness, psychic or physical dependence, or both.

Drugs themselves are only one factor in the agent-host-environmental model discussed earlier in this chapter. The individual (the host) and the setting (environment) are also significant factors that must be considered. An individual's need for drugs can be tackled through treatment and rehabilitation. Environmental factors can be addressed through laws and social policy. The overall goal should be responsible drug use. While solutions to drug problems are not easy, effective methods of dealing with drug use and abuse can be found.

Dealing with People's Need for Drugs

Individuals must ultimately make their own decisions about drug use. The effectiveness of programs to treat dependence and abuse depends a great deal on these decisions and on the individual's willingness to kick the habit.

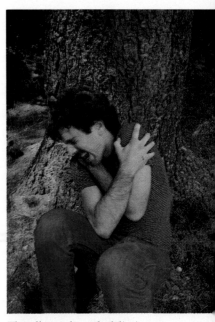

The effects of psychedelics/ hallucinogens are difficult to portray, but they can be very disturbing. (Ken Lax/ MediChrome)

flashbacks—*brief, sudden, unexpected perceptual distortions and bizarre thoughts—similar to those experienced while on an LSD trip—that occur long after the immediate effects of a drug have worn off.*

Treatment and Rehabilitation

For many drug users, treatment and rehabilitation are difficult and subtle tasks that require a great deal of personal strength and conviction as well as support from other individuals or groups.[51] Overcoming drug dependence can be one of the most difficult tasks a user ever faces, and some people do not succeed.[52]

There is little agreement about what constitutes success in treating drug dependence. Some people believe that recovery requires total abstinence from psychoactive drugs. Others define recovery as using drugs in a controlled way or being able to function well without drugs. Thus, it is difficult to generalize about the success rates of different treatment programs.[53]

People seeking help for drug dependence may be treated on an inpatient or outpatient basis, depending on the drugs used and the severity of the symptoms. In either case, the treatment may include participation in self-help groups such as Narcotics Anonymous. It may also involve individual or group counseling and may include the user's family.[54]

People whose drug abuse is fairly recent or who are not greatly dependent on drugs are often treated on an outpatient basis. Therapy generally encompasses a mixture of resources available in the community—perhaps psychotherapy, self-help groups, educational or occupational services, and halfway houses.[55] Drug users with a serious dependence are more likely to be treated on an inpatient basis, which involves spending a period of time in a treatment center. Some inpatients require gradual **detoxification,** or medically supervised withdrawal from drugs. Sudden withdrawal from some drugs, including heroin and alcohol, can be dangerous, and so the treatment may include carefully monitored doses of the drug to help wean the patient from physical dependence. For heroin users, this may include the use of **methadone,** a synthetic drug that removes the desire for heroin and produces tolerance to its effects. Methadone, however, produces its own physical dependence, although without the serious side effects of heroin.

People who seek treatment for drug dependence often have other serious physiological, psychological, or social problems as well.[56] Some experts estimate that up to one-third of people dependent on drugs have psychiatric or personality disorders. Because experts disagree about the relationship between drug abuse and other disorders, drug users with serious problems may be shunted back and forth between psychotherapy and drug treatment, receiving adequate care in neither venue.

Some drug users also face the problem of multiple drug dependence; this is becoming the norm among people enrolled in treatment programs.[57] In one study of cocaine abusers who sought treatment, 83 percent were also dependent on alcohol.[58] As a result, the trend is toward more general treatment of "substance abuse" rather than treatment for the abuse of a specific drug.[59]

Finding Alternatives to Drug Use

There are other ways to obtain relief from anxiety, become more alert, feel excitement, and experience some of the effects offered by psychoactive drugs.

The use of psychoactive drugs usually masks the symptoms of a problem without really solving it or provides only a short-term solution. A stimulant may help a person feel more energetic, but a lack of energy may stem from inadequate diet or insufficient sleep—problems that the drug does not address. Other alternatives to drug use offer more pervasive and longer-lasting benefits, although these benefits may not be felt as quickly. Improving one's diet, for example, may not provide the same quick surge of energy that using a stimulant does, but it may raise a person's energy level over the long run.

There are a number of alternatives to drug use that a person might consider. Stress-reducing methods (Chapter 2) can help relieve anxiety; psychotherapy and counseling can help with emotional problems; and vigorous exercise can provide a natural high. Even simple things such as going to a movie, having dinner with friends, enjoying nature, and helping others can

detoxification—*medically supervised withdrawal from drugs.*

methadone—*a synthetic drug that removes the desire for heroin and produces tolerance to its effects; used in the treatment of heroin addiction.*

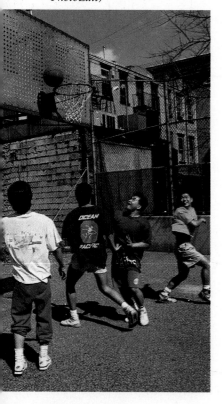

Exercise is a healthy alternative to drugs; people who maintain a regular exercise regimen are likely to live happier, healthier lives. (Robert Brenner/ PhotoEdit)

improve a person's emotional and physical well-being and reduce the desire for the artificially induced feelings provided by drugs. Since people turn to drugs for a variety of reasons, each person needs to discover alternatives that will meet his or her individual preferences and needs.

Societal Solutions to Drug Abuse

Although individuals must ultimately make their own decisions about drug use, the government and society must assume some responsibility for controlling the use of drugs and preventing abuse and addiction. Laws and societal attitudes are important environmental factors that have an impact on the availability and acceptability of drugs.

Society's Concerns and the Law   The greatest drug problem in recent years has been the marketing and use of illegal psychoactive drugs. Not only are these drugs ruining the lives of millions of Americans, they are also at the root of increasing rates of drug-related crimes. The federal, state, and local agencies responsible for enforcing laws against the possession and sale of these substances have stepped up their activities in recent years in response to the growing problem.

Law enforcement efforts are aimed at cutting off the supply of drugs and prosecuting those involved in illegal drug possession and trafficking. Although these efforts have had some notable successes, many experts feel that the real solution to the nation's drug problem lies in reducing the demand for drugs rather than cutting off the supply.

Attacking Demand   One aspect of reducing the demand for drugs is identifying drug users and making available to them opportunities for dealing with their drug use. This issue has become increasingly important because of a growing concern about drug abuse on the job, especially in jobs that affect public safety. Drug testing has become a controversial issue. Some experts point out that drug tests can be unreliable and inconclusive. Others argue that any type of mandatory drug testing infringes on an individual's constitutional right to privacy.[60]

Perhaps a more crucial component in reducing demand is education. Educating people about the dangers of drugs, why people use drugs, ways to avoid drug abuse, and ways to get help with drug abuse problems can reduce the demand for drugs and lead to healthier individuals and a healthier, safer society.

President Richard Nixon established the Drug Enforcement Administration (DEA) in 1973 as part of the U.S. Department of Justice. The DEA investigates the smuggling of narcotics and dangerous drugs into the United States and works with local law enforcement agencies to enforce federal laws on drug abuse and arrest offenders.

Chapter Summary

- People use drugs for a variety of reasons, including to relieve pain and discomfort, escape boredom, escape problems, experience pleasure, and enhance performance.
- Prescription drugs are used to relieve symptoms, prevent illness, control chronic conditions, and treat disease.
- With tolerance, the body becomes adapted to a drug so that larger doses are needed to produce the desired effect. Dependence is a condition in which a person becomes so accustomed to a drug that he or she is unable to function without it. Addiction refers to compulsive use of a drug, including tolerance and psychic and physical dependence.

- The major levels of drug use, which affect the likelihood of dependence, are experimental use, recreational use, situational use, intensified use, and compulsive use.
- The agent-host-environment model views drug dependence as more than just an individual problem; other factors—such as the purity, toxicity, and interactions of the drug (agent factors) and peer pressure, cultural values, and societal laws (environment factors)—also play an important role in drug use and dependence.
- Drugs produce a wide range of effects on the body. Basically, a drug acts only on cells that are compatible with chemical substances in that drug. Drugs can also produce side effects that

are unrelated to their purpose. These side effects can be potentially hazardous.

- Drugs are administered orally, by injection, and by inhalation. The method of administration can be a determining factor in the effect of a drug.
- A drug's effect can be changed by the way in which it is distributed throughout the body, through biotransformation, and by the way it is excreted.
- Effective dose is the standard that physicians use to determine the proper doses of a drug for individuals. This dose differs from one drug to another and from one person to another.
- Drug interactions are a serious and often unpredictable risk of drug use. Because of these interactions, one drug may block the effects of another, heighten potential side effects, or increase the effects of the drugs taken.
- The major categories of psychoactive drugs are sedatives/hypnotics (barbiturates and antianxiety drugs), stimulants (caffeine, amphetamines, and cocaine), marijuana, volatile solvents and other inhalants such as nitrous oxide and amyl nitrite, opiate narcotics (heroin, opium, and morphine), and psychedelics/hallucinogens (LSD, mescaline, psilocybin, and PCP). Each category of drugs entails potentially serious risks.
- Individuals who want to overcome a drug habit can seek help through outpatient or inpatient treatment. This may include counseling, participation in self-help groups, detoxification, or stays in residential treatment centers. People can also seek alternatives to drug use, such as improvement in diet, exercise, social life, and emotional health.
- Societal responsibility for drug use and abuse includes laws to curb illegal drug use and distribution, educational efforts to teach people about the dangers of drugs, and how to get help with a drug problem.

Key Terms

Drug (page 338)

Psychoactive drugs (page 338)

Tolerance (page 339)

Dependence (page 339)

Withdrawal syndrome (page 340)

Addiction (page 340)

Receptor sites (page 343)

Side effects (page 345)

Teratogenic (page 346)

Allergy (page 346)

Anaphylactic shock (page 346)

Cross-sensitivity (page 346)

Route of administration (page 346)

Parenteral (page 347)

Subcutaneous (page 347)

Intramuscular (page 347)

Intravenous (page 347)

Pharmacokinetics (page 348)

Biotransform (page 348)

Metabolites (page 348)

Therapeutic index (page 349)

Synergism (page 349)

Sedatives/hypnotics (page 352)

Barbiturates (page 352)

Anxiolytics (page 352)

Stimulants (page 356)

Amphetamines (page 356)

Cocaine (page 358)

Marijuana (page 360)

Hashish (page 360)

Inhalants (page 362)

Amyl nitrite (page 362)

Butyl nitrite (page 362)

Opiate narcotics (page 363)

Opiates (page 363)

Opioids (page 363)

Opium (page 363)

Morphine (page 363)

Heroin (page 363)

Psychedelics/ hallucinogens (page 364)

LSD (lysergic acid diethylamide) (page 364)

PCP (phencyclidine) (page 364)

Mescaline (page 364)

Psilocybin (page 364)

Synesthesia (page 364)

Flashbacks (page 365)

Detoxification (page 366)

Methadone (page 366)

References

1. Katie E. Cherry and Mark R. Morton, "Drug Sensitivity in Older Adults: The Role of Physiologic and Pharmacokinetic Factors," *International Journal of Aging and Human Development* 28, no. 3 (1989): 159–174.

2. Jerome H. Jaffe, "Drug Addiction and Drug Abuse," in *Goodman and Gilman's The Pharmacological Basis of Therapeutics*, 6th ed., A. G. Gilman et al. (eds.) (New York: Macmillan, 1980): 535–577.

3. Lloyd Johnston, *10th National Survey of Drug Usage among College Students* (Ann Arbor: University of Michigan, Institute of Social Research, February 1990).

4. Dan Sperling, "Teen Drug Use Drops, but Users Get Very High," *USA Today* (undated).

5. Amy Linn, "Of Motherhood," *Philadelphia Inquirer* (September 17, 1989).

6. Ibid.

7. Douglas Martin, "Big Bribe Helps Mothers Fend Off Allure of Crack," *New York Times* (March 7, 1990).

8. Jim Detjen, "Cocaine and Pregnancy: Experts Fear a Holocaust," *Philadelphia Inquirer* (December 15, 1989).

9. Mary E. Guinan, "Women and Crack Addiction," *Journal of the American Medical Women's Association* 44, no. 4 (July–August 1989): 129.

10. Brent Q. Hafen and Brenda Peterson, *Medicine and Drugs*, 2d ed. (Philadelphia: Lea & Febiger, 1978): 28.

11. Cherry and Morton, op. cit.

12. Brent Q. Hafen, *The Self-Health Handbook* (Englewood Cliffs, N.J.: Prentice-Hall, 1980): 77.

13. *FDA Consumer* (December 1980–January 1981): 14.

14. National Institute on Drug Abuse (NIDA), Statistical Series I, No. 4: *Data from the Drug Abuse Warning Network, Annual Data, 1985* (Rockville, Md.: NIDA): 26, 52.

15. Robert Fink et al., "Sedative-Hypnotic Dependence," *American Family Physician* 11 (1974): 116.

16. David Duncan and Robert Gold, *Drugs and the Whole Person* (New York: Wiley, 1982): 71.

17. *Harvard Medical School Health Letter* 7, no. 9 (July 1982): 1–2.

18. *Amphetamine Report*, HEW Series 28, no. 1 (Washington, D.C.: National Clearinghouse for Drug Abuse Information, 1974).

19. T. W. Rall, "Central Nervous System Stimulants," in A. G. Gilman et al. (eds.), op. cit., pp. 592–607.

20. Jill M. VanDette and Laura Cornish, "Medical Complications of Illicit Cocaine Use," *Clinical Pharmacy* 8 (June 1989): 401–411.

21. Frank H. Gawin, "Cocaine Abuse and Addiction," *Journal of Family Practice* 29, no. 2 (1989): 193–197; VanDette and Cornish, op. cit.

22. Norman S. Miller et al., "Cocaine: General Characteristics, Abuse, and Addiction," *New York State Journal of Medicine* (July 1989): 390–394; VanDette and Cornish, op. cit.

23. George R. Gay, "Cocaine," *New York State Journal of Medicine* (July 1989): 384–386.

24. Gawin, op. cit.

25. Miller et al., op. cit.

26. Guinan, op. cit.

27. VanDette and Cornish, op. cit.

28. Miller et al., op. cit.

29. VanDette and Cornish, op. cit.

30. Ibid.

31. Ibid.

32. K. Solomons and V. N. Neppe, "Cannabis—Its Clinical Effects," *South African Medical Journal* 76 (August 5, 1989): 102–104.

33. Ibid.

34. Ibid.

35. Injury Control Research Labortory, U.S. Public Health Service, "Effect of Marijuana on Risk Acceptance in a Simulated Passing Test," HE 20.2859:71–3, March 1972; NIDA, "Marijuana: Research Findings," 1980.

36. Institute of Medicine, *Marijuana and Health*, December 1981 (Washington, D.C.: National Academy of Science Press, 1982): 117–119.

37. AMA Council on Scientific Affairs, "Marijuana: Its Health Hazards and Therapeutic Potentials," *Journal of the American Medical Association* 246, no. 16 (October 15, 1981): 1823–1827.

38. NIDA, "Marijuana: Research Findings," op. cit.

39. AMA Council on Scientific Affairs, op. cit.

40. Katherine Tennes et al., "Marijuana: Prenatal and Postnatal Exposure in the Human," in *Current Research of Maternal Drug Abuse*, NIDA, Research Monograph No. 59, 1985.

41. Solomons and Neppe, op. cit.

42. Ibid.

43. Annabel Hecht, "Inhalants: Quick Route to Danger," *FDA Consumer* 14, no. 4 (May 1980): 19–22; Sidney Cohen, "The Volatile Nitrites," *Journal of the American Medical Association* 241, no. 19 (May 11, 1979): 2077–2078; Phil Gunby, "Nitrous Oxide No Laughing Matter; Nerve Damage Seen," *Journal of the American Medical Association* 239, no. 23 (June 9, 1978); "Here's the Topper: Whipped-Cream Cans May Be Fatal for N2O Abusers," *Medical World News* 20, no. 8 (April 16, 1979): 16; Michela Reichman, "Dentist Urges Colleagues to Cut Occupational Exposure to Nitrous Oxide," (SFGH/UC-San Francisco, August 2, 1981).

44. Cohen, op. cit.

45. Guy R. Newell et al., "Volatile Nitrites: Use and Adverse Effects Related to the Current Epidemic of the Acquired Immune Deficiency Syndrome," *American Journal of Medicine* 78 (May 1985): 811–816.

46. S. Cohen, "Psychotomimetics (Hallucinogens) and Cannabis" in *Principles of Pharmacology*, 2d ed., W. G. Clark and J. delGiudice (eds.) (New York: Academic Press, 1978): 357–369.

47. R. C. Peterson, and R. C. Stillman, "Phencyclidine: An Overview," in *Phencyclidine (PCP) Abuse: An Appraisal*, R. C. Peterson and R. C. Stillman (eds.) (Washington, D.C.: NIDA, Research Monograph 21, Dept. HEW, 1978): 1–17.

48. Cohen, "Psychomimetics."

49. Jerome H. Jaffe, "Drug Addiction and Drug Abuse," in A. G. Gilman et al. (eds.), op. cit., p. 567.

50. P. V. Luisada, "The Phencyclidine Psychosis: Phenomenology and Treatment," in Peterson and Stillman (eds.), op. cit., pp. 241–253.

51. Gay, op. cit.

52. Joan E. Zweben and James L. Sorensen, "Misunderstandings about Methadone," *Journal of Psychoactive Drugs* 20, no. 3 (July–September 1977): 275–281.

53. George W. Bailey, "Current Perspectives on Substance Abuse in Youth," *Journal of the American Academy of Childhood and Adolescent Psychiatry* 28, no. 2 (1989): 151–162.

54. Ibid.

55. Ibid.

56. Miller et al., op. cit.

57. Zweben and Sorensen, op. cit.

58. Miller, et al., op. cit.

59. Zweben and Sorensen, op. cit.; Bailey, op. cit.

60. John P. Morgan, "Employee Drug Tests Are Unreliable and Intrusive," *Hospitals* 63, no. 16 (August 20, 1989): 64.

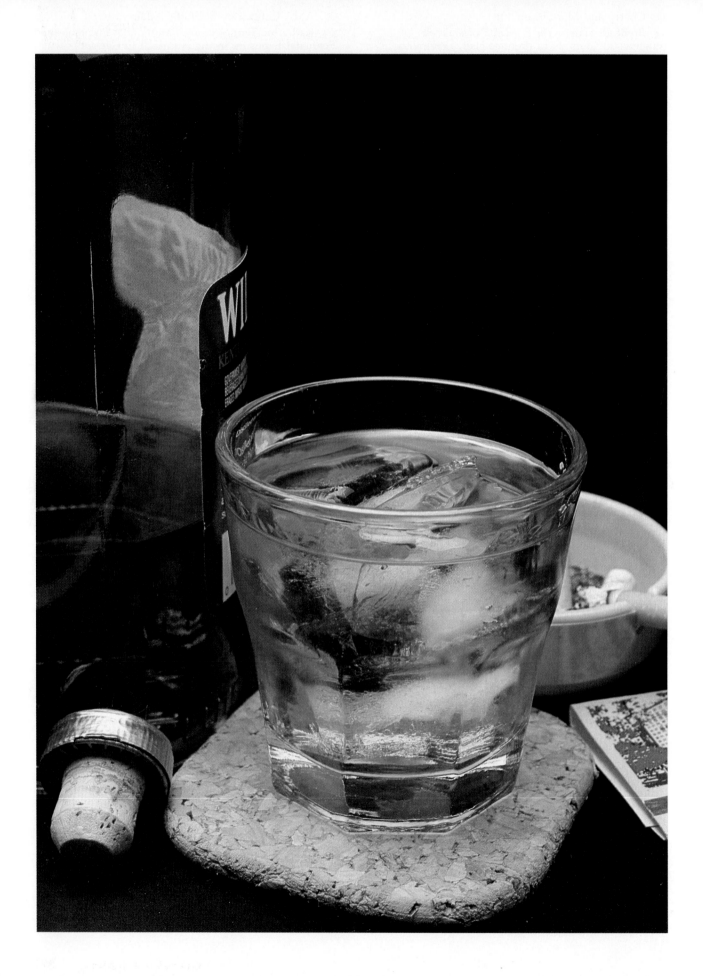

Chapter 14

Alcohol

To Guide Your Reading

When you have studied this chapter, you should be able to:

- Explain alcohol's effects on the body and the factors which lead to alcohol dependence.

- Identify different types of destructive behavior associated with alcohol.

- Describe alcoholism, listing progressive steps in its development and identifying some of the signs which indicate its presence.

- Discuss some of the major health consequences of alcohol abuse.

- Indicate the ways that you can guard against the development of alcoholism and the types of treatment which are available for those who are already problem drinkers.

Sit at the bar in a restaurant and you will see how easily alcohol fits into American society. A romantic meal is warmed by wine and candlelight. The restaurant's host offers a complimentary drink with dinner. A job promotion becomes an occasion to buy a round of drinks for colleagues after work. Alcohol has long been associated with food, celebration, and hospitality.

And yet, at the same time, the steadily increasing consumption of alcohol is causing some of the worst public health problems in our country. Alcohol plays a leading role in highway accidents. It can cause birth defects and infant deaths, and is also responsible for disease and damage to adults. Alcohol-related absences from work and school have reached alarming proportions, and there is a strong association between drinking, violent behavior, financial problems, family conflicts, criminal acts, and mental illness.

This was well understood at the opening of this century. In industrial America alcohol was seen as a source of violence, abuse, and poverty, with women and children as the prime victims. Moral reformers and members of the women's suffrage movement worked to outlaw alcohol at the local level. Employers, who recognized that a sober workforce was more productive, supported their cause. In 1919 a constitutional amendment was ratified by the states, prohibiting the manufacture and sale of alcoholic beverages throughout the nation.

Prohibition did not work, however. Demand remained high, and supplying illegal alcohol made organized crime highly profitable. The prohibition amendment was repealed less than 15 years later, and responsibility for making decisions about the use of alcohol was returned to each individual.

Such decisions cannot be made without accurate information. People need to know how the body takes in alcohol and what changes occur as the alcohol is absorbed. Understanding these facts can help them regulate their consumption so that it does become a problem. People also need information about problem drinking and alcoholism to help them discern whether they, their family, or their friends have a problem and to enable them to decide on which steps to take to get help.

Americans consume about 500 million gallons of alcoholic beverages each year. That is more than 2 gallons for every man, woman, and child.

Alcohol Use and Its Effects on the Body

*Recent research about moderate alcohol use suggests some good news and some bad. Studies have shown that it is associated with lowered risk of heart disease. But other research appears to link use of alcohol in **any** quantities with damage to nerve cells in the brain.*

Because liquor is so accepted and so common in our society, many people do not think of alcoholic beverages as harmful substances. In reality, however, alcohol carries a great risk for the health and well-being of people who use it and of other people around them.

Despite growing public awareness about the dangers, many Americans continue to drink excessively. It is estimated that between 9 and 10 million Americans are either alcoholics or problem drinkers.[1] A first step in saving oneself from a similar fate is to understand what alcohol does.

How Alcohol Works on the Body

Alcohol takes a rather direct route into an individual's system. After it is consumed, alcohol travels to the stomach and small intestine, and from there it is absorbed directly into the bloodstream and distributed throughout the body. Its absorption can be quite rapid, especially on an empty stomach. Since the stomach can absorb fully one-fourth of the total dose (the rest is absorbed in the small intestine), when a drink is taken on an empty stomach the maximum level of alcohol in the blood can be reached in as short a time as 30 minutes (Figure 14.1).

Figure 14.1 Alcohol enters a person's bloodstream through the stomach and small intestine. While it circulates through the bloodstream it affects a wide range of cells. These effects only wear off as the liver metabolizes the alcohol (at a rate of about 2/3 ounce per hour).

Source: Scholastic Science World 39, no. 1 (September 3, 1982): 2.

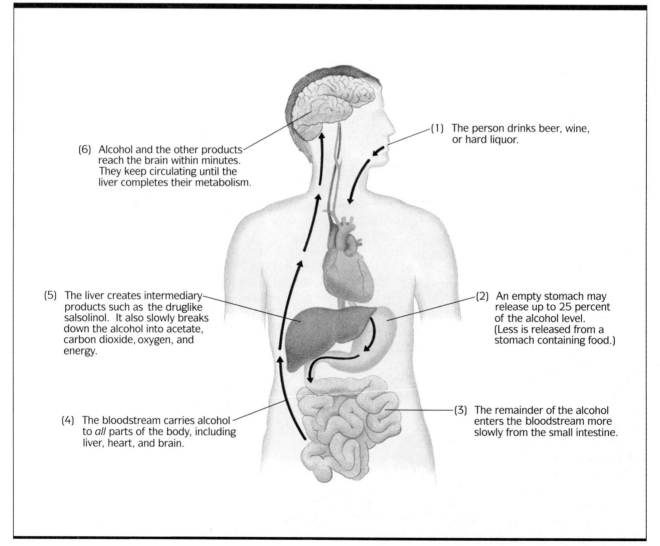

(1) The person drinks beer, wine, or hard liquor.

(6) Alcohol and the other products reach the brain within minutes. They keep circulating until the liver completes their metabolism.

(5) The liver creates intermediary products such as the druglike salsolinol. It also slowly breaks down the alcohol into acetate, carbon dioxide, oxygen, and energy.

(2) An empty stomach may release up to 25 percent of the alcohol level. (Less is released from a stomach containing food.)

(4) The bloodstream carries alcohol to *all* parts of the body, including liver, heart, and brain.

(3) The remainder of the alcohol enters the bloodstream more slowly from the small intestine.

Dose Levels and Time Factors As the blood races through the body, the alcohol travels with it and is distributed fairly uniformly throughout the body tissues and fluids. The more the individual drinks, the more his or her entire body becomes saturated with alcohol, and the more its effects will be felt.

About 10 percent of absorbed **ethyl alcohol** (the active ingredient in alcoholic beverages) is eliminated unmetabolized through the kidneys, lungs, and sweat glands. The rest is metabolized by the liver to form a highly toxic substance known as acetaldehyde. This acetaldehyde is eventually broken down into acetate, carbon dioxide, oxygen, and energy. It also combines with the neurotransmitter dopamine to form an opiatelike substance, salsolinol, which is believed to be highly addictive.

ethyl alcohol—*the active ingredient in alcoholic beverages (distilled spirits, wine, beer) prepared from natural plant products such as fruits and grains.*

The metabolism of alcohol occurs at a fairly constant rate. Depending on the individual, the liver metabolizes about 2/3 to 3/4 ounce of pure ethyl alcohol, or ethanol, per hour. If consumption exceeds this rate, alcohol levels in the bloodstream will rise. Since the brain is seriously affected by alcohol, judgment and motor activity are increasingly impaired as more is consumed.

The effects of alcohol vary from person to person depending on an individual's **blood alcohol level (BAL),** that is, the amount of alcohol that is in the blood at any one time. And the BAL can fluctuate depending on body weight, stress, the contents of the stomach, and other factors. For example, if an individual is drinking a lot of alcoholic beverages quickly and not eating, the alcohol will get into the bloodstream rapidly. Many people find that after a stressful day they are likely to get quite drunk on a single drink before dinner. Yet the very next day, when they are feeling relaxed and happy, they can put away two drinks and hardly feel any effects at all.

blood alcohol level (BAL)— *the concentration of alcohol in the blood at a given time.*

The amount of alcohol a large person can drink with little effect could cause intoxication in a smaller person. There are good reasons for the differences. A smaller, lighter person, with a correspondingly lower volume of blood and a smaller liver, would have a higher alcohol level in the blood that flows to the liver and possibly a higher level in the blood that leaves the liver too. The blood alcohol level also depends on how quickly the alcohol is *removed* from the body; this can vary according to a person's nutritional status, drinking history, and even the time of day he or she drinks.

Effects on the Central Nervous System Alcohol is an anesthetic, a sedative, and a depressant. It is often valued at parties and other social occasions as a stimulant because its sedating action on the brain reduces social inhibitions. If enough alcohol is consumed, the result will be an easily measurable effect—a loss of motor coordination. The person will stagger, slur speech, and drop or spill things. An intoxicated person's vision may also be seriously affected by the alcohol, making it impossible to drive safely. Even small amounts of alcohol can make a drinker relatively blind in the face of bright lights at night and thus a serious hazard on the road.

One bottle or can of beer contains as much alcohol as a glass of wine or a shot of whiskey. And "light" beer contains as much alcohol as regular beer; it is called "light" only because it has fewer calories.

The hangover that follows a few hours' intoxication is usually considered a state of mild withdrawal from alcohol. The sensations are caused, in part, by the drinker's allergic reaction to certain substances found in the drinks. But part of the hangover pain may also be caused by nerve cells in the brain, which become dehydrated by the alcohol. The severity of a hangover is related both to the amount and duration of the drinking and to the physical and mental condition of the drinker. Some people may feel weak and nervous or may become nauseous and vomit. The heart may beat faster, and the individual may have trouble concentrating. Despite what has sometimes been written in popular magazines, there is no cure for a hangover except time. However, rest, the use of aspirin, and the intake of nonalcoholic liquids and solid food will help to relieve the symptoms.

One of the hidden problems with alcohol—as with other depressant drugs—is that while the user gets an initial "glow" of relaxation, an underlying feeling of edginess and agitation also builds up at the same time. This increased

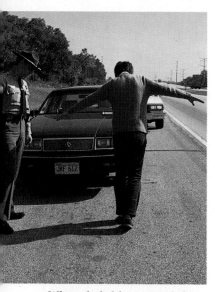

When alcohol has entered the bloodstream, it affects vision and physical coordination in ways that are easily detected. (Van Bucher/Photo Researchers, Inc.)

brain arousal lasts longer than the feeling of relaxed well-being, and it makes the user want another drink to calm down again. That next drink will have its own "edge," possibly setting in motion a vicious circle. Most drinkers simply stop after the second or third drink, so the buildup of brain arousal does not present a problem. But this feature of alcohol's effects may be a factor in alcoholism, discussed more fully later in the chapter.

Factors That Influence Alcohol Use

Despite its increasingly publicized potential for harming health and causing other problems, the use of alcohol remains widespread. People often continue using alcohol even when giving it up could reverse serious health disorders or other problems caused by its use. Alcohol's continued popularity rests on a complex web of physiological, psychological, and social factors.

Physical Addiction   One reason people continue to use alcohol is that they became addicted. Ethyl alcohol is a drug: as with other drugs, users can develop tolerance and become physically dependent (Chapter 13). A person who develops a tolerance to alcohol must consume more and more to achieve the same effects. For example, people who drink to relieve stress must gradually increase their consumption of alcohol to continue experiencing that relief.

Not everyone who develops a tolerance to alcohol develops a physical dependence on it. But it is not unusual for a person with a high tolerance also to have a physical need for alcohol, a chemical dependence that becomes evident when the person stops drinking. In such individuals an abrupt end to drinking will produce painful withdrawal symptoms—ranging from delirium tremens (often called the DTs or the "shakes") to seizures, hallucinations, and other signs of intense disturbance of the central nervous system.

Psychological Dependence   Many people become psychologically or emotionally dependent on alcohol even if they do not develop physical addictions. For example, since alcohol can help a person relax, some people come to depend on alcohol to relieve tension and anxiety rather than take other steps to relieve them. The alcohol makes people feel better without their having to expend any effort. This, in turn, reinforces the apparent value of alcohol for relieving emotionally based mood states. Over time, behavior patterns involving drinking become very familiar and comfortable and are quite difficult to change.

"Chugging" beer or other alcoholic beverages produces a rapid accumulation of alcohol in the bloodstream. This is very dangerous and can lead to acute alcohol poisoning, resulting in coma and even death. Recent incidents of this type of behavior have been reported from campuses, where the practice has sometimes been associated with initiation into fraternities.

Social Pressures   Peer pressure and other social pressures also influence people to use alcohol. The use of alcohol is not the norm in all social circles, of course, but among groups that do use them, the pressure to join in can be strong.

Many social events—parties, dining with friends, socializing at bars, and so on—may involve ritualistic alcohol consumption. People who are drinking frequently urge others to join them. Although each person has the option of drinking or abstaining, peer pressures to drink are often so strong that, for many individuals, it seems as if there is no choice.

Alcohol and Destructive Behavior

A single bout of drinking may cause nothing more harmful than vomiting, a loss of coordination, or other unpleasant physical effects. While these effects are neither serious nor long-lasting, they discourage most people from abusing alcohol through excessive drinking. This is fortunate, because chronic heavy drinking can permanently damage the body. Even the occasional abuse of alcohol can have serious consequences for the people who drink, for those around them, and for the society as a whole.

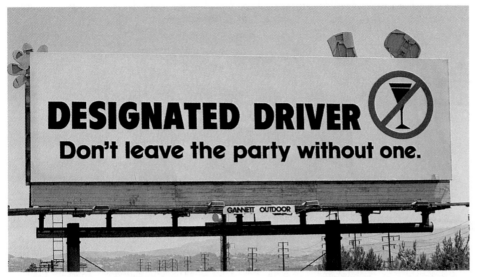

Public service groups use billboard space and other media to emphasize the importance of guarding against the dangers of alcohol abuse. (Tony Freeman/PhotoEdit)

For some people, alcohol abuse can lead to a variety of destructive behaviors including the risk of injury from accidents, violence and criminal behaviors, and domestic turmoil. Such problems do not have to arise from alcohol dependency or addiction; they can be the result of any degree of alcohol use—from occasional drunkenness to chronic abuse.

A combination of alcohol and drugs such as sleeping pills, tranquilizers, antibiotics, and aspirin can be fatal, even when both are taken in nonlethal doses.

Alcohol and Accidents

Drunkenness to the point that it endangers the drinker or others is by no means limited to public offenders locked up in jail. In fact, most intoxication today occurs among men and women who live with their families, hold jobs, and maintain stable community ties. With alcohol such a widely used drug, most of these people have learned to mask the obvious signs of drunkenness. Their perception of time and space may be altered, their judgment faulty, and their reaction time slowed by alcohol, but they try to compensate.

Routine drinking has become all the more ominous as life has become faster-paced and more technological. More and more jobs, such as jobs where the individual is required to operate machine tools, require exacting skill and judgment. Most people cannot avoid these everyday activities that are made impossible or at least extremely difficult by excessive drinking. Alcohol use can lead to serious accidents at work, as well as in the home or at play.

The most vivid evidence of the dangers of alcohol is the daily slaughter of men, women, and children on the nation's highways in alcohol-related accidents. Accidents are the fourth leading cause of deaths in the United States. Motor vehicle accidents account for over half of all these, and they are the highest cause of death among people younger than age 34.[2] Intoxicated drivers have a habit of maiming other people as well: one-third of all people who suffered the loss of arms or legs or other injuries can blame inebriated drivers for their disability.[3]

In most states, a blood alcohol level of 0.10 percent defines legal drunkenness, and it is this figure that is usually used to determine if a person was driving while intoxicated. However, new evidence accumulated by the American Medical Association reveals that almost any measurable blood alcohol concentration interferes with the sharp judgment, coordination, vision, and reaction time necessary for safe driving.[4] Young drivers involved in car accidents are often found to have blood alcohol levels that are quite low, prompting some experts to suggest that even one drink is too much if a person intends to operate a motor vehicle.[5]

Table 14.1 Percentages of Crimes and Injuries Involving Alcohol in the United States

Homicides	74 (70 on weekends)
Beatings	69
Stabbings	72
Shootings	55
Sexually aggressive acts against women	39
Sexually aggressive acts against children	67
Suicides	30
Fatal auto accidents	51
Fatal aircraft accidents (private)	20
Pedestrian accidents	36
Snowmobile accidents	40
Fire deaths	58
Accidental poisonings	71
Drownings	45
Fights or assaults in the home	56
Home accidents	22
Narcotic deaths	20
All arrests	55

Source: James T. Weston, "Alcohol's Impact on Man's Activities: Its Role in Unnatural Death," *American Journal of Clinical Pathology* 74, no. 5 (November 1980): 757.

Alcohol and Violence

While mild doses of alcohol may help people feel less inhibited, drinking does not generally promote social behavior. Quite often, drinkers act in antisocial and sometimes even violent and belligerent ways (Table 14.1).

It is generally agreed that alcohol plays a critical role in violent acts and criminal activity. Alcohol has been consistently correlated with a variety of actions, including disturbing the peace, robbery, rape, assault, and murder. One study of homicides, for example, revealed that alcohol had been used by the victim or the perpetrator, or both, in nearly two-thirds of the cases.[6] Overall, problem drinkers have higher incidences of criminal behavior than the general population. In prison populations the incidence of alcohol problems is high; almost half of all inmates in state prisons claim to have been drinking at the time of their arrest.[7]

Alcohol and Domestic Turmoil

Alcohol abuse can sometimes lead to domestic turmoil, with serious effects on the psychological and emotional health of family members. It can also lead to financial problems if alcohol is allowed to interfere with work or fiscal responsibility. Sometimes the family members of a person who abuses alcohol become so enmeshed in resentment, guilt, and feelings of helplessness that their lives are seriously disrupted. Marriages may be strained by problems relating to employment, finances, and sex. If a drinking problem is especially bad, the family may become socially isolated because of embarrassment over the drinker's behavior and actions.

Alcoholism

Though it is commonly thought of as one of the most common symptoms of severe alcoholism, cirrhosis of the liver actually occurs in fewer than one-tenth of cases. And the prospects for survival from alcoholic cirrhosis are actually better than for other types of cirrhosis.

While occasional drinking may itself be detrimental to the health and well-being of individuals and society, chronic, excessive drinking is an even more serious health threat. Drinking excessively to the point of damaging the body or seriously disrupting one's life is symptomatic of an underlying disease

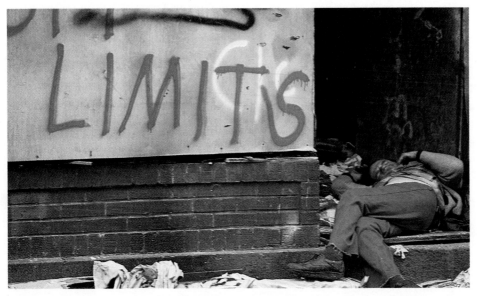

Whether rich or poor, a chronic alcoholic will eventually lose the ability to live life responsibly. (Alan Oddie/PhotoEdit)

known as *alcoholism*. For someone with alcoholism, drinking may lead to mental or physical disorders, such as pancreatitis, malnutrition, anemia, cancer, depression, and psychosis.[8]

The Alcohol Continuum

Alcoholism is a chronic disease characterized by preoccupation with alcohol and a loss of control over its consumption. With alcoholism, an individual becomes dependent on alcohol in a manner similar to other types of drug dependencies. Alcoholism can be envisioned as a progressive disease that develops as a series of stages through which any drinker may pass. At one end of the spectrum is occasional and moderate social drinking with family or friends on special occasions. At the other end is long-term, frequent, uncontrollable drinking with severe physical, psychological, and social complications. The full continuum can be summarized as follows:[9]

1. *Occasional drinker* drinks in small quantities only on special occasions to be sociable.
2. *Light drinker* drinks regularly in small and nonintoxicating quantities.
3. *Social drinker* drinks regularly in moderate and nonintoxicating quantities.
4. *Problem drinker* drinks to intoxication with no pattern to episodes, gets drunk without intending to or realizing it.
5. *Binge drinker* drinks heavily in recurrent episodes, often precipitated by disturbances in work, home, or social life.
6. *Excessive drinker* experiences frequent episodes of uncontrollable drinking affecting work, family, and social relationships.
7. *Chronic alcoholic* is in serious trouble from long-term, frequent, and uncontrollable drinking; experiences physical complications including organic dysfunction, tolerance, and dependence; and develops severe work, home, and social problems.

As a person moves along the continuum toward chronic alcoholism, certain characteristics begin to emerge, including:

- The person drinks to achieve specific effects, such as reduced anxiety, guilt, boredom, tension, or depression.

- The person undergoes drastic personality and mood changes, such as weeping, picking fights, becoming sexually aggressive.
- Others notice and remark on the person's drinking habits; the person's friendships and family life change.
- The person experiences hangovers and stomach trouble or may black out.

Signs of Alcoholism

The diagnosis of alcoholism is not something that can be precise, and it is often difficult for nonprofessionals to make. The disease carries such a stigma that the alcoholic, friends, and family often postpone seeking treatment. Meanwhile, it is not unusual for the alcoholic to deny the problem and rationalize continued drinking. Yet if the problem can be pinpointed and dealt with early, years of anguish can be saved for all concerned. Certain changes in behavior that warn of possible alcoholism include:[10]

- Surreptitious, secretive drinking.
- Morning drinking (unless that behavior is not unusual in the person's peer group).
- Repeated, conscious attempts at abstinence.
- Blatant, indiscriminate use of alcohol.
- Changing beverages in an attempt to control drinking.
- Having five or more drinks daily.
- Having two or more blackouts while drinking. (A *blackout* is an episode of temporary amnesia, in which the drinker continues to function but later cannot remember what happened; this is not the same thing as "passing out" when drunk.)

Causes of Alcoholism

Most authorities now agree that alcoholism stems from a number of interrelated factors, ranging from family life to peer pressure to emotional upheavals. The significance of these factors may vary from person to person in determining whether that person will become an alcoholic.

Legal and readily available in almost every American city and town, alcohol is one of the most widely used and damaging drugs in the United States. (Bernard Asset/Photo Researchers, Inc.)

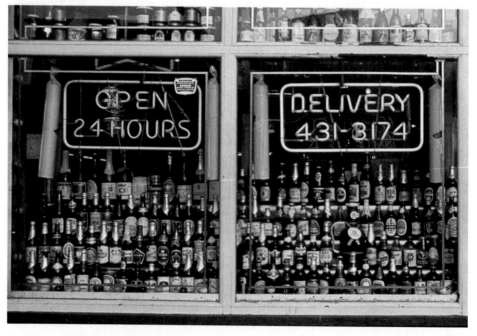

Alcoholism does definitely run in families. Studies in the United States and Europe show that about 50 percent of the fathers, brothers, and sons of hospitalized alcoholics are also likely to become alcoholics. Yet researchers remain uncertain as to whether the family environment, heredity, or a combination of the two determines whether a person will develop alcoholism.[11]

A number of psychological traits have been closely associated with alcoholics. These drinkers tend to have more psychological problems than others, including deep-seated feelings of inadequacy, anxiety, and depression. Researchers also see drinking as a learned behavior that is reinforced by repetition. A person learns to take a drink to relax, for example, and then repeats the behavior in stressful situations until a pattern of heavy drinking has developed.[12]

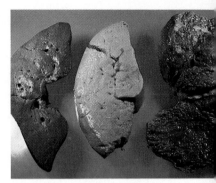

From left to right this picture shows: a normal liver; a fatty liver, which can indicate that cirrhosis is beginning; and a fully cirrhotic liver, with the liver swollen and scarred by excessive alcohol consumption. (A. Glauberman/Photo Researchers, Inc.)

Alcoholism in America

As many as 10 million American adults and 3 million children and adolescents are afflicted with alcoholism. All types of people can develop the disease, although genetic and environmental factors may make some people especially susceptible to it. For example, studies reveal that the incidence of alcoholism is higher for men than for women, although the number of female alcoholics is on the rise. The reason for this increase may be due, in part, to the fact that American women are increasingly adopting work and health-related behaviors more traditionally typical of men. As a result, they are experiencing similar problems and stresses that could contribute to alcoholism. The incidence of alcoholism also differs among religions and ethnic groups. Among Moslems and Mormons, whose religions forbid the use of alcohol, alcoholism is uncommon. Italians and Jews have relatively low rates of alcoholism, although the consumption of alcohol is an accepted practice among both groups. No group, however, is immune from alcoholism. It affects the very old as well as the very young; it affects people at all levels of education, in all occupational fields, and in all socioeconomic strata.[13]

Health Consequences of Alcohol Abuse

Chronic alcohol abuse is linked with many serious health problems that can destroy the body's most important organs and sometimes result in death.[14] Among the problems linked to alcohol abuse are gastrointestinal disorders, liver damage, cardiovascular disease, glandular disorders, damage to the central nervous system, and malnutrition. While chronic alcohol abuse can harm the health of the person who drinks, less excessive alcohol use by pregnant women is associated with birth defects and problems in pregnancy.

Gastrointestinal Disorders

Alcohol stimulates secretion of digestive acid throughout the gastrointestinal system, irritating the linings of the drinker's stomach, esophagus, and intestines. It is not unusual for alcoholics to develop bleeding ulcers in their stomachs and intestines and lesions in the esophagus. Alcohol can give "binge drinkers" diarrhea. It may inhibit the pancreas's production of enzymes that are crucial for the digestion of food. When heavily abused, alcohol can also lead to **pancreatitis** (inflammation of the pancreas).

pancreatitis—inflammation of the pancreas associated with heavy alcohol intake.

Liver Damage

The liver is one of the organs most vulnerable to alcohol abuse. As much as 80 percent of liver disease deaths are alcohol-related.[15] Alcohol changes the way the liver processes important substances; it can also contribute to infections

A Broader View

Alcoholism: A World Problem

Alcoholism is a major problem facing the world today. It affects more lives—and costs nations more money—than drugs, AIDS, or even wars. Last year in the United States alcoholism cost the country $120 billion, roughly double the cost of all other drug addictions combined. With an estimated 10 million alcoholics, the United States ranks 16th in per capita alcohol consumption. The Soviety Union also ranks in the top 20.

Similar steps to combat alcoholism have been taken in the two countries. Both have raised the drinking age to 21 and have increased the legal severity of alcohol-related crimes. In addition to passing new laws, both have established specialized treatment centers for alcoholics. And both agree that the biggest challenge in the international fight against alcoholism is educating the public about its dangers.

In the Soviet Union, an understanding of the international nature of alcoholism is viewed as very important. This involves knowledge of three different factors: the volume and type of alcohol consumption per capita in different countries, the types of behavior induced by typical immoderate drinking there, and the damage that alcohol does to the different economies and societies.

The simplest and most accessible data about alcoholism focus on the volume of different types of alcohol consumed in given countries. From this information three groups of countries can be distinguished: those where hard liquor is the main alcoholic beverage, those where wine drinking does the most damage, and those where beer provides the highest alcohol intake. Here is a typical comparison table:

	Annual Per Capita Consumption[a]		
	Hard Liquor	Wine	Beer
Australia	1.1	2.0	5.9
Canada	3.3	1.0	3.8
France	2.5	9.9	1.9
Italy	1.9	8.1	0.8
Soviet Union	4.2	2.8	1.0
Sweden	2.8	1.1	2.0
Switzerland	2.1	5.3	3.1
United States	3.0	0.9	4.1

[a] *This consumption is based on the straight alcohol content in liters of the three types of alcoholic drink.*

Current research suggests that there is an upward trend in alcoholism that coincides with consumption in many countries: for example, there is a trend toward more wine drinking in both the United States and the Soviet Union. Clearly, both national and international organizations will have to make considerable efforts if alcoholism is to be reduced appreciably.

Finding a solution to the world alcohol problem begins with research into incidence and causes, but it cannot be achieved without more effective treatment programs and, above all, large-scale public education about the disease. People should know the pervasiveness of alcohol problems in the world and in their own countries; and they should also know what types of help are available in their countries and communities.

Based on Don Cahalan, *Understanding America's Drinking Problem* (San Francisco: Jossey-Bass Publishers, 1987); B. and M. Levin, "To Know in Order to Overcome," *Sovetskaya Rossia* (March 13, 1989): 2; B. Walsh and M. Grant, *Public Health Implications of Alcohol Production and Trade* (Geneva: World Health Organization, 1985).

cirrhosis of the liver—*a chronic inflammatory disease in which healthy liver cells are replaced by scar tissue, impairing the liver's function.*

and other disorders. If the liver is disturbed or infected, the body's immune system and ability to flush out poisons are affected. Damage to the liver can also harm other organs because the liver is essential to the production and modification of many substances the body needs, such as a vast array of nutrients necessary for the building, maintenance, and repair of tissues.

Many alcoholics suffer **cirrhosis of the liver,** a chronic inflammatory disease in which healthy liver cells are replaced by scar tissue. Cirrhosis is a

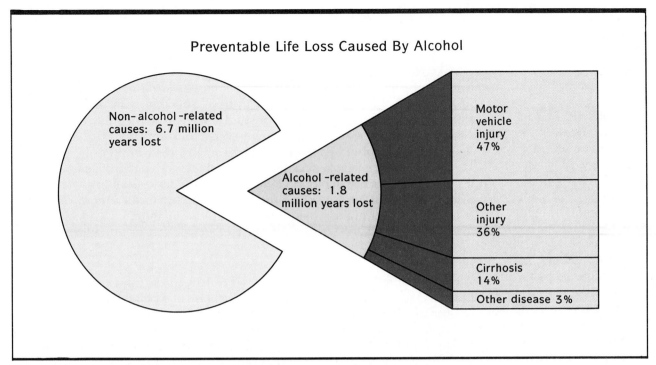

Preventable Life Loss Caused By Alcohol

Non–alcohol–related causes: 6.7 million years lost

Alcohol–related causes: 1.8 million years lost

Motor vehicle injury 47%

Other injury 36%

Cirrhosis 14%

Other disease 3%

Figure 14.2 Preventable deaths are responsible for millions of potential years of life lost. Alcohol is a significant factor in many of these deaths. Of about 1.8 million years of life lost that are blamed on alcohol each year, nearly half are due to motor vehicle injury, and over one-third to other injuries, but even the 14 percent associated with cirrhosis of the liver represent some 250,000 years of life lost.

Source: Adapted from Robert Amler and Donald Eddins, "Cross-Sectional Analysis: Precursors of Premature Death in the United States," in *Closing the Gap*, R. Amler and H. B. Dull (eds.) (New York: Oxford University Press, 1987): 184–185.

leading cause of death among heavy drinkers (Figure 14.2). Drinking can also cause **alcoholic hepatitis,** in which the liver becomes swollen and inflamed.

alcoholic hepatitis—*an alcohol-related disease in which the liver becomes swollen and inflamed.*

Cardiovascular Disease

There is debate in the medical community about whether small amounts of alcohol, such as one drink a day, may actually lower the rates of some heart diseases. There is no question, however, that *excessive* drinking takes a toll on the heart and circulatory system, even causing heart failure in some cases.

Moderate amounts of alcohol can affect the cardiovascular system by altering the heart rate and dilating blood vessels near the skin, which gives the drinker the illusion of feeling warmer. The truth is, however, that the person is actually losing heat from the body *more* rapidly than when alcohol is not present in the bloodstream. Drinking while exposed to cold for long periods of time can reduce a person's resistance to the common cold or even pneumonia.

Glandular (Endocrine) Disorders

Excessive drinking can damage the body's glandular system, which regulates such important functions as moods and sexuality. For example, men who drink too much may suffer impotence and reduced levels of the hormone testosterone; in one study, researchers found that the second most frequent reason for impotence among men was excessive drinking. Women may also throw their hormonal systems out of balance through heavy drinking; recent studies indicate that alcohol abuse can lead to early menopause.

Central Nervous System Damage

Alcohol's most visible and measurable short-term effects are on the central nervous system. Even small amounts of alcohol can change the user's emotional state and physical behavior. Prolonged abuse can have even more damaging and sometimes permanent effects on the central nervous system. Detoxified alcoholics have been found to have difficulty with memory, motor skills, and perception. A number of studies have estimated that 50 to 70 percent of alcoholics who seek treatment suffer problems with the central nervous system: alcohol has literally killed some of their brain cells.

Alcohol abuse is also associated with severe emotional problems. Alcoholics consistently score higher on items measuring depression in psychological tests. And, according to some studies, the risk of suicide among alcoholics runs thirty times higher than in the general population.

Malnutrition

A common myth holds that alcohol, since it is made from fruit or grain, is food. It is not. Alcohol actually starves the body of essential nutrients. It does consist of calories, and so it produces energy; but it contains none of the chemical substances the body needs to build and repair tissue. Alcohol abuse has been reported as the most common cause of vitamin deficiency in America. An alcoholic may undereat or, because the digestive system is disrupted, may be unable to process properly the nutrients that are eaten. Alcoholics may also suffer nutritional imbalances because of the diarrhea, loss of appetite, and vomiting that often accompany heavy drinking. In short, alcoholism can be a form of slow starvation.

Birth Defects

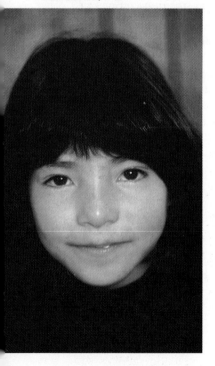

The effects of fetal alcohol syndrome continue long after birth, affecting a person's facial appearance, physical growth, and mental skills. (March of Dimes, Birth Defects Foundation)

Even mild drinking by a pregnant woman can produce adverse effects on a fetus; heavy drinking can cause fetal alcohol syndrome (FAS). Fetal alcohol syndrome consists of three main features—mental retardation; slow growth before and after birth; and a wide range of physical defects, ranging from cleft palate to hip dislocation. Mild to moderate mental retardation is characteristic of the syndrome; in fact, some researchers suggest that maternal alcoholism is the third leading cause of mental retardation in the United States.[16] The physical defects in babies born to alcoholic mothers are believed to be caused by a depletion of zinc in the mother's body, a depletion caused by alcohol.[17]

Some studies show that 74 percent of the infants born to mothers who drink more than ten drinks a day have the syndrome. Alcoholic women are also more likely to abort or give birth to stillborn children.[18]

There is no known safe level of alcohol that a woman can consume during pregnancy. The surgeon general recommends that women who are pregnant or considering pregnancy drink *no* alcoholic beverages and be aware of the alcohol content of certain foods and medicines.[19]

Dealing with Alcohol Abuse

Considering the tremendous harm that alcohol can do, few people knowingly become dependent on it. Many, however, develop alcohol dependency before they are aware of the dangers. Although numerous programs are available for treating this dependency, none can guarantee success.

Perhaps the only certain means of avoiding a dependency on alcohol is not to drink at all. Most people who use alcohol, however, are able to drink safely. For people who already have problems with alcohol, help is available.

Finding Your Own Comfort Level with Alcohol

Social drinking, which encourages alcohol consumption, is widely accepted in the United States; yet alcohol abuse is recognized as a major problem. Not only does abuse lead to violence and accidents; it can also lead to a crippling dependence on alcohol. But how can you tell if you abuse alcohol?

One measure of whether a person is drinking an acceptable amount is whether that person is free of any of the problems that result from drinking. If you are arrested for drunken driving, for example, or if hangovers are affecting your performance in school or on the job, you have been drinking abusively, not socially. A social drinker is able to drink in a way that does not result in such problems. But how can you identify the dividing line before you cross it and get into trouble?

Some experts on alcoholism define social drinking by the amount of alcohol the drinker consumes, but opinions differ as to what amounts are safe. The National Institute on Alcohol Abuse and Alcoholism (NIAAA) says that anyone who consumes at least five drinks on at least one occasion per week is a frequent, heavy drinker, not a social drinker. But other groups give different limits. A recent study concluded that daily consumption of five shots of liquor, three glasses of wine, or four cans of beer will have no harmful effects on someone who weighs 154 pounds (but nevertheless the person might not be sober enough to drive). Another study put the alcoholism cutoff point at four drinks per occasion—as long as the drinker partakes only three days per week.

People clearly differ both in their tolerance for alcohol and in their definition of what constitutes a problem. Everyone would be wise to think carefully about the issue, to be cautious with alcohol, and if they do intend to drink to establish a comfort level which they feel will enhance both their health and their lives. Questions to ask include the circumstances under which you drink and your reasons for using alcohol. As a rule, a social drinker consumes small amounts of alcohol in safe situations. Having a few beers with friends while watching a ball game may be "social"; however, it ceases to be social if the drinking becomes more important than the game or the friends. It is also not social when it involves significant physical or social risk—drinking more than a minimal amount when you will be driving, for example, or drinking in school or at work.

You are not drinking socially when you

- Drink to steady your nerves
- Drink to resolve problems
- Understate the amount that you drink
- Drink when alcohol is likely to harm you
- Drink to the point of intoxication even though doing something that you know requires sober attention, such as driving or performing surgery
- Do something while drinking that you would never have done while sober

Anyone who drinks may abuse alcohol on an isolated occasion, especially someone who is new to drinking and has not yet learned how much alcohol she or he can tolerate. A healthy response to such an episode is to drink more carefully so that it does not recur. However, some people have genetic backgrounds that may render them incapable of this response. People with alcoholic parents, for example, are far more likely than other people to develop alcoholism.

If your drinking ever results in a problem, drink less. If you continue to drink too much despite your efforts, you may be developing a dependency on alcohol and should seek counseling. If you can drink small amounts in safe circumstances, you may never develop a problem with alcohol and you may be able to enjoy a healthy life as a social drinker.

Based on V. M. Jackson et al., "Measurements of Social Drinking: The Need for Specific Guidelines," *Health Values* (January/February 1990): 25; Sandra Mull, "Help for the Children of Alcoholics," *Health Education* (September/October 1990): 42.

Using Alcohol Responsibly

In addition to these points, there are other obvious strategies worth considering:

- *alternating alcoholic and nonalcoholic drinks*
- *arranging to sleep overnight so that you will not have to drive*
- *being ready to take a cab*
- *having a "designated driver" arrangement with your friends*

If you choose to drink alcohol, you must learn to drink responsibly for two reasons: first, doing so will help you guard against losing control and becoming dependent on alcohol; and, second, abusing alcohol is known to be dangerous even if you are not dependent on it, since alcohol abuse can threaten your safety or that of others.

There are several good rules to follow in regard to alcohol:

- Know how much alcohol you can handle and do not exceed this limit, even on special occasions.
- Avoid drinking daily or at other regular intervals; such habits are more likely to lead to dependency.
- Choose drinks that are mixed with nonalcoholic beverages, such as fruit juice or water, instead of drinks that use two or more kinds of alcohol.
- Drink slowly; the faster you drink, the drunker you will get.
- Since food slows the absorption of alcohol, eat before you drink or while you are drinking.
- Accept a drink only if you really want one; when you have had enough, stop drinking and refuse offers for more.

If your drinking seems to be getting out of hand, or if a friend suggests that you may have a drinking problem, seriously consider the situation. Most people with alcoholic tendencies are inclined to deny them. If you even suspect that you may have a problem with alcohol, get help. The sooner you act, the more likely you are to overcome the problem.

The Treatment of Alcoholism

The life expectancy of an alcoholic is 10 to 12 years shorter than that of the average person.

Society has had a difficult time dealing with the issue of whether alcoholism is an illness or simply a weakness and failure of willpower. And if alcoholism is an illness, is it a physical illness or an emotional dysfunction? Treatment has usually approached alcoholism as both a physical and emotional disorder, dealing first with its physical aspects and then with its emotional ones.

Alcoholics Anonymous provides a positive forum for participants to discuss their efforts to deal with alcohol dependence. (Mary Kate Denny/PhotoEdit)

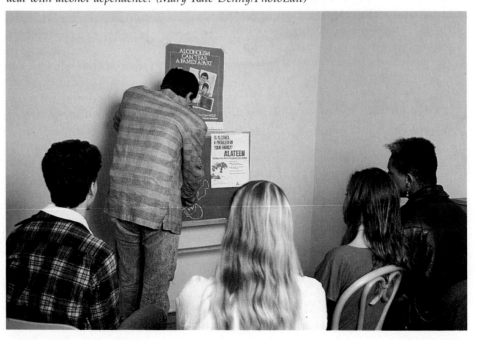

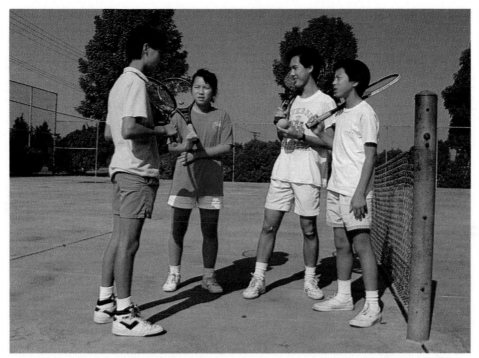

Relaxing, sociable, and health-promoting rather than self-destructive, active exercise with friends is one of the best alternatives to social drinking and substance abuse. (Ron Grishaber/ PhotoEdit)

Detoxification and Counseling

Treatment for alcoholism is likely to start with **detoxification,** the process of weaning the person from physical dependence and repairing the toxic effects of alcohol in the body. In the early stages of treatment, the alcoholic's nutritional needs must also be addressed—as must other health problems created by drinking. After detoxification and attention to the alcoholic's medical needs, many treatment programs provide counseling to address the drinker's psychological and social problems.

Alcoholics Anonymous (AA), founded in the 1930s, is among the most successful of treatment programs. AA members start by admitting that they have lost control over alcohol. They are then encouraged to think about the spiritual dimension of their lives and consider the idea that there is some power higher than themselves (even if they are not "religious" in the formal sense). Then they look closely at themselves, considering where alcohol has led them and what the future might hold.

Throughout the program, individuals receive support from fellow AA members, and eventually they themselves will work to help others through the process. AA's combination of group support, behavior modification, and spiritually oriented thinking has helped many alcoholics recover.

Developing Positive Alternatives to Alcohol Use

Although the use of alcohol is a matter of individual choice, the pressure to drink can be great. At social gatherings and some business events, drinking can be so prevalent that it almost seems required.

Alcohol problems can be prevented by taking responsibility for your drinking behavior *before* your judgment is impaired. Although the effects of alcohol are unpredictable, the fact is that even moderate amounts of alcohol may

detoxification—the process of weaning a person from physical dependence on alcohol or some other drug and repairing the toxic effects of the drug in the body.

Alcoholics Anonymous also sponsors programs for others who are affected by alcoholism:

- *Al-Anon is for adult relatives and friends of alcoholics*
- *Al-a-Teen helps teenage children live with an alcoholic parent or parents*
- *ACOA (Adult Children of Alcoholics) provides similar help for families of older alcoholics*

affect parts of the brain that control inhibitions, judgments, and feelings. The choices and decisions people make can be influenced by these alcohol-induced changes.

It is important to establish your own rules and limits for the use of alcohol. For example, if you are hosting a party, you might limit the amount of alcohol available or limit the time during which alcohol is served. Plan to serve nonalcoholic beverages as well as alcohol.

It is also important to respect an individual's decision not to drink alcohol. Many people abstain from drinking alcohol for religious, health, or moral reasons. Choosing *not* to drink alcohol is another option you can choose.

By developing positive alternatives to alcohol, you can make avoiding alcohol abuse easier for yourself and for others. Depending on your interests, the use of alcohol can be replaced by active pursuits such as walking, biking, tennis, or swimming; by quieter but still absorbing pursuits such as practicing a hobby or reading; and by using direct stress reduction techniques (Chapter 2).

Rather than think about what you might miss by not drinking, think of the benefits: better health, clearer thinking, money saved, and so forth. Your choice to avoid alcohol will be more rewarding if you focus on the things in life you can enjoy without alcoholic intoxication.

Chapter Summary

- After it is consumed, alcohol is absorbed into the bloodstream and distributed throughout the body. Some of it is eliminated unmetabolized through the kidneys, lungs, and sweat glands. The rest is metabolized by the liver, forming a toxic substance that combines with other compounds to form an opiatelike substance that is believed to be highly addictive. Alcohol can impair judgment and motor activity, making it dangerous in certain situations, such as driving a car or using equipment.
- The use of alcohol can be attributed to a variety of factors, including physical addiction, psychological dependence, and social pressures. These factors are often intertwined, making it difficult for a person to avoid alcohol use or stop once use has begun.
- Alcohol use has been linked to a variety of destructive behaviors, including an increased risk of accidents, violent acts and criminal activity, and increased domestic turmoil within a family.
- Alcoholism is a progressive condition marked by a series of stages, including occasional drinking, light drinking, social drinking, problem drinking, binge drinking, excessive drinking, and chronic alcoholism. The signs of possible alcoholism include secretive drinking, morning drinking, repeated attempts at abstinence, indiscriminate use of alcohol, having five or more drinks daily, having two or more blackouts while drinking.
- Chronic, excessive drinking has been associated with a number of serious health problems, including gastrointestinal disorders, liver damage, cardiovascular disease, glandular disorders, central nervous system damage, malnutrition, and birth defects in children born to women who drank during pregnancy.
- People who choose to drink can attempt to use alcohol sensibly by knowing their limits and avoiding habits that may lead to dependency. In addition, people who even suspect they have a problem with alcohol use should seek help.
- The treatment of alcoholism normally begins with detoxification, in which a person is weaned from physical dependence, and proceeds to counseling programs designed to help a person deal with psychological dependence. Alcoholics Anonymous attempts to treat alcoholism through individual introspection, group support, behavior modification, and spiritually oriented thinking.
- People can often avoid the use of alcohol by substituting other, positive alternatives, such as walking, enjoying friends and family, limiting the use of alcohol in their home, and so on.

Key Terms

Ethyl alcohol (page 373)

*Blood alcohol level (BAL)
(page 373)*

Pancreatitis (page 379)

*Cirrhosis of the liver
(page 380)*

*Alcoholic hepatitis
(page 381)*

Detoxification (page 385)

References

1. National Institute on Alcohol Abuse and Alcoholism, *Facts about Alcohol and Alcoholism,* DHHS pub. no. (ADM) (1980): 30–31.

2. National Center for Health Statistics, *Monthly Vital Statistics Report* 34, no. 6, Supplement 2 (September 25, 1985): 5.

3. James T. Weston, "Alcohol's Impact on Man's Activities: Its Role in Unnatural Death," *American Journal of Clinical Pathology* 74, no. 15 (November 1980): 755–758.

4. Council on Scientific Affairs, "Alcohol and the Driver," *Journal of the American Medical Association* 255, no. 4 (January 24–31, 1986): 522–527.

5. Editorial, *Journal of the American Medical Association* 255, no. 4 (January 24–31, 1986): 529–530.

6. National Committee for Injury Prevention and Control, "Injury Prevention: Meeting the Challenge," *American Journal of Preventive Medicine* (1989): 197–198.

7. A. Zeichner and R. O. Pihl, "Effect of Alcohol and Behavior Contingencies on Human Aggression," *Journal of Abnormal Psychology* 88, no. 2 (1979): 153–160.

8. Roland E. Herrington et al. (eds.), *Alcohol and Drug Abuse Handbook* (St. Louis: Warren H. Green, 1987): 181–183.

9. Morris E. Chafetz, *The Alcoholic Patient: Diagnosis and Management* (Oradell, N.J.: Medical Economics Books, 1983).

10. N. J. Estes and M. E. Heinemann (eds.), *Alcoholism: Development, Consequences, and Interventions,* 2d ed. (St. Louis: Mosby, 1982); George Vaillant, *The Natural History of Alcoholism: Causes, Patterns, and Paths to Recovery* (Cambridge, Mass.: Harvard University Press, 1983.)

11. Marc A. Schuckit and Robert M. J. Haglund, "An Overview of the Etiological Theories on Alcoholism," in Estes and Heinemann, op. cit.

12. Jean Kinney and Gwen Leaton, *Loosening the Grip: A Handbook of Alcohol Information* (St. Louis: Mosby, 1978).

13. Herrington et al. (eds.), op. cit., pp. 181–182.

14. This discussion of the impact of alcohol on the body, organs, glands, and central nervous system is based on information and studies cited in Eckardt et al., "Health Hazards Associated with Alcohol Consumption," *Journal of the American Medical Association* 246, no. 6 (August 7, 1981): 648–661.

15. John R. Senior, "Digestive Diseases Information Fact Sheet," *Alcoholic Liver Disease,* vol. 2 (1983).

16. Clair Toutant and Steven Lippmann, "Fetal Alcohol Syndrome," *American Family Physician* 22, no. 1 (July 1980): 113–117.

17. Arthur Flynn et al., "Zinc Status of Pregnant Alcoholic Women: A Determinant of Fetal Outcome," *Lancet* (March 14, 1981): 572–574.

18. Toutant and Lippmann, op. cit.

19. *FDA Drug Bulletin* no. 11 (December 1981): 1.

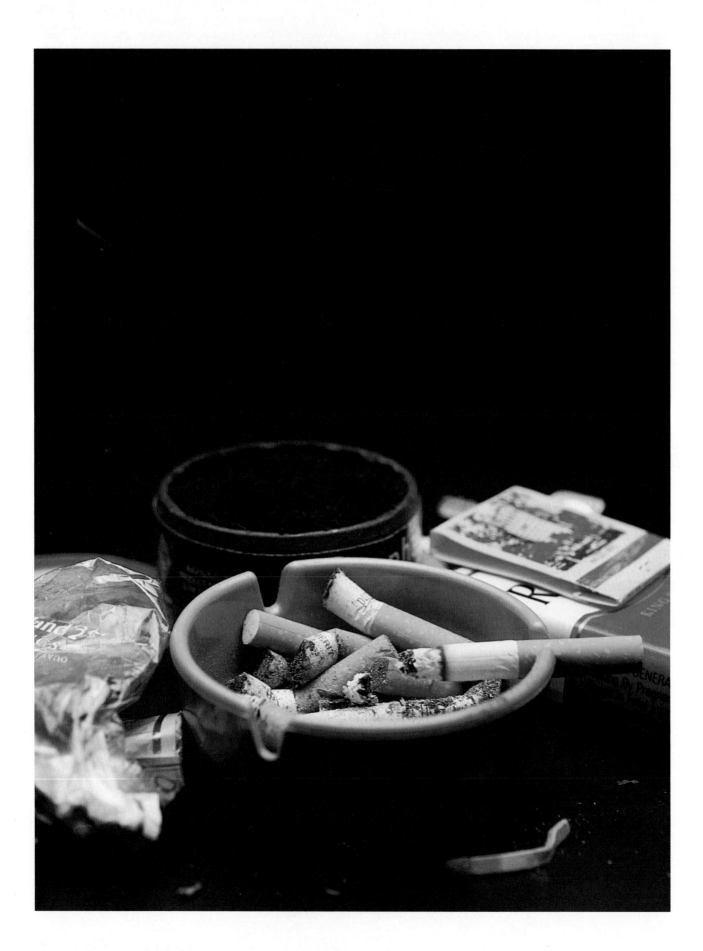

Chapter 15

Tobacco

To Guide Your Reading

When you have studied this chapter, you should be able to:

• Identify the major substances found in tobacco and tobacco smoke and explain the effects of these substances on the body.

• Identify several major diseases associated with tobacco use and discuss the health risks involved.

• Explain how tobacco use can affect not only users, but also infants born to women who smoke during pregnancy and people who inhale the tobacco smoke of others.

• Discuss the factors that influence tobacco use and explain how tobacco can lead to physical and psychological dependence.

• Identify and describe several different types of programs aimed at helping people give up smoking.

One reason that tobacco use is so prevalent today is that commercial interests have made it part of our culture. Tobacco has been an important cash crop since colonial days. When cigarette manufacturing first became a major industry around 1900, the typical smoker was a middle-class working man. With the help of public relations and advertising the tobacco industry extended the smoking fashion to professional men and to women in the 1920s. During World War II advertising conjured romantic images of handsome fighter pilots and beautiful nurses enjoying cigarettes. The "right" cigarette became a sexual lure and a mark of sophistication. One advertiser even conferred a kind of medical certification on smoking, claiming its brand was popular among doctors.

Tobacco promotion successfully targeted the youth market in the 1950s and 1960s. By 1964, when the surgeon general's office published its first report on smoking, more than half of men and one-third of women smoked. Daily smoking among 25- to 34-year-olds was even higher, including 60 percent of men and 44 percent of women.

After the 1964 report, however, the overwhelming facts linking tobacco and disease began to bring results. Congress banned cigarette advertising on television and radio in 1971. Cigarette packages and print advertising were made to carry warning labels. Antismoking information began to be widely distributed.

Although cigarette marketers have kept trying to extend their sales, they are meeting with outraged resistance by some targeted communities. Recently, plans for a new brand (*Uptown*) aimed at black Americans drew the fire of the surgeon general and local leaders, snuffing out the campaign.

The battle against the epidemic of tobacco-caused disease is far from over. Tobacco remains attractive to millions of youths and adults. Nicotine, its addictive agent, strengthens the tobacco habit. But the health community is united in agreement with a recent surgeon general's report which described tobacco as "the chief preventable cause of death in our society."[1]

As a result of the growing determination of health professionals and the growing public awareness about the dangers of tobacco, there has been a major shift in public attitude toward the smoking of tobacco. Smoking is less socially acceptable than it once was—and illegal in many public places. As a result, there has been a substantial decrease in the number of people who smoke: today, about 29 percent of American adults smoke, compared with about 40 percent in 1965. And of some 50 million American men and women who still smoke, most have tried at least once to give up the habit.[2]

However, this means that there are still 50 million Americans who smoke cigarettes. And the recent decline in smoking has been accompanied by a resurgence in the use of smokeless tobacco (chewing tobacco and snuff), especially among young men. Smokeless tobacco users "dip" snuff or chew leaf tobacco. Snuff is a finely ground, moist tobacco that is usually placed between the lower lip and gum, where it is mixed with saliva and absorbed. Chewing tobacco is a rougher-cut tobacco that is placed between the cheek and gum, where the wad (or chaw) is sucked and occasionally chewed.

In 1986, an estimated 8.2 percent of males aged 17 to 19 were using smokeless tobacco. Some of this increase can be attributed to aggressive advertising campaigns that use celebrated athletes to promote a "macho" image and that seem to suggest that snuff and chewing tobacco are "healthier" alternatives to smoking. Despite evidence that these products can also cause deadly diseases, the number of people using smokeless tobacco products continues to increase.[3]

About 23 percent of American college students smoke cigarettes.

Tobacco Use and Its Effects on the Body

Figure 15.1 Tobacco-related deaths account for 18 percent of the 8.5 million years of life lost to preventable causes in the United States each year. This represents 1.5 million years of life lost to tobacco annually. Cancer, heart attack, stroke, and diabetes claim 70 percent of this tobacco-related waste— over 1 million years of life lost.

Unlike alcohol, which has ill effects that can be dramatic and immediate, tobacco's damage becomes apparent only after years of use. This makes it in many ways a more dangerous substance than alcohol. An estimated 390,000 deaths each year—one-fifth of all American deaths—have been attributed to smoking.[4] For each death, figure nearly 4 years of life lost (Figure 15.1).

Source: Adapted from Robert Amler and Donald Eddins, "Cross-Sectional Analysis: Precursors of Premature Death in the United States," in *Closing the Gap*, R. Amler and H. B. Dull (eds.) (New York: Oxford University Press, 1987): 184–185.

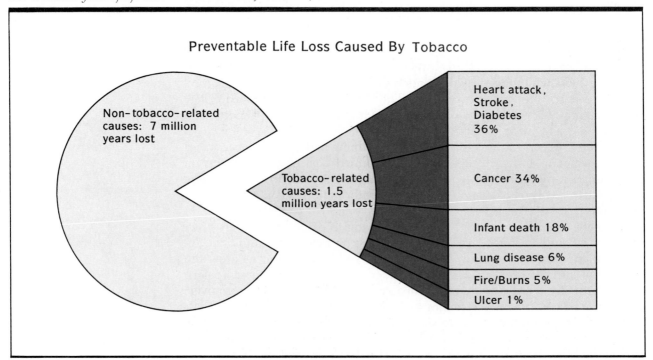

Preventable Life Loss Caused By Tobacco

Non-tobacco-related causes: 7 million years lost

Tobacco-related causes: 1.5 million years lost

Heart attack, Stroke, Diabetes 36%

Cancer 34%

Infant death 18%

Lung disease 6%

Fire/Burns 5%

Ulcer 1%

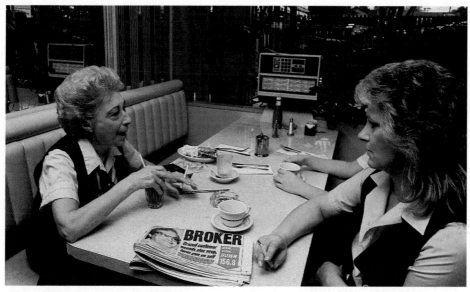

The feeling of well-being that tobacco creates is greatly at variance with its actual effects on the body. (Margot Granitsas/The Image Works)

The Effects of Nicotine

The chemical substance called **nicotine,** a toxic element found in tobacco, is responsible for much of the pleasure people experience while using tobacco. It causes a direct stimulation of the brain cells of the cerebral cortex, affecting brain chemistry and leading to feelings of increased alertness. It also causes muscle relaxation. And, perhaps most important, it has recently been positively identified as a pharmacologically addictive drug.[5]

Unfortunately, these effects come at a very high cost. There are many other chemicals in tobacco which are toxic, causing lasting damage to the human body. And nicotine itself is responsible for many of the harmful effects linked to the use of tobacco.

When nicotine enters the body, it is absorbed into the bloodstream. One-fourth of it soon passes directly into the brain, where it stimulates nicotine receptors, causing the release of chemicals that stimulate the cardiovascular system.[6] As a result, the heart beats faster and blood pressure increases.

Meanwhile, the remainder of the nicotine in the bloodstream travels throughout the rest of the body, where it stimulates other nicotine receptor sites. Not only does nicotine stimulate the gastrointestinal tract, it also causes the adrenal gland to release catecholamines (epinephrine and norepinephrine), which cause the body's fight-or-flight response (Chapter 2). As a result, the heartbeat increases by 15 or 25 beats per minute, the pupils of the eyes dilate, and the blood vessels in the fingers and toes constrict.

> nicotine—*a toxic element found in tobacco that acts as a stimulant and is responsible for many of the harmful effects of smoking.*

Tobacco and Other Toxic Substances

In addition to the addictive drug nicotine, tobacco products contain a number of other toxic substances that can cause harm when they enter the body. Some of these substances are found in tobacco smoke, whereas others are found in tobacco itself.

Toxic Substances in Tobacco Smoke When it burns, the average cigarette produces about 0.5 gram of smoke. To help determine what portions of tobacco smoke are responsible for the various diseases associated with cigarette smoking, chemists have broken down the smoke into its components. More than 80 major toxic substances have been identified in cigarette smoke.[7]

carbon monoxide—*one of the most hazardous gases in tobacco smoke. It impairs the body's capacity to carry oxygen.*

Of all the compounds in cigarette smoke, 92 percent are gaseous—and many of these are toxic. **Carbon monoxide,** one of the gases found in tobacco smoke, is considered to be one of the most hazardous. Carbon monoxide affects the human body in several ways, all of which are related to oxygen deprivation. Carbon monoxide impairs the blood's capacity to carry oxygen, causing serious problems for people suffering from cardiovascular diseases. Some researchers believe that carbon monoxide is partly responsible for the heightened risk of heart attack and stroke among cigarette smokers: it may be the *combination* of carbon monoxide and nicotine that is at fault.[8]

The remaining 8 percent of tobacco smoke consists of solid (nongaseous) matter: ash, a tar-rich condensate, and a "wet particular matter" comprising hundreds of different substances. **Tar,** a sticky residue from burning tobacco, consists of more than 200 chemicals and can be separated into three parts: acidic, basic, and neutral.

tar—a sticky residue from burning tobacco consisting of more than 200 chemicals, many of which are hazardous.

benzopyrene—a chemical found in tobacco smoke, one of the deadliest carcinogens known.

The neutral part of tar shows by far the highest carcinogenic, or cancer-causing, activity: it contains **benzopyrene,** one of the deadliest carcinogens known, and many other chemicals of the same family. The acidic part of the tarry condensate contains phenol and other materials which may be carcinogenic themselves and which may activate "dormant" cancer cells so that they grow and spread. The basic part of tar contains the nicotine itself. It also contains other chemicals that are potent irritants to lung tissue and may play a role in such conditions as chronic bronchitis, chronic obstructive pulmonary disease, and emphysema.[9]

While nicotine affects the body primarily through the bloodstream, many of the other substances directly affect the body's respiratory system. The act of smoking impedes the respiratory system's ability to trap and eliminate air pollutants, including over 2,000 potentially noxious substances found in tobacco smoke.[10] Normally, air pollutants are trapped in mucus secreted by membranes in the nasal cavity, trachea, and bronchi. These irritants are then either eliminated through the mouth or absorbed and eliminated by the lymphatic system. Both of these processes rely on the cilia, or fine hairs, that grow from epithelial cells lining the respiratory passages. The regular intake of smoke can flatten these epithelial cells, causing them to lose their cilia and produce excess mucus. This excess mucus may cause repeated cough reflexes—"smoker's cough"—that clear some of the mucus away. Or the mucus may stay where it is, blocking air passages and causing shortness of breath and wheezing (Figure 15.2).

Cigarette makers are exempt from federal laws that require manufacturers to list the ingredients of their products and have them tested for safety and purity.

Toxic Substances in Smokeless Tobacco In addition to nicotine, the tobacco in snuff and chewing tobacco contains a number of potent chemicals. These include high concentrations of several chemicals known to be carcinogenic. In laboratory studies, animals exposed to some of these chemicals (at levels thought to approximate lifetime daily use by humans) have been shown to develop an excess of a variety of cancerous tumors.[11] In humans, the use of chewing tobacco and snuff has been linked to cancer of the oral cavity, pharynx, larynx, and esophagus.[12]

Tobacco and Major Diseases

Although a tobacco user is unlikely to notice any harmful effects from a single use of tobacco, any sustained use can lead to serious health problems. The facts about the relationship between tobacco and disease are grim, to say the least. About 35 percent of all smokers—40 percent of the men and 28 percent of the women—die prematurely as a result of their use of tobacco.[13] Thirty percent of all cancer deaths are attributable to smoking, as are 21 percent of all coronary heart disease deaths, 18 percent of stroke deaths, and 82 percent of deaths from chronic obstructive pulmonary disease.[14] Smoking is associated with six of the ten leading causes of death.

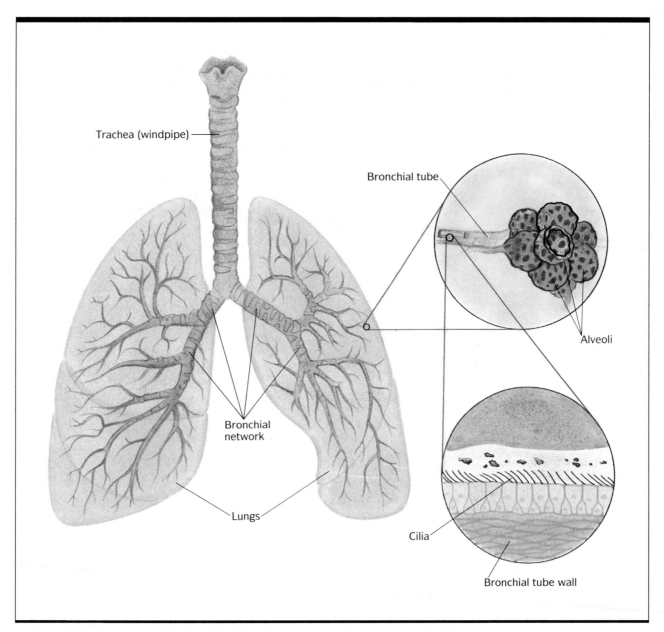

Figure 15.2 The lungs are a network of blood vessels and air passages, where oxygen from inhaled air is transferred to the blood through air sacs called alveoli. *The air passages, or bronchial tubes, can become inflamed by tobacco smoke and narrowed by a defensive secretion of mucus. Normally mucus is transported from the lungs by tiny hairs called* cilia; *but smoking can paralyze these, leaving the lungs with congestion (bronchitis) and reduced defenses against pollution and disease.*

The reduction in a person's life expectancy increases with the number of cigarettes smoked. For example, a man who smokes one pack a day loses 4.6 years of life expectancy; with two packs a day the time lost doubles. The earlier a person begins smoking, the more years of life are lost: if smoking starts before age 25, for example, about 4 years on the average are lost; if it starts before age 15, as many as 8 years are lost.[15]

The range of diseases that are associated with tobacco use is wide (Figure 15.3). Smokers have been shown to have greatly increased risks of premature coronary heart disease, atherosclerosis, aortic aneurysms, cerebrovascular disease, chronic bronchitis and emphysema, asthma, gastric problems, and dental problems (including gingivitis, dental caries, and loss of teeth)—not to mention cancer of the oral cavity, esophagus, pancreas, larynx, lung, kidney, and bladder.

The Tobacco Institute, the lobbying group for the tobacco industry, maintains that evidence linking smoking to increased mortality is inconclusive. It argues that adults have the right of free choice.

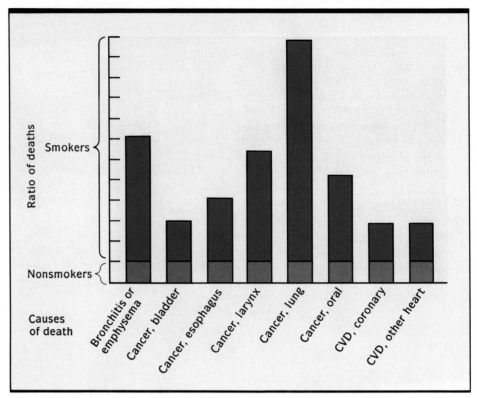

Figure 15.3 Smoking greatly increases the risk of death in a large number of diseases, as shown by this bar chart. For every nonsmoker who dies of bronchitis or emphysema, for example, more than six smokers will die of these same diseases.

Source: Daniel Chiras, *Environmental Science* (Menlo Park, Calif.: Benjamin/Cummings, 1987).

Although most of the research linking tobacco use to death and serious illness has focused on cigarette smoking, the studies that exist suggest that smokeless tobacco users often suffer dire consequences as well. These include decreased ability to taste and smell, gum and tooth devastation, high blood pressure, and cancer of the oral cavity and the esophagus. One study revealed that cancer of the mouth and throat is up to 50 times more common in people who had a lifetime practice of using snuff.[16]

Bronchitis and Emphysema

An earlier section of this chapter described how smoking can cause the epithelial cells of the respiratory system to flatten, causing them to produce excess mucus that can block air passages. If these epithelial cells are continuously assaulted as a result of chronic smoking, they can also become inflamed. This inflammation leads to chronic bronchitis, an inflammation of the mucous membranes that line the bronchial passages of the respiratory tract. Bronchitis is marked by coughing, spitting of saliva and mucus, and some difficulty in breathing.

Over time, chronic bronchitis may extend to other parts of the lungs and severely damage tissues. Breathing becomes more difficult as smooth muscle tissues enlarge and mucus becomes stuck in the passages. As a result, air is trapped in the alveoli, which are the air sacs in the lungs. The thin walls between the alveoli degenerate, which causes them to fuse and create enlarged air sacs. The resulting condition, in which air is taken in easily but is expelled only with great difficulty, is called emphysema, a potentially crippling and debilitating condition that can ruin a person's quality of life and result in death.

Smokers are 13 times more likely than nonsmokers to develop emphysema. A majority of patients develop the disease between the ages of 45 and 65. Next to heart disease, it is the most frequent single cause of permanent disability in the United States.

Cancer

The evidence linking smoking with various types of cancer is now overwhelming (Figure 15.4). According to the U.S. surgeon general, "Cigarette smoking is the major single cause of cancer mortality in the United States."[17] Of all cancer deaths, almost one-third can be linked to smoking.[18]

Even if an individual does not develop cancer after many years of smoking, the risks are still not eliminated. Death from lung diseases is six times more frequent among smokers. In addition, when an individual is exposed to tobacco and other carcinogens, such as asbestos, there appears to be a synergistic effect—the combined effect is greater than the effect of each on its own. For example, the risk of developing lung cancer increases sharply for those who smoke *and* work with asbestos. Blue-collar workers face the greatest danger, because they are the group that is most exposed to toxic agents *and* they also have the highest smoking rates, particularly among men.[19]

Once a rare disease, lung cancer is now considered to be an epidemic. In 1990 it was estimated to have killed 142,000 people. The American Cancer Society estimates that 83 percent of lung cancer—85 percent for men and 75 percent for women—is caused by smoking.[20]

The *way* an individual smokes affects the chances of developing lung cancer: the risk increases depending on how many cigarettes are smoked each day, how deeply the smoker inhales, and how much tar and nicotine are contained in the cigarettes smoked. People who started smoking early in their lives are also at greater risk than those who have only smoked for a few years.

If a person stops smoking, the chance of dying from lung cancer decreases; but it takes 10 to 15 years for the smoker's mortality rate to drop back to the nonsmoker's rate.[21]

Figure 15.4 These cross sections of the wall of a bronchial tube show the early stages of lung cancer. The normal wall has a lining of columnar cells (with cilia) supported by basal cells. First, irritation of the basal cells causes them to multiply. Next, the columnar cells are destroyed. The basal cells become "squamous," or scalelike. And finally they spread unevenly through the connective tissue.

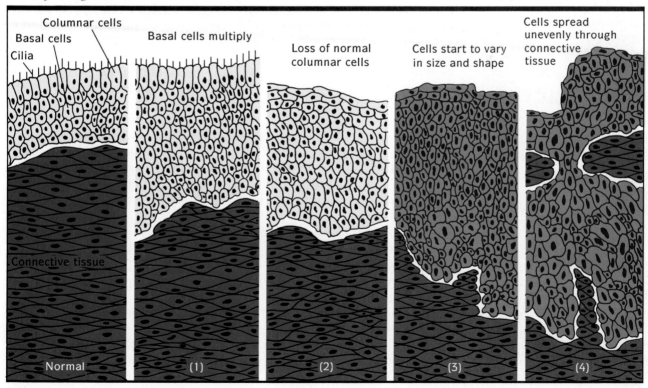

Cardiovascular Disease

The risk of cardiovascular disease in cigarette smokers is one and one-half to two times greater than that of nonsmokers.[22] People who smoke and also have high blood pressure and/or a history of heart disease in their family are in an even higher risk category for having a heart attack at some time in their lives. The more they smoke, the greater the risk of having a heart attack—and at a younger age than nonsmokers. The risk of heart disease will decrease after a person quits smoking, but, as with lung cancer, it takes 10 years after quitting for the risk of heart attack to drop to that of nonsmokers.[23] People who smoke also share a high risk of developing atherosclerosis, and those who have survived a heart attack face an increased possibility of suffering another one.

The combination of smoking and the use of birth control pills also increases the risk of cardiovascular disease. A woman who uses birth control pills and smokes as well is 10 times more likely to suffer a heart attack than a woman who neither smokes nor uses oral contraceptives.[24] (This combination may also be linked to strokes.) According to the Food and Drug Administration, the risks increase further with age and with heavy smoking (15 or more cigarettes a day).[25]

Tobacco and the Lives of Others

The toxins in tobacco and tobacco smoke can harm the health not only of people who smoke, but of others as well. Children born to women who smoke during pregnancy are affected by it, and so are people of all ages who inhale tobacco smoke produced by others.

The Dangers of Tobacco Use during Pregnancy

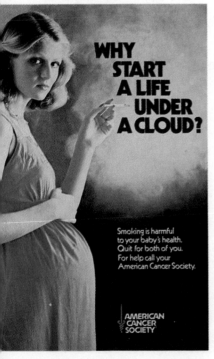

Researchers have established a direct relationship between smoking during pregnancy and adverse effects on the health of the baby. (Courtesy American Cancer Society)

A woman who smokes during pregnancy seriously endangers the health of her unborn child. Several large studies, involving tens of thousands of pregnancies, reveal that pregnant women who smoke have up to ten times as many miscarriages and stillbirths and two to three times as many premature babies as nonsmokers.[26] In one study, researchers calculated that one out of five babies who died would have been saved if their mothers had not been smokers.[27]

Furthermore, babies born to women who smoke during pregnancy are, on average, nearly one-half pound lighter than babies born to nonsmokers.[28] The importance of birth weight cannot be overstated. A newborn's weight is an important index of mortality risk; the lower the weight, the greater the risk of death. While the minimum weight for a healthy newborn is 2,500 grams (5½ pounds), among the infants of mothers who smoke, twice as many weigh less than 2,500 grams at birth as do babies of nonsmoking mothers. And, according to the office of the U.S. surgeon general, "there is abundant evidence that maternal smoking is a direct cause of the reduction of birth weight."[29]

The effects of tobacco do not end when a baby leaves the hospital. Studies have found that smoking during pregnancy may affect the growth, mental development, and behavior of children at least up to the age of 11.[30] In one study, children were examined at birth and then at 7 and 11 years of age. In reading and math, the offspring of women who smoked at least ten cigarettes daily during pregnancy lagged an average of 3 to 5 months behind children born to nonsmokers.[31]

Because of the potential damage to children, both at birth and during their later development, it is recommended that all women stop smoking during pregnancy.

Passive Smoking and the Rights of Nonsmokers

Reports from the U.S. surgeon general's office suggest that tobacco smoke in enclosed indoor areas is an important air pollution problem. This had led to the controversy about **passive smoking**—the breathing in of air polluted by the second-hand tobacco smoke of others. Carbon monoxide levels of side-stream smoke (smoke from the burning end of a cigarette) reach a dangerously high level of 42,000 parts per million. (For purposes of comparison, note that the Environmental Protection Agency sets 100 parts per million as the maximum allowed for air to be considered "clean.") True, the smoke can be greatly diluted in freely circulating air, depending on ventilation, the size of the room, and other factors, but the 1 to 5 percent carbon monoxide levels attained in smoke-filled rooms can be sufficient to harm the health of people with chronic bronchitis, other lung disease, or cardiovascular disease.[32]

Nicotine also builds up in the blood of nonsmokers exposed to cigarette smoke hour after hour. It has been estimated that passive smoking can give nonsmokers the equivalent in carbon monoxide and nicotine of one to ten cigarettes per day.[33]

While most people suffer some discomfort as well from passive smoking, people with allergies to tobacco smoke suffer the most. In one study of people with and without smoke allergies, 69 percent of those without allergies developed eye irritation from passive smoke, 29 percent had nasal irritation, 32 percent reported headaches, and 25 percent developed coughs. For the subjects with smoke allergies, the percentages were even higher.[34]

Passive smoking has also been shown to be harmful to the children of smokers. Children whose parents smoke have a higher incidence of respiratory problems, such as bronchitis and pneumonia, than do children whose parents do not smoke. The effects of such problems may last a lifetime: studies show that respiratory problems in adulthood are related to early childhood respiratory conditions influenced by parental smoking.[35]

Nonsmokers are increasingly successful in campaigns for protection against passive smoking. In recent years, several cities have adopted laws that limit or ban smoking in enclosed public spaces such as restaurants. Many employers, too, have banned smoking in workplaces or have restricted it to designated areas. Moreover, smoking is now entirely forbidden on many airline flights.

passive smoking—the breathing in of air polluted by the tobacco smoke of others.

A National Academy of Sciences study has found that nonsmoking spouses of smokers face a 25 percent greater risk of contracting lung cancer than spouses of nonsmokers.

In 1974 The National Interagency Council on Smoking and Health adopted the Nonsmokers' Bill of Rights. The three basic rights are:

- **The right to breathe clean air** *(air that is free of harmful tobacco smoke)*
- **The right to speak out** *(to express discomfort over tobacco smoke)*
- **The right to act** *(to work to help pass laws against tobacco smoke, especially in public places)*

Factors That Influence Tobacco Use

Despite the increasing opposition to smoking by nonsmokers, and despite the risks, many of which have been widely publicized, smokers continue to light up and tobacco use remains widespread. People addicted to nicotine have been known to continue using tobacco even while undergoing treatment for lung cancer or emphysema. As with alcohol, people appear to do this for a variety of reasons—social as well as physical and psychological.

Social Pressures

Certainly, people start smoking as a result of social pressures. For example, advertising has been highly successful for the tobacco companies, as mentioned at the beginning of this chapter. But the impact of advertising has been considerably lessened by the ban on TV and radio commercials for tobacco and, arguably, by the warning labels carried in print advertising and on cigarette packages themselves. Yet people continue to cling to the smoking habit, and new people take it up, often people for whom television and not the printed word is the most influential medium.

The Fire about No Smoking

During recent years, the percentage of Americans who smoke has steadily declined. As nonsmokers' numbers have increased, they have become increasingly outspoken about their so-called right to clean indoor air. In response, many states and cities have passed laws restricting smoking in public places, including offices, restaurants, theaters, hospitals, and many other enclosed areas. The first speaker argues that the drive against smoking has gone far enough: smokers already have their rights unduly abridged. The second speaker feels that more needs to be done.

Smokers Already Suffer Too Much Smokers are hooked on a legal but extremely harmful and addictive drug. Cigarettes have been found to be as addictive as heroin or cocaine: smoking a cigarette is like freebasing nicotine. Heart attack victims have been seen smoking on their way to the hospital. Many continue to smoke even after major heart surgery.

Most smokers began smoking at an early age, persuaded to start by clever advertisements and by society's tacit approval of cigarettes. Throughout the history of the United States, people have smoked. When Columbus discovered the New World in 1492, he discovered tobacco as well. The southern colonies thrived on the wealth provided by tobacco as they exported it to England and to Europe. Tobacco has been a staple of American life—a sign, in the popular culture, of health, wealth, sex appeal, and status. A hundred years ago no one would have dreamed of telling smokers not to smoke. In fact, during the first decades of this century the tobacco companies were so successful selling the American public on smoking cigarettes that 40 percent of the population became addicted.

Most smokers today are aware of the dangers of smoking, and they have tried to stop—by going "cold turkey," using behavior modification therapy, going to smoking-cessation classes, or trying hypnosis and dozens of other methods. But the addiction is so powerful that most ultimately begin smoking again.

By now—persuaded that one of our pleasures, though legal, is deadly, and finding ourselves unable to give it up—we smokers are offended and annoyed by the demands of those who have been lucky enough not to get hooked. Smokers' rights have already been compromised too much.

Nonsmokers' Rights Should Not Be Ignored The effects of tobacco on smokers have been known since the publication of the 1964 surgeon general's report that linked cigarettes to cancer. Since 1965 warning labels have appeared on packs of cigarettes; since 1971 television and radio advertisements for cigarettes have been banned; and for the last two decades the number of people who smoke has been declining.

However, in 1986 a new surgeon general's report publicized the dangers of passive smoking—inhaling smoke from other people's cigarettes. What nonsmokers had long feared was now proved: people who regularly inhale passive smoke are themselves at risk of contracting serious respiratory disease and even cancer. The 1986 report changed the public debate about cigarette smoking.

Until that report, most nonsmokers had limited their opposition to waving smoke away and coughing conspicuously. After the report was published, we began to see that passive smoke is a matter of health, not just annoyance. This is why we are becoming militant about getting local ordinances against smoking in public places and making sure they are enforced.

But we are protesting for more than our individual health. At stake too is the cost that all people have to bear as a result of smoking. Smokers have more illnesses and thus more days lost from work than nonsmokers. Many health insurance dollars go to pay for treatment of these illnesses. The more that society as a whole can discourage smoking, the better off it will be.

Do nonsmokers always have the right to smoke-free air? Should our society further limit the rights of smokers? Or are the restrictions against smoking now adequate? Have smokers' rights already been compromised too much?

Based on "All Fired Up over Smoking," *Time* (April 18, 1988): 64–71.

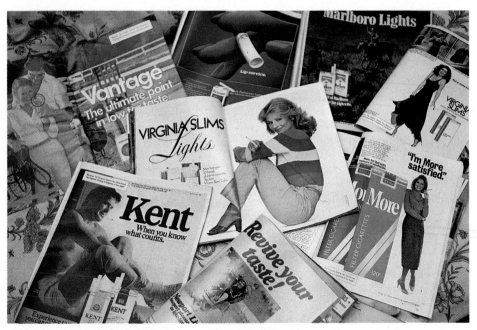

Advertising has played a key role in the hold that tobacco has on much of America. (Van Bucher/Photo Researchers, Inc.)

New smokers are often led into smoking through direct peer pressure. This has always been an influential force. Adults are influenced at work or social gatherings, as evidenced by the fact that people tend to adopt their boss's cigarette brand or the brand favored by their circle of friends. One study, for example, found that 68 percent of young female smokers had boyfriends or husbands who smoke. The surgeon general's 1988 report shows inverse relationships between smoking and educational status and social class: college-educated people employed in white-collar jobs are less likely to smoke than less-educated blue-collar workers, and smoking is less prevalent among people with higher incomes.[36]

For adolescents, of course, social pressure takes on another dimension. Children see many adults smoking, and yet it is illegal for them; this makes cigarettes a forbidden fruit and smoking seem like a rite of passage to adulthood. Smoking behind the barn and in the lavatory at school have been standard images of rebellious initiation throughout this century—but it is only during the last 25 years that the full damage that this can cause has been apparent. Many smokers began their habit in this way, succumbing to social pressures from friends.

Seventy-five percent of all smokers begin smoking before the age of 20.

However, if tobacco did not cause dependence, little harm would be done. Unfortunately, it does cause dependence, and in not one, but two ways. As an addictive drug, nicotine causes a direct physiological dependence. And as a result of this and other factors, it also creates a psychological dependence which makes the habit even harder to break.

Tobacco and Physiological Dependence

One sign that nicotine is addictive is that it can produce a tolerance in the smoker, who must consume more and more to achieve the same effects. For example, people who smoke to relieve stress must gradually increase their daily intake to continue experiencing the same level of relief.

Another typical indication of physiological dependence on a chemical substance is the withdrawal syndrome (Chapter 13). Smokers develop a craving for tobacco, and when they quit, or if they do not have a cigarette for a long time, they may become anxious, irritable, aggressive, and hostile, often experiencing headaches, excessive hunger, nausea, and constipation or diarrhea.

These symptoms appear while the body is going through more basic changes: after a person quits smoking, the heart rate and blood pressure drop, the level of adrenal hormones in the bloodstream drops, and the body's general arousal level decreases.

According to one theory, addiction to smoking creates alterations not only in the chemistry of the body, but also in the functioning of an individual's brain. Whenever tobacco users are not using tobacco, their brains seem to be in a state of hypoarousal—*less* aroused than normal—and they feel *less* stimulated than usual. In order to get their brain's stimulation back to normal, they must use tobacco.

Tobacco and Psychological Dependence

The addictive effect of nicotine on the body is one reason that it is a habit-forming drug. The physiological need itself—the cycle of stimulation and depression caused by nicotine—is also an important factor in creating psychological dependence. Psychological dependence is also created, however, by the pleasurable experiences or rewards that smokers may come to associate with smoking as a result of the particular habits they develop.

Tobacco use can easily become linked with daily routines. The morning cup of coffee, the work break, and the drink at the end of the day can all be occasions for habitual smoking. Smoking can also be a part of involvement in work: as the work intensifies, so does the smoking. Some people reward themselves with a cigarette after they accomplish a task. Thus, learning theory (Chapter 3) can be used to help explain the smoking habit. The chemical factors are made much more powerful because other secondary reinforcers—sights, smells, and aggreeable surroundings—are also present.

In addition, the convenience of tobacco is another reason for its popularity. It comes in unusually handy forms. Cigarettes are convenient to carry, to light, and to hold, and moreover they give nervous people something easy to do with their hands. Smokeless tobacco is tucked into the mouth, leaving the hands totally free. Such ease of use provides very little discouragement, and makes the psychological habit that much easier to acquire.

Vending machines make a hazardous, albeit legal, drug easily available to the public. (Tony Freeman/PhotoEdit)

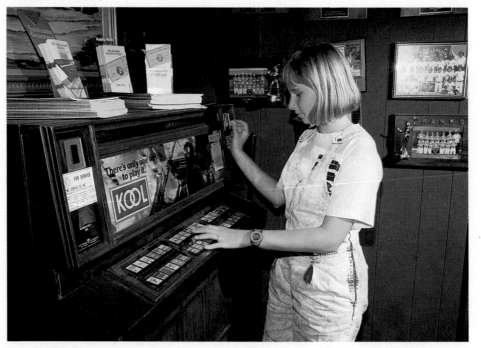

Giving Up Smoking

Although there has been a dramatic decrease in the number of smokers during recent years, the number of people who start the tobacco habit has not shown so great a decrease—and in this lies good news for smokers. Much of the decrease has occurred because many smokers have successfully quit. For more than 20 years, increasing numbers of people have been successful in giving up smoking. According to a number of scientific reports, most people who have successfully quit have done so without professional help.[37] There are, however, a wide variety of treatment programs available for people who cannot quit smoking on their own.

It is estimated that over 30 million Americans have quit smoking.

There are many ways to break the smoking habit, ranging from simply quitting "cold turkey"—which some authorities consider the most effective method—to elaborate, highly structured (and sometimes expensive) group programs that attempt to reduce smoking over a period of many weeks.

Individual Programs

A number of products are available to help people quit smoking on their own. These include books, records and cassettes, over-the-counter drugs, nicotine-containing chewing gum, and sets of graduated filters designed to reduce tar and nicotine intake over a period of time. Two drugs, clonidine and bispirone, have also been used to alleviate withdrawal symptoms. The effectiveness of individual efforts has been difficult to evaluate.

Group Programs

There is also a wide variety of group programs and clinics available to help people stop smoking. Some are sponsored by nonprofit health organizations such as the American Cancer Society, the American Heart Association, and the American Lung Association. Others are run as profit-making businesses.

Group programs usually involve lectures, films, discussions, and practical tips on how to stop smoking. Computers are sometimes used to tailor approaches to the needs of each individual. Many programs pair off participants so that they can bolster each other's determination to quit. Some group programs meet regularly over a period of weeks, and others are concentrated into perhaps a 5-day program. Some hospitals offer intensive, 24-four-hour-a-day, live-in programs.

Professional Therapy

Some programs to stop smoking involve hypnosis, where a professional practitioner induces a mild trance and then coaches the person about how to stop. Other programs rely on aversion techniques—such as using mild electric shocks or having the person breathe stale cigarette smoke or smoke extremely rapidly—in an effort to associate smoking with an unpleasant experience. One form of aversion therapy that has had good results is rapid smoking: once a day, the person chain-smokes as many cigarettes as possible, taking puffs every 6 seconds. No cigarettes are allowed between these daily sessions. Six months after completing this treatment, 60 percent of clients report that they are still not smoking. It should be noted that rapid smoking can be hazardous.[38]

Behavior Modification and Learning Theory

Another approach applies the principles of behavior modification. The idea is simple. People who smoke generally do so at certain predictable times: with a cup of coffee, at a party, after a meal. Instead of smoking at those times, the

What Makes Quitting So Hard?

Giving up smoking is often very difficult. You must analyze the forces and pressures surrounding your struggle. Try to recognize the factors which block your desire to change and to keep clearly in front of you the benefits you expect from quitting. To help you sort out your thoughts and feelings try this two-part questionnaire:

Why Do You Continue to Smoke? Recognizing the rewards you get from smoking is essential if you want to give it up. Below are some of the most common reasons that people give for continuing to smoke. Check off the reasons that apply to you and write any additional reasons in the space provided.

I don't want to quit because:

_____ I'll eat more and gain weight.

_____ Smoking relaxes me more than anything else.

_____ Giving up cigarettes will be painful and difficult because I'm hooked on nicotine. I doubt that I'll be able to quit.

_____ I enjoy my after-dinner cigarette and don't want to give it up.

_____ I enjoy having a cigarette when I'm out with friends.

_____ I truly enjoy smoking, even if it's bad for my health.

_____ Smoking is part of my image; it's cool and sophisticated.

_____ I think the health risks associated with smoking are exaggerated. My grandfather smoked all his life and lived to be 86.

_____ Smoking is one of the few pleasures I have in life.

_____ I'd be at a loss with what to do with my hands if I didn't smoke.

List other reasons of your own here:

_____
_____
_____
_____
_____

person substitutes another behavior, such as taking a walk. Rewards and punishments can also be effective in learning to stop smoking. Researchers have reported good short-term results when people had to forfeit money every time they smoked.

Fostering a Smoke-Free Life

Smoking has become less tolerated in our society during the past few years. It is fast becoming a matter of where smokers will be allowed to smoke, rather than where their smoking will be restricted. Battle lines have been drawn between smokers who want to maintain the freedom to light up and non-smokers who want the freedom to breathe air unpolluted by tobacco smoke.

The price of smoking is high for passive smokers, who are involuntarily exposed to the tobacco smoke of others. They are at increased risk of lung

Why Do You Want to Quit? This part of the questionnaire asks you to focus on the reasons you want to quit smoking. Below are some of the reasons other people have given for quitting. Check off the reasons that apply to you and write any additional reasons in the space provided.

I want to quit because:

_____ I'd like to use the money I spend on cigarettes for other things.

_____ I'm concerned about the effects of smoking on my health, especially the increased possibility of lung disease, heart disease, high blood pressure, bladder disease, circulatory problems, and ulcers.

_____ I don't want my friends and family to worry about my health.

_____ I don't want to have the odor of smoke on my hair, clothes, and breath.

_____ I don't want to contribute to "indoor pollution."

_____ I'm tired of waking up in the morning with a sore throat and a bad taste in my mouth.

_____ I don't want to offend other people, especially nonsmokers.

_____ I want to feel healthier, breathe easier, and have more energy.

_____ I want to provide a good example for my children.

_____ I'm tired of feeling chained to the habit of smoking.

List other reasons of your own here:

_____

_____

_____

Now review both sections and decide how honest your answers were. Are some of them statements you have heard other people make, or do they truly apply to *you?* If necessary, make your answers more personal to yourself. Then think through these questions: Which list is more truthful? Which list is more motivating? Maybe you are not yet ready to quit. Or maybe you have omitted some important reasons for quitting.

   Keep in mind, however, that defining your conflicting motivations is only a part of the battle. The most significant step toward becoming a nonsmoker is taking action.

Adapted from Patricia West Barker, *The Quitting Game* (Hampton, NJ: New Win Publishing, Inc., 1981): 18–21. With Permission.

cancer and other diseases also, especially if they are exposed to tobacco smoke at home.

   But the price of smoking is even higher for smokers. It includes the cost of tobacco and health care—and life. A couple that forgoes a pack-a-day habit could each save over $1,000 a year, a significant contribution toward a child's education fund or a secure retirement.

   Naturally, the best advice for those who smoke is to stop. If you are trying to quit, or have been successful in quitting, there may be actions you can take to help keep you off smoking. A brisk walk after meals will improve cardiovascular and pulmonary function as it diminishes tobacco craving. Gum chewing may help; so may a hobby or craft that is interesting and can occupy your hands. When you host a party, designate a smoking room, or allow smoking only outdoors. Limit contact with smokers and avoid places where people will be smoking. Try one of the individual or group programs mentioned in the chapter.

The best advice for those tempted to take their first puff is—don't. (A large percentage of people who light up for the first time are adolescents and young adults). Abstaining from tobacco use is an individual choice that you can encourage in yourself and your friends. The benefits—keener senses of taste and smell, greater lung capacity, improved physical endurance, greater resistance to disease, and longer healthy life—speak for themselves.

Chapter Summary

- Nicotine, the chemical substance found in tobacco, is absorbed into the bloodstream and passes directly into the brain, where it causes feelings of alertness and relaxation. However, it also releases chemicals that stimulate the cardiovascular system, resulting in a faster heartbeat and increased blood pressure. Nicotine also stimulates the release of other chemicals that activate the body's fight-or-flight response.

- Tobacco and tobacco smoke contain a number of other toxic substances. These include carbon monoxide, which impairs the blood's capacity to carry oxygen; tar, a sticky residue that contains carcinogenic substances; and other carcinogenic substances. Smoking affects the respiratory system by irritating and damaging mucous membrances.

- Tobacco use has been linked to a number of serious diseases, including bronchitis and emphysema, various types of cancer, and cardiovascular disease. The use of tobacco can greatly increase the risk of dying from any of these diseases.

- Tobacco use during pregnancy seriously endangers the health of the unborn child by decreasing birth weight; increasing the numbers of miscarriages, stillbirths, and premature births; and contributing to retarded growth and mental development as the child grows older. People who breathe in the smoke of others (passive smoking) are also adversely affected and are at increased risk for the same diseases as smokers.

- Tobacco use can lead to physical dependence as the brain begins to function differently, vacillating between states of hypoarousal (less aroused than normal) and greater stimulation (as a result of tobacco use). Tobacco use can lead to psychological dependence as users begin to associate it with pleasurable experience and other positive reinforcers.

- Some programs that aim to help people stop smoking recommend going "cold turkey" (simply quitting). Others set up individual programs using books, over-the-counter drugs, and other similar aids, and still others center on group programs. Some approaches also involve professional therapy, including individual counseling, behavior modification, the use of hypnosis, and various aversion techniques.

- By giving up smoking, people can save money and extend their lives. Substituting healthy habits like exercise can help people stay free from tobacco. Limiting tobacco use in the home can encourage friends to do the same.

Key Terms

Nicotine (page 391)

Carbon monoxide (page 392)

Tar (page 392)

Benzopyrene (page 392)

Passive smoking (page 397)

References

1. *Cancer: Report of the Surgeon General* (Washington, D.C.: U.S. Government Printing Office, 1982).

2. American Cancer Society, *Cancer Facts and Figures—1990* (Atlanta: American Cancer Society, 1990): 20; Kenneth E. Warner, "Smoking and Health: A 25-Year Perspective," *American Journal of Public Health* 79, no. 2 (February 1989): 141–143.

3. U.S. Department of Health and Human Services, *The Health Consequences of Smoking: Nicotine Addiction. A Report of the Surgeon General* (Rockville, Md.: U.S. Department of Health and Human Services, 1988): 5–20, 565–587.

4. Warner, op. cit.

5. U.S. Department of Health and Human Services, op. cit., pp. 7–9.

6. *The Behavioral Aspects of Smoking*, NIDA Research Monograph Series, U.S. Department of Health and Human Services pub. no. (ADM) 79-882 (1979): 12–13.

7. *The Changing Cigarette: Report of the Surgeon General* (1981): 33–34.

8. *The Behavioral Aspects of Smoking*, op. cit. p. 12.

9. *Smoking and Health: Report of the Surgeon General* (1979): I-15 to I-17.

10. J. F. Nunn, "Smoking," *Applied Respiratory Physiology* (London: Butterworths, 1987): 337.

11. U.S. Department of Health and Human Services, "The Health Consequences of Using Smokeless Tobacco," *A Report of the Advisory Committee to the Surgeon General*, NIH pub. no. 86-2874 (April 1986).

12. Elbert D. Glover et al., "Just a Pinch between the Cheek and Gum," *Journal of School Health* (August 1981): 415.

13. American Cancer Society, *Cancer Facts and Figures—1989* (Atlanta: American Cancer Society, 1989): 20.

14. Warner, op. cit.

15. *The Changing Cigarette: Report of the Surgeon General*, op. cit.

16. Elbert D. Glover et al., "Smokeless Tobacco and the Adolescent Male," *Journal of Early Adolescence* 2, no. 1 (1982): 1–13.

17. *Cancer: Report of the Surgeon General*, op. cit.

18. *The Changing Cigarette: Report of the Surgeon General*, op. cit.

19. Ibid.

20. American Cancer Society, *Cancer Facts and Figures—1990*, op. cit.

21. *Smoking and Health: Report of the Surgeon General*, op. cit., p. I-16.

22. *The Changing Cigarette: Report of the Surgeon General*, op. cit.

23. *Smoking and Health: Report of the Surgeon General*, op. cit., p. I-15.

24. Jonathan E. Fielding, "Smoking: Health Effects and Control," part 1, *New England Journal of Medicine* 313, no. 8 (August 22, 1985): 496.

25. *Smoking and Health: Report of the Surgeon General*, op. cit., p. I-18.

26. Ernest L. Abel, "Smoking during Pregnancy: A Review of Effects on Growth and Development of Offspring," *Human Biology* 52, no. 4 (December 1980): 593–625; Richard L. Naeye, "Influence of Maternal Cigarette Smoking during Pregnancy on Fetal and Childhood Growth," *Obstetrics & Gynecology* 57, no. 1 (January 1981): 18–21.

27. *Smoking and Health: Report of the Surgeon General*, op. cit., p. I-22.

28. Ibid.

29. Ibid.

30. Ibid.

31. Jean Seligmann et al., "Women Smokers: The Risk Factors," *Newsweek* (November 25, 1985): 78.

32. *The Behavioral Aspects of Smoking*, op. cit.

33. Fielding, op. cit., p. 495.

34. James C. Byrd et al., "Passive Smoking: A Review of Medical and Legal Issues," *American Journal of Public Health* 49, no. 2 (February 1989): 209–215.

35. Steven L. Gortmaker et al., "Parental Smoking and the Risk of Childhood Asthma," *American Journal of Public Health* 72, no. 6 (June 1982): 574–578; D. M. Fergusson et al., "Parental Smoking and Respiratory Illnesses in Infancy," *Archives of Diseases in Childhood* 55 (1980): 358–361; Fielding, op. cit., p. 495.

36. U.S. Department of Health and Human Services, op. cit., p. 571.

37. *Primary Care & Cancer* (November 1986): 22–31.

38. J. Allan Best and Maurice Bloch, *Compliance in the Control of Cigarette Smoking*, NIDA Research Monograph Series no. 17 (1977): 209.

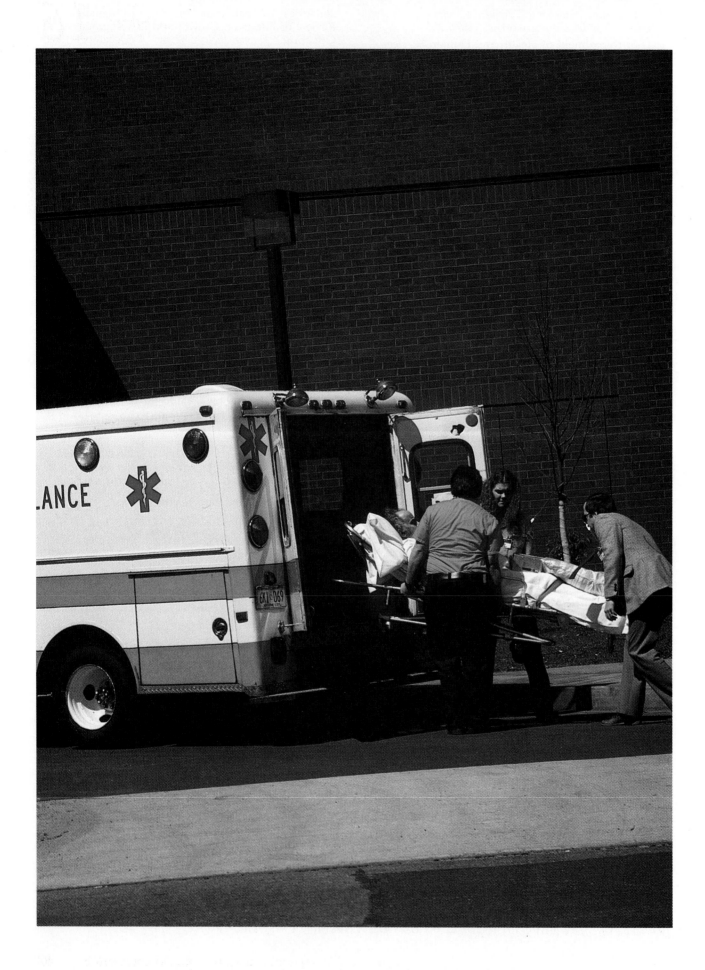

Chapter 16

Injuries and Their Prevention

To Guide Your Reading

When you have studied this chapter, you should be able to:

- Summarize recent thinking about accidental and violent injuries, explaining how the agent-host-environment model is being applied to the occurrence of injuries as well as diseases.

- Identify the most common environments in which injuries occur, typical types of injury for each location, and the people who are likely to be injured.

- Discuss the major types of injuries in the United States, including important factors associated with their occurrence.

- Explain basic strategies for the prevention and control of injuries, specifying particular measures that can be taken against different types of injuries.

- Describe important principles and procedures of emergency care which may be needed at any injury site before professional help arrives.

Injuries are one of the major public health problems facing the United States today. On an average day, more than 170,000 men, women, and children are seriously injured—over 62 million people a year. More than 142,000 of these victims die as a result of their injuries. Indeed, injuries have become the third most common cause of death in the United States after cardiovascular disease and cancer; for people between birth and age 45, they are the single greatest cause of death.[1]

People commonly hear the explanation "It was an accident" in many situations that have led to injury and death. Incidents such as motor vehicle crashes, falls, drownings, burns, and poisonings are often called accidents, as if they were random, uncontrollable acts of fate. However, the term *accident* is often inappropriate: many of the situations in which injuries occur are predictable as well as preventable.

Injury and death also result from violence, which also may seem uncontrollable. However, violence too can result from predictable situations. The real health problem, in violence as well as in accidents, is injury itself—the damage sustained by an individual as a result of an event.

Traffic injuries are second only to cancer in regard to economic cost if medical costs, property loss, legal costs, and lost productivity are included.

Injuries in Perspective

Although injuries represent a serious threat to public health, this need not be the case. Many injuries *can* be prevented. A better understanding of the factors that lead to injury can uncover ways to prevent many of the injuries that people sustain or reduce the seriousness of the injuries that do occur.

Why Injuries Happen

For years researchers tried to explain why injuries occur by focusing on the assumed shortcomings of the victims. They thought that most injuries happen to a few "accident-prone" people.[2] Most researchers, however, have discounted the theory of accident-proneness. Although some individuals may have higher injury rates than others do, current evidence indicates that this is essentially a shifting group of individuals rather than a clearly defined accident-prone group.[3]

Today, investigators attempt to explain injury causation by looking at a variety of factors and the interactions among them. The current view is expressed by the threshold theory and the agent-host-environment model, two complementary explanations of why injuries occur.

Threshold Theory   According to this theory, injuries occur when a force or energy proves to be too great for a person to cope with; in other words, the energy exceeds the threshold of a person's skills and capabilities.

Five basic types of energy are responsible for all injuries: kinetic (mechanical), thermal, chemical, electrical, and radiation. Kinetic, or mechanical, energy includes motor vehicles, firearms, falls, and cuts. A person burned by a stove is injured as a result of thermal energy. Poisoning and injury from toxic substances are attributable to chemical energy. Shock from an exposed electrical wire is an example of an injury due to electrical energy. Injuries due to exposure to x-rays, the ultraviolet rays of the sun, and nuclear radiation result from radiation energy.[4]

For young children and for old people, a major energy source of injuries is gravity: children because they have not yet learned the necessary physical skills and the aged because some of the senses needed to apply those skills may have failed. Gravity also causes injuries to people who take risks, for example, skiers, hang gliders, sky divers, and bungee jumpers.

Whatever the source of energy, injury occurs when the skills needed to handle a particular transfer of energy safely are beyond a person's abilities.[5] Different people vary enormously in their capabilities and therefore in their risk of sustaining injury. Young children, for example, are especially prone to receive certain types of injuries. Their inexperience and lack of knowledge, coupled with less developed physical skills, can be significant factors in this increased risk of injury. Elderly people may also be more prone to sustain injury because of declining physical skills, failing eyesight, arthritis and other diseases, and sometimes impaired mental functioning. Of course, an increased risk of injury is not limited to the very young or the very old. Individuals of any age or group are at increased risk if their knowledge, skills, and abilities fail them in times of need.

Because young children do not understand many of the potential dangers around them, they are often at risk for sustaining an injury. Elderly people, especially those with chronic diseases, can be as accident-prone as children; a short trip across a low-traffic street can become a dangerous journey. (Elizabeth Zuckerman/PhotoEdit; Lawrence Migdale/Photo Researchers, Inc.)

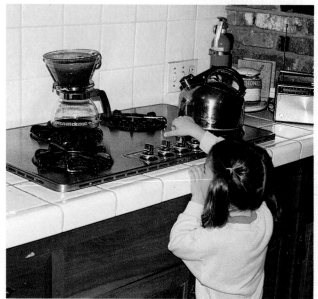
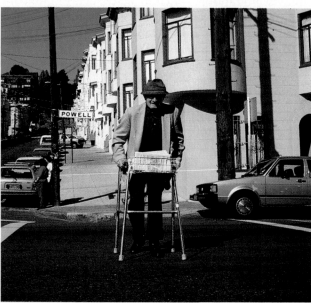

How Much Excitement Can You Take?

Some people are always on the go, trying new experiences and seeking the thrill of accomplishment. Although they take more risks, they are not necessarily involved in more injuries. Other people want more orderly and predictable lives filled with peace, warmth, and tranquillity. This activity will help you find out how stimulating a life you want. If a statement is one that you might easily make, put a check mark in the space. If you would very rarely make the statement, leave the space blank.

_____   1. I would like a job that requires a lot of traveling.

    _____   2. I cannot wait to get indoors on a cold day.

    _____   3. I cannot understand people who risk their necks climbing mountains.

_____   4. I get bored seeing the same faces all the time.

    _____   5. I prefer having a guide when I am in a place I do not know well.

    _____   6. I would prefer living in an ideal society where everyone is safe, secure, and happy.

_____   7. I sometimes like to do things that are a little frightening.

    _____   8. I would *not* like to take up waterskiing.

    _____   9. When I go on a trip, I like to plan my route and timetable fairly carefully.

_____   10. I would like to learn to fly an airplane.

_____   11. I would like to have the experience of being hypnotized.

_____   12. I want to live life to the fullest and experience as much of it as I can.

    _____   13. I would never want to try parachute jumping.

    _____   14. I enter cold water gradually, giving myself time to get used to it.

_____   15. I prefer friends who are exciting and unpredictable.

_____   16. I would enjoy camping out on my vacation.

    _____   17. The essence of good art is its clarity and harmony of colors.

    _____   18. I prefer people who are calm and even-tempered.

_____   19. A good painting should shock or jolt the senses.

_____   20. I would like to drive or ride a motorcycle.

Score your responses. Begin with 100 points. *Add* 10 points for each check in the left-hand column. Then *subtract* 10 points for each check in the right-hand column. Find your score below to see what your ideal level of excitement is.

Scores	Your Ideal Level of Excitement
150 to 200	High
70 to 140	Moderate
0 to 60	Low

Interpretation: People who seek high levels of stimulation often accept higher risks than do those who seek predictable and moderate lifestyles. If excitement is important to you, be sure to double-check your parachute before you take off.

Adapted with permission from Marvin Zuckerman et al., "Development of a Sensation-Seeking Scale," *Journal of Consulting Psychology* 28, no. 6 (1964): 477–482. Copyright 1964 by the American Psychological Association.

The source of energy and the status of a person's skills are not the only factors that contribute to the risk of injury, however. Injuries also may happen because an object fails to function properly. Bicycles malfunction, toys break, and furniture collapses, injuring the children and adults who are using them. Environmental factors also can contribute to injuries, for example, when children's toys are left on a staircase or toxic substances are stored in unsecured locations. Therefore, in determining the cause of injury, it is necessary to consider a variety of factors and the interactions among them. The interaction of all factors is best understood by applying the agent-host-environment model to the subject of injury causation.

Agent-Host-Environment Model The agent-host-environment model was originally used in this book to help explain the causes of disease (Chapter 10). More recently it has been applied to research on injury and has played an important role in explaining why injuries happen.

In this model, the agent, host, and environment are all seen as factors that interact over time to cause injury.[6] Agent factors include the energy source responsible for an injury and the vector, or mechanism, by which that energy is transferred (an automobile is a vector through which kinetic energy can cause injury). Host factors include the person sustaining an injury and the skills, experience, and physical condition of that person. Environmental factors include the site at which an injury occurs and its condition as well as public attitudes and laws that affect the risk of sustaining an injury (Figure 16.1).

With the agent-host-environment model, personal responsibility for injury is only one of three factors that interact to increase or decrease the risk of injury (unlike the threshold theory, in which a person's capabilities are the primary factor). Therefore, a person (host) who takes drugs, is unable to cope

Figure 16.1 The triangular agent-host-environment model, already used to clarify causes of disease and causes of drug use, can also be applied to injuries. People suffer accidental and violent injuries for a number of reasons, many of which can be controlled. In this one-car accident, the brakes on the car (agent/vector) could have been made safer; the driver (the "host" who suffers the injury) should have been persuaded not to drive while intoxicated; and warning signs on the road (environment) could have been made more visible.

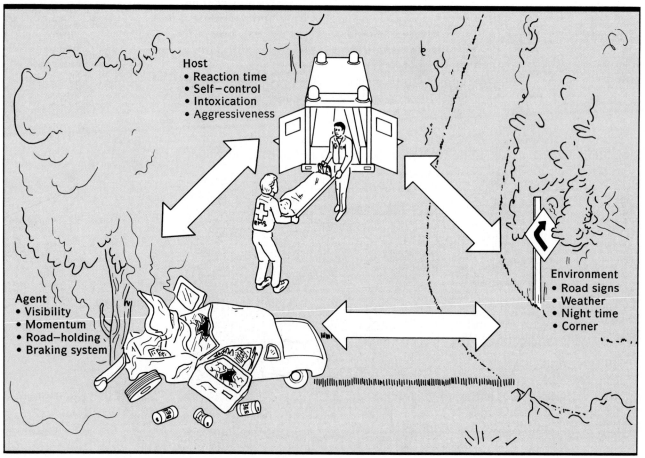

Host
- Reaction time
- Self-control
- Intoxication
- Aggressiveness

Environment
- Road signs
- Weather
- Night time
- Corner

Agent
- Visibility
- Momentum
- Road-holding
- Braking system

with stress, is physically ill, or neglects to wear a seat belt while driving is only one factor affecting the risk of injury. Family and societal stressors, disease organisms, faulty car brakes, unsafe working conditions, and other agent and environmental factors are also important elements.

Of course, a potential change in any of these factors may not necessarily lead to injury if the other factors can compensate.[7] A person driving a car with worn brakes can avoid injury by stopping at the side of the road at the first sign of a problem or by using his or her driving skills to avoid losing control of the car when the brakes fail.

A major advantage of the agent-host-environment model is that by suggesting causal relationships and identifying high-risk characteristics associated with those relationships, it provides a basis for developing strategies to prevent or reduce the risk of injury.[8] (Injury prevention will be discussed later in this chapter.)

Where Injuries Occur

The majority of injuries occur in familiar environments: at home, at work, and at recreational areas. A careful examination of these places can help identify ways to reduce or prevent the risk of serious injury. Certain types of injuries occur more frequently in particular environments primarily because of the types of hazards or safety features that are present.

Injuries at Home   People can be injured at home in a number of ways: falls, burns, poisoning, drowning, severe cuts, and so on. In 1987, 20,500 deaths resulted from injuries sustained at home and on home premises, accounting for 22 percent of all fatal injuries that year. An estimated 3,100,000 persons suffered disabling injuries in the home; among those accidents, 80,000 resulted in permanent impairment.[9]

Home injuries occur more frequently among some groups than others. For example, 22 percent of children under age 6 and 18 percent of adults age 75 or older are injured in the home each year. More men than women die from home injuries, although adult women sustain more nonfatal injuries than do adult men.[10]

Certain home environments increase the risk of injury, and the kinds of injuries people suffer depend a great deal on environmental factors. Deteriorating homes in older neighborhoods may pose a greater risk of injury be-

The lead paint found in some older buildings is just one of several substances that can harm people. (Tony Freeman/PhotoEdit)

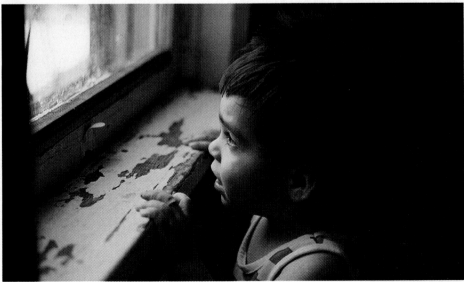

cause of fire or structural hazards. The placement of potentially dangerous substances, including medications, may be a factor in the risk of poisoning and drug overdose.

The most dangerous room in the home is the kitchen: hot stoves and boiling liquids are a danger to everyone, but especially to young children. However, all rooms may contain hazards, such as uncovered electrical outlets, loose rugs or carpeting, sharp or heavy objects, and potentially dangerous substances. The yard and its surroundings also contain numerous hazards, such as unguarded swimming pools, gardening implements, and icy sidewalks.

The fact that knowledge and technology can easily help prevent many home injuries makes their occurrence especially tragic. The use of safety outlets, nonskid carpets, tamperproof bottle caps, and swimming pool enclosures can reduce the risk of certain types of injury greatly. Unfortunately, even though researchers, architects, environmental health workers, and legislators have reduced many of the risks that once were common in the home, residential injuries continue to occur at an unacceptably high rate.

Injuries at Work Every year in this country there are approximately 6,000 work-related deaths and 2.5 million to 11.3 million nonfatal occupational injuries.[11] Many occupations have particular associated injury risks. Sanitation workers are at risk for sustaining lifting injuries, chronic joint conditions, and eye injuries. Fire fighters commonly sustain burns, cuts, sprains, broken bones, smoke inhalation, and eye injuries. Construction workers face a greater risk of having back injuries, cuts, and injuries from slips and falls.

Agriculture, now recognized as one of the nation's most dangerous industries, exposes its workers to risks of tractor rollovers, amputations by machinery, electrocutions, and pesticide poisonings. Workers in forestry, fishing, mining, construction, transportation, and public utilities are among those at greatest risk for sustaining occupational injuries.[12]

While people can be injured on the job in many ways, over 40 percent of all fatal occupational injuries are associated with motor vehicles. This includes highway vehicles and a variety of nonhighway vehicles, such as bulldozers,

In a staircase fall, the agent and energy source is gravity, the vector is the staircase, and the host is the person who suffered the fall (and lacked the skills to negotiate the stairs successfully). What are the environmental factors? They include the design of the hallway, availability of handrails, steepness and straightness of stairs, stair carpeting, and nonslip surfaces.

Construction workers often put themselves in dangerous situations, particularly when they disregard standard safety precautions. (Tony Freeman/PhotoEdit)

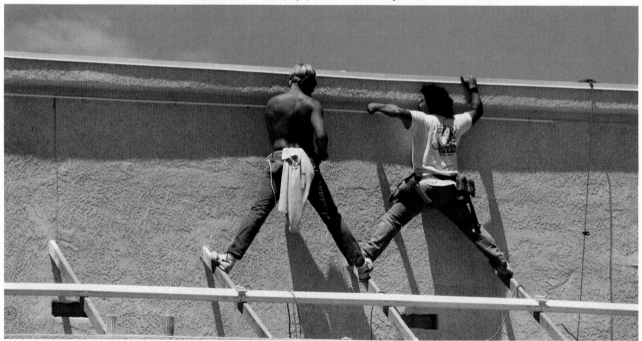

front-end loaders, cranes, forklifts, and tractors. A large proportion of occupational injuries result from falls, especially in construction work.[13]

Age, sex, and race may be factors in the risk of sustaining occupational injuries. There is some evidence that young workers experience a disproportionate number of injuries at work, possibly as a result of inexperience and lack of training. Minority group members also seem to be at greater risk for having occupational injuries. One study found that black workers were more likely to be engaged in hazardous jobs than white workers were. Although men predominate in some of the more hazardous occupations, women in occupations such as nursing and manufacturing frequently sustain serious injuries.[14]

Recreational Injuries Recreational activities such as swimming, boating, hiking, skiing, and tennis are an important part of the lives of many Americans. However, because they are "fun," many people forget that these activities can also be dangerous.

Many recreational injuries go unreported, and many activities are not studied in a systematic way. As a result, it is difficult to determine the full magnitude of the problem. It is safe to say, however, that hundreds of thousands of people are injured in recreational activities every year. Among recreation-related injuries, the highest incidence of death may come from drowning. In 1987, an estimated 4,400 people in the United States died as a result of drowning.[15] Other water-related injuries are associated with boating and diving. Diving, for example, results in approximately 1,000 spinal cord injuries a year, most of which result in permanent paralysis.[16] The typical diving injury occurs when a person hits his or her head on the bottom or side of a swimming pool or shallow body of water.

Playgrounds are frequently the scene of injuries among young children. Although most playground-related injuries are minor, about one-quarter are more severe, involving concussions, crush wounds, fractures, and multiple injuries; a small number of deaths are caused by head injuries. Most playground-related injuries involve falls to the ground (usually from monkey bars, seesaws, or swings), collisions with playground equipment while running, and being struck by moving equipment such as swings.[17]

Competitive sports are another area in which recreational injuries frequently occur. Although serious and disabling injuries may result, the most prevalent injuries are sprains, especially of the limb joints; concussions; and abrasions. Among competitive sports, contact sports such as football and baseball have higher injury rates than do noncontact sports such as tennis.[18]

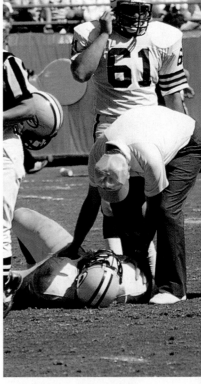

Among all competitive athletes, football players have the highest number of physical injuries annually. (Tony Freeman/ PhotoEdit)

The Role of Violence in Injuries

Violence is defined broadly as the use of physical force with the intent of inflicting injury or death. While some people might question what health professionals can do about violence, it is nonetheless a serious health problem because of the great toll it takes in lives, health, and quality of life. Violent actions are responsible for over 50,000 deaths a year. Information about non-fatal violence is less well reported, but it is estimated that each year at least 800,000 serious assaults result in injury.[19] Moreover, in many parts of the country the fear of violence has a powerful effect on people's lives, resulting in greater levels of stress, increased insecurity, and reduced enjoyment of life.

Injuries caused by interpersonal violence such as homicide and assault are sometimes characterized as "intentional," in contrast to the "unintentional" nature of most injuries. Whether intentional or unintentional, however, the result is the same—injury or death due to a combination of factors involving an agent, a host, and an environment.

Focusing on the injuries caused by violence rather than on the intentionality of the acts allows public health practitioners to analyze violence from the

Injuries due to violence are perhaps the most complex and hard to control, because they derive more from the behavior of the perpetrator (agent) than from the victim's (host's) behavior. However, many experts hold that the behavior of agents of violence may be modifiable in the long run through social and political reform.

perspective of causal factors (such as interpersonal relationships, stress, and availability of weapons). Their findings, combined with the efforts of law enforcement agencies and other groups, can lead to better means of preventing violence. Injury and death rates due to violence *can* be reduced. Indeed, public health officials do not consider violence an inevitable part of life but a concern to be addressed and remedied.[20]

Major Types of Injuries

During the past decade a considerable number of injuries, especially head injuries, have been caused by all-terrain vehicles (ATVs)—three- or four-wheel off-the-road vehicles that can reach 70 miles per hour. Their major problem is instability on turns. The highest-risk group is adolescent males, who receive between 67 and 80 percent of these injuries. Many states have moved to ban or restrict the use of ATVs.

Another way to analyze injuries is to look at the type of injuries that occur when people interact with the environment and with the agents and vectors that cause injury directly. The major types of injuries that occur every year are motor vehicle injuries, falls, burns, drownings, poisonings, and violence-related injuries, including homicides and assaults.

Motor Vehicle Injuries

Every year in the United States, motor vehicles are responsible for almost 50,000 deaths and almost 2 million nonfatal disabling injuries. Among all fatal injuries, motor vehicle accidents are the most common cause of death for people age 1 to 34 and a major cause of death for people of all ages.[21]

Cars are especially dangerous in the hands of people who are intoxicated. Most states have defined a critical blood alcohol level (Chapter 14) which constitutes legal evidence that a person is driving while intoxicated (DWI) or driving under the influence (DUI). Depending on the state, this level ranges from 0.08 to 0.10 percent, as determined by a breath, blood, or urine test. However, even a blood alcohol level of 0.05 percent (which can occur with as few as three drinks in an hour) begins to affect a person's coordination and reflexes: physical skills begin to deteriorate to the point where the risk of sustaining a motor vehicle injury is significantly increased. Moreover, studies have shown that motor vehicle crashes in which alcohol plays a role tend to be much more severe than are nonalcohol-related crashes. The more severe the crash, the greater the likelihood that alcohol is involved. In 1987, an estimated 23,630 Americans were killed in alcohol-related motor vehicle crashes.[22]

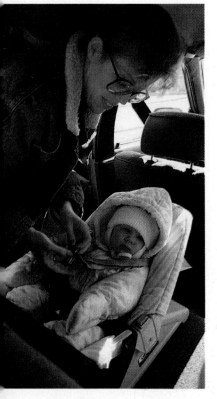

Infant restraining seats are one of the many options that make cars safer. (Rhoda Sidney/PhotoEdit)

Age, sex, and race are other factors in motor vehicle death rates. The death rate peaks in the late teenage years and early twenties and then begins to decline until about age 65, at which point it increases. Men, especially those in their early twenties, are more often fatally injured than are women. The highest death rates associated with motor vehicles are found among Native Americans (51 deaths per 100,000, compared with 24 per 100,000 for whites, 19 per 100,000 for blacks, and 9 per 100,000 for Asians); this may be partly attributable to the high incidence of alcohol use among Native American groups.[23]

A group of factors related to motor vehicle injury which are often overlooked involves the condition of automobiles and their safety features as well as the general safety of the driving environment. The presence of seat belts, padded dashboards, air bags, and other safety features can have a significant effect on the injuries sustained in motor vehicle crashes. Lower speed limits, well-lighted and well-constructed highways, and knowledge of safe driving practices also affect the risk of sustaining a motor vehicle injury.

Injury from Falls

Falls are second only to motor vehicles as a cause of nonviolent fatal injuries in the United States, accounting for over 11,500 deaths in 1987.[24] The group most at risk for fatal falls includes the elderly, especially people over age 75;

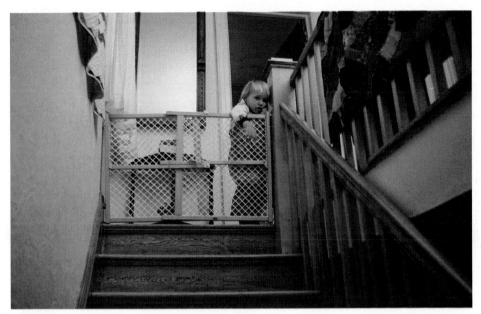

Installing simple devices such as safety gates makes a house safer for small children.
(Richard Hutchings/Photo Researchers, Inc.)

more than half of all fatal falls occur among this group. This is attributed largely to the decline in physical coordination, agility, vision, and balance that characterizes the aging process in many persons.

Children under age 5 are also at increased risk for falls. All children fall as they are learning to walk, and most of these falls do not result in injury. Some falls, however, can result in serious fractures or brain injuries. The incidence of falls is greatest in infancy and then declines throughout childhood, partly as a result of the normal development of physical skills and coordination.[25]

While falls can occur in any environment, over 43 percent of all fatal falls occur in the home. Among children under age 5, almost 67 percent of fatal falls occur there. Among those age 65 and over, about 45 percent of fatal falls occur at home. Environmental factors such as overcrowded furniture, dangerous stairs, poor lighting, loose rugs, and slippery floor surfaces play a major role in the risk of falling among the elderly, accounting for up to 50 percent of falls. Among children, common environmental hazards associated with falls include open windows, open staircases, and playground equipment.[26]

Another factor that contributes to the risk of falling among the elderly is the use of medications. Drugs such as sedatives and barbiturates are often associated with falls, especially in nursing homes, where a large percentage of elderly patients use such medications. Alcohol is also associated with an increased risk of falls among the elderly.

Fire and Burn Injuries

Burns are another significant cause of injury and death in the United States, accounting for over 4,700 deaths in 1987.[27] Burn injuries result from a variety of sources, including fires, scaldings, electricity, chemicals, and ultraviolet radiation. The types of burns associated with each of these sources vary in severity and frequency and are linked to certain age- and sex-related factors.

About 75 percent of all deaths by fire result from house fires; the groups at greatest risk are young children and the elderly. Among the elderly, a large number of nonfatal fire-related burns (about 62 percent) are attributable to the burning of clothing, which often occurs while one is cooking. While clothing-related burns are somewhat common among children, improved flammability standards for children's clothing have resulted in a decreased risk in recent years.[28]

Burns sustained as a result of contact with hot objects (such as a stove) and scaldings from hot liquids are more common among young children. While such burns are seldom fatal, they can result in severe injury and pain. Flammable liquids such as gasoline are a lethal cause of burn injuries among boys from 6 to 16 years of age, and electrical burns are quite common among boys in this age group.[29]

Drownings and Near Drownings

Drowning, by definition, is a fatal injury. "Near drowning," in which a person is submerged long enough to suffer oxygen deprivation, can result in serious injury, including brain damage. As with other types of injuries, certain groups in the population are at greater risk of drowning than are others. For example, the rate of drownings among men is four times greater than that among women. Drowning rates are highest among children under age 5 and between ages 15 and 24.[30] Drowning often occurs among young children who lack proper supervision, because they are not familiar with the dangers of falling into deep water and do not usually call out for help. Among teenagers and young adults, increased risk taking can be a factor in the risk of drowning, as can the use of alcohol.[31]

Environmental factors play a role in the risk of drownings. Although between 50 and 75 percent of all drownings occur in lakes, rivers, and the ocean, a large percentage of drownings among young children occur in swimming pools.[32] This is particularly true in regions of the country where residential swimming pools are common. Proper supervision and safety features, such as fenced enclosures, are important factors in residential drownings of young children. One study found that 72 percent of residential drownings occurred at sites where there was no physical barrier between the house and the pool.[33]

Fences around swimming pools are required by law in many places. They can save lives everywhere. (Jay Foreman/Unicorn Stock Photos)

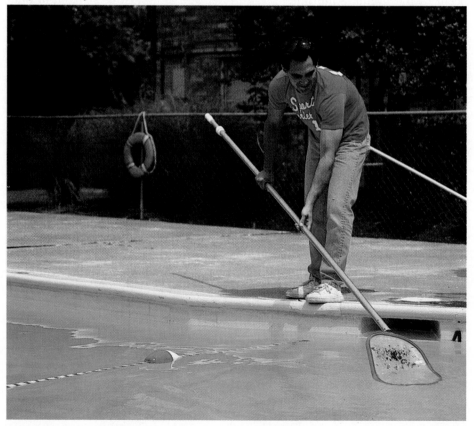

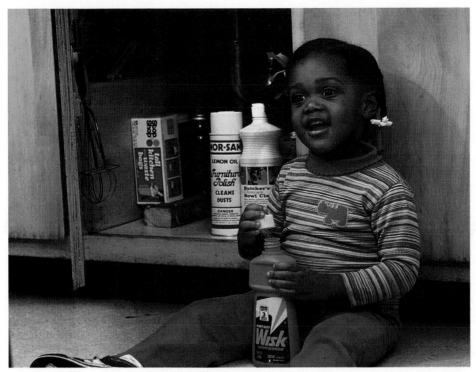

Household cleaners and all other toxic substances should be placed in locked cabinets far out of the reach of children. (Barbara Burnes/Photo Researchers, Inc.)

Injury from Poisonings

In 1987 almost 5,500 deaths in the United States were attributed to poisoning. Poisoning is also responsible for a great number of the nonfatal injuries sustained each year; for example, for each fatal poisoning among children under age 5, an estimated 80,000 to 90,000 nonfatal incidents of poisoning are seen in hospital emergency rooms.[34]

As is the case with many other types of injury, young children and the elderly are at greatest risk for injury from poisoning. For example, studies have shown that children under age 5 have a risk of poisoning 10 times greater than that of elementary-school-age children, and children age 1 or 2 are 17 times more likely to be hospitalized for poisoning than are any other people under 20 years of age.[35] Young children are poisoned by a variety of substances found in the home, from medications to cleansing agents to personal-care products. Fortunately, the rate of ingestion of some potentially hazardous substances has decreased in recent years because of the use of child-resistant safety caps on many products.

In addition to poisoning from liquids and solids, poisoning from gases and vapors is a significant source of injury. The primary cause of such poisoning is carbon monoxide inhalation, most often from motor vehicle exhausts; in 1987, 600 deaths among all age groups were caused by carbon monoxide poisoning.[36]

Childproofing is an example of how the law can operate as an environmental factor: manufacturers and pharmacists may be required to provide childproof tops for certain types of products. Although this has decreased poisoning deaths among younger children, such deaths have increased overall. This appears to result from the misuse of drugs by teenagers and adults; this is an area where laws have thus far failed to affect the environment significantly.

Violence-Related Injuries

In recent years the United States has experienced an ominous increase in injuries and deaths resulting from interpersonal violence. The daily news recounts the latest incidents of homicides, assaults, rapes, and other violent acts. In 1987, for example, nearly 1.5 million violent acts were reported in the United States, a 36.7 percent increase from 1978.[37] This may represent only part of the problem, however, since incidents of assaultive nonfatal violence frequently go unreported.

Assaultive Injuries Every year hundreds of thousands of people in this country are victims of violent assault, from physical disputes among individuals to muggings—street assaults involving robbery—to rape. In 1989, for example, 951,707 aggravated assaults and 94,504 rapes were reported; many more no doubt went unreported. It is estimated that somewhere between 1 in 10 and 4 in 10 rapes go unreported; the number of unreported aggravated assaults is also thought to be substantial.[38]

Most acts of violence are committed by men. Age is another significant factor; during 1986, people under age 25 accounted for 48 percent of arrests for violent crime. Arrest statistics tell only part of the story, however; for every violent act leading to arrest, between 8 and 11 others are committed by juvenile offenders. Another factor associated with aggravated assault and rape is alcohol. Studies have shown that a large number of violent acts occur in places where alcohol is consumed. Another study found that over 50 percent of convicted rapists were under the influence of alcohol when they committed a crime.[39]

Race and socioeconomic status appear to be factors in determining who is victimized by assault and rape. The poor seem to be at greater risk for both assaultive injuries and rape, and blacks are at great risk as well. One study found that rape was 12 times more frequent among blacks than among whites. Age also seems to be a risk factor; studies have revealed that the great majority of rape victims are between ages 13 and 25, predominantly between ages 13 and 19.[40]

Homicide While the great majority of assaultive injuries are nonfatal, homicide represents the fatal end of the spectrum of violent behavior. There were an estimated 21,500 homicides in 1989, a 29 percent increase from 1970.[41]

An increased risk of homicide is associated with various factors. Research has suggested that most homicide victims are young black males; mortality rates are 5 to 12 times greater among young black males than they are among young white males. For black males between ages 14 and 44, homicide is the leading cause of death.[42] Personal relationships are another factor in homicides. It has been estimated that almost half of all homicides are committed by persons either related to or acquainted with the victim.[43]

Homicides frequently arise from arguments rather than criminal activities and usually involve firearms. The use of alcohol and drugs is also frequently associated with homicides.[44] In recent years drug dealing in cities has been linked increasingly to homicides that sometimes involve innocent children and bystanders.

Every year in the United States more than 30,000 deaths and about 150,000 injuries related to firearms occur. Most of them involve men between 15 and 34 years old.

Preventing and Controlling Injuries

Even though injuries pose a major public health problem, widespread misunderstanding of their causation has frequently led to inadequate efforts toward injury reduction and prevention. As long as individuals and their accident-proneness were seen as the primary factor in injuries, efforts to reduce the risk of injury could be only partially successful.

Successful prevention of injuries requires attention not only to host factors associated with individuals but to agent and environmental factors as well. Identifying all the factors that lead to injury and examining their interactions can result in more effective strategies on the part of individuals, organizations, public health professionals, and the government.

Approaches to Injury Control

There are several approaches to preventing and controlling injuries. One is directed at individual behaviors and attempts to change them in ways that will reduce the risk of injury, such as improving driving skills, curbing aggressive behaviors, and stopping the use of alcohol and other drugs. This approach is generally characterized as *persuasion* and includes elements such as education, rehabilitation, behavior modification, and social support systems.[45] Driver education classes, campaigns for stricter gun control, and counseling for drunk drivers are examples of efforts at persuasion. The initiative for such efforts is found at all levels of society, including governmental efforts to develop school health education programs that include an emphasis on injury prevention.[46] Unfortunately, since persuasive methods are aimed primarily at behaviors and attitudes, they are often the least effective method of injury prevention.

Another approach to injury prevention is through legislation. *Laws* approach the prevention of injuries more directly than persuasion can. Some laws are aimed at changing individual behavior, such as laws that require the use of seat belts, infant car seats, and motorcycle helmets. Other laws regulate the possession of handguns, require the installation of smoke detectors, and penalize people who drive while intoxicated.

As few as 10 percent of recreational bicyclists wear helmets. However, helmets are generally required for official races.

While laws requiring behavioral change are generally more effective than educational methods of prevention, they are less effective than laws designed to provide automatic protection through changes in product and environmental design. Automatic protections such as built-in sprinkler systems, automatic seat belts, air bags, and childproof closures on containers have a great potential for preventing injuries and deaths because they require no action on the part of the individual.

Active and Passive Preventive Measures

Preventive measures that require individuals to do something to reduce the risk of sustaining an injury are considered **active prevention.** Examples include the use of nonautomatic seat belts, the use of bicycle and motorcycle helmets, adherence to drunk driving laws, and voluntary compliance with gun laws. The greatest failing of active measures is that they depend on people to act in ways that will reduce their risk of sustaining injury. People forget to use seat belts and helmets, forget to put hazardous substances out of the reach of children, fail to follow the speed limit or comply with other laws, and are often careless or take risks. While education is an important means of changing unsafe attitudes and behaviors and getting people to comply with the law, injury prevention can be achieved even more effectively through the use of passive prevention.

active prevention— *preventive measures that require individuals to do something to reduce the risk of injury, such as use a seat belt or wear a motorcycle helmet.*

Active measures for injury prevention can be effective only when people agree to apply them on a regular basis. (Richard Hutchings/Photo Researchers, Inc.)

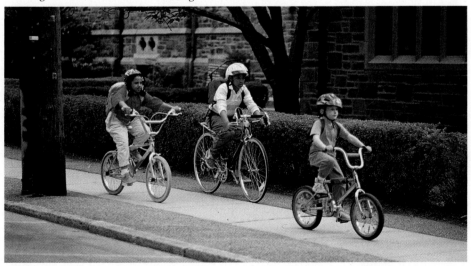

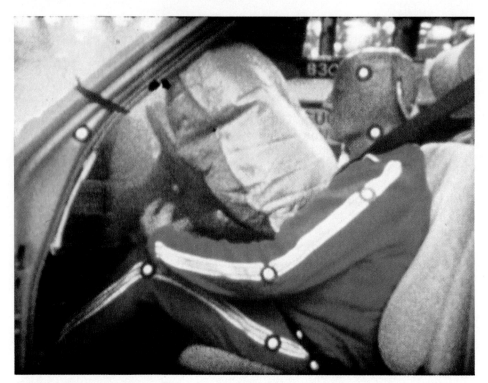

Passive injury prevention measures are designed to work without user participation. To benefit from automobile air bags, car owners need only buy cars that are equipped with them. (Courtesy Mercedes Benz)

Preventive measures that require little or no individual action on the part of those being protected are characterized as **passive prevention.** These measures include seat belts that automatically engage when a person enters a car, automobile air bags, better street lighting, and built-in safety switches on power tools and electrical equipment. Since they require no action by individuals, these measures are directed at agent and environmental factors, modifying them so that they pose less of a risk.

Of course, the best prevention against injury involves a combination of passive and active prevention, of persuasive efforts and laws. Together, the combined efforts of individuals, public health officials, legislators, researchers, manufacturers, and law enforcement officers can eliminate or reduce many of the risk factors that can lead to serious injury or death.

Individual Strategies for Control and Prevention

Despite the progress that has been made in injury prevention in this country, there is still a long way to go. Few states have established comprehensive programs to prevent injury, governments have not always been forceful in legislating injury prevention measures, and some manufacturers have been slow in investigating passive safety features and incorporating them into their products.

Until more passive prevention measures are legislated and incorporated into the design of all products and environments, it is largely up to the individual to act in ways that prevent injury. One should begin by examining one's own behaviors and attitudes to see how they may contribute to the risk of injury. The next step is to identify potential hazards in products and in the environment. Then it is possible to take steps to reduce risky behaviors and eliminate hazards that may lead to injury.

The following are just a few of the many safety tips that can help reduce the risk of injury from motor vehicle crashes, falls, burns, drowning, and poisoning.[47]

Controlling Motor Vehicle Injuries

In addition to observing all traffic laws and driving carefully, people can reduce the risk of injury from motor vehicles by doing the following:

- Avoiding driving while under the influence of alcohol, illegal drugs, or medicines which carry a warning about drowsiness
- Wearing seat belts at all times, whether driving or riding as a passenger
- Using consumer-recommended car seats for infants and requiring older children to use seat belts
- Servicing vehicles regularly and keeping them in good working order
- Maintaining proper tire pressures and levels for gasoline, oil, and system coolants
- Wearing a helmet when riding a bicycle or motorcycle
- Teaching children to cross streets safely and keep away from roads and highways

According to **Public Health Reports,** *the lap-shoulder seat belt restraint system reduces the risk of fatality by 43 percent and that of serious injury by 40 to 70 percent.*

Controlling Falls

Many falls can be avoided, especially those which result from environmental factors. The risk of injury from such falls can be reduced by doing the following:

- Keeping traffic areas in the home well lighted, especially stairs
- Installing stairway gates and window barriers to protect children
- Repairing loose floorboards and floor coverings
- Removing electrical cords from walkways
- Picking up small objects from the floor
- Placing nonskid mats under loose rugs and in bathtubs
- Cleaning up water and grease spills on the floor immediately

Controlling Burns

In addition to using smoke detectors in the home and knowing emergency procedures in case of a fire, people can reduce the risk of burn injuries by doing the following:

- Setting home water heaters no higher than 120 degrees F
- Using flame-retardant clothing for children
- Keeping matches out of the reach of children
- Not buying highly flammable solvents or storing them in safe locations
- Taking care not to overload electrical circuits
- Repairing or replacing worn electrical wires
- Placing guards in front of fireplaces, open heaters, and radiators
- Keeping pots of hot liquids away from the front of the stove and turning pot handles to the rear

Smoke detectors are an inexpensive and reliable early warning system for fires. According to a report by the Federal Emergency Management Agency, smoke alarms reduce the potential for death by 88 percent and the potential for injury by 86 percent. Many states have some form of legislation requiring smoke detectors to be installed in all new constructions.

Controlling Drowning

While the ability to swim is very important in preventing drowning, people can reduce the risk of drowning or near drowning by doing the following:

- Enclosing pool areas or installing fences between the home and wells, ponds, streams, and other bodies of water
- Never leaving a child unattended in a bathtub, pool, or other body of water
- Keeping pails of liquid inaccessible to infants since infants can drown even in small pails
- Knowing and following water safety and boating rules

Appropriate use of personal flotation devices (PFDs) also reduces drownings associated with recreational boating.

Controlling Poisoning

An important breakthrough in reducing the poisoning of children has been the use of safety closures on many bottled products and medications. Some other ways to reduce the risk of poisoning include the following:

- Keeping all medicines and caustic and poisonous household substances out of the reach of children
- Reading the labels on all substances carefully before using them

Violence: You, Society, and Television

Americans are living through a crime wave. Violence fills the towns and cities, no longer confined to "bad" neighborhoods. Public budgets groan under the cost of increased police protection and prison construction. The violence of the times covers the newspapers and enters people's homes through television. Some people believe that many factors contribute to violent behavior and that television viewing provides a safe release from the tensions of modern life. Others support the position that exposure to violence on television is one of the leading causes of violence in American society. Which view do you agree with?

Television Cannot Be Blamed for the Current Crime Wave After several shootings by motorists on a Los Angeles freeway were reported on the news, a comedian quipped that the police were cracking down: a friend had been ticketed for carrying a .45 in a .22-caliber zone.

Violence is obviously part of contemporary life, and it has many causes. Crowding, economic pressure, and frustration with daily life all contribute to the urge to commit violent acts. People who were the targets of violence as children are especially apt to become violent under stress.

Demographics also contributes to the overall trend toward violence. Violent crimes are most often committed by men, young people, and poor people. There is currently a large number of young, poor, males in this country. Furthermore, the fast money people make from selling illicit drugs feeds a frenzy of crime and need.

American society also is stressed by mobility and a two-income lifestyle. Community spirit is hard to build because many people move every 3 to 5 years. Community activities are hard to support because many men and women hold down full-time jobs.

With all these explanations of violence in American society, it seems wrong to place the blame on TV. Too many other factors have contributed to the problem. TV merely reflects the violence in this society. Furthermore, television viewing is voluntary and the selection of programming is greater than ever before.

Moreover, television viewing is in itself a low-risk activity. Some people suggest that viewing violent or horrifying dramas provides a safe release, or catharsis, from the tensions of modern life.

Many strategies can help lessen violence, but avoiding TV is not one of them. Each person should try to foresee conflicts and defuse them, keep a sense of humor, treat people with respect, and avoid pushing strangers—you do not know their frame of mind. If you have violent tendencies, seek counseling. Individuals cause violence; we shouldn't make TV the scapegoat.

- Storing all substances, especially cleaning materials, in their original containers so that the contents are known
- Keeping the telephone number of the local poison control center in a visible and easily accessible location near the phone

Controlling Violence As a cause of injuries, particularly in urban areas, violence continues to be a major problem, not least because several of its many causes are still poorly understood. The major responsibility for violence obviously lies with those who perpetrate it, yet steps can be taken by potential victims that may lessen the likelihood of violence occurring. These steps include the following:

- Taking appropriate cautionary measures such as installing safety locks, avoiding areas known to be dangerous, and traveling with friends rather than alone
- Reporting any violent incidents in the neighborhood and being willing to cooperate with official investigators

Television: Violence and the Plug-In Drug

Many people link the crime wave to the illegal drug trade, but there is another bad habit that spurs people's appetite for violence: television. All you have to do is tally the sensational news stories selected to boost ratings; count the shootings, beatings, and humiliations carried out by cartoon superheroes in the name of justice; and add the mayhem of prime-time dramas and docudramas. The total is a televised parade of negative models for dealing with conflict and stress.

Furthermore, TV dramas encourage little analysis of personal and social problems. Instead, they lure viewers into a glamorous and dangerous world where justice is revenge and power is righteousness.

The escapist experience of television viewing is brought to people's homes by commercial materialism. The symbols of success and happiness, of power and sex, are dangled before people by the creative minds of a multibillion-dollar industry—advertising. Television is a forum for increasing consumer demand for products by pandering to simpleminded fantasies.

The result of the television experience is a populace less able to cope with the stress of contemporary life and therefore more violent. Studies have shown that children who view violent television become more aggressive. Violent criminals report that as children they watched more violent television than does the general population.

A recent study showed that the introduction of television technology predicted a rise in the murder rate 10 to 15 years later. In other words, the TV generation in the United States and Canada committed more murders in parallel with its exposure to television in childhood.

During the same time period (1950 to 1975), murder rates among white South Africans remained low and unchanged because South Africa had banned TV technology. Now, 10 to 15 years after television's introduction there, murder rates among white South Africans are beginning to rise.

If people want to lower the rate of violence in this society, they have to limit the infiltration of violence into their homes through television. It is necessary to limit all TV viewing and completely avoid violent TV. In addition, people must boycott and lobby against violence on television.

What do you think? Do you find that watching a violent show on television provides a release from the tensions of your day? Or do you find the occurrence of violence on television upsetting, creating further tensions that you have difficulty resolving?

Adapted from Brandon S. Centerwall, "Exposure to Television as a Risk Factor for Violence," *American Journal of Epidemiology* 129, no. 4 (April 1989): 643–652.

- Taking care not to escalate situations where there is a danger of violence occurring
- Being aware of potentially dangerous situations among one's acquaintances or family members and being ready and willing to get help from a trusted friend or professional if matters seem likely to get out of control

Providing Emergency Care

Despite efforts at prevention, injuries do happen. Therefore, it is important to know not only how to reduce the risk of injury but also how to deal with an injury when it does occur. Knowledge about basic emergency care procedures can be very helpful in dealing with injuries and other health-threatening conditions. It is also very important to know local medical emergency telephone numbers, such as 911, that provide assistance.

There is a great deal of information available on different types of emergency care procedures. Many communities also offer courses and training at the American Red Cross, American Heart Association, YMCAs and YWCAs, and other community centers on first-aid procedures such as cardiopulmonary resuscitation (CPR) and water safety or lifeguard training. Taking such courses can make you very valuable in an emergency.

Basic Principles of Emergency Care

There are three basic principles for giving emergency care.

1. Always begin by preventing further injury.
2. Do only what is absolutely necessary and get professional help as soon as possible. Certain situations, such as when a person has no heartbeat, is bleeding profusely, or has swallowed poison, require immediate help; others are less life-threatening.
3. Know your limits. Offer help only when you are sure your actions will not cause further injury.

The Good Samaritan law states that "no person who administers emergency care in good faith is liable for civil damages unless such acts are willfully or wantonly negligent."

Basic Procedures for Emergency Care

To be helpful in an emergency, it is essential to act coolly and sensibly. The following sequence of steps applies to any medical emergency. Learning these steps will make you better equipped to use specific emergency care measures.

Try to Remain Calm Injuries and other medical emergencies can be very frightening, and fear can make people do irrational things that make matters worse. In dealing with an emergency, the first thing to do is make sure you are thinking straight. Sometimes this is easier said than done, but it is essential. Keeping calm not only makes you more effective but also reassures the victim that someone sensible is going to try to help. Thus, the first thing to do in an emergency is to take a second or two to calm yourself before attending to the victim. Also, make sure the scene is safe before approaching.

Find Out What Happened Finding out what happened to cause a medical emergency is extremely important. In many instances there are good reasons to use or reject certain emergency care procedures; the only way to determine what to do is to ask what happened. (The method chosen for stopping bleeding from a serious wound, for example, depends on whether a foreign object is embedded in the wound.) While you are finding out what happened, let the victim know who you are and know that you are trying to help.

Examine the Victim In some situations taking time to examine a victim methodically is inappropriate. When the situation is obviously beyond your capability, as with a serious head injury, the best thing is to arrange to have the victim transported to a hospital immediately. In other cases emergency care procedures should begin without delay.

When serious complications may be present, such as after a bad fall, it is very important to make certain that you understand the nature of the injury. Careful examination involves considering the injury in the context of the person's overall condition and includes checking the following:

- *Level of responsiveness.* Observe whether the person is conscious, responsive to what you say, and in pain.
- *Breathing.* Watch the person's chest rise and fall and put your ear close to the person's nose and mouth to listen and feel for breathing. Observe whether breathing is normal (about 12 to 18 breaths a minute) or shallow and rapid, gasping, or absent.
- *Pulse.* Feel for the pulse in the artery at the side of the neck or on the wrist below the base of the thumb (Figure 16.2). Observe whether the pulse is normal (about 70 to 90 beats a minute) or rapid, slow, weak, or absent.

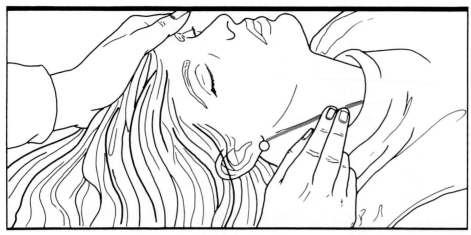

Figure 16.2 To take a pulse at the neck, place two fingers at the victim's Adam's apple and slide them down toward the back of the neck. About halfway down you will feel a groove; this is where the carotid artery runs, supplying blood to the head and brain. Its pulse, if present, will be very noticeable. Be careful not to press too hard or you will stop the flow of blood.

- *Massive bleeding.* The loss of large amounts of blood can cause shock and death. Take immediate steps to control severe bleeding.
- *Pupils.* Check the pupils; they should be of equal size and should get slightly smaller when exposed to a bright light.
- *Deformity.* Compare one side of the body with the other. If one arm or leg is in an unnatural position, it may be fractured or dislocated.
- *Skin.* Look at the victim's face. Check the skin color (flushed, normal, or pale), texture (dry or moist, goose bumps), and temperature (hot, normal, or cool).
- *Neck or spinal cord injury.* Paralysis of the face, arms, or legs is a sign of a neck or spinal cord injury. Avoid moving the person to reduce the chance of causing further injury.

Administer Emergency Care Assessing the victim's condition should take only a minute or two. During that time, you will get a clearer idea of the situation and the injured person will be calmed by your readiness to help. With a better idea of what may be wrong, you will be able to choose the appropriate emergency care procedure and begin applying it.

Common Situations Requiring First Aid

There are a number of situations in which emergency care procedures are required. It is essential for the person providing help to know the proper procedures for each particular situation. What that person does or does not do can sometimes mean the difference between life and death.

Heart Attack and Stroke Cases of cardiac arrest, in which the heart has stopped completely, require CPR. CPR cannot be taught adequately in a brief overview like this, but it is not difficult or time-consuming to learn. A local Red Cross chapter or the local office of the American Heart Association can provide information about courses. Most heart attack victims, however, do not experience cardiac arrest. Emergency care procedures in such cases include the following:

- Arrange for transportation to the nearest hospital.
- Let the victim sit up or lie down as he or she prefers but not move around.
- Watch for nausea and make sure the victim has an open airway.

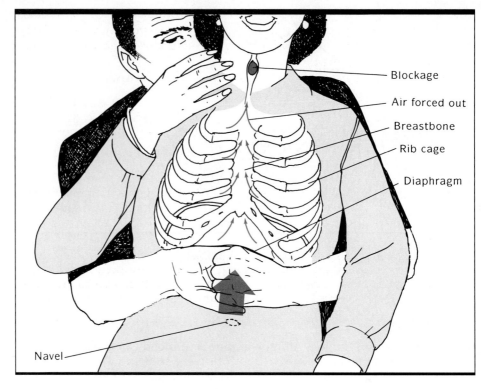

Figure 16.3 The Heimlich maneuver. Pressing inward on the diaphragm forces air out of the lungs, dislodging an object from the airway. Stand behind the victim. Position your fist between the navel and the rib cage to avoid breaking bones. Grasp your fist with your other hand. Pull both hands toward you with a quick upward and inward thrust. Repeat up to four times if necessary.

Blockage

Air forced out

Breastbone

Rib cage

Diaphragm

Navel

According to the American Academy of Pediatrics, back blows are the recommended treatment for choking in infants under 1 year old. Sit down and lay the choking child at a downward angle over one arm. Use the heel of the other hand to give four quick blows to the child's back between the shoulder blades. If breathing does not start, turn the child over, support the child's neck and back, and give four chest thrusts, using two fingers.

shock—a condition in which the body loses control of blood flow.

Choking If a person who seems to be choking on food or a foreign object can speak, do not interfere with that individual's attempts to cough up the object. If the person is unable to speak, it is appropriate to provide emergency care by using the Heimlich maneuver (Figure 16.3). Stand behind the victim and place both arms around his or her waist. Grasp one fist with the other hand and place the thumb side of the fist against the victim's abdomen, slightly above the navel and below the rib cage. Press your fist into the victim's abdomen with a quick inward and upward thrust. Repeat this procedure until the object is dislodged. The Heimlich maneuver should not be used with infants under 1 year of age.[48]

Shock Serious injury, loss of blood, heart failure, severe burns, breathing impairment, and severe emotional upset can cause **shock**—a condition in which the body loses control of blood flow. In shock, the pattern of blood flow is interrupted and the heart cannot circulate blood effectively. Signs of shock include pale, cool, and clammy skin; shivering; a rapid and weak pulse; and shallow and rapid or deep and irregular breathing. A person suffering from shock may also be mentally confused, have drooping eyelids or dilated pupils, experience nausea and vomiting, or collapse.

Shock is a life-threatening condition, and immediate attention is essential. Victims of serious injuries should always be treated for shock. With minor injuries, it is important for the person providing emergency care to watch for signs of shock. Procedures for dealing with shock include the following:

- *Warmth.* Make sure body heat is not lost. Place blankets or extra clothing over and under the victim if necessary.
- *Position.* Do not make the person lie down flat in cases of head and chest injuries, heart attack, and stroke. In these situations the victim may be more comfortable and able to breathe better in a semireclining position. If you are in doubt about these conditions and in all other cases (such as a suspected neck or back injury), keep the victim lying flat. Elevate the feet 6 to 12 inches if no neck, back, or leg injuries are suspected unless the victim is unconscious.

Severe Bleeding Cuts, lacerations, and other wounds may involve damage to both surface and underlying tissue and can bleed profusely. It is always important to determine if foreign objects are embedded in a wound before proceeding with emergency care.

Three basic methods can be used to control severe bleeding.

1. *Direct pressure.* Pressure is applied directly on the open wound with a bare hand or a clean, lint-free cloth or towel. Use just enough pressure to stop the bleeding; too much pressure may cause further injury. If a foreign object is embedded in the wound, do *not* use the direct pressure method and do *not* try to remove the object; both can cause more damage.

2. *Elevation.* The injured site is raised so that it is higher than the heart, using gravity to slow or stop the bleeding. This method should be used in combination with direct pressure. Do *not* use elevation if it entails risking additional injury, as when a fracture is also present.

3. *Pressure points.* Pressure points are locations in the body where arteries pass over bones. If one presses down on a pressure point between the injury site and the heart, the artery can be closed enough to stem the flow of blood (Figure 16.4). The pressure point method is very useful

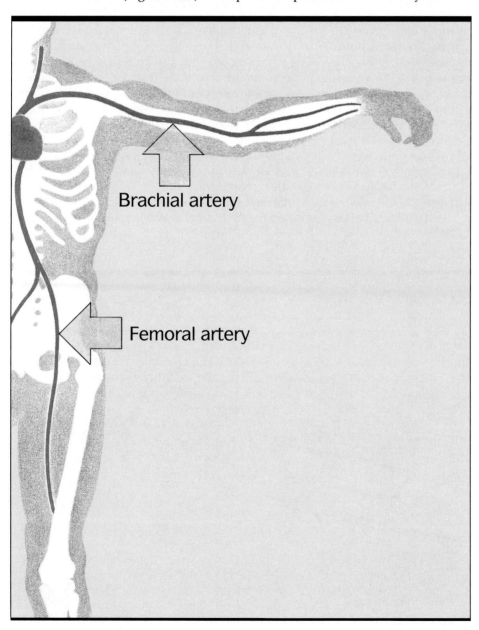

Brachial artery

Femoral artery

Figure 16.4 Pressure points enable you to check arterial bleeding in the arm or leg by applying indirect pressure. When you feel a pulse, you have located the artery. Press the artery against the bone to slow the blood supply. For leg injuries, press the femoral artery (in the groin) against the pelvic rim. For arm injuries, press the brachial artery (inside the upper arm) against the humerus. For hand injuries, find the appropriate artery in the wrist.

when direct pressure and elevation cannot be used or do not suffice; all three techniques can be used in combination.

Unconsciousness Providing emergency care to an unconscious person presents some unusual difficulties. Since the person cannot describe what happened, it is necessary to be particularly careful and conservative in taking action. For example, if there is any evidence that unconsciousness is a result of a severe electrical shock, it is important *not* to touch the person until you have made sure that the electrical contact is broken by using a nonmetal, nonconducting object such as a dead tree branch or wooden handle. General rules to follow include the following:

- Check for breathing, pulse, and pupil size.
- Turn the person onto his or her side if you are sure there is no neck or spinal injury to help breathing and allow fluid to drain out of the mouth and nose so that the person does not choke.
- Help the injury victim maintain body heat by covering him or her with blankets or clothing.
- Never try to give food or liquid to an unconscious or dazed person.
- Arrange for professional medical attention as soon as possible.

Sprains and Fractures A *sprain* is an injury to a joint; a *fracture* is a break in a bone. When a bone is fractured or a joint is sprained, the surrounding tissues swell and sometimes become discolored, the limb may be visibly deformed, and there usually is pain. In addition, if the fracture is *open*, meaning that the skin is broken, there is an added risk of infection. In many cases the victim cannot move a fractured limb, but contrary to popular belief, the ability to move a limb does *not* necessarily mean that the limb is not fractured.

Since only an x-ray can establish whether an injury is a fracture or a sprain, all suspected fractures and sprains should be treated as if they were fractures. The emergency procedures that should be followed include the following:

- Urge the victim to remain still to avoid aggravating the injury.
- The basic rule for emergency care of fractures is to *immobilize the broken bone and both adjacent joints* (Figure 16.5). For example, a suspected fracture of

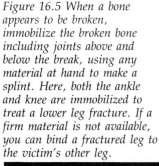

Figure 16.5 When a bone appears to be broken, immobilize the broken bone including joints above and below the break, using any material at hand to make a splint. Here, both the ankle and knee are immobilized to treat a lower leg fracture. If a firm material is not available, you can bind a fractured leg to the victim's other leg.

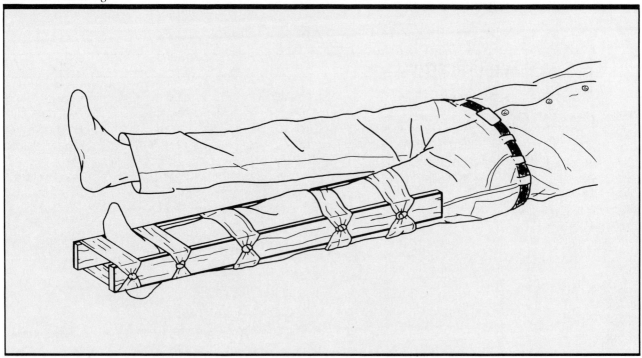

the tibia in the lower leg should be splinted so that the tibia, the ankle joint below it, and the knee joint above it are immobilized. It is relatively easy to rig a splint for a suspected fracture; anything rigid and long enough (such as a pair of skis) will do.

- After splinting, get medical attention for the victim. (*Note:* Special procedures are needed for immobilizing people with head and spinal injuries. Formal training in such procedures is necessary.)

Poisoning and Drug Overdose   People can be exposed to a number of potentially dangerous substances, some poisonous and others nonpoisonous but harmful in large doses (Table 16.1). As a result, information on the appropriate treatment for specific types of poisoning or substance overdose is often difficult to find. Specialized poison control centers have been established in most parts of the country. The telephone number of the nearest center should be easily accessible. General emergency procedures for poisonings and overdoses include the following:

- Keep the victim still; movement spreads the poison through the body.
- Try to identify the poison or substance and determine how much was ingested. If possible, have the container with you when you call the poison control center.
- Call the poison control center as soon as you are sure the victim has a pulse and is breathing. If the victim is not breathing, begin artificial respiration immediately; if the heart has stopped, begin CPR.
- Check for signs of the poison around the victim's mouth, such as burns or other indications that the poison is corrosive. Watch for nausea and vomiting. If the victim vomits, make sure he or she does not choke. Save a sample of the vomit for medical personnel; they may need to analyze it to identify the poisonous substance.
- If the victim is conscious, dilute the poison by having him or her drink water or milk. Try to induce vomiting *unless* there are burns around the mouth or the victim's breath smells like kerosene or gasoline. Such corrosive substances, if vomited, will burn the victim's throat and mouth a second time. If the victim become nauseated, discontinue giving fluids. Never try to give liquids to an unconscious or dazed person.

Table 16.1   Common Household Poisons That Should Be Kept from Children

Cleaning Products	Medicines	Cosmetics	Hobby Supplies	Yard Products
Acids	Antiseptics	Bubble bath	Epoxy glue	Garden sprays
Ammonia	Aspirin	Cologne	Model cement	Fertilizers
Bathroom cleaner	Corn and wart removers	Eye makeup	Paint	Herbicides
Benzene	Cough mixtures	Hair dyes	Paint thinner	Insecticides
Stain removers	Dandruff shampoo	Nail polish	Photography chemicals	Pesticides
Cleaning fluids	Diet tablets	Nail polish	Turpentine	Rodenticides
Metal cleaners	Drugs	remover		
Dishwashing detergents	Eye drops	Permanent wave		
Drain cleaners	Iodine	solution		
Furniture polish	Laxatives	Shaving lotion		
Gun cleaners	Nose drops			
Kerosene	Painkillers			
Oven cleaner	Sedatives			
Pine oil	Vitamins			
Silver polish				
Window cleaner				

Burns Burns are dangerous injuries that can cause extensive damage, and emergency care procedures can be very effective in limiting that damage. These procedures include the following:

- Get the victim away from the source of the burn. If the person's clothing is on fire, smother the flames with a coat or blanket or make the person roll on the ground. Restrain the person from running around in a panic; movement fans the flames.
- Try to determine whether the burn is thermal or chemical. A *thermal burn* is caused by heat, such as fire or steam; the burning will continue as long as the heat remains in contact with the skin. A *chemical burn* is caused by a corrosive substance such as a strong acid or alkali; the burning will continue as long as the concentrated substance remains in contact with the skin.
- Determine the severity of the burn. *First-degree burns* involve surface tissue only; sunburn is a good example. *Second-degree burns* involve blistering, a sign of underlying tissue damage. *Third-degree burns* involve charring and destruction of skin and underlying tissue; such burns are life-threatening.
- For thermal burns, once the source of burning has been removed, cool the burned area immediately by means of immersion or the application of cloths soaked in cool tap water. (Ice water may cause shock.) Do not remove clothing that is stuck to the burn. For anything other than minor burns, seek medical attention promptly.
- For chemical burns, flood the affected area with water for at least 20 minutes, until the burning substance has been washed completely away, and then seek medical attention.
- Do not apply an ointment or cream to any burn unless advised to do so by medical personnel. One of the major dangers associated with burns is infection. Any burn can become infected, but those where the skin is blistered or burned away pose the greatest risk. To prevent both shock and infection, cover burned areas with material that will stick as little as possible, such as a freshly ironed sheet or tablecloth. Get medical help if there is any doubt about the extent of injury or the possibility of infection.

Seizures Seizures, or convulsions, are signs of another underlying problem, a signal that something else is wrong. For example, a child may have seizures as a result of a high fever. Seizures are also a sign of certain chronic diseases, such as epilepsy.

The most important objective of emergency care for seizures is to prevent further injury. Gently lower the person to the floor and do not try to restrain that person's movements. Try to keep the victim on his or her side; this helps keep the airway open by allowing fluid to drain out of the mouth. Do *not* put any object in the victim's mouth to prevent swallowing the tongue; the object itself can injure the victim. After a seizure has passed, consult a physician for instructions on what to do next. People subject to chronic seizures probably know what should be done, so be sure to ask.

Bruises, Minor Cuts, and Lacerations Bruises are closed wounds in which the skin is not broken but damage to tissues under the skin can cause invisible bleeding. The sign of such bleeding is the dark blue skin discoloration associated with a bruise.

If a person with a bruise develops a fever, becomes nauseated, or has red streaks on the skin near the bruise, get medical attention at once. Otherwise, the best procedure is to apply a cold compress to the area. Cold slows the underlying bleeding and reduces the size of the bruise.

While generally not serious, minor cuts and lacerations require emergency care to stop bleeding and prevent infection. The cut and the surrounding skin should first be washed thoroughly with soap and water; there is no need to apply alcohol or other antiseptics. Then blot the area dry and apply a clean bandage.

Infections Sometimes minor injuries become infected. Most infections can be treated successfully if they are recognized and attended to promptly. The main symptoms of infection are skin redness, swelling, fever, tenderness, and swollen lymph nodes. Emergency care involves immobilizing the affected part of the body, applying hot compresses, and getting medical attention.

When Professional Help Arrives

A person providing emergency care can safely relinquish his or her helping role only when professional help arrives. At that point the person should explain the condition in which the victim was found, the emergency care measures already taken, when they were begun, and the victim's response to those measures. Any additional information that may help the professionals deal with the problem should also be discussed. Accurate and relevant information allows professional rescuers to make sure the injured person continues to receive the care he or she needs to recover successfully.

Chapter Summary

- Various factors contribute to the risk of injury. The threshold theory and the agent-host-environment model are used to explain why injuries happen. According to the threshold theory, injuries occur when a force or energy poses a problem that is beyond a person's capabilities. The agent-host-environment model builds on that theory and emphasizes the multiple factors that play a role in causing injuries.
- All types of injuries can occur in the home, including falls, burns, poisoning, and drowning. Home injuries frequently affect the very young and the very old.
- Many work-related injuries are associated with motor vehicles; other significant work-related injuries include falls and burns. Young workers and minority group members also seem to be at greater risk.
- One of the most common recreational injuries is drowning. Another water-related injury is spinal injury from diving. Among young children, falls are a common recreational injury, often occurring in playgrounds. Competitive sports can be quite hazardous, especially contact sports such as football and ice hockey.
- Violence is a significant health problem in terms of the number of people who are killed and injured every year. Unlike injuries which are unintentional, violence-related injuries are often intentional and include such things as assaults, rape, and homicide.
- Motor vehicle injuries are a major cause of death. Young drivers and elderly drivers are at the highest risk for sustaining a motor vehicle injury. The factors involved in many motor vehicle injuries include alcohol and automobile safety features, such as seat belts. The young (under age 5) and old (over age 75) are at the

highest risk for suffering injury from a fall. Environmental factors play a major role in the risk of falling. Burn injuries are also most prevalent among the young and the very old. With drownings, men are at greater risk, as are young children. Many drownings could be avoided through proper supervision of young children. Poisonings are also more common among the young and the old; many are easily avoided by keeping hazardous substances in safe locations. Most violence-related injuries involve young men; race and socioeconomic status seem to be significant factors in determining who is victimized.
- Analyzing agent-host-environmental factors is essential in the prevention of injuries. When the various factors associated with injuries have been identified, steps can be taken to change behaviors, eliminate hazards, and design safer environments.
- The two major approaches to injury prevention are persuasion and legislation. Persuasion includes efforts to change people's behavior through education, rehabilitation, and social support systems. Laws are aimed at encouraging behavioral change and providing safer products and environments.
- Active prevention measures are measures that require individuals to do something to reduce the risk of injury, such as wearing motorcycle helmets or seat belts. Passive prevention measures require little or no action on the part of the individual. They include automatic seat belts and built-in safety switches on equipment. The best form of prevention includes a combination of active and passive measures.
- In spite of the growing concentration on prevention measures, injuries still occur. A practi-

cal knowledge of emergency care procedures is therefore highly valuable. They can be learned from many community sources.

- Important principles of emergency care include knowing one's own limitations, staying calm and reassuring as one assesses the situation, and being able to follow appropriate initial care procedures for different types of problems until professional medical help arrives.

Key Terms

Active prevention
(page 419)

Passive prevention
(page 420)

Shock (page 426)

References

1. Stuart T. Brown et al., "Injury Prevention and Control: Prospects for the 1990s," *Annual Review of Public Health* 11 (1990): 251–266.

2. J. A. Waller, " 'Accident' Proneness: Fact or Fiction?" in *Injury Control: A Guide to the Causes and Prevention of Trauma* (Lexington, Mass.: D C Heath, 1985): 467.

3. Frederick P. Rivara, "Epidemiology of Childhood Injuries," in J. D. Matarazzo et al., *Behavioral Health: A Handbook of Health Enhancement and Disease Prevention* (New York: Wiley, 1984): 1003–1020.

4. Committee on Trauma Research, Commission on Life Sciences, National Research Council, and Institute of Medicine, *Injury in America* (Washington, D.C.: National Academy Press, 1985): 1–21.

5. Rivara, op. cit.

6. National Committee for Injury Prevention and Control, "Injury Prevention: Meeting the Challenge," *American Journal of Preventive Medicine* (1989): 4–18.

7. Judith S. Mausner and Shira Kramer, *Epidemiology— An Introductory Text*, 2d ed. (Philadelphia: W B Saunders, 1985): 26–41.

8. Frederick P. Rivara and Marsha E. Wold, "Injury Research: Where Should We Go from Here?" *Pediatrics* 84, no. 1 (July 1989): 180–181.

9. National Committee for Injury Prevention and Control, op. cit., pp. 145–162.

10. Ibid.

11. Ibid., pp. 177–191.

12. Ibid.

13. Ibid.

14. Ibid.

15. National Center for Health Statistics, *Vital Statistics of the United States, 1987*, Vol. 2A. (Washington, D.C.: Dept. of Health and Human Services, 1989. Pub. no. (PHS) 89-1101).

16. National Committee for Injury Prevention and Control, op. cit., pp. 153–176.

17. Ibid.

18. Ibid.

19. Ibid., pp. 192–203.

20. Ibid.

21. Ibid., pp. 115–144.

22. Ibid.

23. Ibid.

24. National Center for Health Statistics, op. cit.

25. National Committee for Injury Prevention and Control, op. cit., pp. 145–162.

26. Ibid.

27. National Center for Health Statistics, op. cit.

28. National Committee for Injury Prevention and Control, op. cit., pp. 145–162.

29. Ibid.

30. Ibid., pp. 163–176.

31. Carol W. Runyan and Elizabeth A. Gerken, "Epidemiology and Prevention of Adolescent Injury," *Journal of the American Medical Association* 262, no. 16 (October 27, 1989): 2273–2279.

32. National Committee for Injury Prevention and Control, op. cit., pp. 163–176.

33. P. Present, *Child Drowning Study: A Report on the Epidemiology of Drownings in Residential Pools to Children under Age Five* (Washington, D.C.: Division of Hazard Analysis, Directorate for Epidemiology, U.S. Consumer Product Safety Commission, 1987).

34. National Center for Health Statistics, op. cit.

35. National Committee for Injury Prevention and Control, op. cit.

36. Ibid., pp. 145–162.

37. John W. Wright (ed.), *The Universal Almanac—1990* (Kansas City, Mo.: Andrews and McMeel, 1989): 202.

38. Federal Bureau of Investigation, "Uniform Crime Reports for the United States, 1989." (Washington, D.C.: U.S. Dept. of Justice, 1990).

39. National Committee for Injury Prevention and Control, op. cit., pp. 205–212, 243–251.

40. Ibid.

41. Federal Bureau of Investigation, op. cit.

42. Runyan and Gerken, op. cit.

43. National Committee for Injury Prevention and Control, op. cit., pp. 204–221.

44. Ibid., pp. 192–203.

45. Leon S. Robertson, "Behavior and Injury Prevention: Whose Behavior?" in Matarazzo et al., op. cit., pp. 980–989.

46. Harvey F. Davis et al., "The 1990 Objectives for the Nation for Injury Prevention: A Progress Review," *Public Health Reports* 99, no. 1 (January–February 1984): 10–23.

47. Robert A. Dershewitz, "Childhood Household Safety," in Matarazzo et al., op. cit., pp. 1021–1036.

48. American Heart Association, "Management of the Obstructed Airway," in *American Heart Association Instructors' Manual for Basic Cardiac Life Support* (Dallas: American Heart Association, 1981).

PART 6

Caring for Others: Health, Life Span, and Society

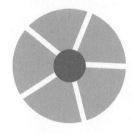

The last part of the book presents broader perspectives on health. It reviews the importance of taking action now to achieve health throughout the life span, considers the experience and meaning of death both to those who die and to those who mourn, surveys personal and societal resources for health care, and stresses collective responsibility for the health of the environment.

Chapter 17 looks at health throughout the life span, including the normal aging process and the effects of lifestyle behaviors on health in people's later years. It stresses the difference that wise health practices now can make in one's old age.

Chapter 18 covers the topic of death: how it affects those who are dying and those who care for them, the steps individuals can take to prepare for their own and other people's deaths, and the process of grief and recovery.

Chapter 19 describes the importance of taking responsibility for one's own health through knowledge about one's physiology and the medical resources available in the United States.

Chapter 20 studies environmental threats to health that have developed during this century, both nationally and globally, and emphasizes the importance of individual and collective action to combat those threats.

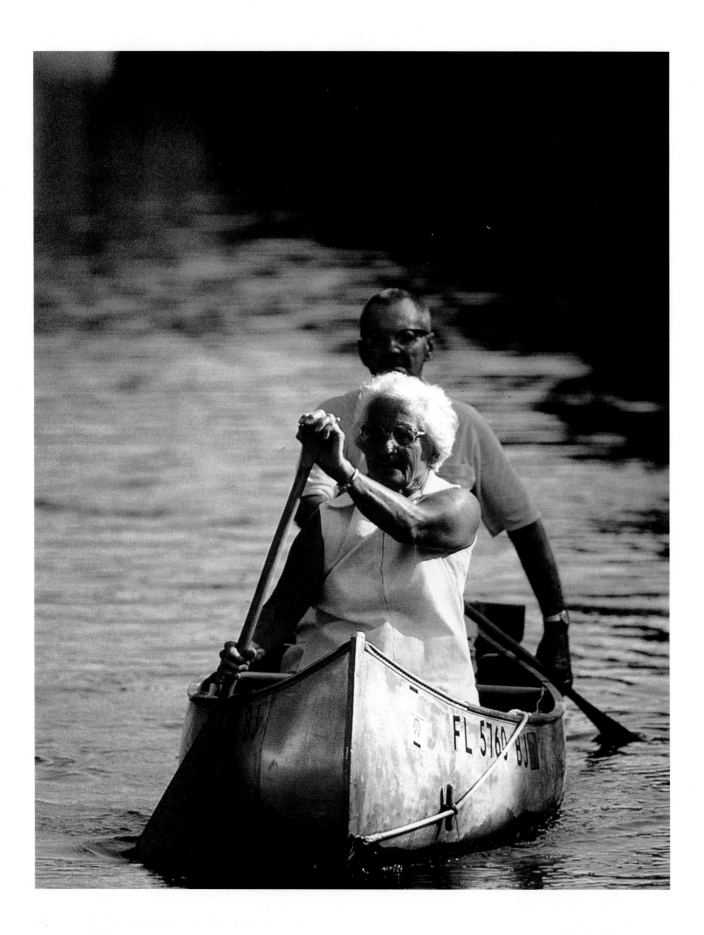

Lifestyle and Growing Older

To Guide Your Reading

When you have studied this chapter, you should be able to:

- Characterize the human life span in terms of healthy aging and pathological aging, and describe the common stages of growth and change in adult life.

- Comment on the concerns of people as they age, both the functions of normal aging and problems associated with disease and other more avoidable disabilities.

- Discuss various constraints on the aging process, including genetic limits to cell reproduction, theories of aging due to physiological damage, and the effects of lifestyle.

- Clarify ways in which people can take actions to lessen the impact of aging on their own lives and on the lives of others close to them.

Growing older is a fact of life; there is no fountain of youth that can stop or turn back the clock. Many people fear the aging process, believing that physical and mental decline is inevitable. Evidence suggests, however, that chronological age is a poor predictor of physical or mental health status and functional ability. While there are age-related changes in physical functioning, it is now thought that many of those changes are related to disuse and to destructive health habits rather than to age.[1] Developing and maintaining a healthy lifestyle throughout your life thus can have a significant effect on how you age.

The thoughts of most younger people are focused on schools, careers, and personal lives; few think seriously about how they will spend their later years. The time to think about this, however, is now; your health at age 64, 75, or older depends to a large extent on your current lifestyle. A healthy old age can be very rewarding, but if old age is marked by pain, disability, loneliness, and fear, it can be unbearable. Developing and maintaining a healthy lifestyle at all periods of life will increase your pleasure not only today but throughout the remainder of your life.

This chapter explores the processes of aging: what is inevitable, what we can affect, and how we can affect it. It looks at the downside of aging—the symptoms that people fear and often expect. And it explores what one can do both for oneself and for the other people in one's life to improve the experiences of growing older.

Some popular misconceptions about older people:

- *Most have serious health problems.*
- *Most end up in nursing homes.*
- *They do not have enough money.*
- *They are not interested in sex.*
- *They are lonely.*
- *They can no longer be efficient at their jobs.*
- *They are absent from their jobs because of illness more than young people are.*
- *They do not get proper medical care.*

Growing Older and Aging

Aging does not begin at age 35 or 55. It is a lifelong process of physical, emotional, intellectual, social, and spiritual changes that occur from birth until death. There is, however, often confusion between normal aging and the aging that may occur during specific periods of one's life because of dis-

normal aging—*certain biological aging processes that seem time-related rather than being a function of disease, injury, or stress.*

ease or poor health. **Normal aging** refers to certain biological processes that are time-related rather than being a function of disease, injury, or stress.[2] After age 40, for example, most people's vision and hearing begin a gradual deterioration which may become quite noticeable as the years go by. Although the rates of change differ from individual to individual, the process of normal aging is inevitable. Within this process, a distinction can be made between *usual aging*, in which factors such as diet and exercise heighten the effects of the aging process, and *successful aging*, in which these factors can play a neutral or even positive role.[3] **Pathological aging** refers to a decrease in functioning caused by illness, stress, injury, and other factors.[4] Some studies have shown that high levels of physical function in old age are associated with the absence of hypertension, a history of never smoking, maintenance of normal weight, and a limited consumption of alcohol.[5]

pathological aging—*a decrease in functioning caused by disease, illness, stress, injury, and other factors.*

Thus, the individual has the ability to control many of the factors that contribute to pathological aging; the human body itself has a great capacity for dealing with some of the other factors; and some health professionals believe that the mind can also contribute to lasting health.[6] Yet, despite its complexity and remarkable resiliency, the human body is not immortal. The normal aging process is built into the human body, and no matter what people do, they cannot avoid the inevitable. They can only affect its course through the activities and habits they develop throughout life.

gerontology—*the study of aging.*

The study of aging—**gerontology**—attempts to shed light on the built-in normal aging process and also to explain other factors which affect how and why people age. Among the things gerontologists study are the human life span and the changes people experience at different stages of their lives.

Human Life Spans

life span—*the maximum amount of time a person lives.*

The length of time a person lives is called the **life span.** There seems to be an approximate limit to the potential human life span; most scientists believe this limit to be about 120 years.[7] Indeed, very few people live past 100 years.

The life spans of individuals vary enormously; some people die very young, while others reach very old ages. In American society today, most people are lucky to reach their eighties, though more and more are doing so. Persons 85 years old and older currently constitute the most rapidly growing portion of the American population (Figure 17.1). The number of people in this age group increased from 2.3 million in 1980 to 2.9 million in 1987, and it is expected to surge to 5.4 million by the year 2000 and reach 7.6 million by 2020.[8]

life expectancy—*the average predicted length of life from birth to death.*

The average predicted length of life is known as **life expectancy.** At present, the average life expectancy at birth in the United States is about 75 years.[9] This means that most children born today can expect to live to the age of 75. At the beginning of this century the average life expectancy at birth was only about 47.3 years.[10] Much of this increase can be attributed to a reduced infant mortality rate, the control of certain diseases, and other medical advances that have helped prolong people's lives. Changes in lifestyle, however, also figure significantly in this increase in average life expectancy.

Life expectancies differ among different groups within the American population. Among white women the average life expectancy is 78.9 years; among black women it is 73.8 years. Among white men average life expectancy is 72.1 years; among black men it is only 65.1 years.[11] Environmental factors play an important part in these disparities. So too do differences in lifestyle.

Growth and Change

As people age, they change in various ways. Their appearance is altered, their physical strength increases and then declines, they can be more prone to injury and disease, and their behavior and concerns may change. Perhaps

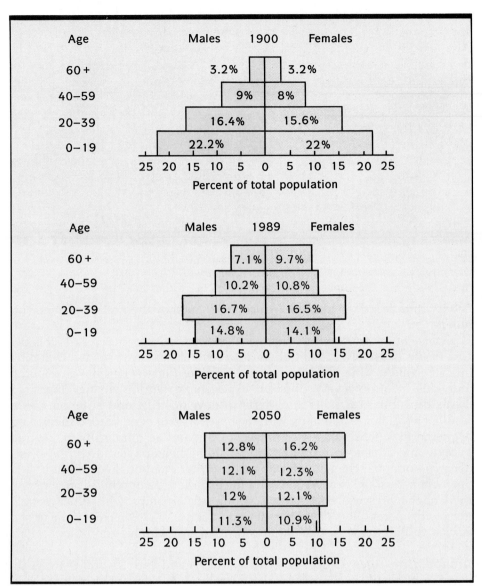

Figure 17.1 Ageism and other problems of aging—physical, psychological, social, and financial—become more urgent as the population gets older. These three population pyramids show how the proportion of older people in the U.S. population is increasing. Younger people predominated in 1900, but the reverse will be true by 2050.

Source: U.S. Bureau of the Census.

most important, they grow in terms of character as a result of meeting challenges and assimilating new experiences.

Psychologist Erik Erikson described life as a series of eight psychosocial stages from infancy to old age, during which the individual encounters certain emotional crises that must be resolved. The resolution of these crises allows the individual to mature and move successfully to the next stage. Erikson's stages are useful in explaining the emotional changes that occur as a person grows older.[12]

Recognizing the characteristics of life's stages and the common reactions to the challenges of each stage can give one a better perspective for shaping one's lifestyle in a way that leads to healthier aging. For the purposes of this chapter, consider the following stages, which are adapted from those of Erikson, and some of the characteristics of each stage.[13]

Preadult (Birth to Age 18) During early childhood and the teenage years, the most obvious form of growth is physical, as the individual reaches physical maturity during this stage. It is also a time, however, when individuals begin to develop the basis for emotional, intellectual, and spiritual development. Much of a person's energies at this stage are devoted to absorbing experiences and shaping a world view. Individuals begin to develop lifelong

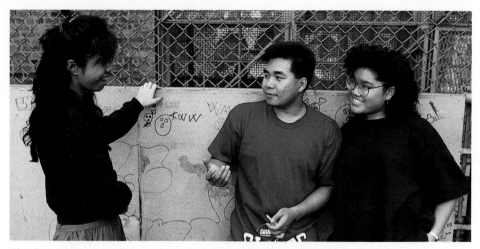

The desire for greater independence from parents and closer bonds with peers is a well-known part of adolescence. (Robert Brenner/PhotoEdit)

habits, attitudes, and behaviors which are shaped by their relationships with others.

Because of the tremendous changes that occur during these years, this period of life is usually broken down into several narrower stages, including infancy, childhood, and adolescence. At each of these stages the developing individual confronts very different experiences. During infancy the child learns basic physical skills and starts to develop trust and autonomy as a result of his or her relationship with the parents. In later childhood the person begins to experience a greater sense of duty and accomplishment. During puberty and adolescence the individual strengthens physically but also undergoes hormonal changes that upset his or her emotional equilibrium, at a time when personal expectations and the expectations of others can generate tremendous pressure. Developing strong relationships with other people during this period helps a person develop a sense of perspective as he or she faces a string of crises involving love, friendship, family, and school.

Adult Entry (Ages 19 to 24)   The late teens and early twenties are years when most people experiment with new roles. It is a time of transition when many people struggle with decisions about the future. During these years most people leave their parents' homes for college or to begin careers. They may select preferred sports and physical activities, or cease formal exercise habits. They begin to develop sexual love relationships and mature friendships; some marry and have children. A person at this stage is secure enough in his or her identity to develop an intimate partnership in which he or she makes compromises for the benefit of another person.

While some people at this stage continue the struggle for individuality and independence that was begun in late childhood, others begin to assert their individuality and independence in a mature way. It is a time when people reflect on the confusing array of options opening before them: intellectual challenges may be greatly expanding, social interactions are widening, and spiritual beliefs are facing serious challenge as they come into contact with other ideas and beliefs.

Young Adulthood (Ages 25 to 39)   By young adulthood many people have married or established a lifelong commitment. Most of them have children, households, and active careers. The timing of childbearing, education, and career is highly variable, however. A large number of people will have divorced and perhaps remarried; a few will be widowed.

In this stage of life individuals may find themselves surpassing their elders in some aspects of life or being surpassed by people younger than themselves. They will probably face the first intimation of aging when younger adults call them sir or ma'am. If they gave up exercise earlier, they may feel the need to start again. Some people at this stage are already the parents of grown children, and they will become conscious role models for these children and for other young people as well. People at this stage frequently begin to choose lifestyles that will shape their later years.

Middle Age (Ages 40 to 59) By middle age most people are liberated by the end of parenting responsibilities. For better or worse, the children are gone. Parents who took primary responsibility for child rearing may return to the work force or seek additional training. Those who focused on a career may begin to assess their achievements. Many are surprised to find themselves the oldest person in a number of settings.

Middle-aged people receive a variety of signals that remind them of advancing age. Society places subtle limits on different age groups in terms of acceptable dress, speech, and style. Since the middle-aged person shows outward signs of aging, dressing or behaving like a younger person may feel inappropriate. Middle-aged people are also reminded of their maturity by their generational relationships; they attend their children's weddings, become grandparents, and begin to take responsibility for their own parents.

During this stage of life people are also reminded of their mortality by the death of friends and family members. When someone dies, the grieving individual sees himself or herself in a new light; when parents die, a person feels like an orphan regardless of his or her age. Despite the increasing reminders of mortality, most people in middle age have reached only the halfway point of their life span. Health can remain strong, especially if people have followed sound health practices, and life experiences engender a perspective that can help prepare an individual practically and psychologically for older life. Middle-aged people may become introspective, reflective, and even "wise."

Older Adulthood (Ages 60 to 74) Older adults usually face a number of role transitions. Spouses frequently die during these years, and some people face serious health crises. Most people retire from work during this stage, and with retirement come major changes in economic and personal status as well as lifestyle. While many older adults are financially well off, others have to manage their money very carefully. Those who have always seen themselves in terms of their work have to adjust their self-image.

Some elderly people do face financial problems. Retirement can cut a person's income by as much as half, and inflation can reduce the value of fixed-income pensions. Some elderly people also face high medical bills, and their contributing payments for Medicare seem to increase at a regular pace.

During middle age and later, people find they have time to contribute to society in many ways, for example, by volunteering their services to the community or to other enterprises. (Bob Daemmrich/The Image Works)

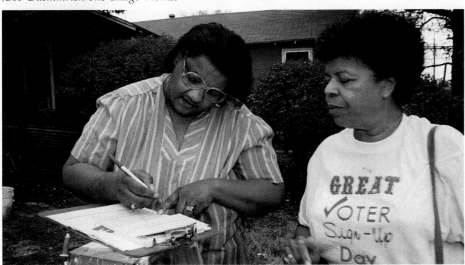

Sporting activities, hobbies, and social relationships can become the new focus of daily living during older adulthood, but people generally find it difficult to begin entirely new pursuits and change long-standing habits. Retirement can also change the relationship between spouses. The additional time spent together causes relationships between some couples to flower, while other people encounter difficulties brought on by unaccustomed closeness.

With careful planning, older adulthood can be a comfortable plateau—the "golden years" of life. A study of intellectually gifted men begun in 1921 revealed that in 1981 the surviving men were generally happy and well adjusted. The researcher found that the seventh decade of life can be a time of fulfillment, with a greater focus on oneself, increased opportunities for self-actualization, continued productivity, and freedom from the responsibilities of earlier adulthood.[14]

Old Age (Ages 75 and Over) If older adulthood represents the golden years, what of the later years of life? Since the potential human life span is over 100 years, old age can represent the longest of life's stages. The quality of life in these later years depends a great deal on the characteristics of lifestyle during a person's earlier years. Some individuals may be lucky in that they are genetically protected from certain diseases that can contribute to decline or disability in the later years. Others may have enough money to buy companionship, better health care, and more physical comfort. For most people, however, the later years are the legacy of an earlier lifestyle. Your habits and behaviors play a significant role in shaping not only the person you are but the person you will become.

The Concerns of Growing Older

The most rapid increase in the older population is expected to occur between the years 2010 and 2030, when the baby boom generation reaches age 65.

While some of the concerns people have about growing older are justifiable, a great deal can be done to maximize health and human potential in the later years of life. Lifestyle when younger plays an important part in determining whether old age will be productive and healthful or painful and limiting. There is no need for fears of deterioration, decline, and loneliness to overshadow positive thinking about growing older. Aging is a normal process; disease and disability are not inevitable parts of it.

Good exercise habits can help ensure a lifetime of physical activity, but physical neglect often leads to debilitating problems later in life. (Tom Davis/Photo Researchers, Inc.; Tony Freeman/PhotoEdit)

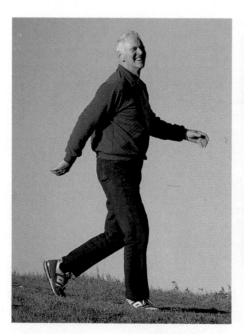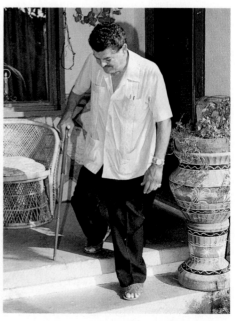

However, disease and disability can occur: and there are several other areas of concern about aging, including changes in appearance, decline in the immune system and in bodily functions, increased susceptibility to injury, and reduced mental functioning.

Appearance and Body Tissues

As adults grow older, their physical appearance gradually changes. Such change is inevitable, although the degree and rate of change vary among individuals. For example, two people of the same chronological age may appear to be of quite different ages.

One of the reasons for changes in appearance during the later aging process is the body's increasing inability to produce new cells to replace dead or worn-out tissue. There is also a decrease in the efficiency of the processes by which cells burn fuel and use the energy produced. Not all tissues in the body appear to be equally subject to these changes: the liver and kidneys, for example, usually are not affected as early as are the skin and certain muscle tissue.

Research has suggested that up to 30 percent of the body's cells may disappear between the ages of 35 and 75.[15] This results in various changes in appearance. Most people shrink physically as they get older. Posture can become stooped because of bone and muscle deterioration. The skull tends to thicken, and nose cartilage tends to grow. Hair often thins and loses its color; some men go bald. The skin loses much of its elasticity and begins to stretch and wrinkle. Skin tissue may also thin and become translucent, especially in places that have been exposed to excessive sunlight, such as the back of the hand.

Older people generally have diminished physical strength. Muscle cells gradually die and are not replaced; the condition of the remaining muscle tissue deteriorates gradually. The ratio of fat to muscle also tends to increase with age—caused both by the built-in aging process and by lifestyle factors. Generally, as people grow older, their bodies become stiffer. Most bones lose density, and joints become less lubricated and more prominent. Since these conditions are often accompanied by pain, older people become less active, and this can accelerate the deterioration.

Body Functions

With age, many of the body's basic functions slow down. The body's metabolism decreases, and less food is needed to supply energy. A 70-year-old, for example, may need only 70 percent of the calories he or she required during youth.[16] The body's ability to return to a state of homeostasis also slows, as does its ability to regenerate cells and fight disease. The immune system, especially when under too much accumulated stress, gradually loses its ability to fight disease, partly because of the decline of the thymus gland, which contributes to the development of the immune system.

In women, the onset of *menopause* (the point when ovulation and menstruation cease; see Chapter 9) is accompanied by hormonal changes that may affect the body's functions. A recent study showed that early natural menopause is associated with reduced life expectancy.[17] Aging also affects the body's sexual functioning. Women remain fertile only until menopause. As men age, their ability to produce viable sperm decreases, though it does not cease entirely. These changes need not interfere with the ability of older people to enjoy sex, however. While health problems or lack of a partner may detract from sexual functioning, research shows that many older men and women continue to lead active sex lives.[18]

As the body ages, internal organs also decrease in efficiency and lose some of their function. Heart rate and pumping capacity decrease, as does the ability of the kidneys to filter blood. The lungs lose some of their elasticity; consequently, the ability to move air in and out decreases. The nervous system slows, resulting in slightly decreased reaction times.

Caring for Aged Parents

Modern medical technology has greatly increased life expectancy, but up to 50 percent of people over age 65 will at some point depend on others for care. Such care is often provided by adult children, who may visit a parent frequently and arrange for social service professionals to make visits. It also is provided at nursing homes, which usually impose a greater financial burden on the elderly individual and his or her family. Both speakers advocate additional support for the frail elderly. However, the first speaker urges that money should be spent to upgrade help for families who provide their own care, whereas the second suggests that increased nursing home care would be preferable.

Family Care Gives the Elderly Independence
Most people in our culture value independence, and older people are no exception—they prefer the autonomy and comfort of their own homes and neighborhoods. As the years advance, elderly people sometimes grow fearful as they gradually trade independence for the assistance they require. When nursing home care looms as a possibility, they feel particularly threatened.

Even when aging brings handicaps or illness, it is preferable for elderly people to maintain their independence by receiving care in their own homes. Families can provide most personal services. They can take parents to different places; help with their finances, household chores, and errands; offer emotional help; and include them in family get-togethers. Families can provide an intimacy that institutional help often lacks.

Outside aid is a vital resource, however. Even today, under provisions of the Older Americans Act, most states have an agency on aging that provides information and referral, transportation, home health and visiting services, and legal aid. Outreach clinics staffed by social workers and nursing assistants can also put families in touch with necessary services such as visiting nurses, physical therapists, and medical or paramedical specialists who make home visits. Support services such as family counseling, respite care, selected in-home service, voluntary support groups, and adult day care do much to help families with the tasks of care giving.

The high cost of alternatives is another argument for care at home. Nursing home costs averaged $22,000 a year at the beginning of the 1990s. Less than 40 percent of older households have that kind of money. Private and government funds would be best spent

Certain cognitive, or learning, functions may change as a person grows older, but these changes do not seem to be an inherent part of the aging process. In fact, most adults maintain *fluid intelligence*—the ability to solve abstract problems and generate new ideas—at normal levels throughout the life span. *Crystallized intelligence*—the ability to use accumulated knowledge and learning—actually increases throughout adulthood and declines only slightly in old age. Any change in these abilities cannot be explained in terms of factors intrinsic to the aging process but may result from nutritional or other factors.[19] Memory also continues relatively unchanged throughout the life span. Early memories usually remain intact, though some older people have difficulty recalling particular recent events.

Advanced age does seem to affect both the quality of sensory perception and the ability to receive, process, and act upon that information, leading to slower responses to various stimuli.[20] The functioning of the sensory organs usually fades with age. Taste and smell may become less acute. Hearing loss at higher sound frequencies commonly begins during the twenties or thirties and continues as a person becomes older. Visual impairment also increases. Older people need more time to adjust to changes in light and to change focus between near and far objects. These changes in vision are partly due to shrinkage of the pupils and loss of elasticity in the lenses.

providing additional services to families, giving tax advantages to care givers, and encouraging other informal supports for the aging.

In the End, Nursing Home Care Is Better and More Economical Caring for the frail elderly can become an impossible burden for a family, affecting the lives of care givers and patients alike.

The care givers are often still coping with the demands of their own growing children. They may need to hold tiring jobs to provide the needed money. When these demands are added to the responsibilities of caring for a sick elderly person, care givers may experience enormous stress, which may damage their relationship with the aged relative.

Many older parents say they want their children to care *about* them, not care *for* them. Frequent friendly visits in a nursing home may be preferable to harried everyday contact. And in a nursing home professional care is available 24 hours a day.

The cost of good nursing home care may actually be lower than the alternatives. Working care givers often find that their jobs are affected: they may be absent more often than before, have trouble concentrating, or perform their jobs poorly. This is a hidden cost to the economy. By contrast, nursing care is actually more efficient when offered at a central location than it is when provided by traveling nurses. For this reason, aid for the elderly would be better offered by providing increased aid to these kinds of facilities and to the families which must make use of them.

Both points of view appear to have some merit. However, on the national level it may be necessary to favor one point of view or the other. And individuals may need to make a decision about caring for older people in their own lives. What are your thoughts about this matter? Any decision must take into account the well-being and security of the older person, the ability of relatives to assume their responsibilities comfortably, and the costs to society. How would you vote? And how would you cope?

Ideas drawn from Marjorie George, ''Caring for Older Americans: Who Will Help You When You Help Your Parents?'' *Aide* (December 1989): 14–19; Priscilla Ebersole and Patricia Hess, *Toward Healthy Aging*, 3d ed. (St Louis: C V Mosby, 1990): 459–463.

Injuries

Since people experience a gradual loss of various abilities as they age, older adults are generally more prone to sustain injuries than are young and middle-aged adults. Poor night vision, slower reflexes, and reduced strength may contribute to a fall down a poorly lit staircase, and damage from such an accident is likely to be more severe in an older person whose bones are more brittle and whose protective musculature is weaker than it was in youth. Furthermore, recovery from a serious injury, such as a broken hip, may be longer and more painful for an older person than it is for a younger one. Older adults can, however, minimize the risk of having accidents by exercising to keep in good condition and by improving the safety of the home. Adequate lighting, secure handrails, and floors and steps that are kept in good repair can help prevent serious injury.

Infectious Diseases

Everyone is subject to acute infections, but such infections may have more serious consequences in people of advanced age. An older person may be less attentive to sanitation and body cleanliness than he or she was in earlier years; older people often contract digestive ailments such as gastroenteritis by eating food contaminated by bacteria. Moreover, since older people are more prone to have accidents, they are more likely to get skin and mouth cuts, scrapes, and other abrasions that enable disease-carrying organisms to enter the body. Because the cleansing mechanisms in their respiratory and urogenital tracts no longer function as well, the consequences of these infections are likely to be more serious.

As was mentioned earlier, the body's ability to repair and renew itself lessens with age and the immune system becomes less efficient. As a result, older people have less resistance to attack by disease-producing organisms. This is why physicians routinely recommend that older people receive preventive inoculations against certain infections, particularly pneumonia and influenza.

Chronic Diseases

About 80 percent of Americans over 65 suffer from at least one chronic disease. About 48 percent suffer from arthritis; 39 percent suffer from hypertension.

In terms of both death and disability, the highest toll among older people results from *chronic conditions*—disorders that persist or worsen gradually as the body's resist-and-repair capabilities decrease.[21] As was pointed out in Chapter 1, these conditions are frequently a delayed result of a person's life-style during earlier years. Some of the most common chronic diseases affecting older people are disorders of the cardiovascular system, cancer, osteoporosis, and diabetes.

Disorders of the Cardiovascular System

Cardiovascular disorders, including heart disease, stroke, hypertension, and atherosclerosis, rank first among chronic diseases of the aged, accounting for more than 60 percent of deaths in people over age 65. The primary cardiovascular disorder is atherosclerosis (Chapter 11), which in turn may result in angina, myocardial infarction (heart attack), stroke, and kidney problems. While cardiovascular disorders are a great concern of older people, a recent study found only a tenuous relationship between aging and cardiovascular disease.[22] These disorders are much more dangerous if an older individual has certain other chronic conditions as well.

Cancer

The second most common chronic disease among older people is cancer. Cancer is actually many different diseases that vary widely in seriousness and treatability (Chapter 12). Approximately half of all cancers are found in people over age 65. This may be due to a number of reasons. One is that certain cancers can be traced to long-term exposure to risk factors such as sunlight. A second reason may be that the immune systems of older people are less efficient. Other reasons include long-term use of alcohol and tobacco and exposure to various toxic substances.

Osteoporosis

osteoporosis—a chronic condition, most common among older women, that is marked by thin, brittle, easily fractured bones.

Another chronic condition common to older people, especially women, is **osteoporosis**, a condition marked by thinning, brittle, easily fractured bones. In patients with osteoporosis, the bones most often affected are the weight-bearing ones of the lower spine and hip and the ones in the wrist. Twenty percent of women with hip fractures die of complications such as pneumonia, making osteoporosis a leading cause of death among older women in the United States.[23]

Osteoporosis affects 25 to 30 percent of women over age 65.

Osteoporosis accelerates the normal process by which bone density and mass decrease with age. Since women have smaller bones to begin with, its effects are more severe for women. The condition rarely produces symptoms—except for mild, chronic lower back pain—until the bones become so thin and weak that they snap just from the weight of the body or break in a simple fall. The vertebrae may disintegrate spontaneously, resulting in severe back pain, loss of height, and ultimately the classic "dowager's hump," characterized by a rounded spine and a shortened chest area.

The cause of osteoporosis is unclear, but the loss of estrogen that accompanies menopause or surgical removal of the ovaries seems to be a factor. (Estrogen apparently plays a role in protecting and preserving bone.) Other contributing factors are inactivity (exercise builds bones as well as muscle), cigarette smoking, excessive alcohol intake, and a family history of osteoporosis. The most likely reason for the loss of bone, however, is prolonged calcium deficiency, a dietary problem which can be avoided (Chapter 5).

Diabetes **Diabetes** is a condition in which the body is unable to regulate the level of sugar in the blood efficiently. The condition is caused by an insufficiency of insulin, a hormone produced in the pancreas. One form of diabetes—type I—strikes early in life. However, another form—type II—generally does not appear before age 40 and is more prevalent among older populations, occurring in about 10 percent of people over age 65.[24] Diabetes poses a special threat to older persons because it can result in blindness and loss of limbs (due in part to poor circulation and nourishment of body cells). It can also lead to neurological problems, kidney problems, and heightened susceptibility to infection. Fortunately, diabetes can be controlled with diet and medication.

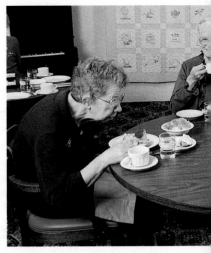

The "dowager's hump" symptomatic of osteoporosis is clearly visible in the posture of the woman on the left. (Blair Seitz/Photo Researchers, Inc.)

Disability

A person's ability to perform personal-care activities is a common measure of minimal physical vitality. Among the typical activities that may be curtailed among older people are walking, bathing, going outside, getting in and out of bed or a chair, dressing, using the toilet, and eating. Among people who experience disability, some have trouble with more than one of these activities. The total number of disabled people over age 65 is not as great as one might expect. Among the entire population 65 and over (not including those in institutions), over 77 percent have no difficulties with personal-care activities. Among people 85 and older, fewer than half have any disability in these areas.[25] Furthermore, disability is more reversible than was previously thought. In a 2-year study of approximately 4,000 older persons, 22 percent of those who were severely disabled at the beginning of the study had improved 2 years later.[26]

One condition that can be disabling for older people is **arthritis**. According to some sources, it is the most common disease among older people; more than 35 percent of men and 56 percent of women over age 65 suffer from some form of this disease.[27] Arthritis is actually a collective term for several diseases—including rheumatoid arthritis and osteoarthritis—that affect the tendons, ligaments, cartilage, and other tissues of the joints. The symptoms of arthritis include pain and stiffness in the joints; as a result, sufferers often become less active, miss work, and lose sleep. Some research has suggested that the symptoms of arthritis are caused by the production of certain chemicals (superoxidants or free radicals) in the immune system which damage body tissue, including joint fluids and membranes, resulting in friction and stiffening.[28] Various treatments, including antioxidant agents and vitamins, have been tried with unclear success. Other treatments focus on reducing inflammation and pain.

diabetes—a condition, caused by an insufficiency of insulin, in which the body is unable to metabolize sugars and other food materials efficiently.

Arthritis—*name for several diseases that affect the connective tissues of joints.*

Alzheimer's Disease

It is a myth that severe memory loss is an inevitable part of growing old. However, there is a condition that involves progressive deterioration of memory and other mental functions and is associated with advancing age: **Alzheimer's disease.**

Alzheimer's disease—*a progressive, irreversible loss of mental and physical capacity associated with advancing age; the symptoms include severe memory loss, confusion, and depression.*

A Broader View

The Role of the Aged in Different Cultures

The challenge of defining a clear role for elderly people is being brought into sharp focus by the aging of the world's population.

Our society tends to see elderly people in the past and those in less developed cultures as role models looked up to as well as looked after by close, loving families. These are, however, rather idealized pictures. While American leaders of state and industry were respected (though the leaders of the new republic were often quite young), most older people did not enjoy this advantage.

Available data indicate that in both colonial and nineteenth-century America, the healthy elderly and their children preferred the independence of separate residences if they could afford them. Sick older relatives were rarely cared for by their families if institutions or hired helpers were available. Perhaps even more than now, there was little community respect for older people who lacked wealth or prestige.

Modern anthropologists suggest that the idea of humane primitive societies is also somewhat mythical. Of course, families that care lovingly for their older relatives are found in primitive cultures, but while the family often acts as care giver, such care is given with varying degrees of humanity. Tribal elders command respect because they still have power, but other old people rely on tribal customs for their care and may not fare so well. They may have assigned care givers (in one culture, the youngest son and his wife; in another, a young grandchild), but the care is not always given with good grace. In some nomadic societies it is customary to abandon the frail elderly if they are unable to move on with the group.

The situation for old people in modern Western societies is in many ways better. Those who cannot finance their own care and are not cared for by their families are able to benefit from volunteer organizations and government programs. Great Britain, for example, provides the elderly with helpers who shop, cook, and clean for them. Government mail carriers in Denmark check on elderly people along their routes, sometimes dropping off library books or groceries along with the mail. In Sweden more than 70 percent of the elderly are able to live in their own homes, thanks to extensive social and health services.

In patients with Alzheimer's disease, the brain's medium-sized and small blood vessels degenerate. A common early symptom is severe difficulty with short-term memory. As the condition worsens, the patient may display personality changes, have difficulty reading or speaking, and become extremely disoriented. Ultimately, those suffering from Alzheimer's disease become completely helpless and dependent on the support of others—at tremendous emotional cost to those who care for them.

Progressive, with no known cause or cure, Alzheimer's disease is now believed to have a gradual onset, beginning well before an individual grows old. Recent studies have linked the disorder with head injuries sustained earlier in life and with thyroid disease. Some experts think that it may be related to the individual's genetically determined background and may be associated with a specific biochemical defect (this would mean that it is potentially treatable).[29] Using the few clues that are available, researchers are trying to devise a test to identify Alzheimer's disease early and to develop a drug that will halt or reverse the cognitive difficulties and memory deterioration that characterize the condition.[30]

The proportion of older people afflicted with Alzheimer's disease is quite low—only 6 to 8 percent. Memory loss, confusion, and other symptoms often displayed by older people may in fact be caused by a wide range of disorders, many of which are treatable. Emotional problems such as depression—caused by loss of family ties, anxiety over money, and loss of independence—

Although Western societies provide some excellent care-giving systems—and the United States is not the most advanced nation in this respect—much still needs to be done if the growing population of old people is to feel cared for and valued. A tendency remains for only a few prominent older people to be recognized as contributing to society. The rest, if they have enough health and money, are urged to spend it playing out a somewhat isolated retirement, and those who are not so lucky must make do as they can, benefiting from social services but no longer able to feel valued for themselves and their work.

However, the elderly can often find a valued place in society. Although poor families may not always take aged relatives into their homes by choice, many find valued help with the children and household chores, to the economic and social advantages of all: grandparents and grandchildren can give each other care and attention that the middle, working generation does not have time to provide. In Africa's poverty-stricken cultures, too, the elderly have recently found a vital though tragic role, caring for children and grandchildren who have become afflicted with AIDS.

In the public arena, too, there are opportunities for the elderly to use their experience and abilities to contribute to society. Some agencies specialize in finding jobs for people over age 60, while others focus on finding volunteer work—and not only work to help the other aged. The Foster Grandparents program, for example, employs older women to prevent child abuse by helping young mothers cope with their babies.

As the percentage of older people in American society increases, the challenge is not only to care for seniors but also to realize their value as a resource for the rest of the community. Not only will this benefit the younger generation, it also will benefit the aged, giving them a sense of purpose traditionally accorded only to leaders and elders.

Ideas included from Corinne Nydegger, "Family Ties of the Aged in Cross-Cultural Perspective", in Beth B. Hess and Elizabeth W. Markson, *Growing Old in America,* 3d ed. (New Brunswick, N.J.: Transaction, 1985): 71–85.

can lead to symptoms that resemble those of Alzheimer's disease. So can overconsumption of alcohol, accidents, poor vision and hearing, and physical disorders such as malnutrition, glandular problems, drug toxicity, infection, dehydration, and atherosclerosis. Brain tumors, small strokes, epilepsy, and other cerebral disorders can also produce symptoms that mimic those of Alzheimer's disease.

People who suffer from Alzheimer's disease should be encouraged to maintain their daily routines, physical activities, and social contacts for as long as possible. Medication is available to relieve some symptoms, such as depression and severe agitation. Behavior therapy may slow the process of mental deterioration, and exercise and proper nourishment may help delay the loss of physical mobility.[31] The children of people with Alzheimer's disease seem to have an increased risk of developing the condition. Symptoms usually develop before age 65 in these people, and the progress of the disease is likely to be rapid and severe.[32]

Depression and Suicide in the Elderly

Depression and suicide are other potential threats to people as they grow older, although the risks are greater for some groups than they are for others. Rates of suicide among men increase with age, while the rates for women remain relatively unchanged. The risk of suicide is highest for white males;

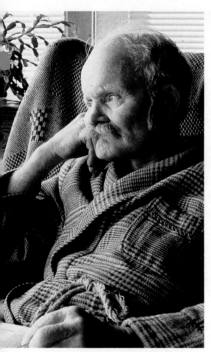

about 25 white men in 100,000 kill themselves by age 40. This rate rises dramatically after retirement age to over 50 suicides per 100,000 men beyond age 80. Although nonwhite males commit suicide at a much lower rate than do whites, the rate for this group increases in later years from about 10 in 100,000 at age 70 to about 20 per 100,000 above age 85.[33] Furthermore, suicide attempts among older persons are more likely to be fatal compared with attempts by adolescents, who succeed only about 1 percent of the time.[34] These statistics do not include "silent suicide," or the attempt to kill oneself by passive means such as refusing food or medical treatment. Silent suicide occurs not among the terminally ill but among otherwise healthy older people.[35]

Depression seems to be the leading cause of suicide, and it may be underdiagnosed among older persons because of the belief systems of family members and health care providers. People just do not want to believe that another human being, especially a respected elder, may have developed an emotional disorder such as depression.[36] Furthermore, the symptoms of depression can be confused with those of organic brain disorders such as Alzheimer's disease.

Although most older people live happy lives, a small percentage of the elderly are plagued with severe depression. (Myrleen Ferguson/PhotoEdit)

The Causes of Aging

Considering the wonder of human procreation, the body's inability to maintain itself indefinitely seems ironic. A single cell grows into an astonishingly complex organism that is well adapted to foster survival and further procreation, and then this organism ages and dies. Why? Several theories have been proposed to explain this phenomenon.

Cellular Aging

Clues to the causes of aging can be found at the cellular level. In the 1950s and 1960s researchers discovered that human cells tend to duplicate themselves only about 50 times, after which they stop reproducing and begin to die.[37] The cells in effect seem to "run out of time." Researchers also discovered that cells seem to "remember" how many times they have reproduced. When cells were removed from a conducive medium, they stopped dividing; when they were returned to that environment, they continued to divide up to a limit of about 50 doublings. Clearly, the number of cell divisions completed, not chronological time, seems to be the crucial factor in cellular aging.

Later research showed that cells from older individuals tend to reproduce fewer times than do cells from younger ones. Senescent (aged) cells showed signs of change and decay and a reduced sensitivity to a variety of growth factors and hormones. Once their healthy functions were reduced, these older cells did not work as well as younger cells. Research also showed that cells from individuals with premature aging diseases have greatly reduced life spans in laboratory culture dishes. Such limits to life span, as seen in cellular reproduction, are as evident in people as they are in laboratory cultures.[38]

Recent research on certain animals has suggested that life span may be increased by a low caloric intake. For more information, see the material on body composition and physical health in Chapter 6.

Genetic Limits

Based on research on cellular aging, many experts believe that there is a genetically programmed limit to life. The fact that each species lives out its existence within certain limits suggests that genes may have an effect on life span. There is already some evidence to support this hypothesis. Studies have located a gene that affects the life span of one species of worm. When the gene is removed, the worms live 70 percent longer than normal.[39]

Research has also suggested the existence of "longevity-determining genes" that may affect the body's ability to cope with damage.[40] In mice, a complex of genes has been identified that seems to play a role in the ability of a mouse's body to repair damaged genes.[41]

It has also been suggested that human cells contain certain genes that may be beneficial up to a certain age (through procreation or afterward) but become harmful later in life. Evolution would have no way of selecting against these harmful genes since they express themselves only after the childbearing years.

With increasing knowledge of genetics, scientists believe they will be able to identify the genes that affect aging and longevity in humans.

Theories of Aging

In addition to a genetically linked limit to the human life span, various theories have been suggested to explain the causes of aging. Some of these theories suggest that aging is dependent on the hereditary factors contained in genes and chromosomes. Others look to physiological causes related to basic bodily functions.

Although genetics may predispose people to some of the changes that occur during the aging process, following a healthy lifestyle in one's younger years can delay the onset of many of these changes.

The Error Theory It has been postulated that as cells divide and redivide, they introduce errors into the genetic material. These errors, compounded over many cell divisions, eventually result in an "error catastrophe" in which the cells can no longer function normally. Recent research, however, has shown that a stable rate of errors can be maintained indefinitely without causing harm to later cells.[42] Thus, while errors created during cell regeneration may play a role in aging, an error catastrophe is not inevitable.

The Free Radical Theory Another theory of aging involves free radicals, which were mentioned earlier in connection with arthritis. These chemically unstable oxygen-containing molecules are produced when food is metabolized. Free radicals are scavengers that travel throughout cellular material, causing problems. They attack deoxyribonucleic acid (DNA), the macromolecules that contain genetic material. They also bond with fats and leave pigments that impair cell function and may cause mutation of chromosomes. During youth, antioxidant enzymes bond with free radicals and prevent damage. As people age, however, their bodies produce fewer antioxidants and thus sustain more cell damage. Proponents of this theory believe that the use of antioxidants such as vitamins C and E can prevent or reduce the production of free radicals and thus reduce cell damage and extend the life span.

The Somatic Mutation Theory This theory postulates that cellular substances and compounds are routinely manufactured incorrectly, or mutated. The mutations may be spontaneous, as suggested in the error theory, or may result from environmental factors such as exposure to radiation. The mutated cells are then replaced by new cells that have a high incidence of abnormal chromosomes.[43]

The Cross-Linkage Theory This theory suggests that the irreversible aging of certain proteins is responsible for the failure of tissues and organs to function properly, as is seen in hardening of the arteries. The accumulation of these compounds causes problems with normal protein synthesis and the immune response.[44]

The Effects of Lifestyle on Aging

While the various theories of aging may help explain why the human organism eventually breaks down, another important factor is involved in the aging process. That factor is lifestyle—the attitudes, habits, and behaviors that people follow in daily life. Science has no way of extending the human life span beyond the limits set by evolution and genetics. Each individual can, however, live a healthier and longer life by adopting a healthier lifestyle. Such a lifestyle will help a person cope with the challenges of growing older and forestall or prevent some of the conditions that can shorten life or cause disability (Table 17.1). The next section will briefly examine how you can make a difference for yourself as well as others in extending life and achieving greater health and fulfilment.

Making a Difference

Everyone can shape a life that is longer and healthier as well as satisfying and rewarding. The key is to develop healthy behaviors now and maintain them throughout your life.

In shaping a better life, most people struggle to balance various competing interests: immediate needs and long-term health and happiness, their own well-being and that of their children, family concerns and the needs and demands of society, and even their nation's well-being and that of the rest of the world. The way people resolve these issues can make a difference in the quality of their life and health as well as the life and health of others. In addition to taking action for their own lives, people can help others through community or political involvement, volunteerism, and relationships with family members and friends. For many people, the act of helping others plays an important role in their own health and well-being.

Making a Difference for Yourself

Ultimately, individuals are responsible for their own health and well-being. The description of a healthy lifestyle that appears throughout this book offers guidance in shaping habits and behaviors which can maximize health, prolong life, and promote physical, mental, and social well-being.

To achieve long and healthy lives, people must assess their strengths and weaknesses and then adjust their life patterns accordingly. There are many options for improving health; knowledge of these options coupled with sound planning can help each person make decisions that are best for himself or herself.

Maintaining Physical Health   Exercise plays an important role in the maintenance of physical health as a person ages. Regular exercise can help reduce the loss of muscle mass that accompanies the aging process. Between the ages of 30 and 70 years, the average person loses 30 to 40 percent of the body's muscle mass. Exercise can retard these changes by as much as 20 years.[45] There is also substantial evidence to link exercise with a reduction in the risk of developing cardiovascular disease and with improved general well-being and morale.[46] One longitudinal study showed that even among people age 80 or older, the most physically fit were the least likely to have health problems 2 years later.[47] A program of regular exercise would thus seem to be essential for maintaining physical health as one grows older (Chapter 4).

Diet and nutrition also have an important impact on physical health. Research in nutrition has shown that lifelong dietary habits affect a person's health in old age. Dietary factors such as an excess caloric intake, a high salt intake, and a high fat intake can predispose individuals to various health-

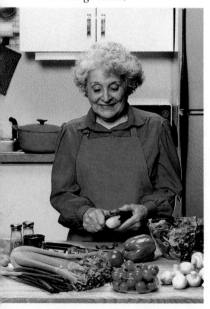

The eating habits that people develop when young affect their food choices and their health throughout life. (Benn Mitchell/ The Image Bank)

Table 17.1   The importance of lifestyle in good health: Estimated contribution (percent) of lifestyle compared to other important factors to the 10 leading causes of premature mortality

Leading Causes of Death	Lifestyle	Environment	Human Biology/Genetics	Health Care System
Cancer	37	24	29	10
Heart disease	53	9	27	11
Motor vehicle accidents	69	18	1	12
Other accidents	51	31	4	14
Homicide	66	30	4	0
Suicide	60	35	2	3
Stroke	50	22	21	7
Cirrhosis of the liver	70	9	18	3
Influenza/ pneumonia	23	20	39	18
Diabetes	26	0	68	6
All	53	21	16	10

Source: Adapted from G. E. Alan Dever, *Epidemiology in Health Services Management* (Rockville, Md.: Aspen, 1984): 37.

threatening conditions, including obesity, diabetes, hypertension, and atherosclerosis. Although the negative effects of a poor diet may become evident slowly, they accumulate with age. Thus, eating habits that contribute to a healthy old age must begin in youth and middle age (Chapter 5).

Other factors that have an impact on physical health include the use of dangerous substances such as alcohol, tobacco, and drugs; the risk of accidents; and exposure to infectious diseases. All these factors have been discussed in detail throughout this book.

For people concerned about their physical health, regular visits to professional health practitioners can help point out potential problems early and prevent the complications that may accompany a neglected condition. Various types of checkups are recommended for different stages in a person's life, as the risk of developing certain conditions becomes greater with age (Chapter 9). Health professionals can also advise people about emerging ideas and new findings on medical treatment and healthy lifestyle.

Health care is a special concern of some elderly members of minority groups. Linguistic and cultural differences as well as lower income make finding and using health care services difficult for some of these people.

Maintaining Intellectual and Emotional Health

There is a reciprocal relationship between physical health and intellectual and emotional health. Good physical health contributes to good intellectual and emotional health and vice versa.

Developing an optimistic outlook toward life is an important factor in good health. A positive attitude can help guard against destructive behaviors that may threaten a person's health. The ability to put life crises in perspective can also improve an individual's decision-making ability. An active mind can improve the quality of life at all ages, especially in retirement or old age, when illness may deprive a person of stimulation.

Some positive aspects of retirement: more time for family, travel, and hobbies; no more job stress. Some negative aspects: boredom, loss of self-worth, missing fellow workers, loss of sense of being needed.

The habits, general activity, and coping strategies associated with good intellectual and emotional health can help people adjust to the changes that come with age. A recent study showed that while older people tend to use fewer coping strategies, they adjust to the stresses of health problems better than do their younger counterparts. Although the coping strategies older people use—taking responsibility for their own health, nurturing healthful emotions such as love and self-esteem, feeling accepted by others, achieving goals, and finding amusement—tend to be less active than those used by younger persons, these strategies work well for them.[48]

Intellectual and emotional health can have an important impact on stress, which affects a person's overall health and well-being. Attitude can greatly affect an individual's reaction to events that may be stressful. For example, people with so-called Type A personalities are at greater risk for developing heart disease and stroke than are those who react to stress less intensely. Learning how to cope with stress and resolve feelings such as anger and frustration can thus help preserve health (Chapter 2).

Intellectual and emotional well-being is also enhanced by keeping active. Hobbies and interests that provide stimulation throughout life by helping to balance rest and work cycles can be pursued during retirement as well. Some older persons stimulate their minds by going back to school. Others travel through educationally affiliated programs designed to meet their needs. Still others may begin new careers rather than accept a nonworking retirement.

Another important factor in maintaining intellectual and emotional health is the development of strong family and social ties. The maintenance of active networks of family members and friends contributes to emotional health by providing emotional support and companionship.[49] The feeling of belonging that people get from these ties also makes them feel wanted, needed, and loved.

Good intellectual and emotional health can best be nurtured by keeping interested in the world and abreast of the times, caring about and reaching out to others, developing a sense of independence and self-efficacy, developing new interests and hobbies, and treating oneself with dignity.

A healthy and productive old age depends on health habits acquired early in life and carried on through the years. Getting involved in hobbies and social activities and planning ahead financially also help make the retirement years more rewarding.

Maintaining Social and Spiritual Health

A recent study showed that men and women both seek and maintain meaningful friendships in their later years.[50] Such relationships help maintain an individual's social health and well-being.

As people grow older, the social relationships provided by friends and family members play a more important role as other activities decrease. Women who have been central care givers in their families find that their roles change with age. People who retire must find replacements for the social interactions that were once part of their daily routine. A study of unemployed workers over the age of 50, for example, showed that they experienced long and difficult periods of adjustment.[51]

Generally, people feel better within networks of friends and loved ones. The loss of an intimate relationship can be devastating and is sometimes associated with declining health or a shortened life span. In one study, the immune systems of recently widowed men declined during the 2 months after the deaths of their wives and their recovery from this lost capacity was slow.[52] Stories of one spouse dying shortly after the death of the other are common. Other studies have shown that widowed women do not live as long as married or single women, and one study comparing Protestant ministers and Catholic priests showed that marriage seems to be associated with a longer life expectancy.[53]

People develop and maintain social relationships in various ways. Many people choose to live in retirement communities where they can enjoy the company of people with similar needs and perspectives. A recent study showed that middle-income adults residing in age-segregated retirement communities tend to be more sexually interested and active than are their peers in mainstream communities.[54] Since intimacy and companionship can enhance health, retirement communities may offer a health advantage to older adults. For some older people, community senior centers can be good places for meeting peers. Such centers usually offer programs that include recreation, entertainment, educational and fitness classes, and meals. Churches, synagogues, and many other community institutions often provide similar services for older people. Other older people find greater fulfillment within groups that are less age-restricted, allowing them to develop relationships with people of various ages. These people may find satisfaction tutoring school-age children, working in a variety of community organizations, and providing companionship to the very elderly disabled.

As the number of older persons in American society grows, the focus may shift from the separation of age groups to intergenerational social arrangements. With their experience and wisdom, older persons can be an important resource for their communities. Volunteer organizations provide one way to help channel their talents toward the needs of the community. For instance, the Service Council of Retired Executives provides free consulting services to new businesses. Participation in such volunteer efforts can benefit older persons as well as the communities they serve; the volunteer can regain the status that once came from a job or a role within the family. Volunteerism also provides an opportunity to develop friendships and social relationships while serving others.

Spiritual health is a more elusive quality. It can come from formal or informal religious beliefs and affiliations or from a strongly held personal philosophy and world view. While spiritual health is an essential part of well-being, it may become more important as a person ages and begins to experience feelings of personal mortality. It brings an inner peace that helps the individual cope with the inevitability of death as well as with the challenges still left in life. A belief in organized religion is not an essential factor in maintaining spiritual health. A recent study showed that personal morale was helped also by nonorganized religious activity and intrinsic religiosity.[55]

Making a Difference for Others

People nurture themselves as they help others. As parents, grandparents, friends, lovers, neighbors, and citizens, they can improve their own lives and health by helping to improve the lives and health of others. It is important to consider the autonomy of others, however, before imposing oneself on them. To be most effective, one must understand the diverse needs and interests of the people being helped.

Making a Difference for Children
Attitudes toward food, exercise, conflict, friendship, love, work, religion, and every other aspect of life begin to develop during childhood and continue developing as one matures. Adults take full responsibility for shaping their own lives, but children are helped by their parents, and are also guided by the influence of others.

One way children learn is by example. By adopting a healthy lifestyle, parents can help their children develop habits that will maximize their health and prolong their lives. Good habits developed early are more likely to carry over into adulthood. Moreover, by becoming healthier themselves, parents are less likely to become a burden to their children in later years (Chapter 7). In a more direct way parents play a crucial role in their children's health by ensuring that they receive proper medical care when necessary.

While parents play an essential role in shaping the lifestyles of their children, they are not alone in the process. Children also learn from other family members, friends, and teachers. Grandparents can play an especially important role in children's lives. They are often a respected source of support for children, people to whom the children can turn during times of tension with their parents.

Through their association with older persons, children learn respect for others. Furthermore, the wisdom and experience of older people can help children prepare for the challenges of growing older, for example, by helping them learn strategies for coping with problems and avoiding the risk factors associated with poor health. By working together and discussing options before crises arise, both the old and the young can face future challenges more effectively.

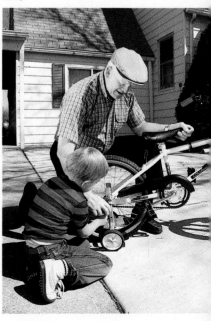

Close intergenerational relationships can play an important part in the lives of the old and the young alike. (Blair Seitz//Photo Research, Inc.)

The Generation Gap: A Two-Way Street

As individuals move from one stage of life to the next, their ability to communicate with people of different ages may change. Think for a moment about how you communicate with your parents, your grandparents, and other people older than yourself. What about children—your own if you have them—or other people who are younger than you? How easy is it to talk about matters of importance to you? How good are you at giving their ideas a fair hearing? Are you able to discuss your relationship with each other? Communicating involves both sides understanding the other's priorities, values, and beliefs—not always an easy task in a rapidly changing world.

Children and parents often have difficulty communicating about important matters. One major problem is that there is often conflict in regard to dependency and control. For example, teenagers want the power to make their own decisions, while parents may fear their children are becoming too independent. Young marrieds pride themselves on resolving the challenges of their new life, while their parents still wish to help them out. Older people want to remain independent and look after themselves, while children sometimes feel they should play a larger role in caring for their aging parents.

Most people are continually seeking a comfortable level of dependency with their families. While it is nice to be taken care of, too much of it can make people feel oppressed. Taking care of oneself is a point of pride; people need to feel self-reliant and in command of their lives. While this is true in any relationship, establishing this balance is especially important to parents and children. Poor communication about these issues can result in a considerable degree of tension and unhappiness on both sides.

As parents age, good communication becomes particularly important. Fortunately, there are ways for parents and children to create communication that is a two-way street leading to improved understanding and mutual respect. To begin with, it is helpful to talk about matters of concern before they become urgent. A candid discussion, initiated by the children or parents, about the potential problems of aging can make dealing with these difficulties much easier if they do occur.

A younger person might handle this while discussing a friend's situation—someone's father appears to be growing forgetful, for

Making a Difference for Friends and Family Individuals can help older friends and family members in a number of ways. It may be as simple as being available to listen to their problems and concerns, or it may take the form of more organized approaches: friendly visitor programs that match home-bound older persons with volunteers who stop in regularly, volunteer programs to assist in nursing homes, or community meals-on-wheels programs to help feed homebound older persons of limited means.

Adult children are often responsible for taking care of their aging parents. Studies show that adult children provide 80 percent of the health and social services needed by their parents.[56] Taking care of an aging parent or older relative can be very rewarding. However, it can also be very stressful and financially draining, and may lead to abuse. A recent study showed that abuse of aging adults may result when the abused and their care givers become increasingly interdependent because of the loss of a family member, increased social isolation, and increased financial dependency of the care giver on the elderly person.[57] An awareness of the dangers of these conditions can help reduce the occurrence of such abuse. At the same time, it is important to emphasize that adult children can be effective care givers without threatening their own well-being or that of their parents.

Some older adults may require the more special care that can be found in continuing care or life care centers. Among those requiring special care, some may prefer home care arrangements, which allow a person to remain in famil-

example, or an aunt or a great-aunt has suffered a fall. The conversation could be brought around to the younger person's apprehension about what to do if his or her own parents have problems. While the parents may start by asserting that nothing of the sort is likely to happen, they may still be willing to discuss what should be done *if* such an event occurs.

Similarly, parents can help prepare their children for a time when they may be unable to make decisions for themselves. They might discuss what the options would be if they became unable to maintain their home. They could perhaps come to live with one of their children, or they might hire live-in help or move to a community for older people. It is important for each to listen carefully to the other, even though the situation has not occurred yet—and may never occur. There are two parties involved in any such decision, and each should try to understand the other person's wishes and seek common ground.

These topics are difficult to discuss. As parents age, they may be afraid of burdening their children with their fears or angry about the prospect of losing their independence. They may even resent the children's comparative youthfulness and be reluctant to

admit it—even to themselves—if they feel their abilities are diminishing. Children may fear that they will insult, embarrass, or anger their parents if they mention the topic of old age, especially if they suspect that their own suggestions will be different from those of their parents.

Yet it is better to open the dialogue before the situation becomes critical. Although many people remain alert and physically and mentally competent throughout their lives, many people, children and parents alike, tend to deny the dangers of advancing years. Even though the initial conversations may be awkward, they will become easier if they are not a one-time event. Parents and children will be more able to cope during a crisis if the channels of communication are already open.

Based on information from Jane Synge, "Avoided Conversations: How Parents and Children Delay Talking about Widowhood and Dependency in Later Life," in *Aging and Society*, John B. Williamson (ed.) (New York: Holt, Rinehart & Winston, 1980); Marjorie George, "Caring for Older Americans: Who Will Help You When You Help Your Parents?" *Aide* (December 1989): 14–19.

iar surroundings. Relatively few older persons use the services of nursing homes for long-term care; only about 5 percent of the older population is in a nursing home at any given time.[58]

Making a Difference for Humanity Since lifestyle and aging issues affect everyone, they are the subject of much public debate. How can society create a healthier environment for all its people? What should be done to cope with the burgeoning numbers of older people? What resources should be directed toward the needs of the elderly, and what implications might this have on other groups with special needs, such as poor children and the homeless? Can and should public policy promote healthy lifestyles, or is this solely the responsibility of the individual? Tackling these and related issues takes knowledge, perseverance, and a sense of perspective. Answers will not come easily, but individuals can make a difference in determining the outcomes.

Chapter Summary

- Normal aging refers to a biological process that is time-related; pathological aging refers to a decrease in functioning caused by illness, stress, injury, and other factors.

- Several factors contribute to the body's resilience and ability to maintain health. These include a natural equilibrium called homeostasis, an array of mechanisms to combat disease and injury, the ability of certain cells to regenerate, and a connection between psychological hardiness and physical well-being.

- The human life span seems to have a maximum limit based on biological evolution. Few people reach the human maximum; life expectancy varies considerably, depending on numerous factors.
- Successful growth and emotional development can be conceptualized as a positive progression through a series of emotional stages, each with unique characteristics. Stages discussed in this chapter are preadult, adult entry, young adulthood, middle age, older adulthood, and old age.
- As people grow older, they often are faced with concerns such as changing appearance and body functions, a greater risk of accidents, a higher susceptibility to certain infectious diseases and chronic conditions, and the threat of disability. While some of these concerns are unavoidable, others may be ameliorated by changes in lifestyle during the course of a person's life.
- Clues to the causes of aging can be found at the cellular level. Research suggests that aging is built into human genetics and that there is a genetically programmed limit to life.
- Several theories, including the error theory, the free radical theory, the somatic mutation theory, and the cross-linkage theory, are cited as the causes of aging based on genetic and other physiological factors.
- Individuals can shape a longer and healthier life by developing a healthy lifestyle and maintaining it throughout their lives.
- There are various ways people can maintain their physical, intellectual, emotional, social, and spiritual health as they grow older. One of the main purposes of this book is to examine the ways in which people can improve their lifestyles.
- Individuals can help improve the lives and health of family members and friends in a number of ways: listening to their problems and concerns, becoming involved in volunteer programs, caring for aging parents or other relatives, and so on.
- Individuals can have an impact on the life and health of their children by providing good role models and helping the children develop good health habits.

Key Terms

Normal aging (page 436)

Pathological aging (page 436)

Gerontology (page 436)

Life span (page 436)

Life expectancy (page 436)

Osteoporosis (page 444)

Diabetes (page 445)

Arthritis (page 445)

Alzheimer's disease (page 445)

References

1. M. W. Riley and K. Bond, "Beyond Ageism: Postponing the Onset of Disability," in *Aging in Society: Selected Reviews of Recent Research*, M. W. Riley et al. (eds.) (Hillsdale, N.J.: Erlbaum, 1983).

2. Nancy L. Wilson and Rosanne Trost, "A Family Perspective on Aging and Health," *Health Values* II, no. 2 (March–April 1987): 53.

3. John W. Rowe and Robert L. Kahn, "Human Aging: Usual and Successful," *Science* 237 (July 10, 1987): 143–149.

4. Wilson and Trost, op. cit.

5. J. M. Guralnik and G. A. Kaplan, "Predictors of Healthy Aging: Prospective Evidence from the Alameda County Study," *American Journal of Public Health* 79, no. 6 (June 1989): 703–709.

6. Bernie Siegel, "How to Heal Yourself! The Curing Power of Hope, Joy, and Inner Peace," *Redbook* (June 1989): 110–160.

7. Emily T. Smith et al., "Aging—Can It Be Slowed?" *Business Week* (February 8, 1988): 60.

8. Charles F. Longino, "Who Are the Oldest Americans?" *The Gerontologist* 28, no. 4 (1988): 515–523.

9. Population Reference Bureau, *1989 World Population Data Sheet* (Washington, D.C.: Population Reference Bureau, 1989).

10. U.S. Department of Commerce, Bureau of the Census, *Statistical Abstract of the U.S.* (Washington, D.C., 1966).

11. National Center for Health Statistics, *Health, United States, 1989* (Hyattsville, Md.: Department of Health and Human Services, March 1990), DHHS pub. no. (PHS) 90-1232, p. 106.

12. Sandra Scarr and James Vander Zanden, *Understanding Psychology* (New York: Random House, 1987): 377.

13. Ibid., p. 394.

14. Edwin Shneidman, "The Indian Summer of Life: A Preliminary Study of Septuagenarians," *American Psychologist* 44, no. 4 (April 1989): 684–694.

15. E. Fritz Schmerl, *The Challenge of Age* (New York: Continuum, 1986): 6.

16. Victor Showers (ed.), *World Facts and Figures,* 3d ed. (New York: John Wiley, 1989): 371.

17. David A. Snowdon et al., "Is Early Natural Menopause a Biological Marker of Health and Aging?" *American Journal of Public Health* 79, no. 6 (1989): 709–714.

18. W. H. Masters, V. E. Johnson, and R. C. Kolodny, *Human Sexuality,* 3d ed. (Boston: Little, Brown, 1988).

19. Rowe and Kahn, op. cit.

20. Geri Maas Burdman, *Healthful Aging* (Englewood Cliffs, N.J.: Prentice-Hall, 1986).

21. The discussion is based on Howard C. Hopps, "Pathologic versus Nonpathologic Aspects of Senescence," in National Research Council, *Panel on Aging and the Geochemical Environment* (Washington, D.C.: National Academy Press, 1981): 25–41.

22. T. Bennett and S. M. Gardiner, "Physiological Aspects of the Aging Cardiovascular System," *Journal of Cardiovascular Pharmacology* 12 (suppl. 8) (1988): S1–S7.

23. "The Calcium Craze," *Newsweek* (January 27, 1986): 48–49.

24. Beth J. Soldo and Emily M. Agree, "America's Elderly," in *Population Bulletin* 43, no. 3 (Washington, D.C.: Population Reference Bureau, Inc., September 1988).

25. Soldo and Agree, op. cit.

26. Kenneth G. Manton, "Planning Long-Term Care for Heterogeneous Older Populations," *Annual Review of Gerontology and Geriatric Psychiatry* (New York: Springer, in press), from Soldo and Agree, op. cit., "America's Elderly," p. 20.

27. Soldo and Agree, op. cit., p. 20.

28. Durk Pearson and Sandy Shaw, *Life Extension* (New York: Warner Books, 1982): 296–301.

29. John M. Last (ed.), *Maxcy-Rosenau's Public Health and Preventive Medicine,* 11th ed. (New York: Appleton-Century-Crofts, 1980): 1338.

30. James A. Mortimer et al., "Alzheimer's Disease: The Intersection of Diagnosis, Research and Long Term Care," *Bulletin of the New York Academy of Medicine* 61, no. 4 (1985): 334–337.

31. David A. Lindeman, *Alzeheimer's Disease Handbook* (Washington, D.C.: U.S. Department of Health and Human Services, April 1984).

32. Marsha F. Goldsmith, "Steps toward Staging, Therapy of Dementia," *Journal of the American Medical Association* 251, no. 14 (April 13, 1984): 31.

33. Robert I. Simon, "Silent Suicide in the Elderly," *Bulletin of American Academic Psychiatry Law* 17, no. 1 (1989): 83–95.

34. Ibid.

35. Ibid.

36. Ibid.

37. L. Hayflick, "Recent Advances in Cell Biology of Aging," *Mechanisms of Ageing and Development* 14 (1980): 59–79.

38. J. Fred Dice, "Cellular Theories of Aging as Related to the Liver," *Hepatology* 5, no. 3 (1985): 508–513.

39. Smith et al., op. cit., p. 62.

40. R. C. Adelman (ed.), *Testing the Theories of Aging* (Boca Raton, Fla.: CRC Press, 1982): 26–27.

41. Smith et al., op. cit., p. 62.

42. Dice, op. cit.

43. Howard J. Curtis, *Biological Mechanisms of Aging* (Springfield, Ill.: Charles C Thomas, 1966).

44. Johan Bjorksten, "The Cross Linkage Theory of Aging: Clinical Delay of Aversive Stimulation," *Biological Psychology* 3, no. 2 (September 1975): 113–120.

45. Smith et al., op. cit.

46. Susan B. Gilbert, "Health Promotion for Older Americans," *Health Values* 10, no. 3 (May–June 1986): 38–46.

47. Tamara Harris et al., "Longitudinal Study of Physical Ability in the Oldest-Old," *American Journal of Public Health* 79, no. 6 (June 1989): 698ff.

48. Suzanne Meeks et al., "Age Differences in Coping: Does Less Mean Worse?" *International Journal of Aging and Human Development* 28, no. 2 (1989): 127–140.

49. Jay Meddin and Alan Vaux, "Subjective Well-Being among the Rural Elderly Population," *International Journal of Aging and Human Development* 27, no. 3 (1988): 193–206.

50. Karen A. Roberto and Priscilla J. Kimboko, "Friendships in Later Life: Definitions and Maintenance Patterns," *International Journal of Aging and Human Development* 28, no. 1 (1989): 9–19.

51. John C. Rife and Richard J. First, "Discouraged Older Workers: An Exploratory Study," *International Journal of Aging and Human Development* 29, no. 3 (1989): 195–203.

52. E. Fritz Schmerl, *The Challenge of Age* (New York: Continuum, 1986).

53. Ibid., pp. 79–81.

54. Stellye Weinstein and Efrem Rosen, "Senior Adult Sexuality in Age Segregated and Age Integrated Communities," *International Journal of Aging and Human Development* 27, no. 4 (1988): 261–270.

55. Harold G. Koenig et al., "Religion and Well-Being in Later Life," *The Gerontologist* 28, no. 1 (1988): 18–28.

56. Marjorie George, "Caring for Older Americans: Who Will Help You When You Help Your Parents," *Aide* (December 1989): 14–19.

57. Michael A. Godkin et al., "A Case-Comparison Analysis of Elder Abuse and Neglect," *International Journal of Aging and Human Development* 28, no. 3 (1989): 207–225.

58. National Center for Health Statistics, "Use of Nursing Homes by the Elderly: Preliminary Data from a 1985 National Nursing Homes Survey," *Advance Data* (May 14, 1987): 1.

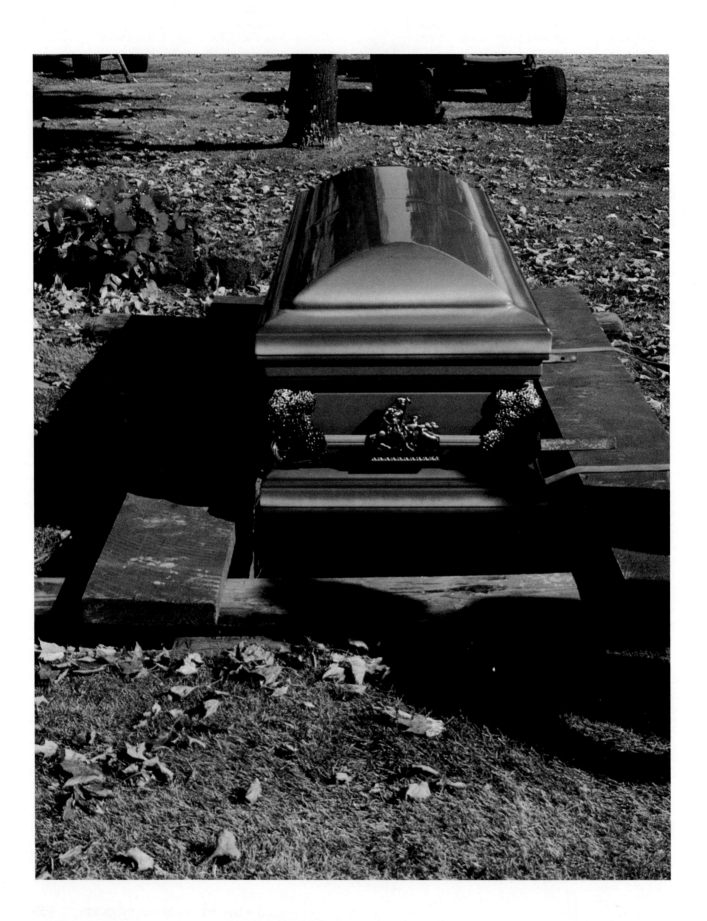

Chapter 18

Dying and Death

To Guide Your Reading

When you have studied this chapter, you should be able to:

- Describe different views of death held in different cultures and by people of different ages in our own culture.

- Discuss the stages people may go through when confronting the fact that they are about to die and the various reactions of different individuals, depending on situational and personal factors.

- Explore ways that others may respond to the fact that a relative or friend is about to die, including practical considerations of medical and emotional care.

- Enumerate several preparations that people can make for their own deaths to save their loved ones from difficult dislocations and decisions during a period of grief.

- Review the typical responses of those who are bereaved, the ways in which funeral ceremonies may help them, and other factors that may enable them to cope with and lessen their sadness over time.

Although death is a natural part of the life cycle, for many people it is a difficult subject to talk or even think about. When it is discussed, euphemisms such as "passed away" or "departed" are often used to avoid referring to death directly. Increasingly, however, the subject of death is discussed more freely, and **thanatology,** a Greek word meaning "the study of death," has become an important field of research.

thanatology—*the study of death*

Modern changes in disease patterns and technological advancement have made research into death and its implications all the more essential. People in this country today are increasingly less likely to die from short, acute illnesses or injuries. While death was in the past considered to occur with absence of heartbeat and cessation of breathing, these are now only evidence of **clinical death:** a period during which—although these life signs have stopped—all the vital cells of the body may still survive. With quick medical intervention, a "clinically dead" person may be revived or put on a life-support system until treatment can be provided.

clinical death—*the brief period after heartbeat and breathing have stopped, but before vital body cells decay irreversibly.*

Such advances have led physicians, lawyers, and religious leaders to reconsider what death is. A concept has been developed, **brain death,** defined when an electroencephalogram (EEG) detects no brain activity for at least 24 hours, even though breathing and circulation are artificially maintained. But there is still uncertainty whether this can be accepted as evidence of true death. Thus, new philosophies of death are emerging, and new forms of care for people who are near death.

brain death—*this occurs if an EEG (electroencephalogram) detects no brain activity for 24 hours, even though breathing and heart circulation are artificially maintained.*

The problems of survivors are also a concern. For the first time, researchers are objectively studying how people react to the death of a loved one and how such a loss may upset people's emotional and physical well-being. While everyone must face death—their own or the death of others—at some point in their lives, the study of death may, ironically, help people gain a greater perspective on the meaning of life.

The Meaning of Death

People who have had near-death experiences describe a variety of sensations, such as seeing their own body from another point in physical space, seeing or moving through a dark tunnel, seeing some sort of bright light, and seeing or hearing a deceased person they recognized.[1] Despite such descriptions, no one knows for sure what death is really like, and there are almost as many opinions and theories about death and dying as there are people.

From the earliest times, people have given special meanings to death, defining it not only as the end of biological function but also as a state of being in itself. Views about death are deeply influenced by questions concerning the meaning of life, the existence of a soul, and what happens to the spiritual self after death. Human cultures from the most primitive to the most technologically advanced—and individuals within those cultures—grasp toward their own religious and mystical answers to these questions.

Human societies have typically developed rituals to bury the dead; in the past these have included burying objects to be used by the person in a further existence. Evidence of some kinds of burial go back to the Old Stone Age.

Differing Views of Death

Not all people or cultures have viewed death with fear. Although some have viewed it as a state of eternal misery, others have viewed death in a neutral or even positive light—as a state of peace or a sleeplike trance. In many modern cultures, the human body has often been compared to a machine, with death the ultimate and final breakdown.

A common view of death among some people and cultures is that it is a diminished state, one in which people simply do not function as well as when they were alive. Children often hold this view, believing that dead people can both think and feel, but do neither very well. The ancient Mesopotamians held a similar view, believing that the dead gradually submerged to an underworld, slowly sinking into an unhappy state with no capacity for pleasure. Such a concept, if it survives in present cultural attitudes, may tend to make people afraid of a dead body, seeing it as a form already plunged into some other and more frightening world—a world that might also pull the living downward into its shadows. As a result, the deceased may be seen as alien and terrifying, and survivors may even be afraid to touch the body.

The fear of death and dying can sometimes sentence a dying person to a kind of "social death" that makes his or her final days very difficult. Friends, relatives, and others may turn away from the dying person, acting almost as if he or she were invisible or already dead. Family members may talk about the person as if he or she were not in the room; or they may be reluctant to touch the person, thus withholding ordinary expressions of love and emotion. Medical professionals may also be less attentive, feeling that there is little more they can do and that their services would be better used on other patients who are not terminally ill.

It is not unusual for relatives and medical personnel to behave as if the dying person were incapable of making decisions. Yet dying individuals are often just as aware as a healthy person—fully alert to their surroundings until the final moments, and able to hear, see, and feel as always. Sentencing dying people to a premature "social death" can plunge them into a debilitating depression that makes their situation all the more painful.[2]

Most of us have strong feelings about death, and rightfully so, since it is a critical part of life. It is good to stand back, however, and look at these feelings to better understand them and decide whether they are based on humane ideas or cultural superstition. In some cases, it is a good idea to examine one's attitudes, perhaps changing them in order to be kinder to oneself as well as to those who are dying.

Individual Responses to Death

The meaning of death varies from individual to individual. For some people, the thought of death may be joyful if they believe it will bring a reunion with a

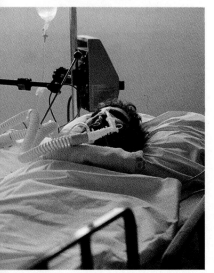

Even though society can now provide fine technological care on a level unavailable until recently, this does not alter the fact that death can still be a lonely experience. (Larry Mulvehill/Science Source/Photo Researchers, Inc.)

loved one who has already died. For others, death means a painful separation, the absence of someone central to their everyday lives. For still others, death is seen as the ultimate solution—a way out of difficult problems. Suicide may thus be seen as a way to resolve a sense of failure or as a way to express pent-up anger and hostility.

Since few people discuss death, individuals often are not aware of what others think and feel about it, and they often assume that everyone feels the same way they do. A person may assume, for example, that a terminally ill friend or relative is longing for death to bring relief from prolonged suffering. The friend or relative, however, may be dreading death because it will cut short a life he or she still finds precious. In making such assumptions, people may offend or hurt others for whom death has a different meaning.

Responses to death vary not only from individual to individual, but also from one age group to another. Sometimes, however, these responses are not what people might expect.

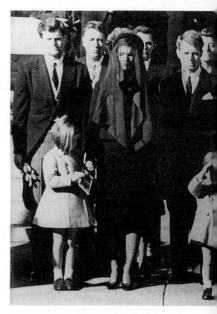

In a famous photograph from the 1960s, John Kennedy, Jr., salutes at his father's funeral. The national tragedy brought everyone together, but each person had to deal with his or her own private understanding of death. (Keystone/Sygma)

The Response of Children In the early 1900s, many people in America died before age 50, and most died at home surrounded by family and friends. Children of all ages were thus exposed to death and were encouraged to view it as a natural part of the human experience. Today, on the other hand, most deaths occur among a more elderly population, with two-thirds dying in hospitals and nursing homes.[3] Consequently, children are less directly exposed to death in their formative years when they have the security and comfort of their family to help them deal with it. It is not surprising, therefore, that these children may have difficulty coping with death when they become adults.

Even though children usually associate death with old age, it appears that anxiety over death has roots in early childhood. Psychologist M. H. Nagy identified three stages of conceptual awareness of death. Before the age of 5, children do not perceive death as an end of life but rather as a separation, which results in a separation anxiety. Between the ages of 5 and 9, this separation anxiety gives way to fears of being taken away by death and of experiencing pain, burial, and perhaps some form of life after death. Children at these ages tend to personify death as a ghost, a skeleton, or the bogeyman. After age 9, children begin to recognize that death is final, inevitable, and irreversible and that it is the end of bodily life.[4] While more mature understandings of death develop as people grow older, some forms of death anxiety persist throughout adulthood, although such anxieties carry different attitudes about mortality than those held in childhood.[5]

Children's fears of their own death develop in a similar manner. When children are still very young (2 to 4 years), their perception of what is happening to them is a reflection of the behavior of parents and loved ones rather than a fear of death. Before they can understand the idea of their own death they must have a concept of their own uniqueness; a sense of past, present, and future; and the ability to imagine change in their physical selves. These concepts are usually developed by the age of 9. By that age, children understand that their physical being may cease to exist, and they begin to become afraid of their own death.[6]

Adults often assume that children cannot cope with or understand death, and they try to shelter the young from even hearing about a death. Yet there is abundant evidence that even preschoolers are quite aware of death; children are certainly exposed to death on television. However, these are impersonal deaths and do not have the same emotional impact as the death of a pet or the death of a parent, sibling, or other relative.[7] Children will not necessarily be traumatized by references to death; indeed, research shows that they are *more* likely to be disturbed by death if it is treated like a dark, terrible secret than as a natural part of living.[8]

With death a part of children's lives and awareness, adults need not be afraid to broach the subject. Talks about death and what it means can be integrated into everyday conversations prompted by the death of a pet or a death on a television show; having just one dramatic discussion of the subject can be unnatural and scary. It is also better to discuss death in relaxed situations rather than wait for the death of a relative or family member. An adult overwhelmed by grief may give a child a distorted and more fearsome impression of death.

When a death does occur, children may react in ways that adults do not always easily comprehend at first. Even in their own grief, parents should try to be patient and understanding and observe their children's reactions carefully. Some experts believe that a reason children may not show grief is that their personalities are not fully developed; instead of mourning, they may become anxious or use defense mechanisms, such as rationalizations.[9] At a young age, children cannot verbalize their feelings, and so they may act them out. A child may express grief, for example, by reenacting familiar activities of the deceased, such as going for a walk or working in a toolshed. These are the child's way of reminiscing and may be a clue that the child wants to talk about the dead person.

For a while, children may also be irritable, argumentative, or have trouble concentrating or sleeping. As time goes by, sad feelings seem to lessen and children adjust. A relaxed and patient adult can usually help a child explore his or her feelings and aid the child in returning to more normal moods. Adults should remember that grieving is a normal process; adjustment to loss from death takes time, and individuals must proceed at their own rate. However, excessive and persistent preoccupations with death on the part of children should be considered signals of distress.[10]

The Response of Adults Reaching adulthood does not necessarily guarantee a mature attitude toward death; many adults have problems dealing with the subject. Fears of their own vulnerability may cause some people to ignore symptoms, such as a persistent weight loss or cough, which may be signs of serious medical problems. Such individuals may accept the idea that others die but may not be able to face their own mortality. Such denial can keep them from seeking necessary medical care.

Some studies suggest that men and women may differ in their response to death. In one study, for example, women reported a greater concern over death than men, a finding that might be related to a tendency among some women to feel that they have comparatively less control over their own lives.[11] Such differences are not accepted by all experts, however; many other studies find little or no difference between the sexes. All that can be stated conclusively is that a fear of dying is a recurring theme among both men and women.

The Response of the Elderly Older people—who are often assumed to be "ready for death"—may, nevertheless, have a difficult time facing it when the time grows near. It is often assumed that elderly people gradually disengage themselves from life by reducing their responsibilities and emotional involvements. They may retire, for example, and live a less active life. They may reevaluate their activities to decide what to do during the remainder of their lives; an older person may suddenly take a long trip or develop a new hobby. Friends and relatives may assume that these activities signal a slow withdrawal from life, even a preparation for death. But many older people cling to life, cherishing it no less than a younger person. It is incorrect to assume that an elderly person will automatically accept death or a serious, terminal illness as timely.

Remembering that others may feel differently about death than we do should help us to refrain from making awkward remarks about it before we have a solid idea of how others are feeling. It is often most helpful to begin by listening.

How Anxious Are You about Death?

Most people claim to be comfortable talking about death in the abstract, but the prospect of one's own death or that of a loved one may make a person nervous. For other people, however, death is a preoccupation or an unfaced fear.

This activity will help you assess your own anxiety about death. If a statement below is one that applies to you, check the left-hand column. If you would very rarely make the statement, check the right-hand column.

Applies to me	Doesn't apply to me		
_____	_____	**1.**	I am very much afraid to die.
_____	_____	**2.**	The thought of death seldom enters my mind.
_____	_____	**3.**	It does not make me nervous when people talk about death.
_____	_____	**4.**	I dread thinking about having to have an operation.
_____	_____	**5.**	I am not at all afraid to die.
_____	_____	**6.**	I am not particularly afraid of getting cancer.
_____	_____	**7.**	The thought of death never bothers me.
_____	_____	**8.**	I am often distressed by the way time flies so rapidly.
_____	_____	**9.**	I fear dying a painful death.
_____	_____	**10.**	The subject of life after death troubles me greatly.
_____	_____	**11.**	I am really scared of having a heart attack.
_____	_____	**12.**	I often think about how short life really is.
_____	_____	**13.**	I shudder when I hear people talking about World War III.
_____	_____	**14.**	The sight of a dead body is horrifying to me.
_____	_____	**15.**	I feel that the future holds nothing for me to fear.

To start, give yourself a score of 60 points. For questions 1, 4, 8, 9, 10, 11, 12, 13, and 14, *add* 10 points to your score for each check in the left-hand column. For questions 2, 3, 5, 6, 7, and 15, *subtract* 10 points each time you checked the left-hand column.

Scores	Anxiety about Death
130 to 150	Extreme
90 to 120	Moderate to high
80 or less	Reasonable

Interpretation: High anxiety about death can reflect depression or a loss of enjoyment of life. Extreme anxiety about death can be almost paralyzing. If you find yourself troubled about death, consult a counselor; also see the references at the end of this chapter.

Adapted from Donald I. Templer, "The Construction and Validation of a Death Anxiety Scale," *Journal of General Psychology* 82 (1970): 167. Reprinted with permission of Heldret Publications, Washington, DC.

The Process of Dying

It is difficult to define the point in time when a person begins to die. The exact moment that a disease becomes terminal can rarely be pinpointed, for illness is a process of gradual deterioration. Doctors cannot even easily agree on what constitutes a terminal illness, and the prognosis changes for certain illnesses as progress is made in treating them. Certain types of cancer, for example, are less deadly today than in the past, because they can now be detected and treated early.

Stages of Acceptance

Doctors also recognize the limits of medical knowledge. Many patients have unexplained, seemingly miraculous recoveries or remissions in their diseases. Until these are understood, defining terminal illness will be nearly impossible.

Because the exact moment when the unalterable movement toward death begins is so elusive, dying arrives in several stages for most people. The initial news usually comes when a doctor or other health professional tells a patient that he or she is dying. With that news, the individual begins to move from the psychological position of a living person to that of a dying one. The process is rarely simple. It is not unusual for people to take some time to accept the news that they are dying. Some are not psychologically ready to hear such news, so they distort facts and information. At times, too, doctors are disturbed by having to relay unpleasant news, and so they may garble the message in clinical terms that are not readily understood. As a result, it often takes time for an individual to understand a terminal diagnosis and accept it. And many people slip in and out of accepting their fate.

The Stages of Kübler-Ross   Based on interviews with hundreds of patients, psychiatrist Elisabeth Kübler-Ross concluded that many dying people go through five specific stages[12]:

1. There may be a *denial* of the diagnosis: a terminal patient will often assert that the news cannot be true.
2. The dying individual may grow *angry* at the world, asking "Why me?"
3. The person may try to *bargain* with fate, asking to be allowed to live long enough for an important event, such as a child's graduation or wedding.
4. He or she may grow *depressed*, drained by stress and physical suffering, and may withdraw from friends and family.
5. Finally, the dying person may *accept* fate. This final stage is rarely a happy or blissful one; but the individual does grow more peaceful and becomes resigned to a foreseeable death.

Kübler-Ross found that some people may not get to every stage: some stop along the way, never accepting their death. Some may go back and forth among various stages or may experience more than one stage at the same time.

One of the hardest tasks for any doctor is to tell a patient that an illness may be terminal. (Blair Seitz/Photo Researchers, Inc.)

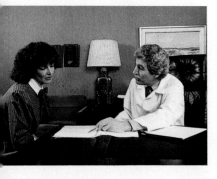

Other Viewpoints   The research of Kübler-Ross has been helpful for its compassionate exploration of what dying people experience, and she has offered useful strategies by which people can cope with their feelings when a loved one is dying. (For example, people must be patient when a dying person grows angry and must understand that such anger is not directed at them but at the thought of dying.)

However, as more studies have been made of death and dying, it has become clear that not every dying person goes through the stages described by Kübler-Ross. It has also become increasingly clear that no one facing death should feel that he or she necessarily *should* go through five stages—or any series of stages—to adapt to the situation. Indeed, researchers are finding that most often an individual's distinctive attitude and conduct during dying simply reflect his or her attitudes and conduct throughout life.[13] Some studies show that a patient's age, particular disease, environment, cultural background, personal temperament, and even lifestyle affect the way he or she copes with dying.[14] What researchers *do* find to be a nearly universal fact is that the emotional needs of a dying person are not much different from anyone else's: like everyone else, dying people crave the love and esteem of others.

Responses of the Dying

The prospect of death sometimes prompts new insights and emotional growth on the part of the dying person. Some people use the time they have left to examine their lives and long-held beliefs. For the first time, they may be able to cope with and solve problems that have plagued them for years. Driven by a clearer sense of time limits, they may try to resolve past conflicts and smooth over estrangements with family and friends.[15] Such an attitude, however, is not universal and should not necessarily be anticipated as an integral part of the process of dying.

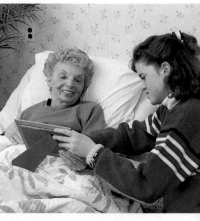

For someone who is dying, human companionship, love, and respect are as important as they are to all of us. (Tom Dunham)

The primary psychological state of most dying patients can best be described as ambivalence—a constant wavering between opposites, in which the individual sometimes needs other people and sometimes abhors their presence; is sometimes angry and sometimes serene; sometimes openly confronts death and sometimes denies it; sometimes struggles to survive and sometimes appears resigned to die.

The Problem of Pain For some people, one of the most significant concerns about dying is the thought of the pain that may accompany it. Pain is a two-part phenomenon. One part is a person's perception of the physical sensation of pain, and the other is the person's psychological reaction to it. Thus, factors such as anxiety, depression, and fatigue can add to a dying person's pain, causing an unreasonable amount of suffering in the final days or weeks. A person who is angry, depressed, or feeling isolated may feel much more pain than one who is given sympathy and understanding. Indeed, studies show that simple emotional support, sleep, and diversions can help alleviate pain that might otherwise become intractable and intolerable over time.[16]

*The term **pain threshold** is sometimes used to account for psychological factors in pain. If one's pain threshold is high due to positive factors such as rest, love, and entertainment, a physical sensation may be perceived as an ache and the pain may be successfully disregarded. Negative factors, however, such as fear and loneliness can actually lower the pain threshold so that the same sensation is experienced as agony.*

As Death Approaches What happens to people as they get closer to death? One study found that terminally ill patients close to death may have a decreased ability to integrate external stimuli and may begin to pull away from the people around them. It has been suggested that this pulling away occurs in an attempt to hold themselves together—to avoid reminders of their condition or to reduce what they perceive as the chaos of their surroundings.[17]

As actual death approaches, people are likely to feel increasingly drowsy and may be quite unaware of what is happening around them. Drugs, the disease, and the psychological distancing done by the patient tend to contribute to this drowsiness. Only about 6 percent of dying patients are conscious immediately before death, and so the moment of dying is rarely distressful. There is even some evidence that as death approaches, the brain releases a chemical that makes the moment of death pleasant instead of painful. For most people, death comes as they would wish it—quickly, painlessly, and peacefully.

The Will to Live There appears to be a phenomenon of emotional state—a "will to live"—which can be a crucial variable in the process of dying. The role of such an emotional factor has been a topic of interest in research for some time. Studies of prisoners of war (POWs) in North Korea, for example, observed that POWs who died more rapidly than their physical conditions alone would warrant were more likely to express feelings of helplessness and despair than those who survived longer.[18] Similarly, it was observed that a

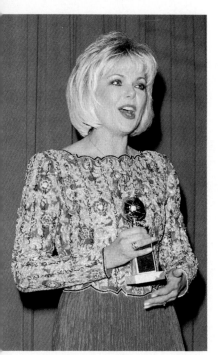

Celebrities, such as Ann Jillian, who have managed to recover from deadly disease, can provide great encouragement to people who feel hopeless in the face of a threat to their lives. (Trapper/Sygma)

lack of meaning in life was often predictive of death among inmates in Nazi concentration camps during World War II.[19]

Such evidence seems to suggest, therefore, that the extent to which people are in control of themselves and their environment may be an important factor in determining how long they will live.[20] Thus, feelings of helplessness and hopelessness may hasten the onset of death, whereas feelings of self-efficacy or control and a strong "will to live" may increase a person's chances of survival. Some therapeutic approaches have attempted to marshal a person's will to live and sense of self-efficacy in order to extend life expectancy. For example, one approach claims that a remarkably high number of cancer patients have outlived their initial prognoses.[21]

Suicide — When the Will to Live Falters

Unfortunately, some people who lose their will to live, who find life unbearable, and who are unable to cope decide to take matters into their own hands. Each year, thousands of Americans attempt suicide; many succeed. In 1988, there were a reported 30,260 deaths from suicide[22]; and it is estimated that suicide attempts are eight times more common than completed suicides. Certain groups seem more susceptible to suicide than others. For example, the rate of death from suicide is more than three times greater for males than for females, although females are reported to attempt suicide more often. Age also seems to be a factor; among persons age 15 to 24, suicide is second only to accidents as the leading cause of death.[23]

The people who attempt suicide are not necessarily those who face a terminal illness or serious disability; many are physically healthy. In fact, suicide is normally treated as a mental health concern, and suicide prevention focuses on identifying individuals at high risk due to mental illness, especially depression.

Studies have helped shed some light on why people attempt suicide. In one study of college students, researchers found that a majority of the students believed that suicide is a cry for help and that people who try to kill themselves do not really want to die but are just trying to get the attention of others. They believed that people who attempt suicide are not acting rationally at the time but are responding to feelings of loneliness or depression or to other painful circumstances. A large majority of the students felt that a more open expression of feelings would result in a substantial decrease in the suicide rate.[24]

Other studies, including a 100-year retrospective study of a Pennsylvania Amish community, suggest that heredity may significantly influence the likelihood of suicide. The findings indicate an increased risk of suicide for persons with a strong family history of suicide.[25] Suicide may also result from culturally supported beliefs (as in the Japanese tradition of committing ritual suicide, or *hara-kiri,* when one has been dishonored) or from an overwhelming desire to end extreme suffering or infirmity (as in terminal illness or very old age).

Suicide is a significant cause of death among college students. Review Chapter 3 for the warning signs for suicide, which include severe depression and extreme mood swings, accompanied by the person's giving away previous possessions, obvious anxiety in facing a crisis, and talking about suicide and death.

Suicide is a self-destructive act, but its effects are felt most by the victim's loved ones, who must deal with the pain and grief of loss. Since suicide is usually an unexpected death, survivors may be particularly unprepared to cope. In addition to their grief, they may blame themselves for not knowing that something was wrong or for not helping in some way. The loss of a child by suicide can be particularly painful to parents, who feel responsible for the health and well-being of their children.

Unlike deaths due to terminal illness, suicide can, in many instances, be prevented. Knowing the warning signs of a potential suicide (Chapter 3) and reaching out to people who are troubled can often make the difference between life and death.

Care of the Dying

Although dying is essentially an individual, personal experience, it can be affected by the actions and attitudes of others. The type of care a dying person receives and the responses of loved ones and care givers can make a great difference in the person's happiness and comfort during the time that remains.

The Responses of Other People

The way both medical professionals and loved ones treat a dying person depends very much on the circumstances. Sometimes the quality of care they provide depends on how certain death is and on how far off it is thought to be. A cancer patient who lingers for days, weeks, or months is sometimes left isolated, with medical professionals and family allowing him or her to "fade away." No heroic efforts are made to keep the person alive; and the patient typically loses control over his or her care and becomes a low priority to medical personnel.[26]

Medical personnel respond to their perceived ability to cure the patient. When a cure is not possible, the standards for decision making become murky and unclear—the type of care needed (supportive or palliative care) is not yet well defined.

By contrast, the medical system rallies all of its resources to rescue a patient in a sudden emergency, such as a heart attack, a premature birth, or a motor vehicle crash. The person is often surrounded by people intent on ensuring his or her comfort and welfare. The family is jolted into sudden concern and spends much time with the dying person.

The ambulatory dying—those not confined to a bed during their illness (such as some terminal cancer patients)—have the same needs as people dying in hospitals, but they also have other concerns. On the surface, their daily lives may be changed very little; thus, death and dying may seem especially unreal. They may hesitate to talk about their condition, for fear of losing friends or jobs. As death approaches, these people may feel particularly isolated, partly because of their own fears and partly because of the uneasiness that family and friends may display in their presence. It is important for people to realize that their support and concern for a dying person can make a great difference in that person's experience. More sensitive care can, and should, be given to all dying patients.

Over three-quarters of the deaths in the United States each year are from chronic degenerative diseases that involve a period of illness before death occurs.

Practical Issues of Care

In facing death, a terminally ill patient and his or her loved ones must not only adjust to emotions about dying, they must also deal with a number of practical issues. For example, should the patient be kept at home, be put in a hospital or nursing home, or receive a combination of home, hospital, and nursing care? Which environment offers the best care at a cost the family can afford?

Decisions on these issues are just as critical to the final experiences of the dying patient as the emotional adjustments he or she must make. They can play a significant role in making the last days more pleasant and comfortable for everyone. Although most people die in a hospital, in recent years there has been an increase in other alternatives to care for the terminally ill, including hospices and home care.

Other cultures have often done a better job at helping and understanding the dying than ours does. The hospice movement, for example, began in England.

Hospices The word *hospice* refers as much to a philosophy of care as to a type of health care service. It encourages patients to take more control over the care they receive and to participate as fully as possible in life until death occurs.

Hospices offer a variety of services, including personal care for dying persons and emotional support for them and their families. Many also offer support services for the bereaved after the death of a hospice patient. Some hospices are affiliated with hospitals, some work with home health agencies, and

Communicating with Someone Who Is Dying

Communicating with a friend or relative who is dying can be a real service to a person one cares about. It can also be a comforting experience for you. Being with, talking with, hugging, and listening to someone who is dying can give you both a chance to say things you always meant to say, clear up unresolved issues, and begin to deal with your feelings.

Talking with someone who is terminally ill is disturbing to many people. It can seem awkward; you do not know what to say and are afraid of saying the wrong thing. You may worry about talking about feelings in a way that is unnatural to you. In the face of something as serious as death, people often do not know how to behave. As a result, many people put off communicating with a dying relative until it is too late, even though they know that they will regret their procrastination later. It is important to realize that a person who is sick or terminally ill does not expect or want you to be any different from the way you usually are.

Many people are afraid of expressing their sadness while talking to someone who is dying. Whether the person knows about his or her condition or not, you do not need to hide your feelings or stop yourself from crying. The person will see your tears as a sign of concern and love and even end up taking the positive role of comforter.

When you are faced with the reality that a friend or relative is dying, you need to face your own feelings honestly. Losing someone you care about is very hard, and dealing with someone else's death reminds everyone of his or her own mortality. Most people are frightened of death, but recognizing that fear and trying to keep it in perspective may help you communicate with a dying relative more easily.

Some people are afraid that they will hurt a terminally ill person by reacting negatively to his or her appearance or behavior. It may be easier to be supportive if you are prepared in advance. Ask someone else what to expect— how does the person appear, what is his or her mood, how easily does he or she tire? You should also find out in advance how much the ill person knows about the true chances for recovery. You do not want to upset the patient by revealing information he or she is not aware of.

There are no real rules for communicating with someone who is dying, but there are guidelines you may find helpful. First of all, just be yourself. If you are naturally a very physically expressive person, hug or touch your relative as much as usual. If you have always joked with this person, do not lose your sense of humor now. If you have never talked easily about your feelings with this person, you may want to work up to doing so gradually.

A large part of your role in communicating with a terminally ill person will probably be to listen. Let the person talk about whatever he or she wants to discuss. It may be about his or her illness or fears; it may be about plans for family members after he or she is gone; it may be about outside events or interests. Let the person guide you in what you discuss when you are together.

The person you are talking to may never bring up the subject of his or her impending death. Many people who are dying do not want to talk about death. Other people may not be aware that the sickness is terminal. Follow the person's lead. Do not feel you have to bring up the subject or offer reassurance or consolation. It is better to provide support with comments that tell the person you care about what he or she has to say. Comments such as "I'm sorry that's painful" and "It sounds as if you're lonely here in the hospital" tell the person you are willing to listen to his or her concerns.

When you communicate with someone at the end of his or her life, it is a chance for you to say some of the things that have been left unsaid over the years. A simple statement such as "You know how much I have always loved you" can make both you and the person who is dying feel much better.

Based on Lynne Ann DeSpelder and Albert L. Strickland, *The Last Dance: Encountering Death and Dying* (Palo Alto, Calif.: Mayfield, 1983); Elisabeth Kübler-Ross, *On Death and Dying* (New York: Macmillan, 1970).

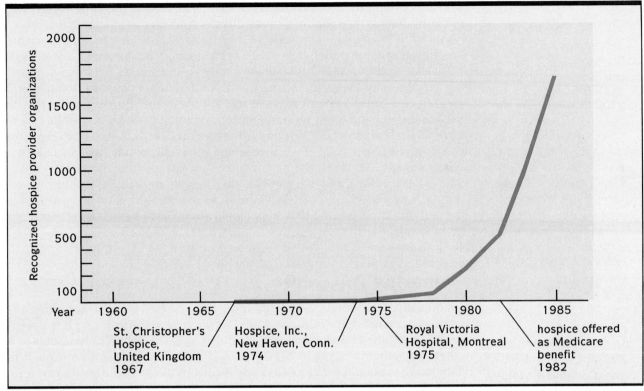

Source: Vincent Mor, *Hospice Care Systems* (New York: Springer, 1987): xiii, 1–4.

others are independent. In addition to inpatient care, hospices arrange for their services to be brought to the patient's home through a system of professional and volunteer care providers.[27]

Hospice care is distinguished by its emphasis on meeting the needs of the dying patient and often the family. The primary goal is to allow patients to be as free from physical pain and discomfort as possible and to meet their psychological, social, and spiritual needs by providing a comfortable, caring environment in which loved ones can actively participate in the patient's care.

The highest priority of hospice care is to make the dying patient comfortable without using devices for prolonging life, such as respirators, intravenous feeding apparatus, and so on. Instead, pain and other distressing symptoms are controlled by the skillful use of medications. Although almost 80 percent of terminal patient care is still provided by hospitals and nursing homes, hospice care is becoming increasingly important[28] (Figure 18.1).

Home Care   Another common alternative to institutional care is home care (in which hospice care may or may not play a role). Home care for the dying is seen as a particularly good option if the family is able and willing to provide care. With the patient at home, family members can take active roles in providing care and can offer a level of emotional and psychological support that is not available in an institutional setting, such as a hospital. One study, for example, found that mutually responsive relationships had a positive effect on patients' length of survival.[29] Another study revealed that dying persons who were surrounded by supportive families had not thought much about suicide, whereas dying patients who were abandoned by support systems not only had thoughts but also actual plans for suicide.[30]

Studies show that home care can prove beneficial not only to the dying person but to the family as well. Patients generally experience more dignity and comfort at home than in the hospital, and families adjust with less difficulty. Home care costs the family a fraction of what a hospital stay would

Figure 18.1 The philosophy and methods of hospice care have gained popularity in the United States because they provide dignified and humane care for the terminally ill and their families. Hospice care is also less costly than conventional hospital treatment. The first hospices in North America were established in the middle 1970s after pioneering work had been done in Great Britain. Surveys of hospice providers indicate a rapid rise in this approach to care for the dying, especially after 1982 when hospice was introduced as a Medicare benefit.

cost, and programs encouraging such care also benefit the community as a whole by freeing hospital beds for patients requiring acute care.[31]

Yet, while home care can provide a humane way to die, it can also create strain among family members. It is not unusual, for example, for several relatives to feel that they must take primary responsibility for the dying person. So the family members must sort through their various abilities and relationships to find an appropriate role for everyone. Some may be able to provide the dying person with intensive psychological support, while others may feel more comfortable attending to practical details, such as paying bills. Relatives also frequently find themselves uncertain about how to talk to a dying relative. At times they try to reassure the person that he or she is getting better. But the dying patient often knows death is near and may resent such pretense, desperately wanting to talk about his or her true status and perhaps to be assured that all personal affairs have been taken care of and are in good order.

Preparing for Death

Since death is an emotional experience, the practical side of preparing for death and doing what needs to be done is often very difficult. Yet it is important to think ahead and consider critical issues such as the preparation of a will, the possibility of organ donation, and the decision at a certain point to employ life-sustaining measures. Early decisions about these issues can forestall future problems and can play a role in making the last days of life more pleasant, comfortable, and free of worry.

Legal Preparedness: Making a Will

A *will* is a legal document that specifies how a person wishes his or her property to be distributed after death. Everyone should have a will. Without one, a person's property will be distributed not as he or she would want, but according to the laws of the state of residence. In addition, the absence of a will may provoke disputes among family members over claims to the person's possessions in the event of death.

Although a valid will can be written on a simple "do-it-yourself" form (Figure 18.2), it is usually wiser to seek the advice and assistance of an attorney. In either case, the following information may be helpful[32]:

- The *testator* (the person making the will) names an *executor* to supervise the distribution of property after death.
- One or more witnesses (the number depends on the testator's state of residence) must sign the will. To prevent coercion and fraud, witnesses may not be beneficiaries of the will.
- Upon death, the executor files the will as designated by the county or state (typically, in the office of the clerk of the probate court). The executor also has the witnesses called in to verify the deceased's signature and their own and to swear that they have witnessed the proper execution of the will.
- Property that is titled (such as a jointly owned home bearing the right of survivorship) and insurance benefits (where the surviving spouse or other individual has been designated as beneficiary) will be passed along automatically, independently of the will. If no additional property is bequeathed under the will, administration of the estate is unnecessary; but the will may be filed and become a matter of public record, available if it is ever needed.
- A person who dies without a will is said to have died *intestate*. If the person owned any property, the court appoints an administrator to distribute it in accordance with the state's laws.
- A will should be kept in a place that is safe but readily available to spouse, parent, or other next of kin. A safe-deposit box may not be the best place.

FIRST CODICIL TO THE WILL
OF
(YOUR NAME)

I, **(your name)**, as a resident of **(county, state)**, declare this to be the first codicil to my will dated **(day, month, year)**.

FIRST: I revoke the provision of Clause **(number)** of my will which provided **(include the exact language you wish to revoke)** and substitute the following: **(add whatever is desired)**.

SECOND: I add the following provision to Clause **(number)**: **(add whatever is desired)**.

THIRD: In all other respects I confirm and republish my will dated **(day, month, year)**.

Dated: **(day, month, year) (your typewritten name)**

I subscribe my name to this codicil this **(day)** day of **(month, year)**, at **(city, county, state)**, and do hereby declare that I sign and execute this codicil willingly, that I execute it as my free and voluntary act for the purposes therein expressed, and that I am of the age of majority or otherwise legally empowered to make a codicil and under no constraint or undue influence.

(your signed name)

On this **(day)** day of **(month, year)**, **(your name)** declared to us, the undersigned, that this instrument was the codicil to **(his/her)** will and requested us to act as witnesses to it. **(He/She)** thereupon signed this codicil in our presence, all of us being present at the same time. We now, at **(his/her)** request, in **(his/her)** presence, and in the presence of each other, subscribe our names as witnesses and declare we understand this to be **(his/her)** codicil and that to the best of our knowledge **(he/she)** is of the age of majority, or is otherwise legally empowered to make a codicil and under no constraint or undue influence.

We declare under penalty of perjury that the foregoing is true and correct.

(witness signature) residing at **(witness address: street, city, county, state)**

(witness signature) residing at **(witness address: street, city, county, state)**

(witness signature) residing at **(witness address: street, city, county, state)**

Figure 18.2 Here is a part of a will, set up in a do-it-yourself format. It is actually a codicil, used to amend an existing will so that the whole document does not have to be prepared over. This codicil, like a do-it-yourself will, needs to be typed, dated, signed, and witnessed to become legal. For anything but a simple will, however, experienced legal advice is recommended.

Source: Denis Clifford, *Nolo's Simple Will Book: How to Prepare a Legally Valid Will* (Berkeley, Calif.: Nolo Press, 1987): 14: 6–7. Reproduced with permission.

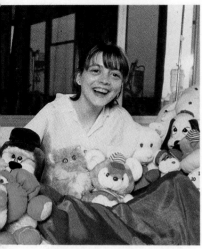

This young French girl has a fresh lease on life because she received a pair of lungs from a dying child. Imagine the feelings of a donor's parents, whose permission is required for such an operation. (Bamberger/Figaro/Gamma-Liaison)

Information regarding transplants, donor cards, and referrals to local agencies can be obtained toll-free at 1-800-ACT-GIVE or through ACT (the American Council on Transplantation) Dept. 21, Box 1709, Alexandria, VA 22313-1709.

euthanasia—*allowing or helping a person to die.*

passive euthanasia—*a situation in which no action is taken to prolong life even though action might enable a person to live longer.*

active euthanasia—*a situation in which something is done to a patient to cause death.*

(In some jurisdictions, safe-deposit boxes must be sealed upon a person's death and are not released until audited by the tax authorities.)
• A will should be reviewed periodically to make sure that it is up to date. If the testator moves to a new state, the will must meet the legal requirements of the new place of residence.

Organ Donation

Modern medical technology and surgical techniques have made it possible to transplant a variety of body parts from dead donors to live patients. Donated organs can be used to save another person's life, as with a kidney or liver transplant, or to help the person live more productively, as with a corneal (the cornea of the eye) transplant.

Today, it is fairly widely accepted that an individual has a right to decide what will be done with his or her body after death. People may choose to bequeath their entire bodies or specific body parts for use in transplants, medical treatments, or medical research and education. While the right of organ donation is widely accepted, one study found that only about 3 percent of the respondents had actually made preparations for the use of their organs.[33] Those who have chosen to become donors often carry donor cards, which are legal documents stipulating what parts of the body may be used in the event of death.

All 50 states have enacted some form of legislation providing for the donation of the body or designated body parts upon the death of the donor. Despite this legislation and the legal decisions of donors, organ donations are sometimes not utilized because of objections by the deceased's family. Hospitals are unlikely to take an organ from a dead person if the family objects, even though the deceased person legally chose to be a donor.[34]

The Right to Die and Euthanasia

While the right of organ donation is quite widely accepted, there is less general acceptance of the idea that any means should be used to prolong the life of a person with a debilitating and terminal medical crisis. There is also much less acceptance of the idea that a person has the right to take steps to end his or her life should the pain and problems of a serious illness become unbearable. The basic question underlying these ideas is whether people have the right to control their own fate—whether they have the right to control how they die or when death will occur. This is known as **euthanasia**—allowing or helping a person to die.

The issue of euthanasia can be considered from several perspectives. **Passive euthanasia** refers to situations in which no action is taken to prolong life even though action might enable a person to live longer. An example of passive euthanasia would be *not* hooking up a respirator to a person who is unable to breathe unassisted. In contrast, **active euthanasia** refers to situations in which something is done to a patient to directly cause death. An example of active euthanasia would be the removal of an already functioning life-support system (such as a respirator or intravenous feeding tube) from a vegetative, comatose person. Another, more extreme, example of active euthanasia would be giving a dying person a lethal injection to hasten death, thus ending pain and suffering.[35]

While many people might agree that people have the right to control their own fate, and might also agree that people should not have to endure unbearable pain and suffering, the issue of euthanasia is not that simple. Death affects not only the deceased, but also family, friends, and others. Their "right" to have the person live may be just as valid as the person's "right" to die. Therefore, while euthanasia might be merciful to a dying person, it places a difficult burden on others.

Several landmark court cases are helping establish some precedents in the issue of euthanasia. The case of *In re Quinlan* involved a request by the parents of Karen Ann Quinlan, who was bedridden and comatose, to have a life-sustaining respirator shut off, arguing that their daughter no longer had a life worth living. The *Quinlan* case prompted a public debate over just what right people have to decide the circumstances of their own dying days, and what rights others may have. The final ruling of the New Jersey Supreme Court was in favor of the parents' request—2 years after their daughter first went into a coma.

Shortly after the Quinlan case, the Massachusetts Judicial Court deliberated in the case of *Superintendent of Belchertown State School v. Saikewicz*. This case involved a request by the legal guardian of Joseph Saikewicz, a 67-year-old leukemia patient, to discontinue chemotherapy treatments. The decision of a lower court was upheld, permitting discontinuation of the treatment.[36] In both the *Quinlan* and the *Saikewicz* cases, the courts recognized the right of people to refuse medical treatment under certain circumstances and extended that right to the families and guardians of individuals unable to make the decision for themselves.

The issue is far from settled, however. In a more recent case in Missouri, that state's supreme court denied Nancy Cruzan's parents the right to ask that a feeding tube be disconnected from their comatose daughter, saying that there was not adequate evidence under state law that Nancy herself would have wished this. This decision signaled a retreat from the principles established in the *Quinlan* and *Saikewicz* cases, leaving the final "right" of a person to die still unresolved.[37] The *Cruzan* case was appealed to the U.S. Supreme Court, but there it was asserted that this was a matter for state law not covered by the United States Constitution. (In the end, more evidence was produced in Missouri, and Cruzan *was* finally allowed to die.)

At the current time, several states have "natural death" laws, allowing patients to refuse treatment in terminal illnesses. Others have statutes allowing patients to appoint surrogates, who can act on their behalf if they are unable to make such decisions themselves. Some states also recognize "living wills," which are legal documents that contain directives about withholding life-sustaining medical treatment in certain circumstances.[38]

The idea of euthanasia raises many questions. When would it be appropriate or inappropriate to request or provide assistance in euthanasia? What would the distinction be between killing a person and allowing the person to die? Does the state have a valid role in deciding when and how a terminally ill person can die? Some people argue that if society helps terminally ill patients die because it agrees that death is preferable to intense pain and suffering or to a prolonged vegetative state, it will be difficult to draw the line as to who should be allowed to die. Others argue that respect for human dignity demands respect for individual freedom and the right to decide freely about one's own fate.

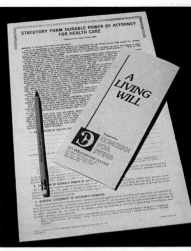

Living wills are becoming an accepted way for people to ensure that after a near-fatal accident with no prognosis for recovery, they will be allowed to die rather than be kept alive in a vegetative state. (Tony Freeman/PhotoEdit)

After Death: Responses of the Living

After someone dies, the impact of death is felt by the living. Survivors mourn the loss of parents, children, spouses, friends, and other loved ones. As difficult as it may be, these survivors can and do learn to cope with their loss. Among the first things that help in the coping process are funerals and mourning.

Funerals and Mourning

After death comes **mourning**—all those culturally reinforced patterns of thought, feelings, and behaviors that individuals experience as a result of

mourning—all the culturally reinforced patterns of thought, feelings, and behaviors that individuals experience as a result of losing a loved one.

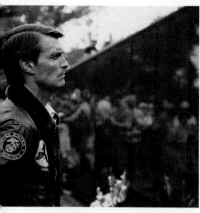

War memorials not only serve as a patriotic memorial to those who died for their country, they also provide a tangible solace for every individual who mourns their loss. (Owen Franken/Sygma)

One custom that is observed in many religions and cultures, but not in the United States, is the final funeral ceremony, which commonly marks an end to mourning. A public ceremony like the initial funeral, this final ceremony is held after some time has elapsed, and it appears to help the bereaved in these cultures to come to terms with their grief. After the ceremony they may be free, or even encouraged, to marry again.

It is not unusual for people to plan ahead for their own funerals. This takes a major burden off the shoulders of a grieving family and shows a very practical and caring acceptance of the inevitability of death.

losing a loved one. Part of mourning is the larger society's support for survivors and the rituals and expectations with which society responds to death.

When death finally arrives, it brings a need for a parting ceremony, a rite of passage, that can help friends and relatives absorb and comprehend their loss. This ritual occurs, in one form or another, in every human society and like other rituals, satisfies deep-seated human needs.

Funeral Customs   In the United States, funeral customs vary widely, depending on such factors as religion, geographic region, personal preferences, and finances.

In some places, for example, people view the deceased's body at a funeral home the night before the funeral service. In other places, there are two viewing nights, one for the immediate family and one for others. In some religions, it is traditional to prepare a meal at the church for after a funeral; in others, neighbors bring food to the home of the deceased and visit with the family. Among some groups, friends and relatives may hold a "wake" in which they stay up all night in the room with the deceased's body.

The funeral ceremony itself may be religious or secular in nature. In some cases, family members may participate by helping plan the funeral or by writing parts of the funeral service. The decision for either cremation or burial also varies widely depending on custom and religion.

The Purpose of Funerals   Funerals are of major psychological value to survivors. The funeral provides an important emotional release in the first few days after death, giving the survivors something concrete to do. It also helps confirm the reality of the death and provides a network of people who may be called on for support. Funerals also seem to fulfill several important societal functions, such as bringing families together, thus affirming the importance of family networks and helping reinforce the social order through public ritual.

Postfuneral rituals are also helpful to survivors. Sending out acknowledgments for kindnesses expressed at the time of death and sorting out and disposing of the deceased's personal effects can be a healthy indication that the death is being accepted.[39]

Planning for a Funeral   The traditional funeral is often a sizable expense. As a ceremonial expense it ranks second only to weddings. An increasingly elaborate array of choices is available in planning a funeral.

Extravagant and elaborate practices have brought the funeral industry under attack for inducing people to spend large amounts of money in their most vulnerable moments. In some instances, certain practices of funeral directors have been attacked as deceptive and unscrupulous. In recent years, the Federal Trade Commission (FTC) has drawn up proposals to regulate the funeral industry with the aim of protecting consumers from exploitation. One practice targeted by the FTC is the automatic embalming of the deceased's body without prior permission from the family. Contrary to popular belief, embalming is not required by law; the underlying motive for embalming appears to be financial gain, since a funeral with a body maximizes the funeral director's services and usually means that the family will buy a more expensive casket for the body. The FTC has also suggested changes in the way caskets are marketed, that no casket be required for cremation, and that all funeral homes offer low-cost containers for cremation.[40]

Families are advised to plan ahead for funerals, so that the costs can be anticipated and kept within reasonable limits. The Better Business Bureau suggests that families treat funeral services like any other service and shop around; a family can visit funeral directors to get information about the kinds of arrangements available and their costs, including an itemized price list for all services and arrangements. In some areas, nonprofit, nonsectarian groups

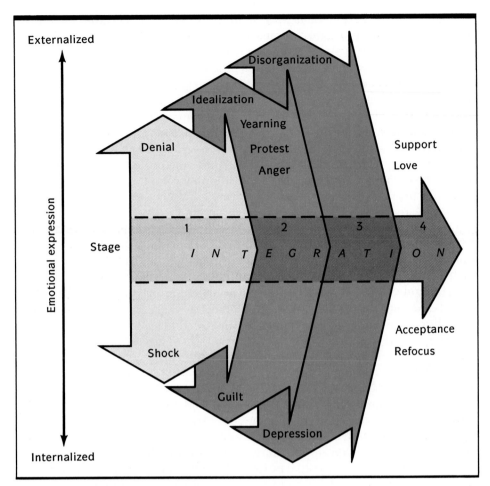

Figure 18.3 The grieving process. During the grieving process the mourner may pass through several stages characterized by different ranges of emotional expression. In Stage I denial may accompany the initial shock at the loss of a loved one. In Stage II the mourner yearns for an idealized loved one. Anger at abandonment may turn to guilt. In Stage III the mourner may be disorganized and depressed. Finally, in Stage IV the mourner integrates the loss. Love and support of friends help the mourner accept the loss and refocus his or her ongoing life.

called "memorial societies" have been established to provide assistance in planning a funeral.

Bereavement

The death of a loved one causes a great deal of stress, which can have a profound effect on the survivors. There is the stress that comes from **bereavement**—the loss of a loved or valued person—and from the change in one's own status (as from spouse to widowed person) that results from the death. Then there is the stress of **grief**—the subjective, emotional response to bereavement. When people grieve, they may experience symptoms of distress in both their minds and bodies. Grief can sometimes become so intense that it causes biochemical and physiological reactions that can precipitate physical illness and even death.[41] The psychological and behavioral responses to grief can cause loss of memory and difficulty in mental concentration—sometimes even to the point where the grieving person questions his or her sanity.

Many experts believe that survivors go through various stages as they attempt to deal with their loss and work through their grief; these stages are part of the process of mourning (Figure 18.3). The stages a bereaved person may experience include shock, a yearning for the deceased and protest that the death occurred, a period of disorganization and despair, and finally, an integration and adjustment to a realistic view of life without the deceased. People may progress through the stages in that order, regress to previous stages, skip stages, or experience different stages simultaneously.[42]

Patterns of Bereavement The way someone reacts to a death depends, in part, on the way the loved one died. When death comes as a surprise, the bereaved spouse, child, or other loved one may feel that there are no limits to

bereavement—*the loss of a loved or valued person.*

grief—*the subjective, emotional response to bereavement.*

the grief and that it may never ease. A sudden death can be especially devastating for the survivor because he or she usually lacks time to assemble a support system.[43] On the other hand, studies have shown that a lingering illness before death gives survivors a chance to anticipate the death and to begin to come to terms with it.[44] With such "anticipatory grief" a person begins to feel the loss and to grieve before the actual death of the loved one; after the death, the person may even express some relief that the loved one's suffering is over. When there is time for anticipatory grieving, the survivor does not usually suffer as intensely at the moment of death and immediately after as do people confronted with sudden and unexpected loss. Yet, even for those who anticipate it, the sense of loss and desolation are still strong when the death actually occurs.[45]

This explains the phenomenon popularly called "dying of a broken heart." Spouses frequently do lose their lives within a year of each other—the surviving partner has essentially "lost the will to live."

Researchers have found certain patterns among the bereaved. While these patterns may not emerge in every case, they do arise often enough to warrant attention. Soon after the death, a survivor often tends to idealize the deceased; the person may remember the deceased as the best mother, father, wife, husband, or friend who ever lived. Over time other, repressed memories emerge, often followed by surges of anger, which can be quite unexpected and intense. A wife, for example, may be angry that her husband has "left" her alone, especially if she has to care for children. This reaction can be confusing to the survivor and may lead to feelings of guilt, especially since the deceased has perhaps been idealized. Generally, this anger passes; it is only one step toward coming to a more realistic view of life without the deceased.

Survivors may experience loneliness long after the funeral. The death of a spouse, for instance, has immediately removed the source of most of the survivor's social interactions. There may be a loss of companionship, a loss of a primary source of love and caring, a changed and often-worsened financial situation, and a reduced opportunity for physical and sexual contacts.[46] Although there is usually an initial burst of concern and caring from friends and family, these other people often return rather quickly to their daily lives, and the widower or widow is left alone to face days and months of readjustment.

For at least 1 year, and possibly more, the bereaved person is an individual at risk; the highly emotional state of grief and mourning can actually jeopardize a person's physical health and well-being. For example, a deterioration in health and an increase in physical illness may result from the bereaved person's neglecting him- or herself. The bereaved may also suffer from psychosomatic illnesses, including headaches, low back pain, frequent bouts with colds and flus, excessive fatigue, and sleep disturbances.[47]

Certain situations may have a special effect on the bereaved. Some evidence, for instance, suggests that bereavement after a suicide differs from bereavement after other causes of death. The survivor may deny that the cause of death was suicide because the idea is too painful. He or she may also engage in a prolonged search for the motives that the deceased may have had for committing suicide.[48] A different situation involves a bereaved person who was in a "secret" relationship that was never socially sanctioned. These "secret survivors" have a tendency to view the loss as retribution or justice. People involved in a long-term extramarital affair, for example, may be especially vulnerable to feelings that they and their deceased partner are being punished for their behavior. In addition, since the relationship was secret, the bereaved may lack normal channels for expressing grief and receiving support. Their grief may be misunderstood or even resented by some people, and sources of support are limited to perhaps only a few very close friends.[49]

Bereavement in Children The impact of a death on children can be intense and long-lasting. At one time it was assumed that children under the age of 5 were too young to be affected by death. Studies have shown, however, that young children are *very much* affected by the death of people close to them. For example, although children between 2 and 5 years of age do not fully

My Story

Coming to Terms

It has been almost 4 months since Laura died. I look at photographs of my 28-year-old cousin's beautiful face and still cannot believe that she is gone.

Just 6 months ago we stood together, talking in my aunt's living room. I was admiring a stained-glass jewelry box Laura had made. She was so talented, so bright. There will be no more glass jewelry boxes now. We'll share no more conversations. She is gone.

I found out in March that Laura had lymphoma. "It's the worst kind of blood cancer," my aunt told me. "Things do not look good." My face dropped. I froze, silent and stunned from this tragic news. "No, not Laura," I thought. "She'll fight it. She'll pull through."

Laura and her parents lived far from me. After I spoke to my aunt, I tried to phone Laura but got her answering machine. I found out later that she was not taking any calls because she did not want to talk to anyone. So I wrote to her.

What do you say to someone with a life-threatening illness? I wrote and rewrote several letters but mailed only two. "Please let me know if there is anything I can do," I said in the first letter. "Things will get better," I said in the second.

My aunt kept me posted on Laura's progress. She told me that Laura was undergoing chemotherapy. She was still working during the week but reserved her weekends for treatments. Despite the fact that she had lost her hair, it sounded as if things were going well. Laura and her parents were attending a support group at their local hospital. Their "I Can Cope" group was set up to help the terminally ill and their families.

Then, all of a sudden, things changed. My aunt called me to tell me that Laura was getting worse and that there was talk of her getting a bone marrow transplant. I decided that I needed to see her. I took some time off from work and made travel arrangements. By the time I arrived at my aunt's, Laura had been admitted to the hospital with an infection. Fluid was building up in her lungs.

I'll never forget the day I visited Laura in the hospital. She did not wake up. She lay in her bed, gasping bravely for breath. She was virtually comatose, and at times, when her eyes opened, I prayed for her recovery. But immediately her eyes glazed over, and she dozed off again. Later, as my aunt and I changed Laura's position so she could breathe and drain her lungs more easily, I found myself praying again—but this time for Laura's painless and immediate death. Her mouth dripped mucus, and her breathing came in fits and starts. Then, as her mother held her, she simply stopped breathing.

I wondered why this had happened to a kind, gentle woman whose life should have been unfolding before her, not ending. I felt angry at whoever or whatever had robbed her of a chance to marry, raise a family, and live a long and happy life. I wanted cancer to be a dragon so that I, with my sword, could save her by slicing off its huge, ugly head. But now there was nothing I could do.

Although it hasn't been easy, I've managed to go on. I remember Laura the way she looked in one of her photographs, smiling and happy. I have learned to cope, and my outlook on life has changed. I now think of life as a series of fleeting but wonderful moments, like that moment captured in her photo. And I vow to myself to make the most of each one.

I still feel the pain of death—the hurt of Laura's and that of others I have loved. Yet I know that there is a world full of people just like me who feel this pain. Somehow, knowing that I am not alone helps. And for now I will try to learn to live with the grief and remember to experience the joy of living every day.

Ideas based on information from Richard A. Kalish, *Death, Grief, and Caring Relationships*, 2d ed. (Belmont, Calif.: Brooks/Cole, 1985); Anne M. Brooks, *The Grieving Time: A Year's Account of Recovery from Loss* (New York: Harmony, 1985).

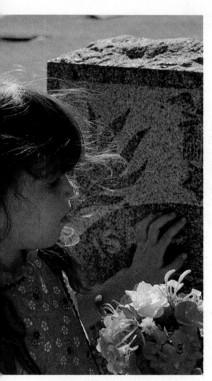

The impact of death on little children can sometimes be very severe. They need many opportunities both to understand their loss and to sense the loving support of others. (Alan Oddie/PhotoEdit)

understand the meaning of death, they ask for the deceased person, express anger and confusion, and sometimes regress to bed-wetting, using baby talk, and drinking from a baby bottle.[50]

Loss of an important person in childhood can have lingering effects, too: there is some evidence that people who as a child have lost someone dear to them are more likely to suffer physical or mental illness as adults.[51] Some studies, for example, have suggested that childhood bereavement may be related to depression and schizophrenia in later life.[52]

Not only do children feel the loss of the loved one who has died, but they may also suffer from lack of attention from grieving family members. Although some bereaved mothers or fathers may become more attentive to their children, many find it difficult to cope with both their own sorrow and their children's needs. For most children, the greatest difficulty is not knowing or understanding what is happening. Taking the time to explain can help to ease the child's anxiety, confusion, and pain.

Bereavement in Parents   The most devastating kind of bereavement is often that of a parent over the loss of a child. Not only is there a feeling of loss over a very intimate relationship, but there is also a feeling of loss over an unfulfilled life full of potential. The death of a child is often seen as hideously unnatural, and many parents refuse to accept the death until they are actually confronted with the body.

Accepting the death is often only the beginning of a grieving period filled with intense longings for the youngster and tremendous guilt. (Guilt may be particularly intense if the sudden, unexplained death of an infant is involved.) Parents ask what they could have done to prevent the death, and even the slightest reminder of the child—a toy in a neighbor's yard—may set off waves of yearning and grief. These feelings can upset the family's normal relationships: a surviving child may feel neglected or afraid, or try to act (or be pushed into acting) as a replacement for the deceased. The strains on the family can become all the more intense because there are few social supports available, especially if a child is stillborn or dies shortly after birth.

The death of a daughter or son is very disorganizing and difficult for both parents, whether the child was young or had reached adolescence or adulthood. However, studies have found some differences in the way that mothers and fathers react to a child's death. It has been found, for instance, that mothers tend to grieve more than fathers. In the case of an infant's death, mothers tend to feel the loss more acutely and to experience a greater degree of anger, despair, and guilt than fathers. As they cope with the death, mothers tend to talk about their feelings with others, while fathers cope by increasing involvement in outside activities.[53] There is also some evidence to suggest that the status of the child may have an effect on parental grieving: healthy children are grieved more than unhealthy children, male children are grieved more than female children, and children that are more similar to a parent are grieved more than those who are dissimilar.[54]

Such differences, however, should not discount the trauma caused by the death of a child. Parents may have more difficulty coping with a child's death than with the death of other loved ones. Psychological healing after the death of a child takes a long time; the grief following the death of a child may continue for several years and then may only be alleviated, rather than healed.[55]

Coping with Grief   No one can predict exactly how long a person will grieve for the loss of someone dear. "Normal" grief seems to begin with a period of acute mourning immediately following or soon after a death and then diminishes gradually over the course of 2 or more years.[56] Too little grieving soon after a death or too much grieving too long after, or both, are considered abnormal.

In order to cope with death, a grieving person has to come to terms with certain "tasks of bereavement," including the need to detach him- or herself from the deceased, maintain relationships with others who can be supportive, and hold on to a satisfactory self-image.[57] Researchers have also found that there are ways of coping with grief that can lessen the stress and help people come through the experience intact. Perhaps most important of all, studies show that it is crucial for people to "allow" themselves to grieve and to verbalize the feelings that accompany grief. The simple act of expressing feelings about oneself, the death, and the person who died can help a person survive the most desolate moments. Talking helps to release negative emotions such as hatred and guilt: if such feelings are left unattended, they can make a person feel desperate and confused; if discussed, they can help the bereaved come to understand that the feelings are the natural outgrowth of a sense of abandonment and loneliness. Grief is an expression of the conflict between the longing for the deceased and the recognition that the person is truly gone forever; talking helps to bring the reality of death into focus. Talking also, however, helps to reinforce the feeling that, although a loved one may be gone forever, his or her memory will live on as a permanent part of those who remain.[58]

People of past generations seem to have come to better terms with death than we in modern society have. Because of modern medicine, we may actually harbor a greater fear of death: we have become less inclined to see death as natural and more and more to view it as alien and a defeat of medical powers.

Chapter Summary

- Views of death differ among individuals and among cultures. Some view it as a negative state, perhaps one of misery or diminished function. Others view it in a positive light, as a state of peace or bliss.
- Although the response to death differs from individual to individual, there are certain typical responses among different age groups. Young children often do not understand death, but it does cause anxiety because of a fear of separation. As children grow older they begin to form mature understandings. Yet many adults still have problems dealing with death, due to fears of their own vulnerability. Although many people assume the elderly are ready to accept death, that is often not the case.
- Kübler-Ross identified five stages of dying: denial, anger, bargaining with fate, depression, and acceptance.
- People's attitudes about dying may be affected by cultural background, age, personal temperament, and lifestyle.
- One of the most significant concerns about dying is the fear of pain. As death approaches, people may pull away from people around them. As actual death approaches, people are likely to feel drowsy and may be unaware of what is happening around them.
- A "will to live" may be an important variable in a person's survival. People who are in control of themselves and their environment and who have a strong will to live often survive longer than those who have lost the will to live. Some people who lose the will to live attempt suicide

as a way of escaping problems or unbearable illness.
- Hospice care encourages patients to take more control over their care and to participate fully in life until death occurs. Hospice care provides emotional support for patients and their families and tries to free the patient from pain without the use of life-sustaining devices. Home care can also be emotionally satisfying for patients because of the familiar environment and the presence of loved ones.
- Euthanasia—allowing or helping a person to die—is a controversial issue. In passive euthanasia, no actions are taken to prolong a person's life. In active euthanasia, something is done to cause death. Some court cases have upheld the right of people and their guardians to determine their own fate by declining or removing life-support systems; others have denied this right. Euthanasia raises various ethical and moral questions such as: What is the distinction between killing a person and letting him or her die? Should the state be allowed to determine a person's fate?
- Funerals provide an emotional release for survivors and confirm the reality of death. Funeral customs vary; some provide for viewing the deceased before the funeral, sometimes friends or family bring food to the survivors' home, sometimes families participate in the funeral service.
- People in mourning often experience shock, a yearning for the deceased and a protest that the death occurred, a period of disorganization and

despair, and finally, an integration and adjustment to a realistic view of life without the deceased.

- If death is a surprise, grief is often very intense because the survivors have not been able to prepare themselves. If death is expected, "anticipatory grief" often allows a person to feel the loss and come to terms with it a little before death actually occurs. Soon after death, survivors often idealize the deceased; then repressed memories may surface, sometimes followed by anger; eventually a more realistic view emerges. Bereaved children may express confusion or anger and sometimes may regress to infantile behavior; they may also suffer more long-lasting effects, such as depression. Bereaved parents are normally devastated by the loss of a child; the death is seen as unnatural, and parents may sometimes blame themselves and feel tremendous guilt.

- To cope with grief, a person has to come to terms with certain tasks of bereavement, including detachment from the deceased, maintaining other supportive relationships, and holding on to a satisfactory self-image. It is crucial for people to allow themselves to grieve and to verbalize their feelings with friends and other loved ones.

Key Terms

Thanatology (page 459)
Clinical death (page 459)
Brain death (page 459)

Euthanasia (page 472)
Passive euthanasia (page 472)

Active euthanasia (page 472)
Mourning (page 473)

Bereavement (page 475)
Grief (page 475)

References

1. Ian Stevenson et al., "Are Persons Reporting 'Near-Death Experiences' Really Near Death? A Study of Medical Records," *Omega* 20, no. 1 (1989–1990): 45–54.

2. R. J. Kastenbaum, *Death, Society and the Human Experience*, 2d ed. (St. Louis: Mosby, 1981): 10–20, 25–26, 32, 45.

3. P. B. Friel, "Death and Dying," *Annals of Internal Medicine* 97, no. 5 (1982): 721–767, cited in Kenneth R. Crispell and Carlos F. Gomez, "Proper Care for the Dying: A Critical Public Issue," *Journal of Medical Ethics* 13 (1987): 74–80.

4. M. H. Nagy, "The Child's Theories concerning Death," *Journal of Genetic Psychology* 73 (1948): 3–27.

5. J. Conrad Glass, "Changing Death Anxiety through Death Education in the Public Schools," *Death Studies* 14 (1990): 31–52.

6. W. M. Easson, "Management of the Dying Child," *Journal of Clinical Child Psychology* 3, no. 2 (1974): 25–27; C. M. Binger et al., "Childhood Leukemia: Emotional Impact on Patient and Family," *Northeast Journal of Medicine* 380 (1969): 414–418.

7. R. A. Kalish, *Death, Grief, and Caring Relationships*, 2d ed (Belmont, Calif.: Brooks/Cole, 1985).

8. Nagy, op. cit.

9. Kastenbaum, op. cit., pp. 10–20, 25–26, 32, 45.

10. Cynthia R. Pfeffer, "Preoccupations with Death in 'Normal' Children: The Relationship to Suicidal Behavior," *Omega* 20, no. 2 (1989–1990): 205–212.

11. Andrew R. Dattel and Robert A. Neimeyer, "Sex Differences in Death Anxiety: Testing the Emotional Expressiveness Hypothesis," *Death Studies* 14 (1990): 1–11.

12. Elisabeth Kübler-Ross, *On Death and Dying* (New York: Macmillan, 1970).

13. Kastenbaum, op. cit., p. 191.

14. A. D. Weisman and R. J. Kastenbaum, *The Psychological Autopsy: A Study of the Terminal Phase of Life* (New York: Behavioral Publications, 1968).

15. Russell A. Meares, "On Saying Good-bye before Death," *Journal of the American Medical Association* 246, no. 11 (September 11, 1981): 1227–1229.

16. Robert G. Twycross, "The Assessment of Pain in Advanced Cancer," *Journal of Medical Ethics* 4 (1978): 112–116.

17. Robert J. Baugher et al., "A Comparison of Terminally Ill Persons at Various Time Periods to Death," *Omega* 20, no. 2 (1989–1990): 103–115.

18. H. D. Strassman et al., "A Prisoner of War Syndrome: Apathy as a Reaction to Severe Stress," *American Journal of Psychiatry* 112 (1956): 998–1003.

19. V. E. Frankl, *Man's Search for Meaning: An Introduction to Logotherapy* (New York: Washington Square Press, 1963).

20. Kalish, op. cit.

21. O. C. Simonton et al., *Getting Well Again* (Los Angeles: Tarcher, 1978).

22. National Center for Health Statistics, *Monthly Vital Statistics Report* 39, no. 12 (April 14, 1990): 13.

23. National Committee for Injury Prevention and Control, "Injury Prevention: Meeting the Challenge," *American Journal of Preventive Medicine*, 1989, pp. 252–260.

24. George Domino et al., "Collegiate Attitudes toward Suicide: New Zealand and United States," *Omega* 19, no. 4 (1988–1989): 351–364.

25. Fanice E. Egeland and James N. Sussex, "Suicide and Family Loading for Affective Disorders," *Journal of the American Medical Association* 254, no. 7 (1985).

26. Barrie R. Cassileth and James L. Stinnett, "Psychosocial Problems," in *Clinical Care of the Terminal Cancer Patient*, Barrie R. Cassileth et al. (eds.) (Philadelphia: Lea & Febiger, 1982): 108–118.

27. Kalish, op. cit.

28. L. A. DeSpelder and A. L. Strickland, *The Last Dance: Encountering Death and Dying* (Palo Alto, Calif.: Mayfield, 1983).

29. A. D. Weisman and J. Worden, "Psychosocial Analysis of Cancer Death," *Omega* 6, no. 61 (1975).

30. A. Gielen and K. A. Roche, "Death Anxiety and Psychometric Studies in Huntington's Disease," *Omega* 10, no. 2 (1979).

31. Barbara Ward, "Hospice Home Care Programs," *Nursing Outlook* (October 1978): 646–649; S. Malkin, "Care of the Terminally Ill at Home," *Canadian Medical Journal* 115 (July 1976): 129–130; Anthony Amado et al., "Cost of Terminal Care," *Nursing Outlook* (August 1979): 522–526; R. G. Benton, *Death and Dying: Principles and Practice in Patient Care* (New York: Van Nostrand Reinhold, 1978): 64–66.

32. Harry Hayman, "Some Legal Suggestions—Your Will," *Help Your Widow While She's Still Your Wife: A Guide to the Rights and Benefits of Widows* (Alexandria, Va.: Retired Officers Association, 1983).

33. R. A. Kalish and K. K. Reynolds, *Death and Ethnicity: A Psychocultural Study* (Farmingdale, N.Y.: Baywood, 1981).

34. DeSpelder and Strickland, op. cit.

35. Patrick Nowell-Smith, "Euthanasia and the Doctors—A Rejection of the BMA's Report," *Journal of Medical Ethics* 14 (1989): 124–128; J. Fletcher, "Ethics and Euthanasia" in *To Live and to Die*, R. Williams (ed.) (New York: Springer-Verlag, 1973).

36. Colleen Galambos, "Living Wills: A Choice for the Elderly," *Social Work* 3 (March 1989): 182–185.

37. Susan M. Wolf, "Holding the Line on Euthanasia," *Hastings Center Report*, special supplement (January–February 1989): 13–15.

38. Galambos, op. cit.

39. Christopher Bolton and Delpha J. Camp, "The Post-Funeral Ritual in Bereavement Counseling and Grief Work," *Journal of Gerontological Social Work* 13, no. 3/4 (1989): 49–59.

40. Rebecca A. Cohen, "The FTC Assault on the Cost of Dying," *Big Business and Society Review* 27 (Fall 1988): 48–53.

41. G. L. Engel, "A Unified Concept of Health and Disease," in *Life and Disease*, D. Ingle (ed.) (New York: Basic Books, 1963); J. Frederick, "Grief as a Disease Process," *Omega* 7 (1976): 297–306; W. E. Rees and S. G. Lutkins, "The Mortality of Bereavement," *British Medical Journal* 4 (1967): 13–16.

42. Jan Van Der Wal, "The Aftermath of Suicide: A Review of Empirical Evidence," *Omega* 20, no. 2 (1989–1990): 149–171.

43. Robert Weinbach, "Sudden Death and Secret Survivors: Helping Those Who Grieve Alone," *Social Work* 34 (January 1989): 57–60.

44. C. M. Parks, *Bereavement* (New York: International Universities Press, 1972).

45. I. O. Glick et al., *The First Year of Bereavement* (New York: Wiley-Interscience, 1974).

46. Dale Lund et al., "Stability of Social Support Networks After Later-Life Spousal Bereavement," *Death Studies* 14 (1990): 53–73.

47. Susan J. Souter and Timothy E. Moore, "A Bereavement Support Program for Survivors of Cancer Deaths: A Description and Evaluation," *Omega* 20, no. 1 (1989–1990): 31–43.

48. Van Der Wal, op. cit.

49. Weinbach, op. cit.

50. J. Bowlby, "Childhood Mourning and Its Implications for Psychiatry," *American Journal of Psychiatry* 118 (1961): 481–498; B. Raphael, *The Anatomy of Bereavement* (New York: Basic Books, 1983); M. W. Speece, "Research Plan: Preliminary Investigations—A Study of Young Children's Death and Death-Related Experiences," unpublished paper cited in DeSpelder and Strickland, op. cit.

51. E. F. Furman, *A Child's Parent Dies* (New Haven, Conn.: Yale University Press, 1974); Robert Bendiksen and Robert Fulton, "Death and the Child," *Omega* 6 (1975): 45–60.

52. Kalish, op. cit.

53. Nancy Feeley and Laurie Gottlieb, "Parents Coping and Communication following Their Infant's Death," *Omega* 19, no. 1 (1988–1989): 51–67.

54. Christine H. Littlefield and J. Philippe Rushton, "When a Child Dies: The Sociobiology of Bereavement," *Journal of Personality and Social Psychology* 51, no. 4 (1986): 797–802.

55. Sarah Brabant, "Old Pain or New Pain: A Social Psychological Approach to Recurrent Grief," *Omega* 20, no. 4 (1989–1990):273–279.

56. Brabant, op. cit.

57. Van Der Wal, op. cit.

58. Charles E. Hollingworth and Robert O. Pashaw, *The Family in Mourning: A Guide for Health Professionals* (New York: Grune and Stratton, 1977): 145–147; Benton, op. cit.

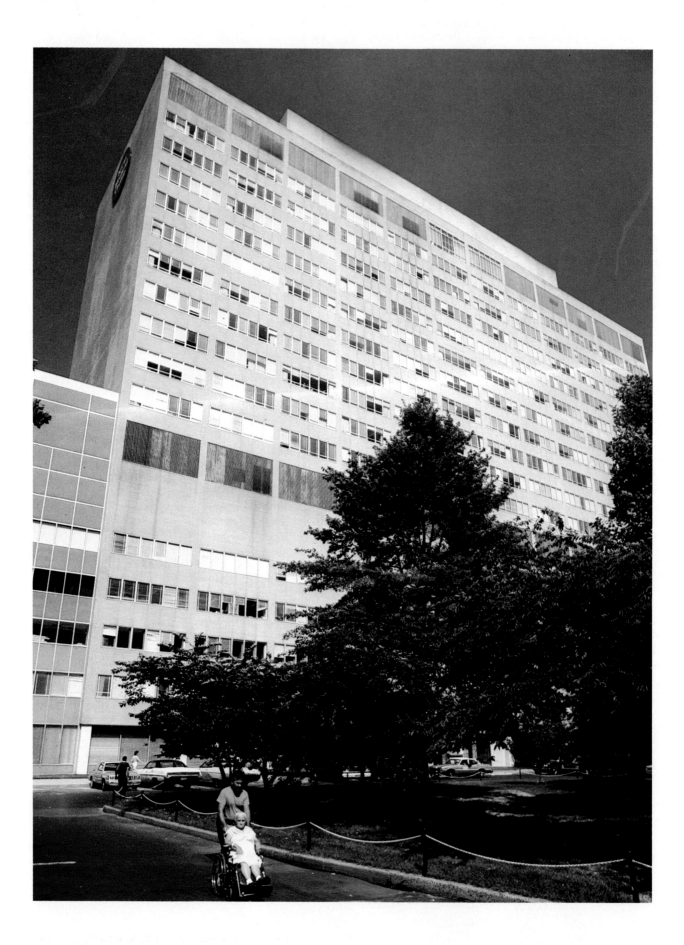

Chapter 19

Medical Care in America

To Guide Your Reading

When you have studied this chapter, you should be able to:

- Explain the importance of being health-activated and describe some of the basic attitudes, judgments, and types of action characteristic of health-activation.

- Describe important information needed for medical self-care, such as normal physiological data, the way to organize a medicine chest, the importance of physical examinations, and criteria for seeking medical help.

- Compare and contrast the different types of medical help available in the United States today, indicating factors to consider when choosing among them.

- Discuss different ways in which health care is financed in the United States and analyze some of the advantages and disadvantages of the available systems.

The saying "History repeats itself" may be appropriate in comparing the development of health care with the development of society in the United States. In the pioneer days, when many people were isolated from doctors because of an undeveloped system of transportation, self-reliance got them through most medical problems. At the turn of the twentieth century, with the development of modern transportation and medicines to cure or control many diseases, people began to rely passively and unquestioningly on doctors for medical treatment and cures for ailments. Today, a return to the earlier pattern is in evidence—a trend toward taking greater responsibility for one's own health and health care.

This greater self-responsibility has come about in part because more and more Americans are beginning to understand the value of good health and realize that they can do a great deal to promote their own health and well-being. People realize that their own actions can play an important role in preventing many health problems and in dealing with the minor problems that may arise.

Becoming Health-Activated

Although many people still equate health care with health professionals, increasing numbers of individuals want to become more active participants in their own care and treatment. Health care is no longer seen as the exclusive domain of doctors, nurses, and dentists but rather as something that each person has an interest in.[1]

This trend toward more active participation, or health-activation, reflects a spirit of self-reliance similar to that of the early pioneers. People are again taking some of the responsibility for health care into their own hands. They are becoming more confident about their own self-efficacy—their ability to take actions that affect their own lives and health.

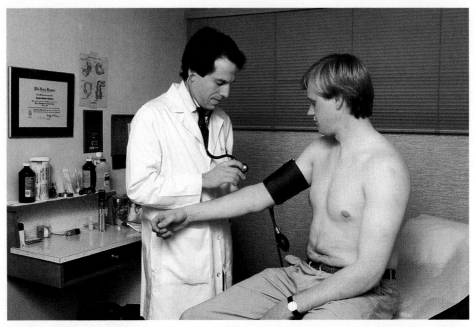

Health-activated people have regular physical examinations and seek the advice of a qualified doctor when health problems arise. (Hank Morgan/Science Source/Photo Researchers, Inc.)

While health-activated individuals assume more responsibility for their overall health, the goal is not to eliminate the role of health professionals. Rather, it is to know when to use those professionals, who to consult, and how to make the best use of medical advice and expertise.

Realizing the importance of what they can do for themselves, health-activated people want to learn what steps they should take to stay healthy, deal with medical problems that do not require professional attention, and manage small medical problems so that they do not become major ones. Some people regularly engage in aerobic exercise, eat low-fat and low-cholesterol foods, avoid tobacco, do not abuse alcohol and drugs, and practice stress management techniques. They are aware of the risk factors associated with lung cancer and cardiovascular disease and modify their health behaviors to reduce those risks and to enhance the quality of their lives. Health-activated people understand that many of the factors that affect health are under their control and that a healthier lifestyle is often the most effective way to ensure good health.

Judging Health Care Problems

People could save substantial amounts of time and money if they were able to distinguish between medical problems that require professional care and problems that can be treated at home.

Consider the time and money spent on professional treatment of minor ailments such as headaches, stomachaches, diarrhea, muscle aches and pains, mild fevers, and the common cold. These ailments usually run their course within a short period of time despite what a doctor may prescribe. Furthermore, some of these problems are caused by viruses that cannot be killed by antibiotics or other medicines. Doctors cannot cure such problems; they can only tell a patient what to do for himself or herself, such as rest or drink plenty of fluids. Health-activated people know what they can do for themselves to deal with the symptoms of such minor illnesses.

Being health-activated also includes using one's judgment to determine when to seek professional help. When a medical problem exceeds a person's skills, the tools or information available, or the support to deal with it, it is time to consult a health professional.[2] For example, a person with occasional indigestion—a feeling of stomach irritation, a burning sensation in the throat, or hyperacidity—has a common health problem that can be treated at home with over-the-counter antacids. However, repeated indigestion over a long period and additional symptoms such as blood in the stool constitute a cause for concern. A health-activated person recognizes unusual, uncommon, or truly alarming symptoms and acts promptly to get appropriate professional treatment or advice.

Health-activated people know when to seek medical advice, but they are also aware that the final decision on health matters is their own. They have an understanding of health matters and are ready to question the advice and recommendations of health professionals, and they do not commit themselves in advance to follow a doctor's orders. If they are unsure about a doctor's opinion on a serious matter, they are not afraid to seek a second opinion from another practitioner.[3]

Second opinions are required by some insurance companies before expensive procedures are performed.

Judging Health Products and Treatments

Today's health-conscious consumer is inundated with information on a broad range of health care topics and issues. While this plethora of information is useful in helping people become health-activated, it may also cause confusion and indecision. Various and often conflicting studies and opinions make it difficult to know what to believe about health care issues. A major goal of this text is to help provide insight into many of these issues.

The same is true regarding health care products and methods of treatment. When seeking an over-the-counter (OTC) drug to relieve cold symptoms, a consumer may feel overwhelmed by the vast array of medications for sale. People face similarly difficult choices when they consider alternative methods of treatment. In treating a backache, for example, a person can choose among rest, exercise, various medications, and a variety of relaxation techniques.

A health-activated individual considers the various alternatives and chooses what seems to be most appropriate for his or her needs, based on as much information as possible. This may mean choosing among several OTC medications or taking no medications at all, treating oneself or seeing a doctor, and seeking a second opinion or getting advice from a practitioner of an alternative method of treatment.[4]

Many newspapers and periodicals carry regular features about the human body and health care. New discoveries are continually made in medical science. Reading reports about them can be especially valuable after you have developed a basic understanding from courses such as this one.

People with colds usually do not need to see a doctor unless the symptoms are severe or persist for a long time. If you have confidence in your ability to recognize minor illnesses, it is usually possible to cure yourself at home. (Mary Kate Denny/PhotoEdit)

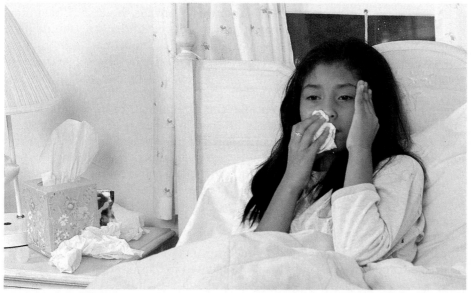

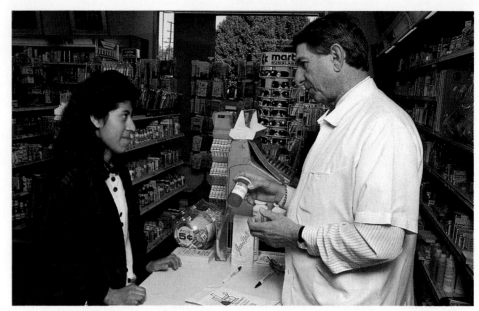

A wise consumer consults a pharmacist about the helpful and harmful effects of drugs and possible interactions with other medicines. (Bill Aron/PhotoEdit)

Selecting Medications One area of choice for consumers concerns OTC medications. With so many brands and varieties available, the health-activated individual considers carefully before choosing a medication to relieve the symptoms of a minor illness. This means thinking about the symptoms to be relieved, reading labels on medications, and perhaps speaking to a pharmacist or consulting a reference book about drugs and medications. Taking these steps allows an individual to choose the OTC medication that is most likely to meet his or her needs.

Another area of choice concerns the use of prescription drugs, specifically the use of brand-name versus generic drugs. When a company develops a new drug, it is given the exclusive right to market that medication under its brand name for up to 14 years. During this time the drug is available only in the brand-name form. When this period ends, other companies can begin producing the drug under a **generic name**—the name of the chemical ingredient in the drug—or under their own brand names.

generic name—*the name of the chemical ingredient in a drug.*

While generic drugs are supposed to meet the same federal standards for safety, purity, and effectiveness that apply to brand-name drugs, there have been recent controversies about whether this is always the case. Consumers should be wary of any drugs that are not produced under strict guidelines.

Since generic drugs are often less expensive than brand-name drugs, they can save consumers money. However, the decision whether to use them instead of brand-name drugs requires some research by the consumer. The primary resource, of course, is the physician who prescribes the drug, but health-activated individuals often take the time to gather information from other sources as well. Pharmacists, with their knowledge of drugs and access to drug information, are an excellent source of information and advice. A trip to the public library to glance through reference books on drugs and medications can provide the consumer with important information for making a decision. With this information in hand, the health-activated individual is better able to question a physician about the benefits of a particular brand-name versus generic drug.

"Caveat emptor" (buyer beware) is as good a motto for the health-activated consumer as it is for anyone planning to purchase goods or services in the United States.

Avoiding Medical Quackery Sometimes people's fear of pain, illness, or death leads them to seek help from unqualified practitioners who sell miracle cures or treatments that are painless and fully guaranteed. Driven by the desire for profit, these medical quacks urge patients to trust them rather than rely on competent health professionals.

Evaluating information about types of medical treatment can help people avoid quackery and save them not only money but their lives. While most quack cures are harmless, some of the products and treatments offered by quacks are harmful; some are deadly. All are expensive and represent a needless cost.

The best way for people to protect themselves against quackery is to learn what *does* work and learn how quacks work, too. Quackery often follows certain patterns. People should beware of the following:

The most troubling problem with quackery is that it delays access to the health care that is needed. Such delays can worsen the course of a disease or even turn out to be fatal.

- A product or service that claims to be battling the medical profession, which is supposedly suppressing the discovery
- A remedy sold door to door, advertised at public lectures, or promoted in sensational magazines or by crusading organizations
- People who employ scare tactics in trying to promote their products or treatments
- The use of unsubstantiated "testimonials" that claim that a product or service has done wonders for others
- A product or service that claims to be good for a vast array of illnesses or is guaranteed to provide a quick cure

A health-activated person does not rely on such self-serving claims. Good and reliable information on products and types of treatment is available from licensed physicians; the U.S. Food and Drug Administration (FDA), which was created to protect consumers against unsafe and ineffective products; the Federal Trade Commission (FTC), which warns consumers about false advertising; the U.S. Postal Service, which guards against the sale of fraudulent products by mail; and the Consumers Union, which impartially tests and rates consumer products.

Of course, no agency is infallible. The FDA approved certain food additives and preservatives that were shown later to have carcinogenic properties (Red Dye No. 2 and nitrites added to smoked meats).

Medical Self-Care

In addition to judging health care problems and making choices about the use of medications and medical treatment, health-activated people are able to take care of some of their own medical needs. Through caring for themselves, people gain greater knowledge about their bodies and how they function. This helps them develop a sense of power over their bodies and makes them realize that health is largely a matter of how they care for themselves.[5]

Medical self-care allows people to utilize skills, information, and insight to deal with minor medical problems that do not require a physician. Carrying out medical self-care responsibly includes monitoring one's own health, being prepared to deal with minor problems at home, and knowing when to suspend self-care and seek the help of a health professional.[6]

An important outgrowth of self-care is the self-testing items available to interested consumers. Devices to measure blood pressure, analyze blood sugar levels, diagnose pregnancy, predict ovulation, and test for colorectal cancer are available. Pharmaceutical companies are testing others, including one for calculating cholesterol levels. Self-tests should be performed in conjunction with regular medical care, not used as a substitute for it.

Measuring Your Body's Physiological Data

How does a person know when he or she has a medical problem? One indication is whether the person's condition seems different from "normal." This can be determined by measuring some basic physiological data. Each individual has certain normal, or baseline, measurements, including temperature, respiration, pulse, and blood pressure. When these measurements differ from what is normal, it is an indication that something may be wrong.

Temperature, Respiration, and Pulse The 98.6 degrees Fahrenheit (37 degrees Celsius) body temperature that is usually considered normal is only a statistical average. A person's normal temperature can vary a degree or two on either side, depending on the individual, the time of day, and other fac-

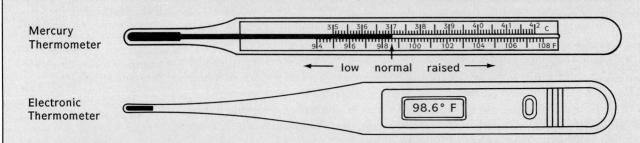

Mercury
Thermometer

Electronic
Thermometer

98.6° F

← low normal raised →

Figure 19.1 Always compare temperatures taken by the same method. Axillary (under the arm) readings are lower than oral readings, which are lower than rectal readings. To measure oral temperature with a mercury thermometer, do the following: 1. Clean the thermometer. 2. Shake it down below 95°F (35°C). 3. Place it under the tongue and hold it in place with the tongue and lips. Allow 3 to 5 minutes to register. 4. With the light to your back, slowly turn the thermometer until the silver band of mercury is magnified against the white background. Read to the nearest 0.2°F or 0.1°C.

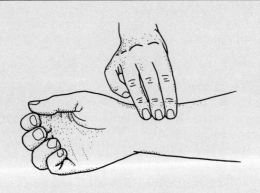

Figure 19.2 Measure pulse rates at rest. 1. Place the index and middle fingers along the line of the artery, on the thumb side of the wrist. (Never use your own thumb to measure someone else's pulse; you may feel your own pulse instead.) 2. Count the beats of the pulse for half a minute and multiply by two.

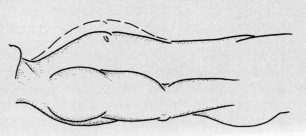

DESCRIBING ABNORMAL BREATHING
Unusually deep breathing
Unusually shallow breathing
Difficulty in breathing when lying down
Waking up unable to breathe
Excessive sighing and yawning
Noisy, wheezy, or bubbly breathing
Wheezing with difficulty exhaling (a sign of asthma)

Figure 19.3 Respiration rate is the number of times the chest rises and falls in 1 minute. The normal adult rate is 12 to 19 breaths a minute; the normal infant rate is 30 to 40. Observe respiration rates at rest for consistency. Also note any abnormal breathing and be prepared to describe the condition and onset to your doctor.

tors, such as a woman's menstrual cycle. A variation greater than that, however, usually suggests infection (Figure 19.1).

Pulse, or heartbeat, is affected by age, physical exertion, stress, and, of course, cardiovascular disease. The pulse rate also may be affected by emotions, pain, sex, and body composition. In nearly all people, the pulse rate tends to rise with fever. In a healthy adult at rest, the heart normally beats 60 to 90 times a minute. For athletes the rate may be as low as 40 to 60 beats a minute, and for young children it may be as high as 90 to 120 beats a minute (Figure 19.2).

The normal range for an adult's respiration is 12 to 19 breaths a minute; this rate can change as a result of strenuous activity or emotional tension as well as illness. It is also important to learn the *sound* of one's normal respiration. If respiration seems to be shallower or deeper than normal or if unusual noises are associated with it, this is an indication that something may be wrong (Figure 19.3).

Blood Pressure Blood pressure is affected by several factors, including the strength and speed of the heartbeat, the total blood volume, and the condition of the arteries. Blood pressure measurements consist of two figures, the systolic and diastolic rates, which are expressed as a fraction, with the systolic pressure on top. (A reading of 120/80 is read as 120 over 80.)

Blood pressure can vary considerably depending on the individual and on age; pressures generally increase as people age. Normal systolic pressure ranges from about 110 or lower to about 140 or higher; diastolic, from about 60 to 90. A reading of 120/80 is considered ideal in a healthy young adult.

Blood pressure can also vary with the time of day and with circumstances. Tension, excitement, weight gain, kidney disease, hormonal malfunction, and other events may cause blood pressure to rise; malnutrition, injury, extensive bleeding, and a number of illnesses can cause it to fall.

Among all physiological data, blood pressure is perhaps the most important item to measure regularly. As stated in earlier chapters, hypertension has been called the silent killer because it rarely produces noticeable symptoms before the damage is done.

The Home Medicine Chest

One aspect of medical self-care is administering OTC medications or employing simple treatments when one is dealing with minor illnesses or injuries. In these instances, people generally reach into the medicine chest to find what they need.

A properly stocked medicine chest should contain medical supplies for treating minor ills that do not require a doctor's care (Table 19.1). In stocking a medicine chest, however, it is important to consider individual health care needs as well. A person who has never had a problem with constipation probably has little need to keep a laxative on hand. Such considerations are especially important when one is purchasing medications that have an expiration date or may be hazardous to children. It makes little sense to purchase items that may lose their effectiveness before they are used or may be dangerous.

The FDA recommends the following safety measures for the safe storage of medications:

- Date all OTC drugs to indicate when they were purchased.
- Buy medicines and health supplies in realistic quantities—only enough for your immediate needs.

Table 19.1 Basics for the Home Medicine Chest

Nondrug Items	Drug Items
Adhesive bandages (assorted sizes)	Analgesic (aspirin, acetaminophen, ibuprofen); all reduce fever and pain, but only aspirin reduces inflammation
Sterile gauze (pads and a roll)	
Absorbent cotton	
Adhesive tape	Emetic to induce vomiting (syrup of ipecac and activated charcoal)
Elastic bandage	
Small, blunt-end scissors	Antacid for stomach upset
Tweezers	Antiseptic solution for cleaning minor wounds
Fever thermometer (rectal for young child)	Cortisone cream for skin inflammation and rash
Hot water bottle	Calamine lotion for poison ivy, insect bites, and other skin irritations
Heating pad	
Eye cup (for flushing objects out of the eye)	Petroleum jelly for dry skin and diaper rash
Ice bag	Antidiarrhetic
Dosage spoon (household teaspoons are rarely the correct size)	Cough syrup (nonsuppressant type)
Vaporizer or humidifier	Decongestant
First-aid manual	Burn ointment
Plus other supplies and medicines as common sense and family needs dictate	

Source: Adapted from *FDA Consumer.*

In the case of prescribed antibiotics, there should be no leftovers. Although people may stop taking them once they feel better, this is unwise because the infection may recur unless the medication is finished.

- Store all drugs out of the reach of small children, locked up if necessary.
- Read labels carefully and observe all warnings and cautions.
- Do not use medicine from an unlabeled bottle. Transparent tape over a label will keep the label from wearing or washing off.
- Do not administer medicine in the dark; the label may be difficult to read clearly.
- Pay attention when measuring drugs.
- Do not take several drugs at the same time without consulting a physician or asking a pharmacist about possible drug interactions.
- Remove leftovers regularly, especially prescription drugs used for a prior illness.
- Flush discarded drugs down the toilet and dispose of their containers so that children will not have access to them.

Always take special care before administering drugs or other products from a medicine chest, especially to young children or elderly persons. A small mistake in dosage can be very harmful to a child or older adult. It is best to ask a doctor before giving medicine to young children or the elderly, a pregnant or nursing mother, or anyone who has a chronic health condition. Also, always ask a doctor or pharmacist about possible drug interactions with other medicines or foods before administering any type of medication to someone who is already taking another drug, whether prescription or nonprescription.

Physical Examinations

An occult blood test detects hidden blood in the stool, indicating a need for further testing for colon cancer. The test results can also indicate ulcer formation, hemorrhoids, inflammation of the bowels, diverticulitis, and polyp and tumor growth.

While "norms" such as temperature, pulse, and blood pressure can be monitored by individuals, other norms can be established only through physical examinations by a physician. Moreover, taking responsibility for scheduling regular physical examinations is an important activity done by health-activated individuals who monitor their health.

Physical examinations can vary considerably in complexity, from those involving extensive screening, questioning, and laboratory and monitoring tests to much simpler exams involving only a few key tests and observations (Table 19.2). The nature of the exam depends on variables such as age, current

Table 19.2 Typical HMO Procedures. A thorough health screening identifies potential risks. Periodic physical examinations add and update information

Health Screen		Physical Examination Schedule[a]		
Medical history	Assesses past and present health status	Age	Interval	
Health risk appraisal	Lifestyle screening identifies controllable health risks	19–29	6 years	
		30–39	4 years	
Height, weight, blood pressure, and pulse rate	Determines current status	40–49	3 years	
		50–59	2 years	
Noncontact tonometry	Screens for glaucoma	60+	Physician's discretion	
Electrocardiogram (ECG)	Records heart function			
Analysis of body composition	Determines muscle, fat, and water mass	**Routine Tests for Women**[a]		
Laboratory testing		Mammogram	Age	Interval
Blood work	Measures cholesterol, glucose, hemoglobin, hematocrit, and factors which reflect liver and kidney function		35–39	once
			40–49	2 years
			50+	yearly
Urinalysis	Reflects kidney, bladder, and systemic functioning	Pap test	all	yearly
Stool analysis	For patients over 40: assesses risk of colon cancer			

[a] *Examination intervals recommended by HIP/Rutgers Health Plan, a health maintenance organization in New Jersey.*

Source: Wellness Works, RCHP Health Screen Rutgers Community Health Plan, A Division of HIP/Rutgers Health Plan ©1986.

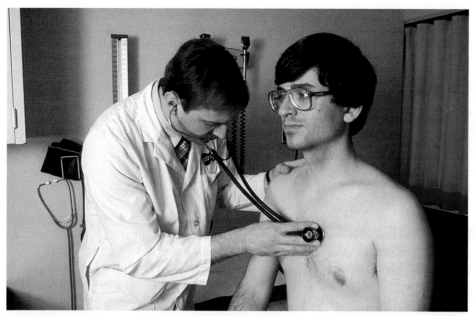

An annual physical examination by a qualified physician is a necessary aspect of maintaining good health. (SIU/Photo Researchers, Inc.)

health, and symptoms or problems. For example, people over age 50 should have an annual colorectal test for occult blood. Periodic examinations are very important because of their greater potential for spotting adverse conditions before they become serious.

Frequency of Physical Examinations   There is little agreement among physicians and professional medical associations about the optimum frequency of physical examinations.

A general rule of thumb is that as people grow older, regular physical examinations have a greater potential for detecting adverse health conditions. While young, people should have enough physical examinations to establish what is normal for them. The American Medical Association recommends an examination every year or two between ages 2 and 20. Between ages 20 and 30, routine annual examinations rarely reveal a new illness. In these age groups, it is probably better to wait until unusual symptoms appear and then respond promptly by visiting a physician. Exceptions include pregnant women and people with chronic diseases. At all ages, people who have abnormal symptoms, have existing medical problems, or are taking a prescribed medication should have physical examinations as often as recommended by their physicians.

What Is Tested   A basic part of a physical examination is a blood pressure test to check for hypertension, which usually does not manifest itself with overt symptoms. The physician may also request a urine sample to test for signs of bladder and kidney infection or diabetes and a blood test to determine the blood count and cholesterol, glucose, and triglyceride levels. In addition, during a physical examination the doctor will generally listen to the heart and lungs, look in the throat and check the thyroid and neck area for enlarged or tender lymph nodes, and feel the abdomen to detect tumors, enlargement of organs, or tender areas.

Beyond those basic procedures, the tests performed depend on factors such as sex, age, medical history, and risk factors for developing a particular disease. A woman with a family history of breast cancer may be a candidate for an annual *mammogram* (breast x-ray); a person who smokes may see a doctor more frequently for diagnostic tests to detect lung cancer.

For people past age 40, an electrocardiogram may be included in examinations to diagnose heart problems. An ECG is also recommended for people who experience shortness of breath, chest pain, or faintness and people starting a strenuous exercise program.[7]

The American Cancer Society recommends that women age 20 to 40 with no abnormal symptoms have a breast exam by a physician every 3 years, a self-exam every month, and a baseline mammogram between ages 35 and 39. In addition to monthly self-exams, women age 40 and over and women who have had a hysterectomy and are taking estrogen supplementation should have a professional breast exam every year and a mammogram every 1 to 2 years for those 40 to 49 and every year for those age 50 and over (when the risk of developing breast cancer is increased).[8]

Women who are or have been sexually active or have reached age 18 should have an annual pelvic exam and Pap test to check for cervical cancer. If a woman has had three or more consecutive satisfactory annual exams, the Pap test may be performed less often at the discretion of the physician.[9]

To help reduce the risk of prostate cancer, it is recommended that men receive an annual rectal exam beginning at age 40. These exams are also recommended for both men and women over age 40 to test for colon and rectal cancer. Men should also have a testicular exam as part of a regular physical examination in addition to monthly testicular self-exams.[10]

Apart from regular physical examinations, regular dental checkups and eye examinations are an important aspect of medical care. Dental exams are necessary to take care of routine dental concerns and detect gum disease and oral cancer. Regular eye exams, while important for testing visual acuity, can also reduce the risk of contracting *glaucoma,* a condition of increased pressure within the eyeball that can lead to blindness. The eyes should be checked for glaucoma every 2 years after age 35.

When to Seek Professional Help

Remind yourself of the warning signs of particular diseases, for example, cancer (Chapter 12). Look for the following signs:

- *Change in bowel or bladder habits*
- *A sore that does not heal*
- *Unusual bleeding or discharge*
- *Thickening or lump in the breast or elsewhere*
- *Indigestion or difficulty in swallowing*
- *Obvious change in a wart or mole*
- *Nagging cough or hoarseness*

The need for routine physical examinations varies, but people should not delay in seeking professional help if they experience persistent, severe, or unusual symptoms or medical problems. Greater self-reliance should *not* lead individuals to ignore such things or try to deal with them themselves. Certain symptoms are associated with potentially serious problems, such as cardiovascular disease, stroke, and cancer (Chapters 10 through 12). A health-activated person recognizes these symptoms and responds to them quickly by seeking professional medical help.

In addition to the symptoms associated with certain diseases, there are certain emergency situations in which a person should see a physician immediately. Aside from obvious situations such as massive bleeding that cannot be stopped, major burns, suspected broken bones, and suspected poisoning, immediate medical help is necessary if a person:

- Is in severe pain
- Has cold sweats, particularly if combined with light-headedness or chest or abdominal pain
- Is short of breath at rest (if not because of simple exertion)
- Is unconscious or in a stupor
- Is so disoriented that he or she cannot describe what has happened or say his or her name or whereabouts

Knowledge about when to see a physician and when and how to treat minor medical problems at home is an important aspect of medical self-care, but it is not the only one. Health-activated individuals are also very familiar with the professional health care system and are concerned about evaluating the health care providers and institutions they go to for help.

Health Care Providers and Institutions

The body is a resilient organism. In some situations it can gather all its resources to heal itself or set things right again. At other times individuals can help restore or maintain their own health through medical self-care. Sometimes, however, people and their bodies need the kind of help that only health care professionals or institutions can provide.

Physicians and Dentists

There has been a significant trend in the United States toward a decline in the number of physicians in general practice and a rise in the number specializing

Figure 19.4 People usually start by going to a primary-care physician, who may refer them to a specialist if necessary. In addition to those shown below, there are pediatric specialists, geriatric specialists, and physicians who focus on particular types of testing and treatments. To qualify as experts in particular areas, doctors need additional years of training.

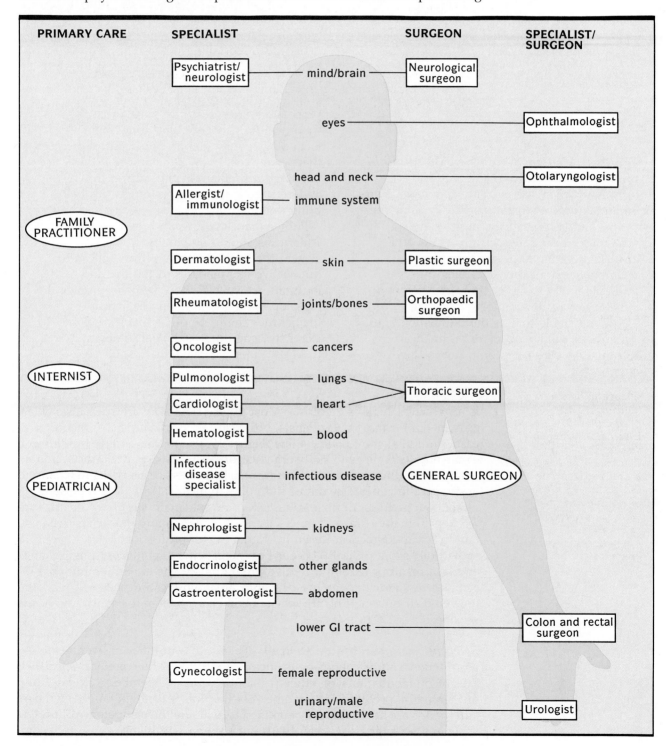

Can the United States Afford High-Quality Health Care for Everyone?

Health care costs have been rising at a rate of two and a half to three times the rate of inflation, resulting in sharp increases in medical insurance costs and a swelling number of uninsured Americans. This has caused a growing ethical debate about the use of expensive medical technologies. Two sides of this debate are presented below. The first speaker argues that a patient's health must be of paramount concern and that cost should not influence when and to whom health care services are available. The second speaker disagrees, arguing that it is time for the medical community and society to establish criteria that limit the use of costly procedures.

The Best Medical Care Must Be Available for Everyone Advances in medical technology over the past 40 years have been breathtaking—neonatal, pediatric, pulmonary, cardiac, and surgical care units; genetic screening; renal dialysis; transplants and artificial organs. Although these new technologies are expensive, they must be available to everyone or there is a risk of developing an unfair medical system.

It is inevitable that as the population ages, Americans will spend more on medical resources to care for people late in their lives.

Medical writers are already discussing "successful cost-containment strategies" that consider health care for the elderly in light of what society can "afford." That is not equitable, since health is a basic right of all people. No one should have the right to withhold care for any reason, including a person's age. Medical decisions must rest with the patient.

Instead of curtailing the use of medical technology, Americans should use it for all it is worth so that the level of health in this nation can be improved. After all, new procedures often result in substantial savings by preventing surgery, and innovative technologies may identify and control diseases that would cost many times more if they remained a problem in the future. In addition, greater use of resources can help bring down costs.

Rather than focusing on how to limit care, Americans should streamline a wasteful system that has too many redundant and duplicative technologies in too many locations. Hospitals often compete to have the most up-to-date equipment; as a result, in major cities there are often seven or eight expensive computerized axial tomography (CAT) scanners or magnetic resonance

in a particular type of medicine. Most physicians today are specialists: allergists, pediatricians, gynecologists, obstetricians, cardiologists, surgeons, and gastroenterologists, to name a few (Figure 19.4). The same trend is often true of dentists as well, with oral surgeons, orthodontists, periodontists, and so on. This trend has resulted in fewer medical professionals who are willing to deal with the general health of the population.

Another trend is an increasing lack of an adequate supply of health care workers in many rural and inner-city areas, where many physicians are hesitant to set up a practice. Recently, young health professionals have begun to spread out geographically because of increasing competition in major cities and as a result of federal incentive programs. However, until additional incentives are provided for moving into areas where the need is great, the uneven distribution of health services will be a problem for many Americans seeking access to health care.

Selecting a Physician or Dentist There are a number of avenues to explore when you are choosing a doctor, dentist, or other medical specialist. The recommendations of others, including family members, friends, and other medical professionals, can be very helpful. (Although family members and friends are not necessarily qualified to evaluate the competence of professionals, their suggestions can be useful.) When one is receiving the recom-

imaging (MRI) systems within blocks of one another.

As a democratic and caring society, the United States must focus on the aspects of health care reform that will guarantee equal access to medical care for all its citizens.

It Is Time to Limit the Use of Expensive Medical Procedures Health care costs exploded 51 percent between 1984 and 1989, largely because of the use of new technologies in medicine. It is time to admit that this country cannot afford everything that medical science has invented and make some hard choices about how available technologies should be used.

The trustees of a Boston hospital made such a choice several years ago when they decided not to establish a heart transplant program. They weighed the value of saving an estimated six lives per year against the economic effect of the program on all other hospital patients and the effect on cardiovascular death in the entire society. They correctly evaluated a new and costly technology on the basis of the greatest good for the greatest number and allocated their resources guided by conscious social policy rather than emotion.

As the population grows older, Americans must recognize that many procedures, such as providing chemotherapy for 90-year-old patients with metastatic cancer, prolong dying without prolonging life and merely provide expensive deaths. Health economist Victor Fuchs calls this "the flat curve of medicine" and believes that money is better spent for prenatal care and preventive health care.

Although Americans can take great pride in the array of medical technologies they have developed, it is time to be realistic and develop a policy that allocates resources in a way that provides the most health care for the most people at a reasonable cost.

Costly high-tech care has been described as both a boon and a curse to this society because although it performs miracles, it prolongs dying and consumes resources desperately needed in other parts of the health care system. As a society, how can the United States reconcile this dilemma? Do you agree that there should be guidelines for the use of certain expensive procedures? In a rapidly aging society, should there be limits to health care for the elderly. Why or why not?

Ideas based on Richard Lamm and Duane Bluemke, "High-Tech Healthcare and Society's Ability to Pay," *Healthcare Financial Management* (September 1, 1990).

mendations of another person, it is important to ask why that person has recommended a particular professional. What one person may consider a good quality in a physician or dentist is not necessarily something another person will find appealing.

In some places, free referral services offer the names of physicians on staff at affiliated medical centers. This can be an important source, especially for people who have already chosen a medical center to use in case of illness. Some referral services also provide information about the qualifications of particular doctors, including their medical education and number of years in practice.

Inquiries at the nearest accredited hospital or dental school can uncover a list of the names of qualified physicians and dentists who practice there, as can talking to the nurses and staff physicians (residents) at those institutions. County medical and dental societies often provide the names (but no evaluations) of local doctors or dentists.

Directories available in most libraries can be used to find out about a physician's educational background, training, and other credentials. The *Directory of Medical Specialists*, published by the American Medical Association, lists physicians, by state, who are certified by the professional boards of their specialties. The American Dental Association publishes a similar directory of dentists.

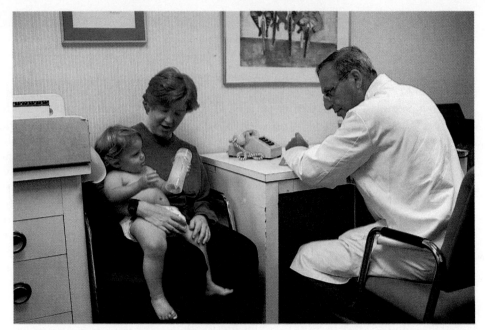

Found mostly in rural areas, single-doctor clinics can provide excellent basic medical care, though they do not provide the extensive medical services available at larger medical groups with several specialists. (Robert Brenner/PhotoEdit)

After you have compiled a list of possibilities, the next step is to call the physicians' or dentists' offices and ask questions about fees, the average waiting period for a visit, board certification, and the availability of the doctors or dentists in case of emergency.

The last step in selecting a health professional is to make an appointment. After that visit, a person can decide whether he or she would feel comfortable entrusting his or her health care to the doctor or dentist. The visit can also reveal something about the professional's philosophy of health care and professional manner, including provider-client interactions. If the doctor or dentist does not seem right, it is always possible to choose someone else.

It is much better to be vigilant before receiving treatment than to discover problems afterwards. Medical malpractice suits can provide only compensation to a patient, never a cure. Others are also hurt because doctors and hospitals must buy malpractice insurance and will often call for more tests and documents to guard against litigation. All of these are factors in the rising cost of medical care in the United States.

Assessing Medical and Dental Care Although many people do not agree with whatever a doctor or dentist says, health-activated people use professional medical advice as one of many sources of guidance.[11] If they are not satisfied with a doctor or dentist's performance or attitude, they consider finding another one. Health-activated people evaluate the care their medical professionals are providing, taking into account that a good doctor or dentist should do the following:

- Emphasize preventive medicine, ask about lifestyle, and make suggestions for improvement
- Take a careful medical history, listen to complaints, and answer questions and explain procedures in nontechnical language
- Take the time to do a thorough exam
- Welcome a second opinion, especially if surgery or an extensive procedure may be necessary
- Not keep the patient waiting for a long period
- Maintain a courteous and nonjudgmental attitude

Communicating with Doctors and Dentists People naturally prefer medical professionals who communicate clearly and respectfully, avoid jargon, explain things well, and keep interruptions to a minimum. They want medical professionals to show respect by listening without interruption, making eye contact, and responding directly to spoken and implied questions.[12] Communication is a two-way street, however. The way in which a patient responds is also important in building a working relationship with a doctor or dentist.

Patients have a responsibility to provide accurate information and communicate clearly with a doctor or dentist. For example, describing symptoms concisely and clearly is very important, as is providing information about allergies, medications being taken, and changes in habits or behaviors that may be associated with the health problem being investigated.

Patients also have a responsibility to ask questions so that they understand the diagnosis and treatment. This includes asking about the medications prescribed, how and when to take them, and what side effects may exist. It also includes asking what a particular treatment involves, why it may be necessary, and whether there are alternatives.

Be prepared for a meeting with a doctor, perhaps with a list of detailed symptoms, current medications and allergies, and questions to ask. It is vital that patients understand what a medical professional has said before leaving the office, clinic, or hospital. However, do not hesitate to call back with other important information or questions at a later time.

Hospitals and Clinics

Hospitals and clinics play a crucial role in the health care system. With their large staffs, high-tech diagnostic equipment, advanced life-support systems, and great variety of services, most hospitals can provide every type of medical care. Medicenters and clinics, while usually not as well equipped as hospitals, can provide specialized care from same-day minor surgery to treatment of emergencies such as broken bones. However, since medicenters and clinics usually lack advanced life-support systems, high-risk patients are probably better off going to a hospital even for a minor procedure.[13]

Assessing Health Care Institutions Just as with health professionals, it makes good sense to evaluate a health care institution before using it. Brochures and other materials describing services, staff, and policies are available from many health care institutions; they can be an important source of information in making an evaluation. The opinions of personal doctors, family members, and friends can also be useful.

Many medicenters specialize in a particular branch of medicine. For example, sports medicine centers are being established in many communities, offering a full range of orthopedic services. (Alan Felix/Medical Images, Inc.)

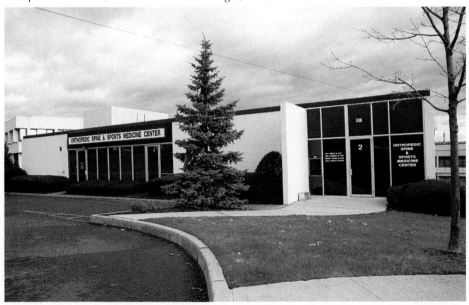

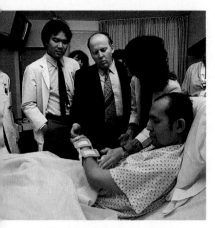

Teaching hospitals attract students and give them superior training, and so medical care in such hospitals is usually the best. (Tom Tracy/MediChrome)

When you are trying to evaluate an institution, there are a number of issues to consider. The care received at a clinic, medicenter, or hospital has much to do with the medical professionals who work there. Therefore, in selecting a health care facility, it is important to find out about the physicians on staff. Hospital affiliation is an important consideration, since having hospital privileges is a sign of professional achievement and trust.

Another important consideration in selecting a health care facility is the fee structure. Some clinics require patients to pay for services and submit their own claims for insurance reimbursement. Others wait for insurance reimbursement and then bill for noncovered expenses.

Evaluating the safety of health care institutions is also important. Some hospitals have a history of patients becoming ill from doctor-caused (iatrogenic) or hospital-originated (nosocomial) infections. In others, doctors may be more likely to perform nonessential surgery or may be less experienced in performing the type of surgery a patient requires.[14]

One of the first things a person should find out about a hospital is whether it is accredited by the Joint Commission on Accreditation of Hospitals (JCAH). The JCAH is a professional group that sets minimum standards for hospital performance and confers accreditation only to institutions that meet those standards. There are a number of additional guidelines for choosing a good hospital, among which are the following:

- The best hospitals are often teaching hospitals that are affiliated with respected medical schools and have full "house staffs" of interns and residents.
- Good hospitals offer a wide range of services, including an x-ray laboratory, intensive care units, coronary care units, a postoperative recovery room, an emergency room, an outpatient department, a blood bank, and a pathology laboratory.
- Good hospitals have board-certified physicians in a broad range of specialty areas, such as internists, surgeons, neurologists, and psychiatrists.
- Good hospitals regularly assess the quality of their own care; for example, a committee of physicians regularly reveiws the hospital's surgical cases to make sure that all surgery performed is necessary and appropriate.

It was not until the beginning of the twentieth century that hospitals came to be regarded as places where sick people could get proper care and have a chance to recover. Before that time hospitals served primarily as havens for the homeless, the destitute, and people with diseases considered hopeless and were generally run by religious organizations. Patients usually were placed two or three to a bed, and sanitation was virtually unknown, so infection was common. Medical discoveries such as the germ theory of disease, antisepsis, and anesthesia led to safer methods of practicing medicine, and the view of a hospital as a place for healing emerged.

Dealing with Health Care Institutions One major mistake a hospitalized patient can easily make is to give up control over his or her health care. The patient should be sure to maintain an active role in making decisions about hospital care. If the patient is unable to speak for himself or herself, a family member should act on his or her behalf.

Probably the most common complaint about the quality of medical care today concerns the dehumanization of treatment. Patients are sometimes annoyed by curtness on the part of the hospital staff, complaining of being treated as a diseased organ rather than a whole person. There are instances when patients who want to know are not given adequate explanations of their condition, the procedures being used to diagnose it, or the risks involved in a certain course of treatment. Directions for taking drugs and information about their side effects may be inadequate as well. In an effort to improve these aspects of patient care, the American Hospital Association has issued a "patient's bill of rights," which lists the rights hospital patients should demand (Table 19.3).

Complementary Approaches to Health Care

What can a patient do when conventional medical techniques and procedures have not been successful? What can someone do to enhance the care received from a doctor? For some people, the answers to these questions may be found in the growing trend toward the use of nonconventional therapies such as osteopathy, chiropractic, homeopathy, and acupuncture. Because the trend is

Table 19.3 Patient's Bill of Rights

1. The patient has the right to considerate and respectful care.

2. The patient has the right to obtain from his or her physician complete current information concerning his or her diagnosis, treatment, and prognosis in terms the patient can reasonably be expected to understand. When it is not medically advisable to give such information to the patient, the information should be made available to an appropriate person on the patient's behalf. The patient has the right to know, by name, the physician responsible for coordinating his or her care.

3. The patient has the right to receive from his or her physician information necessary to allow for informed consent before the start of any procedure or treatment. Except in emergencies, such information for informed consent should include but not necessarily be limited to the specific procedure and/or treatment, the medically significant risks involved, and the probable duration of incapacitation. Where medically significant alternatives for care or treatment exist or when the patient requests information concerning medical alternatives, the patient has the right to such information. The patient also has the right to know the name of the person responsible for the procedures and/or treatment.

4. The patient has the right to refuse treatment to the extent permitted by law and to be informed of the medical consequences of his or her action.

5. The patient has the right to every consideration of his or her privacy concerning his or her own medical care program. Case discussion, consultation, examination, and treatment are confidential and should be conducted discreetly. Those not directly involved in his or her care must have the permission of the patient to be present.

6. The patient has the right to expect that all communications and records pertaining to his or her care will be treated as confidential.

7. The patient has the right to expect that within its capacity a hospital must make a reasonable response to the request of a patient for services. The hospital must provide evaluation, service, and/or referral as indicated by the urgency of the case. When medically permissible, a patient may be transferred to another facility after he or she has received completed information and an explanation concerning the need for and alternatives to such a transfer. The institution to which the patient is to be transferred must first have accepted the patient for transfer.

8. The patient has the right to obtain information about any relationship of the hospital to other health care and educational institutions insofar as his or her care is concerned. The patient has the right to obtain information about the existence of any professional relationships among individuals, by name, who are treating him or her.

9. The patient has the right to be advised if the hospital proposes to engage in or perform human experimentation affecting his or her care or treatment. The patient has the right to refuse to participate in such research projects.

10. The patient has the right to expect reasonable continuity of care. He or she has the right to know in advance what appointment times and physicians are available and where. The patient has the right to expect that the hospital will provide a mechanism whereby he or she is informed by his or her physician or a delegate of the physician about the patient's continuing health care requirements after discharge.

11. The patient has the right to examine and receive an explanation of his or her bill regardless of the source of payment.

12. The patient has the right to know what hospital rules and regulations apply to his or her conduct as a patient.

to use these therapies in partnership rather than in competition with conventional medicine, such therapies may be called complementary approaches to health care.[15]

Do such therapies work? This is a difficult question since medical research is funded primarily by the government and the pharmaceutical industry, neither of which has been inclined to invest in research on unconventional therapies. Some studies have shown that complementary medicine is at least as successful as conventional medicine for the short-term treatment of certain conditions. The few studies on long-term treatment of certain conditions have suggested that they may on occasion be more successful. For example, some studies have shown that acupuncture or hypnosis is as effective as painkillers in relieving pain and can be more effective in the long term.[16] This is not to say, however, that there are no complementary health practitioners whose certification is dubious, who are fraudulent, or who dupe their clients. The crucial issue is to separate the quacks from those who are competent and offer real possibilities for healing.[17]

Some people consider all complementary medicine to be quackery. As a result, the Coalition for Alternatives in Nutrition and Healthcare (CANAH) was founded in 1984 to defend complementary medicine and holistic, or integrative, health care. According to CANAH, many conventional health practitioners call complementary approaches quackery to discourage competition. CANAH is proposing a health care rights amendment to the U.S. Constitution, which would provide that no government can pass laws interfering with the people's right to choose the type of health care they prefer for themselves or their children for the prevention or treatment of disease, injury, or illness.[18]

While there are a variety of different complementary health care approaches, some of the most common and well-known are osteopathy, chiropractic, homeopathy, and acupuncture.

Osteopathy   Osteopaths are the most accepted alternative health care practitioners, largely because of the versatility of their training. The idea behind osteopathy is that the structure and function of the body are interdependent; if the structure of the body becomes altered or abnormal, the function is altered and illness results. Doctors of osteopathy receive an education similar to that of doctors of medicine (MDs), but they also learn manipulative skills and may use them in their treatments, trying to manipulate the bones and muscles to bring the body back to normal. Because of their training, osteopaths are accepted by most institutions that accept MDs.[19]

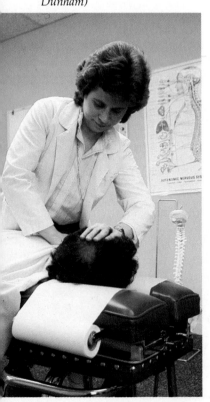

Many people have benefited greatly from the skills of qualified chiropractors. (Tom Dunham)

Chiropractic   Chiropractors are concerned with the function of the muscles and bones. Chiropractic is the largest of the complementary healing professions. It is based on the theory that subluxations, or misalignments of the spinal vertebrae, interfere with the proper functioning of the central nervous system and ultimately cause disease. Chiropractors treat patients by adjusting the vertebrae to restore proper alignment of the spine. In addition to their adjustment techniques, chiropractors may use exercise, advice, nutritional guidance, and changes in work position in their treatment.[20] Chiropractic is generally considered to be useful in treating problems such as stiffness and pain in the neck or back. Its theory of disease causation is considered very controversial, as is the scope and quality of chiropractic education.

Homeopathy   Homeopathy is an approach to healing that is based on the principle that "like is healed by like." Homeopathic practitioners hold that diseases and symptoms can be cured by treating the patient with tiny doses of the substance that is causing a problem. For example, a person suffering from nausea and vomiting may be treated with tiny doses of ipecac, a drug that *causes* vomiting. This is supposed to stimulate the body's natural defense mechanism to fight whatever is causing the ailment.

Acupuncture   Acupuncture is an ancient Chinese method of healing and relieving pain. Needles are inserted into the body at strategic points along invisible lines, or meridians. The needles do not draw blood. Once the acupuncturist knows the nature of the complaint, the patient is examined to find the points along the meridians that correspond to the problem. The needles are then inserted into those points for about 20 minutes. At times they are connected to an electrical current to produce further stimulation.

While the effectiveness of acupuncture in curing disease has not been documented, there is evidence to support its effectiveness in treating pain. Studies have shown that acupuncture eases pain by causing the release of endorphins, the naturally occurring opiatelike chemicals that suppress the transmission of pain signals in the brain. This success also seems to depend on changes in energy fields and electrical circuits that flow within the body.[21]

One of the most dramatic uses of acupuncture occurs during surgery. Acupuncturists can anesthetize a patient during major surgery, yet the patient remains awake and feels no pain. Acupuncture is also being used to treat addictive problems such as smoking, compulsive eating, and drug abuse.[22]

There is little scientific evidence to support the effectiveness of most alternative approaches to medicine, and many conventional health practitioners question their use. They have proved helpful to some people, however. In general, people should not rely on a nonconventional approach *instead* of a conventional one, although they may wish to try such approaches *in conjunction with* conventional health care.

Because it is known that AIDS is spread by contaminated needles, people who consult acupuncturists should make sure that strict standards of antisepsis and hygiene are maintained.

The Cost of Health Care

Every year in the United States an enormous amount of money is spent on health care—over $500 billion in 1987 (almost $2,000 per person.)[23] Soaring health costs caused by increasing hospital and doctor fees, expensive technology, and the increased use of medical services have put a tremendous strain on the medical system and have led to growing concern about the future of health care in this country (Figure 19.5). The nation may soon face a difficult choice: whether to provide adequate health care at any cost or to contain costs by rationing services. At stake is the health of all Americans, but especially those who cannot afford the high cost of health care or do not have health insurance.

Figure 19.5 Since 1970 American spending for health care has risen nearly sevenfold. Spending for nursing home care, hospital care, physician services, and dental services has risen faster than has spending in other categories.

Source: U.S. Bureau of the Census, *Statistical Abstracts of the United States, 1990,* 110th ed. (Washington, D.C.: U.S. Government Printing Office, 1990): Table 136.

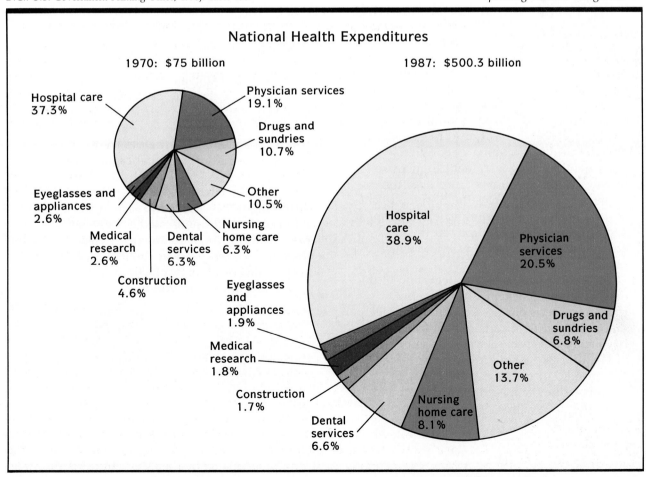

National Health Expenditures

1970: $75 billion

1987: $500.3 billion

Hospital care 37.3%
Physician services 19.1%
Drugs and sundries 10.7%
Other 10.5%
Nursing home care 6.3%
Dental services 6.3%
Construction 4.6%
Medical research 2.6%
Eyeglasses and appliances 2.6%

Hospital care 38.9%
Physician services 20.5%
Drugs and sundries 6.8%
Other 13.7%
Nursing home care 8.1%
Dental services 6.6%
Construction 1.7%
Medical research 1.8%
Eyeglasses and appliances 1.9%

World Health Care Systems

Americans tend to think of themselves as world leaders in medical care. American hospitals have, after all, pioneered many of the most advanced medical treatments. However, third world nations tend to adopt health care systems based on socialized medicine rather than on the private insurance-based system in use here. In socialized systems, providing health care is ultimately the government's responsibility. Medical care is available to all citizens regardless of age or illness, and money to pay for it comes from taxes.

The Canadian system has emerged in recent years as a model socialized system. Looking at its basic structure can provide some important insights about the benefits and weaknesses of such a system. To begin with, a division of the Canadian government distributes all the money necessary to pay for the medical care of its citizens. Although this money comes primarily from taxes, the Canadian people are not taxed excessively; the government has avoided this by creating an efficient medical system whose backbone is the medical community. Costs are kept down by placing a cap on the incomes of doctors and nurses, who work long hours and serve many patients.

This does not mean that people who live in countries with socialized medical systems receive the best medical care. In Canada, if a hospital wants to adopt a new technology, it must petition the government to increase its budget. If the government approves the petition, it usually forces the hospital to cut costs elsewhere. Budgeting is left to hospital department heads, who are not involved enough with patient care to know which procedures could save money.

The British health care system, one of the earliest socialist systems, has different problems. Decisions are based on the idea that the benefits of certain technologies do not justify the cost. As a result, some people in Great Britain do not receive the treatment they need. For example, elderly patients with chronic kidney failure are not treated and often die. In addition, some treatments that affect the quality of life more than they affect life expectancy are relatively rare or not done at all. As a result, people in Canada and Great Britain—and in many other nations—do not have the freedom of choice and individual liberty that those in the United States do.

For all its faults, though, even the British system appears to have some advantages over the U.S. system, as you can see in the following table:

	United States	Great Britain
Infant mortality rate (males)	12.8	12.2
Life expectancy (males)	70.9	71.3
Physicians per 1,000 persons	1.9	1.3
Hospital admission rate (% of population)	17.0	12.7
Hospital beds per 1,000 people	5.9	8.1
Average hospital stay (days)	9.9	18.6
Hospital expenditure per day	$360	$140

As you can see, the United States does not have an extensive hospital capacity. The 5.9 beds per 1,000 statistic is 27 percent below Great Britain's, but the percentage of people in U.S. hospitals each year is one-third higher than in Great Britain.

U.S. hospital administrators try to compensate for low hospital capacity by keeping the average hospital stay short; however, the cost of $360 a day remains one of the highest in the world. The medical establishment in the United States seems to prefer shorter, high-technology-based treatment programs over the longer therapy approaches commonly practiced in Europe, Japan, and the third world.

Based on Victor R. Fuchs and James S. Hahn, "How Does Canada Do It? *New England Journal of Medicine* (September 27, 1990); Ed Rubenstein, "The Health of Nations," *National Review* (September 1, 1989); David Holzman, "A Severe Case of Swelling Expenses," *Insight* (February 9, 1987).

Health Insurance

Most Americans have some form of health insurance, though the adequacy of coverage varies widely. However, about 33 million people (almost 14 percent of the population) have no health insurance at all, a situation that is one of the most urgent health policy issues today. Most of the uninsured are working poor people whose job benefits do not include health insurance or who earn too much to qualify for government health insurance programs and cannot afford to pay insurance premiums themselves.[24]

Unlike most two-party transactions, in which a buyer purchases goods or services directly from a seller, most health care payments are handled by a third party—the insurance carrier. This insurer may be billed directly by a health care provider who either accepts the amount received as full payment or bills the patient for the difference. Alternatively, the patient may pay the health care provider first and then be reimbursed by the insurance carrier.

Several kinds of health insurance coverage are available. **Basic health insurance** pays benefits for hospitalization and for medical and surgical expenses. This means that *part* of the hospital bill and *part* of the physicians's and surgeon's fees—but only up to a given amount—are paid by the insurance company. **Major medical insurance** is designed to protect a person from the high medical expenses that can accumulate if he or she is seriously injured or ill for a long time. Typically, major medical coverage is purchased for an extra fee to complement basic medical coverage. **Disability insurance** pays benefits to a person who is unable to work because of injury or illness.

Private Insurance Plans Most private health insurance is provided by nonprofit corporations such as Blue Cross–Blue Shield and by commercial insurance companies. Since the mid-1970s, self-insured plans have been gaining in popularity, as have prepaid plans such as health maintenance organizations (HMOs). All these plans offer insurance with two kinds of policies: group and individual.

Group policies account for the majority of private insurance plans; most are offered by employers to groups of employees. These policies usually offer basic coverage for cheaper rates than are charged for individual policies. Some companies have begun taking steps to limit group health insurance coverage, something that would have been unthinkable several years ago. Some have given employees the choice of receiving health care through a company-designated network of doctors and hospitals or paying a greater share of the expenses out of their own pockets.[25] More and more group plans are including features to help manage costs, such as incentives for getting a second surgical opinion, outpatient surgery, and testing on an outpatient basis.

Individual policies are bought primarily by single persons, couples, and families who are self-employed and do not have access to group plans. With individual policies, the cost of comparable coverage is generally substantially higher than it is with group policies.

Government Insurance Programs The government subsidizes some health coverage for the elderly, disabled, and poor through Medicaid and Medicare. **Medicare,** a federal health insurance program designed to benefit people age 65 or older and the disabled, has two parts: Part A and Part B.

Part A Medicare is an insurance program for compulsory hospitalization. It pays a large part of the hospital bill when a senior citizen on Social Security has to be admitted. Alternatively, it may cover skilled nursing services, part time home health care, or, for the dying, hospice care. There is, however, a deductible amount that the patient must pay for hospitalization; and if the

According to the U.S. Bureau of the Census, the age group least likely to have health insurance coverage is the 16- to 24-year-old group. Almost one-third of the people in this age group lack health insurance at some time during a given year. Many lose coverage under a parent's policy when they reach age 18.

basic health insurance—*insurance that pays for hospitalization and for medical and surgical expenses.*

major medical insurance—*medical insurance designed to protect against the high medical expenses that may accumulate if a person is seriously injured or ill for a long time.*

disability insurance—*insurance that pays benefits to a person unable to work because of injury or illness.*

group policy—*a kind of insurance policy offered by employers to groups of employees.*

individual policy—*an insurance policy bought primarily by single persons, couples, and families who are self-employed and do not have access to group plans.*

Medicare—*a federal health insurance program for people 65 and older and those who are disabled.*

Deciding on a Type of Medical Plan

The escalating costs of health care make medical coverage a necessity for everyone. Many people subscribe to a particular medical plan because their employer provides it as a fringe benefit. If that is your situation, it is helpful to understand as much as possible about your medical coverage.

In other companies employees are offered a choice between traditional health insurance, such as Blue Cross–Blue Shield, and a health maintenance organization (HMO). If you have to make a choice because your employer offers several plans or if you have to secure your own coverage, you can make a better decision if you are well informed about both types of health insurance.

Traditional health insurance protects people from major medical expenses and loss of income caused by health-related problems. There are three basic kinds of policies that provide different types of coverage. The first— major medical policies—are the most comprehensive. They cover hospital stays and physicians' services in and out of the hospital. The second—hospital-surgical policies—cover only hospital services and surgical procedures. The third—hospital-indemnity and dread-disease policies—offer the most limited benefits. Hospital-indemnity policies pay a fixed amount each day you are in the hospital. Dread-disease policies pay benefits only if you contract a specific illness, such as cancer.

Most employers that offer traditional health insurance require employees to pay a deductible each year before benefits begin to be paid. Sometimes the deductible is quite high.

Health maintenance organizations cover the same things traditional health insurance does but operate differently. HMOs are prepaid health care plans with predetermined fixed benefits. An HMO requires that people enroll, become members, and agree to use only its services. In return, the HMO provides a defined set of services from participating health care professionals at a predetermined price. Most HMOs require people to pay a small copayment fee when they use these services.

There are two types of HMOs. The most familiar type—the prepaid group practice— has doctors either on salary or working under contract. These plans often have their own outpatient facilities, which members must use except in extreme circumstances. Hospital admission is strictly controlled.

The other type of HMO—the independent practice association—contracts with doctors who maintain a private practice in addition to seeing HMO members. These plans usually use hospitals for inpatient services, and so their costs may be higher. However, it is possible to enroll and not have to change doctors if your doctor participates in the plan.

When a consumer compares specific plans, he or she needs to ask what each one does and does not cover. For example, many major medical and hospital-surgical policies do not cover routine prenatal care or routine deliveries. Subscribers have to buy a separate rider to pay the cost of routine maternity care.

The next question consumers need to ask is: How does the policy pay? For example, does it only pay the usual and customary fee? If that is the case, when a bill is greater than the insurance company's "usual" figure, subscribers may have to pay for part of it.

Finally, consumers need to ask how much the policy costs. What are the deductibles, premiums, or copayments? If two policies are comparable in every way but cost, it makes sense to choose the one that is less expensive.

Personal preferences and priorities are the main considerations in deciding which type of health insurance to choose. For some people, being able to stay with a particular doctor is the most important factor. For other people, the premiums charged or the benefits offered play the key role in this decision. To some people, the most important features may be convenience, a relaxed atmosphere, and the ability to get an appointment quickly. No one plan will have everything you want, but you probably can find a plan that meets enough of your personal needs so that you feel comfortable with it.

Based on *Choosing an HMO: An Evaluation Checklist* (Washington, D.C.: AARP Health Advocacy Services Program Department, 1986); "The Crisis in Health Insurance," *Consumer Reports* (August 1990): 533–547.

illness lasts more than two months, patients or their families must begin to contribute to the costs.[26]

The main physician's charges are not covered; these can be lessened by Part B, a voluntary program that involves an additional monthly fee. Part B also covers other medical services not covered by Part A, but usually it pays only 80 percent of an "approved charge"—a charge that may often be considerably less than the full bill.[27]

In 1988 Congress passed a Catastrophic Coverage Act, increasing the fee and providing improved coverage; this was repealed in 1989 because of objections to the increase. Currently, private insurance companies sell "Medigap" policies, which cover costs Medicare does not pay.

Medicaid is a federal-state health insurance program to assist people of any age who cannot pay for medical care. Under Medicaid, those who can meet the standards of "medical indigence" are wholly or partly covered for hospital stays and other medical expenses. During the last decade, tightened eligibility rules have eliminated thousands of poor women and children from the program.[28]

In 1990 the Medicare deductible was equivalent to about one day's stay in the hospital—just under $600.

Medicaid—a federal-state health insurance program to assist people of any age who cannot pay for medical insurance.

Health Maintenance Organizations

Some critics of fee-for-service care believe that the traditional system of payment for services encourages physicians and hospitals to give more care (such as tests and surgery) than is really needed and to charge for that care. Partly in response to this problem, health maintenance organizations were developed. An HMO is a type of group practice plan in which consumers pay a set fee every month in return for complete health care at little or no additional cost.

More than 31 million Americans are currently enrolled in HMOs.[29] There are two major types: group practice and individual practice plans. Group practice plans provide medical services at centers staffed by salaried physicians. Laboratories, x-ray facilities, and pharmacies are all on the premises, and so members can obtain outpatient care at one location. Individual practice plans offer medical care in the private offices of doctors under contract to an HMO. In an individual plan, patients have a wider choice of physicians.

HMOs have some advantages over traditional health care systems. For one thing, they are structured in a way that encourages patients to "think preventive." Since various services are offered at one location and since most costs are covered, patients may be more likely to come for preemptive tests, which can help catch health problems early and prevent them from becoming more serious. Moreover, some studies have shown that HMO patients have less frequent hospitalizations, shorter periods of hospitalization, and less surgery than do patients under the care of fee-for-service practitioners.

Some people feel that there are disadvantages to HMOs. With an HMO, a patient relinquishes much of his or her freedom to choose physicians and can be shuffled between rotating doctors. Furthermore, HMO physicians are not independent professionals but employees of an HMO, with a duty to serve not only the interests of their patients but the demands of the HMO as well.[30]

Before deciding to join an HMO, it is important to find out what membership includes. Does it include drugs, dental care, and/or eyeglasses? Are there any extra costs? How many of the HMO's doctors are board-certified? How are doctors reimbursed, and are there incentives that enable or allow them to skimp on care? Can patients choose the doctors they prefer? How long does it take to get an appointment? Is the HMO affiliated with accredited hospitals? Who pays for emergency treatment by an unaffiliated physician? In addition to finding the answers to these questions, people investigating HMOs should evaluate their own health care needs and expectations to see if they are compatible with an HMO's services and philosophy of health care.

Controlling the Cost of Health Care

There are no simple ways to control the ever-increasing costs of health care. For its part, the government might try to regulate fees and provide incentives for quality care at a more reasonable cost (but without limiting patient care). Health care providers might do more to encourage preventive care and avoid the use of expensive and unnecessary testing and procedures. Most important, individuals can take steps to help keep their medical costs down and bring about changes in the health care system. While individual actions may not solve the problem, they can make a difference.

The best way for individuals to keep health care costs down is to become health-activated and health-conscious. By taking charge of their own health, people are better able to distinguish between medical problems that require professional help and those which can be dealt with less expensively through self-care. Health-activated people are willing to gather information about health problems, methods of treatment, and the medical services provided by physicians, hospitals, and clinics—information that can save them time and money. They are prepared to ask questions of health professionals and assume greater control of their own health care needs, including making decisions about treatment options and medications. Most important, they practice prevention by adopting the principles of a healthy lifestyle. By focusing on prevention, people can eliminate much of the need for expensive medical care and ensure optimal health and well-being.

Chapter Summary

- Becoming health-activated regarding health allows individuals to increase their sense of control over their health and assume basic responsibility for many of their health care needs.

- Health-activated people take steps to remain healthy, deal with medical problems that do not require professional attention, and manage small medical problems so that they do not become major ones. They judge health care problems and are able to decide when to care for themselves and when to seek professional help. They are also able to make informed choices regarding health care products and treatments.

- Normal body temperature is 98.6 degrees Fahrenheit, normal adult respiration is 12 to 19 breaths a minute, the normal pulse rate for healthy adults is 60 to 90 beats a minute, and normal blood pressure for healthy adults is 120/80. However, these norms may vary in accordance with a variety of factors, including age, sex, time of day, stress or emotional tension, and, of course, general level of health.

- A home medicine chest is useful in dealing with minor injuries and medical problems. A well-maintained medicine chest includes medications and supplies to deal with emergency situations as well as the individual needs of family members. Safety measures for a medicine chest include maintenance of the freshness of all drugs, realistic amounts of all supplies, carefully labeled supplies and medications, storage

out of the reach of children, and proper use of all supplies.

- Regular physical examinations allow medical problems to be detected early, before they become more serious. Physicians generally check blood pressure, the heart and lungs, the lymph nodes, and the abdomen for signs of tumors, enlarged organs, and tender areas. The frequency of examinations varies with age, sex, and medical history. Various health organizations recommend particular schedules of examinations to test for certain diseases.

- A person should seek professional help if he or she experiences persistent, severe, or unusual symptoms or medical problems. Certain symptoms are associated with various diseases, such as cancer and cardiovascular disease, and should receive prompt professional attention.

- In selecting a health professional, a person should consider the professional's qualifications, philosophy of care, credentials, and demeanor. Recommendations from family members, friends, and other medical professionals may be helpful in selecting a doctor or dentist; hospitals, referral services, and reference directories can also be useful in judging qualifications.

- In assessing health care institutions, a person should consider the services offered, the qualifications of the staff members, the fee structure, the safety record of the institution, and accreditation.

- In addition to conventional methods of treatment, people may seek treatment with a variety of alternative, or complementary, approaches, including osteopathy, chiropractic, homeopathy, and acupuncture. Osteopathy is similar to standard medicine, though its practitioners place more emphasis on manipulations to adjust body structure. Chiropractic involves less rigorous training but is also based on manipulating muscle and bone. Homeopathic practitioners treat diseases by using tiny amounts of the same substance that caused the problem. Acupuncture uses needles to relieve pain and heal certain medical problems.
- The basic kinds of health insurance coverage are basic health insurance, major medical insurance, and disability insurance. All these types of insurance can be provided through private insurance plans (group or individual policies) or government-funded programs (Medicare and Medicaid).
- An HMO is a type of group health practice in which consumers pay a set fee every month for complete health care at little or no additional cost. One advantage HMOs have over traditional systems is that they encourage prevention, since people can receive routine screenings and examinations at no extra charge. A disadvantage is that patients must choose among the participating doctors and thus lose some freedom of choice concerning health professionals.
- The best way for individuals to control the cost of health care is to practice prevention and take steps to adopt healthier behaviors and a healthier lifestyle.

Key Terms

Generic name (page 486)

Basic health insurance (page 503)

Major medical insurance (page 503)

Disability insurance (page 503)

Group policies (page 503)

Individual policies (page 503)

Medicare (page 503)

Medicaid (page 505)

References

1. Tom Ferguson, "Self-Care in the Information Age," *Medical Self-Care* 39 (March–April 1987): 77, 80.

2. Tom Ferguson, "The Power of Self-Care," *East West* (October 1986): 58–60.

3. Tom Ferguson, "The Rise of the Medical Prosumer," *Medical Self-Care* 45 (March–April 1988): 52, 64.

4. Tom Ferguson, "Toward Self-Responsibility for Health, Part II," *Medical Self-Care* 38 (January–February 1987): 67, 72.

5. Kirk Johnson, "A Medical Lab in Every Home," *East West* (October 1986): 61–65.

6. Keith W. Sehnert, *Selfcare-Wellcare* (Minneapolis: Augsburg, 1985): 147.

7. "Road Signs," *Vim and Vigor* (Summer 1988): 71–72.

8. American Cancer Society, *Cancer Facts and Figures—1990* (Atlanta, Ga.: American Cancer Society, 1990): 18.

9. Ibid.

10. Ibid.

11. Bill Thomson, "Are You Your Own Best Doctor?" *East West* (October 1986): 54–57.

12. Ferguson, "The Rise of the Medical Prosumer," op. cit., pp. 52, 64.

13. Jon Hamilton, "Shopping Mall Medicine," *American Health* (March 1988): 106–110.

14. Victor Cohn, "How to Survive the Hospital," *American Health* (March 1987): 99–108.

15. Stephen Fulder, "A New Interest in Complementary (Alternative) Medicine: Towards Pluralism in Medicine?" *Impact of Science on Society* 143, vol. 36, no. 3 (1986): 235–243.

16. Ibid.

17. Mark Blumenthal, "Crashing the Quackbusters," *East West* (November 1988): 81–84.

18. Michael Davis, "Medical Freedom Fighters," *East West* (November 1988): 65–68.

19. Material on osteopathy and homeopathy from Sehnert, op. cit., pp. 112–131.

20. Fulder, op. cit.

21. Sehnert, op. cit.

22. Fulder, op. cit.

23. U.S. Bureau of the Census, *Statistical Abstract of the United States: 1990,* 110th ed. (Washington, D.C., 1990): 92.

24. Ibid., p. 100.

25. Malcolm Gladwell, "Health-Insurance Rates to Rise 20%–30%, Experts Say," *Arizona Republic* (October 28, 1988): 1, 6.

26. *1990 Medicare and Medicaid Benefits* (Chicago: Commerce Clearing House, 1990): 6–12.

27. Ibid., pp. 13–16.

28. Donald Robinson, "Who Should Receive Medical Aid?" *Parade* (May 28, 1989): 4–5.

29. Donald Robinson, "How Well Do You Know Your HMO?" *Parade* (February 5, 1989): 17–18.

30. Nancy Gibbs, "Sick and Tired," *Time* (July 31, 1989): 48–51.

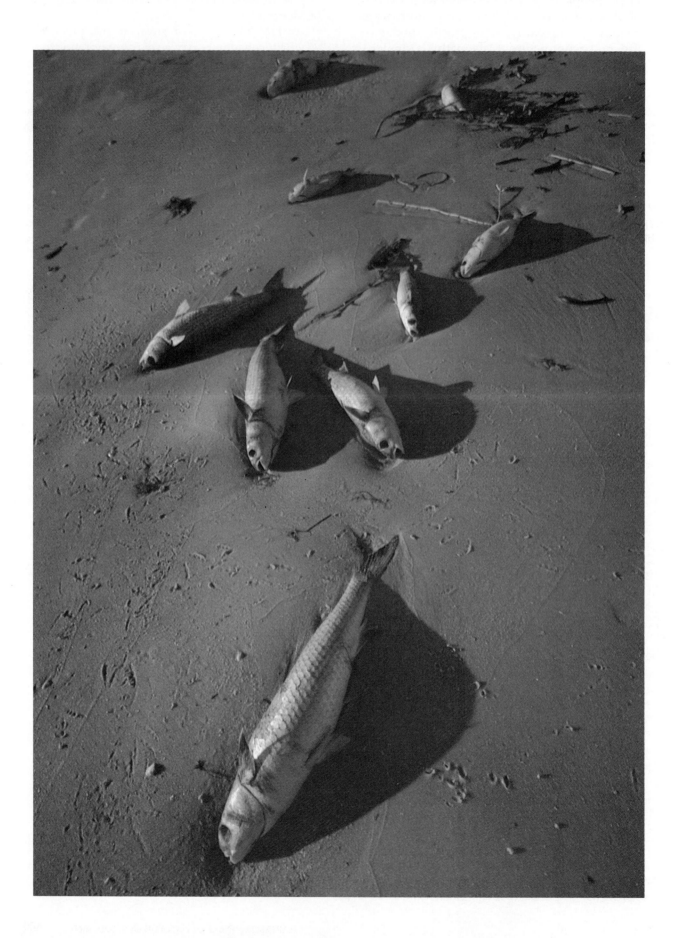

Health and the Environment

To Guide Your Reading

When you have studied this chapter, you should be able to:

- Describe the major types of atmospheric pollution that affect local environments and the measures that are being taken and can be taken to alleviate them.

- Describe the different types of pollution that affect the nation's water resources and explain how society is currently attempting to deal with them.

- Describe the problem of solid waste, how to clean up sites that were polluted in the past, and how to

prevent these problems from occurring in the future.

- Assess the problems being caused by pollution and poor use of resources on a global scale and describe ways in which these problems might be addressed.

- Explain and evaluate types of individual and collective action which can be taken to address environmental problems.

Detergents, dyes, food additives, drugs, synthetic fibers, pesticides, fertilizers, plastics, and fuels—the list is endless. These and other products of the twentieth century's technological revolution line cupboards, refrigerators, and medicine chests; hang in closets; cover lawns; furnish homes; and propel machinery. In many ways such technological innovations have been an undeniable boon to humanity. Agricultural technology has increased food production and made more food available at reasonable prices. Medical technology has conquered many diseases and brought others under control. Industrial technology has improved the working lives of millions of people and raised their standard of living. Overall, technology has brought better lives to millions of people throughout the world.

Although modern technology has proved beneficial in many ways and has become an integral part of modern life, many of its products and the processes used to create them are being blamed for one of the major ills of the modern world—environmental pollution. **Pollution** includes not only undesirable substances but also forms of energy, such as heat, that have destructive effects on the physical environment.[1]

pollution—*any substance or energy that contributes to the development of undesirable environmental effects.*

Pollution has become a problem of critical dimensions not only because of its effects on the physical environment but also because of its effects on the health of the people who live in that environment. One of the worst examples of its potential effects occurred in Bhopal, India, in December 1984, when more than 2,500 people died and 80,000 to 90,000 were seriously injured after a deadly gas escaped into the air from a Union Carbide plant. Less dramatic examples occur every day as people are exposed to environmental pollutants that gradually erode their health.

While the greatest effects of pollution are on people's physical health, pollution can affect other aspects of health as well. Concern over the environment may affect people's emotional health as fears, pessimism, and a sense of

The human body can handle a certain amount of pollution because of built-in systems for self-cleaning, such as the cilia, *which clear the bronchial tubes, and* enzymes, *which help break down chemicals at the cellular level. Only when exposure exceeds the body's ability to handle a particular pollutant is a person likely to suffer ill effects.*

helplessness produce despair and mental anguish. Social health may be affected by the dehumanization of lives and jobs caused by machines and other technological advances; it also may be affected when pollution interferes with economic and social planning. Spiritual health may be affected as people struggle to reconcile their values and desires with the conditions created by environmental pollution and the need to control it.

The Quality of the Local Environment

The most noticeable effects of pollution have involved the local environment. A city's air is fouled with smog; a region's lakes, streams, and rivers carry sewage and industrial wastes; hazardous chemicals are seeping into the water from an abandoned landfill; and mounds of garbage blot the landscape. Towns, cities, states, and nations have felt the negative effects of such pollution and have had to deal with problems of air quality, water quality, solid waste disposal, and the storage and treatment of hazardous wastes.

Air Pollution and Protection

People once believed that the earth has an unlimited supply of breathable air. It is now clear, however, that air is a vital natural resource that must be protected before it is irreversibly fouled by automobile exhaust and industrial waste.

Pollution of the Atmosphere *Air pollution* refers to the presence in the air of contaminants that do not disperse properly and interfere with human health.[2] A certain amount of air pollution is caused by natural events such as volcanic eruptions, forest fires, and the decay of plants and animals. This natural pollution, however, is not as serious a threat to the environment as is the pollution caused by human activities.[3]

Every year manufacturing plants throughout the United States release billions of pounds of pollutants into the air, including known or suspected carcinogens (cancer-causing agents) such as methylene, chloride, benzene, and butadiene.[4] Industrial and manufacturing processes also release sulfur dioxides, nitrogen dioxides, particulate matter, and other substances.

Tempting though it may be to put most of the blame for pollution on industry and large corporate manufacturing, most air pollution is caused by individuals and small businesses. Forty percent of the pollutants in the smog (smoke and fog combined) that periodically blankets cities such as Los Angeles comes from automobile exhausts, and another 40 percent comes from dry cleaners, bakeries, and consumer products.[5]

Consequences of Atmospheric Pollution Air pollution poses its most immediate threat to the respiratory system, but over time it can also harm other parts of the body, including the brain and heart (Table 20.1). The following are the principal contaminants responsible for air pollution:

- *Sulfur oxides.* Produced primarily by the burning of fossil fuels (coal, oil, and natural gas), sulfur oxides are thought to be a principal cause of excessive deaths during major smog incidents. They irritate the eyes, throat, and upper respiratory system, causing coughing and choking.
- *Carbon monoxide.* A colorless and odorless gas, carbon monoxide is released from motor vehicle exhausts and constitutes more than half of all human-made air pollution. Exposure to significant doses of carbon monoxide causes oxygen deficiency in the blood, resulting in impaired respiration and malfunctioning of the brain and heart; impaired hearing, vision, and thought; and even unconsciousness or death.
- *Hydrocarbons and nitrogen oxides.* Released into the air as a result of motor vehicle emissions and the burning of fossil fuels, hydrocarbons and nitro-

Table 20.1 Major Air Pollutants and Their Health Effects

Pollutants	Major Sources	Characteristics and Effects
Carbon monoxide (CO)	Vehicle exhaust	Colorless, odorless poisonous gas; replaces oxygen in red blood cells, causing dizziness, unconsciousness, or death
Hydrocarbons (HC)	Incomplete combustion of gasoline; evaporation of petroleum fuels, solvents, and paints	Although some are poisonous, most are not; react with NO_2 to form ozone or smog
Lead (Pb)	Antiknock agents in gasoline	Accumulates in the bones and soft tissues; affects blood-forming organs, kidneys, and nervous system; suspected of causing learning disabilities in young children
Nitrogen dioxide (NO_2)	Industrial processes, vehicle exhausts	Causes structural and chemical changes in the lungs; lowers resistance to respiratory infections; reacts in sunlight with hydrocarbons to produce smog; contributes to acid rain
Ozone (O_3)	Formed when HC and NO_2 react	Principal constituent of smog; irritates mucous membranes, causing coughing, choking, impaired lung function; aggravates chronic asthma and bronchitis
Total suspended particulates (TSP)	Industrial plants, heating boilers, auto engines, dust	Larger visible types (soot, smoke, and dust) can clog the lung sacs; smaller invisible particles can pass into the bloodstream; often carry carcinogens and toxic metals; impair visibility
Sulfur dioxide (SO_2)	Burning coal and oil, industrial processes	Corrosive, poisonous gas; associated with coughs, colds, asthma, bronchitis, and emphysema; contributes to acid rain

Source: Environmental Protection Agency.

gen oxides combine to form smog. Nitrogen oxides in particular are thought to contribute to respiratory difficulties and reduce the oxygen-carrying capacity of the blood.

- *Ozone.* **Ozone** is a form of oxygen that is created when sunlight reacts with gasoline fumes, other hydrocarbons, and nitrogen oxides. It is a powerful oxidizing agent that can irritate or damage mucous membranes, especially in the respiratory system. In addition to causing tissue damage, it can cause headaches, fatigue, coughing, and eye problems. Nearly 80 million Americans are breathing unhealthy levels of ozone.[6]

- *Particulate matter.* Particulate matter includes dust, ash, and other fine solid particles that are by-products of fuel combustion, other types of burning, and abrasion milling. These particles irritate the eyes, throat, and lungs; some, such as asbestos, can cause cancer.[7]

ozone—a form of oxygen created when sunlight reacts with gasoline fumes, other hydrocarbons, and nitrogen oxides; also present in the ozone layer of the upper atmosphere.

Individuals vary considerably in their sensitivity to air pollutants. People with heart disease or respiratory ailments such as asthma, bronchitis, and emphysema are more likely to feel the effects of air pollution. However, even those who do not have these problems may be affected to some degree: although there is no proof that air pollution *causes* disease, people in heavily polluted areas suffer more short-term respiratory ailments and chest infections than do people in clean-air zones. Smokers are at especially high risk for developing pollution-related ailments because cigarette smoke and air pollution seem to have a synergistic effect.

Improving Atmospheric Air Quality The Clean Air Act of 1970, a federal law designed to restrict air pollution in the United States, has established strict air quality standards based primarily on health considerations rather than economic ones. It empowers the U.S. Environmental Protection Agency (EPA) to set limits on major pollutants and mandate reductions in automobile and factory emissions.

The EPA's enforcement of the Clean Air Act has been more vigorous at some times than it has at others. Enforcement was most active in the 1970s, a time of widespread public distrust of big business. (Even then, however, deadlines for meeting pollution limits were routinely missed.) In the 1980s, the EPA took a more pro-business stance and let up on enforcement. As a

Particulate matter is in general the easiest form of air pollution to combat. Among the techniques used are fabric filters, water sprays, and static electricity. To remove specific polluting gases, chemical converters can sometimes be used, but expensive changes in fuels and industrial processes are sometimes the only viable methods.

How Knowledgeable Are You about the Environment?

Growing environmental awareness has helped teach people that many lifestyle choices can make a big difference in improving the health of the planet. In fact, the things people buy and the way they live can have a profound effect on the environment.

The following questionnaire asks about your lifestyle and explores how well you understand the environmental impact of the choices you make. Respond yes or no to each question and then jot down in a few words what you think the result of your choice would be. The answers provided below will help you evaluate whether your choices have a positive or negative impact on the environment, and the accompanying explanations will help you assess your understanding of how personal choices can contribute to a cleaner, safer world.

Yes   No   **1.** I make sure the tires on my car are properly inflated, balanced, and rotated every 6,000 to 8,000 miles.

Environmental impact: _____

_____

Yes   No   **2.** I dispose of leftover paint by flushing it down the drain with lots of water.

Environmental impact: _____

_____

Yes   No   **3.** I use rechargeable batteries.

Environmental impact: _____

_____

Yes   No   **4.** I make sure my pet wears a collar that discourages fleas.

Environmental impact: _____

_____

Yes   No   **5.** I use an alternative to incandescent light bulbs.

Environmental impact: _____

_____

Yes   No   **6.** I would vote for a "bottle bill," which requires consumers to pay deposits on bottles and then refunds the deposit when the bottles are returned.

Environmental impact: _____

_____

Yes   No   **7.** I purchase and ask for organically grown fruits and vegetables when I shop.

Environmental impact: _____

_____

Yes   No   **8.** I wash dishes by hand instead of in the dishwasher.

Environmental impact: _____

_____

Self-Assessment (continued)

Answers:

1. Yes. Tires that are underinflated have a shorter life and can waste up to 5 percent of a car's fuel by increasing "rolling resistance." Regularly balancing and rotating your tires will help extend their life, conserving resources that go into making new tires and reducing disposal problems, and will help conserve fuel.

2. No. Dispose of latex paint by letting it evaporate outdoors and then discarding the remaining solid waste with normal garbage. Oil-based paint is toxic and a dangerous pollutant. Check with local authorities in your area to see if they accept it or call the EPA hot line (1–800–424–9364) for more information.

3. Yes. Rechargeable batteries last much longer and contribute less to hazardous waste. Disposable alkaline batteries contain mercury, a highly toxic substance that has become a major source of contamination in some waste dumps.

4. No. Most flea collars contain dangerous pesticides that may harm pets and can threaten the environment through their manufacture and disposal (Americans throw away approximately 50 million flea collars a year). Use a citrus oil spray or another natural alternative.

5. Yes. Compact fluorescent bulbs, although more expensive, last longer and use about one-fourth of the energy that incandescent bulbs use.

6. Yes. Bottle bills have a positive environmental impact. In the nine states that already have such bills, a 90 percent compliance rate has reduced solid waste by 8 percent and litter by 50 percent.

7. Yes. Supporting organic growers and demanding their produce can help reduce the use of herbicides and pesticides. Consumer demand increased organic food production in California from $20 million to $100 million in just 4 years.

8. No. A dishwasher is generally more efficient, especially if you leave the water running when you wash or rinse dishes by hand.

Evaluating How Your Choices Affect the Environment:

Score one point for answering yes to questions 1, 3, 5, 6, and 7. _____
Score one point for answering no to questions 2, 4, and 8. _____

Evaluating Your Knowledge about the Effect of Your Choices:

Score an additional point for each answer in which you correctly described the environmental impact of your choice. (If your answer was close or partially correct, score half a point.) _____

Total: _____

If you scored 11 to 16 points: Your choices are having a positive environmental impact, and you have a good understanding of the relationship between personal choices and environmental quality.

If you scored 6 to 10 points: You could make better choices to help improve the environment and increase your knowledge about the impact of your choices.

If you scored below 6 points: You could definitely do more to help the environment and increase your knowledge about the impact of your choices. Reread the questions and explanations carefully to understand how you could make better choices.

Based on ideas from Earthworks Group, *50 Simple Things You Can Do to Save the Earth* (Berkeley, Calif.: Earthworks Press, 1989).

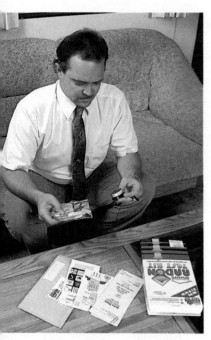

Radon levels in houses can be measured with a simple, inexpensive test kit. Information on radon is readily available from the Environmental Protection Agency. (David Young-Wolff/PhotoEdit)

result, many large U.S. cities regularly exceeded the mandated standards for air quality and received no penalties or fines for doing so.[8] In the late 1980s and in the early 1990s environmental issues again began to be debated more prominently, an indication that stricter regulation may lie ahead.[9]

Air Pollution at Work and at Home While the focus of concern about air pollution is on the atmosphere outside, air pollution is also a problem in many American workplaces and homes.

The problem of second-hand cigarette smoke has already been discussed (Chapter 15). During the last two decades many workplaces have reduced considerably the concentration of other airborne toxins in the work environment. However, air pollutants found in the workplace—such as inorganic arsenic, asbestos, benzene, beryllium, mercury, and vinyl chloride—can still be hazardous to one's health; some substances have been found to cause disease among people who have only minimal daily exposure.[10] Exposure to even small amounts of asbestos is associated with an increased risk of developing lung and intestinal cancers.

Air pollution may also be a problem in the home. Airborne toxins can come from a number of sources, including household cleaning solutions, paints, varnishes, paint removers, aerosols, pesticides, and other consumer products. Some of these toxins, such as benzene and carbon tetrachloride, are suspected carcinogens. Many homes are also exposed to a natural air pollutant—radon, a colorless, odorless gas produced by the natural decay of radium in the soil. Radon seeps into homes through cracks in foundations and through pipes and water pumps; it can be released into the air from drinking water, especially in rural homes that draw water from wells rather than municipal water supplies. Experts are monitoring people exposed to radon to determine whether it increases the incidence of lung cancer.

Water Pollution and Protection

carrying capacity—*the ability to support a human population of a certain size.*

The **carrying capacity** of a given region of the world—its ability to support a human population of a certain size—depends on that region's supply of water. Unfortunately, the world's water supply is limited and cannot keep pace with current population growth.[11] Of perhaps greater concern is the fact that the water available—surface drinking water, groundwater, and even the oceans—is becoming increasingly polluted.

Water pollution—any physical or chemical change in water that can adversely affect organisms—is not a new phenomenon. Some water pollution occurs naturally, especially bacterial pollution, which results when decaying plant and animal matter enters the water supply. Human societies have always had to contend with diseases such as cholera, dysentery, and typhoid fever, which can be contracted when a person drinks unclean water. However, while modern technologies have helped improve these problems of the water supply in many places, toxic substances, acids, and heat have increasingly begun to threaten water resources in many parts of the United States and throughout the world.

Chemical Pollution The type of water pollution that may have the most serious consequences for human health is *chemical pollution*. Canadian and U.S. researchers have found that the levels of toxic chemicals in the bodies of the 37 million people living around the Great Lakes are about 20 percent higher than they are in other North Americans.[12]

chlorinated hydrocarbons—*a group of chemicals that includes dangerous pesticides such as DDT, chlordane, and Kepone.*

Among the most persistent and dangerous water pollutants are the **chlorinated hydrocarbons,** which include dangerous pesticides such as DDT (now banned in the United States), chlordane, and Kepone. These chemicals may enter the food chain or affect people more immediately. For example, workers at a Virginia chemical plant where Kepone was manufactured suffered from a variety of illnesses, and some of them became sterile.[13]

Another dangerous group of chemicals are **polychlorinated biphenyls (PCBs),** which are used in the manufacture of electrical equipment. In recent years the increased presence of PCBs in the water supply has become a matter of concern. PCBs have been linked to reproductive disorders, kidney damage, liver ailments, and eye irritation.

Mercury is another dangerous substance that finds its way into the water supply. Mercury is a naturally occurring element distributed widely in the earth's crust. Certain microorganisms can convert it into an organic form, methyl mercury, which produces devastating symptoms when consumed in sufficient quantities.

The effects of mercury poisoning were illustrated most dramatically in Japan in the 1970s. From the early 1930s until 1971, certain Japanese factories released industrial wastes containing substantial quantities of mercury into the Pacific Ocean. Marine microorganisms converted this mercury into methyl mercury, which became progressively more concentrated as it moved up the food chain to humans. The people most severely affected were the residents of a fishing village in Minamata Bay, whose diet consisted almost solely of fish. Mercury poisoning resulted in 52 deaths; more than 100 other people experienced serious symptoms, including inability to speak, mental retardation, and numbness of the arms and legs, followed by deterioration of muscle tissue, gradual loss of vision and hearing, disruption of equilibrium, loss of coordination, and emotional disturbance. Many of the victims became permanently disabled, and children born to mothers who had eaten contaminated seafood were severely deformed.

As a result of the Minamata episode and other mercury-related disasters, most industrialized nations have instituted strict regulations prohibiting mercury pollution. Acute mercury poisoning from contaminated food is far less likely to occur than it was in the past.

Acid Rain   Another type of water pollution is **acid rain**—rain containing nitrogen and sulfur oxides discharged from motor vehicles and coal-burning power plants and factories. Rising into the atmosphere, these pollutants circulate, react with moisture, and turn into nitric and sulfuric acids, which eventually fall back to earth as precipitation that is as acidic as lemon juice or vinegar. When this acidic rain gathers in lakes or streams or falls on forests, it can damage and even destroy plant and animal life. The effect of acid rain on humans is unclear, but acid sulfate particles—bits of "acid dust" that float down independent of rain, snow, and sleet—are thought to contribute to a number of respiratory ailments.[14]

The effects of acid rain on the environment can be disastrous. Data compiled by the EPA show that at least 75 percent of the lakes in New Hampshire and Rhode Island, 60 percent of the lakes in Maine and Massachusetts, and 43 percent of the lakes in the upper Midwest may soon be so acidic that they will no longer be able to support plant or animal life.[15]

Acid rain illustrates clearly the links between various parts of the environment and demonstrates how pollution of one part of the environment causes harm in other parts. Acid rain occurs as a result of pollutants discharged into the air, but its greatest effects are on the water in lakes and streams, although it can damage forests and human-made structures as well. Moreover, the effects of acid rain are often felt hundreds of miles away from the original source of the pollution.[16] Many of the towering industrial smokestacks that were designed to minimize local air pollution have apparently *increased* acid rain and spread it over a wider area. These smokestacks eject pollutants higher into the atmosphere, where they form acidic compounds more easily and are carried farther before falling as precipitation.

Acid rain also illustrates the global nature of pollution. Pollutants from industries in the midwestern section of the United States rise into the atmo-

polychlorinated biphenyls (PCBs)—*a group of hydrocarbons that, as water pollutants, have been linked to reproductive disorders, kidney damage, liver ailments, and eye irritation.*

acid rain—*rain containing nitrogen and sulfur oxides discharged from motor vehicles and coal-burning power plants and factories, which react with moisture in the atmosphere.*

Every year in the United States acid rain destroys thousands of acres of forests by destroying the roots and leaves of ground foliage and trees. (Gilbert S. Grant/Photo Researchers, Inc.)

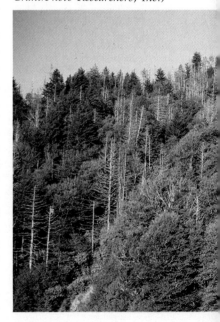

Besides its effects on living organisms, acid rain has been implicated in the deterioration of metal bridges and stone buildings.

eutrophication—*the depletion of oxygen in a body of water caused by an increase in its temperature, as by thermal pollution, which diminishes the ability of the water to support aquatic plant and animal life.*

thermal pollution—*an undesirable increase in the temperature of a body of water, as by the introduction of warm waste water from a factory.*

sphere and fall as acid rain in Canada. Similar conditions occur among the countries of Europe. Recognizing the international scope of this problem, 21 nations have signed a Protocol on the Reduction of Sulfur Emissions aimed at limiting damage from acid rain. While the United States has acknowledged that something must be done about this problem, as of 1989 it had not signed the agreement.[17]

Nutrient Pollution   One of the classic forms of water pollution is the discharge of sewage and other organic matter into lakes, rivers, and streams. This organic matter accelerates the growth of bacteria, which consume oxygen and leads to **eutrophication,** or decreased oxygen dissolved in the water. As oxygen levels fall, fewer plant and animal species are able to survive. In addition to damaging or destroying aquatic species, sewage may contain microorganisms that pose a risk to human health. While the use of water treatment facilities has reduced the risk of nutrient pollution in much of the United States, problems still exist in some areas. In other parts of the world, particularly in developing nations, this type of pollution poses a serious health threat.

Thermal Pollution   Another type of water pollution that is destroying plant and animal life in lakes and rivers is **thermal pollution**—the release of water that, because of its industrial uses, is too warm. Sharp changes in water temperature cause *thermal shock*—a sudden death of aquatic animals and plants that cannot tolerate the temperature change. Less severe changes may interfere with the reproduction of aquatic species and can increase their susceptibility to parasites and certain toxins.[18] Increased water temperature can contribute to eutrophication, with all its attendant dangers. Thermal pollution is a problem that even the best-intentioned companies are not yet able to prevent.

Improving Water Quality   Some efforts to reverse the effects of water pollution may take generations, but the steps taken so far to clean up American waters have demonstrated that dramatic results can occur in only a few years. Lake Erie, which was too polluted to support life in the 1960s, is now markedly better. Water quality is improving in the Chesapeake Bay, as it is in the Cuyahoga, Potomac, and other rivers once severely polluted by agricultural, urban, and industrial wastes.

Such improvements continue to be made thanks to public awareness and governmental efforts. For example, under the National Pollution Discharge Elimination System (NPDES), fluids may not be pumped into a river or lake without a permit specifying which substances the discharge may contain. Contamination from a specific source is thus easier to trace, and any company caught discharging an unauthorized substance can lose its permit. As a result, most deliberate industrial pollution of water has stopped. However, pollution from other sources, such as runoff from farms, roadways, and homes, is more extensive and difficult to stop.

Most U.S. cities today have modern sewage treatment plants which have improved water quality, yet several others with antiquated sewage treatment systems continue dumping sludge (the material left after sewage is treated) into the sea. As of 1990, Boston, New York, and a number of New Jersey communities were still dumping sewage treatment residue into the Atlantic Ocean at a discharge point approved by the EPA.[19]

In 1986 Congress revised the Safe Drinking Water Act to protect *aquifers*— the underground supplies that provide water for about half the U.S. population. The act now provides funds for protecting any aquifer that is the sole source of drinking water for an area, and it requires state governments to draft plans for protecting other public water supplies as well. Despite such efforts, conservationists say that further efforts by the federal and state governments are needed to protect the nation's water supplies.[20]

Lake Erie had productive fisheries during the 1950s; they were destroyed by water pollution less than 20 years later. Today, however, water quality in the lake is clearly on the mend. (Martin Rogers/Stock Boston)

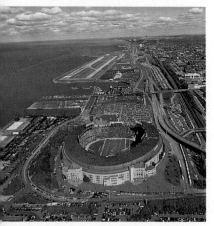

Table 20.2 Common Hazardous Wastes

Chemical	Use	Hazard
C-56	Bug and insect killer	Acutely toxic, suspected carcinogen
Trichloroethylene (TCE)	Degreaser	Suspected carcinogen
Benzidene	Dye industry	Known human carcinogen
Curene 442	Plastics industry	Suspected carcinogen
Polychlorinated biphenyls (PCBs)	Insulators, paints, and electrical circuitry	Acutely toxic, suspected carcinogen
Benzene	Solvent	Suspected carcinogen
Tris	Fire retardant	Suspected carcinogen
DDT	Bug and insect killer	Acutely toxic
Vinyl chloride	Plastics industry	Known human carcinogen
Mercury	Multiple uses	Acutely toxic
Lead	Multiple uses	Acutely toxic, suspected carcinogen
Carbon tetrachloride	Solvent	Acutely toxic, suspected carcinogen
Polybrominated biphenyls (PBBs)	Fire retardant	Effects unknown

Source: Council on Environmental Quality.

The Land: Pollution and Protection

Many pollutants are disposed of legally on the ground in landfills constructed for the purpose; others are dumped illegally. These pollutants include hazardous wastes—toxic substances generated primarily by industry—and non-hazardous wastes—numerous types of garbage and discarded materials generated by industry, municipalities, and private households. In recent years solid wastes have become a major pollution problem and health problem in the United States and other countries (Table 20.2).

Hazardous Wastes Every year the United States produces more than 255 million metric tons of hazardous waste, or about 1 ton per person. This does not include household hazardous wastes such as dead batteries, painting supplies, and cleaning fluids. According to the EPA, only about 10 percent of these wastes are disposed of safely. The rest end up in municipal landfills, abandoned warehouses, fields and forests, and lakes, rivers, and streams, where they pose an increasingly serious health threat.[21]

Uncontrolled dumping of hazardous wastes can have tragic consequences. Between 1947 and 1952 the Hooker Chemical and Plastics Corporation dumped 21,800 tons of pesticides, cleaning solutions, and other toxic wastes into the Love Canal near Niagara Falls, New York. In 1953 Hooker covered the site with dirt and sold it to the Niagara Falls Board of Education, which then built a school on the site and sold adjoining home lots.

In 1978, after flooding in the neighborhood, residents reported noxious odors permeating homes, slime oozing into basements, children experiencing painful rashes and watering eyes, and, most alarming of all, unusually high rates of miscarriages, birth defects, liver ailments, nervous disorders, epilepsylike seizures, genetic damage, and cancer.

Eventually the landfill's topsoil began to wash away, revealing corroded and leaking metal casks. Analysis by the EPA revealed that the dump contained more than 80 chemicals, including 10 potential carcinogens, solvents that damage the heart and liver, and pesticides so dangerous that their commercial sale had been restricted for years.[22] President Jimmy Carter declared a state of emergency in the area, and 237 families were evacuated in August 1978.

Another hazardous waste disaster occurred in Times Beach, Missouri, a suburb of St. Louis. In 1971 road crews began spraying recycled waste oil on the dirt roads of Times Beach to keep down the dust. As it turned out, the oil had been mixed with sludge from a chemical plant. This sludge contained dioxins, which, according to some scientists, are among the most dangerous

Baking soda, vinegar, soap, ammonia, and borax are substances that, when mixed properly, provide safe, efficient alternatives to toxic household cleaners. For instance, baking soda and water alone can clean many surfaces. Baking soda is an excellent deodorizer and can be sprinkled in corners. Vinegar and water are good for cleaning glass. A simple damp rag can be used for dusting.

chemicals known. Dioxins are notorious for producing dramatic health problems even in incredibly small doses. Although no human deaths have been directly attributed to dioxins, they have been associated with a host of diseases, including cancer and kidney and liver diseases. In 1982 the EPA bought the entire town of Times Beach and evacuated its residents at a cost of $26.3 million in government funds.

Similar problems are sure to surface in the future. Chemical wastes may be dangerous for hundreds of years, and learning to dispose of them safely must therefore be a high priority.

Cleaning Up Yesterday's Poisons: Superfund

In the 1970s Congress created the Superfund to provide funds for cleaning up old, often abandoned hazardous waste dump sites (Figure 20.1). In 1986 Congress extended the Superfund for 5 years and provided an additional $9 billion.[23]

Under the Superfund law, the EPA can clean up a dump site and then file lawsuits to recover the cost from those responsible, including the site's present or past owners, anyone who arranged for hazardous waste disposal or treatment at the site, and anyone who transported wastes to the site. The Superfund law also allows the EPA to impose civil and criminal penalties for injuring natural resources. In addition to the federal law, 33 states have passed Superfund laws.[24]

One social obstacle to waste management is known as the NIMBY (not in my backyard) syndrome. Some communities have organized to resist the placement of new disposal or incinerator sites in their neighborhoods.

Many environmentalists are disappointed with the Superfund's cleanup record. Only 27 of the 1,224 dump sites on the federal Superfund cleanup list have been declared completely clean. Rather than being used to clean up sites, much Superfund money has been spent on consultants and studies of the sites.

Dealing with Hazardous Wastes

Hazardous wastes can be treated in a number of ways to make them less toxic or at least reduce their bulk.[25] One method is *incineration*, or burning at a very high temperature under controlled conditions for a prescribed time. Incineration is an effective means of destroy-

Source: U.S. Bureau of the Census, *Statistical Abstracts of the United States, 1990,* 110th ed. (Washington, D.C.: U.S. Government Printing Office, 1990): 205.

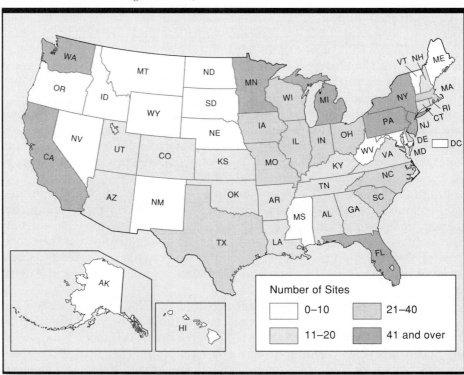

Figure 20.1 The national priorities list for the Superfund program includes over 1,200 sites to be cleaned up. Notice the high concentration of sites in the Northeast—more than one-quarter of all sites are east of Ohio and north of Maryland, where U.S. industry is located.

ing the toxins in wastes, but it is very costly. Another method is the use of chemical treatments, which can neutralize some hazardous wastes by breaking them down into nontoxic substances. Other hazardous wastes can be treated chemically to make them less soluble in water or neutralize their acidity or alkalinity.

Under a law enacted by Congress in 1984, certain deadly toxins, such as PCBs and dioxins, must be neutralized or destroyed in incinerators. Other toxic wastes can be disposed of through a relatively inexpensive "cap and contain" method in which the toxic substances are enclosed within clay and synthetic barriers and then buried. Although this method does not eliminate toxic substances from the environment altogether, the clay, which is highly resistant to water, and synthetic barriers help keep them from spreading through the soil into the water supply and food chain.

A handful of landfills around the United States are authorized to accept treated toxic wastes for burial in this manner. One of the largest sites is in Pinewood, South Carolina. Every year 135,000 tons of hazardous wastes are hauled to the Pinewood dump to be contained and buried. A state health inspector is on the site at all times to ensure that all required procedures are carried out.

Despite its stringent security measures, Pinewood has been the focus of protests by environmental groups, and the number of such high-security dump sites is dwindling. Today a mere 4 percent of industrial hazardous wastes is sent to such burial sites. The remaining wastes are treated and disposed of at the sites where they were produced.[26]

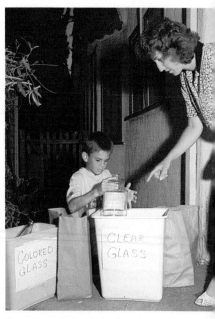

Recycling paper and glass is one way for everyone to take an active stance on the issue of waste control. (Mary Kate Denny/PhotoEdit)

Solid Nonhazardous Waste and Recycling The amount of garbage and trash produced by American households swelled by 80 percent over the last two decades, and before the turn of the century it may increase another 20 percent. Dealing with this refuse has become a formidable and growing problem.

As of 1988, about 80 percent of household refuse in the United States was going to landfills, another 10 percent was being incinerated, and the remainder was being recycled. Meanwhile, the nation's landfills are being rapidly filled to capacity, and many are shutting down. The number of active landfills dropped from 18,000 in the late 1970s to only 6,000 in 1988; by the mid-1990s the number may be below 4,000.[27] The nation is quickly running out of acceptable places to dispose of refuse.

To help deal with the problem, in 1988 the EPA set forth a plan that called for Americans to recycle 25 percent of their household trash by 1992. *Recycling*, or processing for reuse, can reduce the amount of trash sent to dumps and prevent the waste of natural resources and energy. Producing recycled aluminum, for example, takes only 5 percent as much energy as producing aluminum from its ore, bauxite. Recycling paper uses 64 percent less energy than does producing paper from virgin pulpwood and helps preserve forests.[28]

In addition to voluntary and mandatory recycling, the waste disposal problem may be reduced in part by action on the part of manufacturers to reduce the amount of packaging they use for their products. The use of more biodegradable materials—materials that decompose in the environment—could also reduce the bulk of garbage in landfills and extend their use.

Hints for garbage recycling:

- *Use fewer disposable products, for example, razors, cups and plates, and diapers. Instead, buy products designed for reuse and repair.*
- *Try to avoid buying products in Styrofoam and plastic containers. Paper and cardboard are less damaging to the environment.*
- *Reuse bags and other packaging materials whenever you can.*
- *Favor products with less packaging. Some products contain more layers of packaging than are necessary, for instance, several small boxes inside a larger box.*
- *Support recycling efforts in your home, neighborhood, community, and state.*

Global Environmental Issues

Leading ecologist Barry Commoner pointed out in his book *The Closing Circle* that the earth, like health, is a system in which every part is linked to all the others in an incredibly complex network of interconnections and interdependencies. Any pressure placed on one component of this system will ultimately have effects on the system as a whole. This notion helps explain why

Ecological relationships are often so complex that they negate the effects that planners intended. For example, despite the increased use of pesticides, the amount of crops damaged by insects has nearly doubled in the past 40 years. Some insects develop resistance to pesticides. On occasion pesticides have even helped harmful insects by killing their natural enemies.

pollution, while most noticeable within a local environment, can nevertheless have serious consequences on the global environment as a whole and why efforts to reduce pollution locally can have a broad beneficial effect. Human-made pollution, which is unnatural to the system, puts a stress on the other parts of the system and accumulates to the point where it is harmful not only to the local environment but to the global environment as well.

If present trends hold, by the turn of the century the world will have more people and more pollution than it does today. As a result, the environment may become dangerously unstable and more vulnerable to disruption. Already pollution appears to be having many dangerous worldwide effects, such as an apparent thinning of the ozone layer, a protective barrier that has helped make the earth hospitable to life for millions of years. If left unchecked, other conditions, such as global warming, deforestation, food shortages, and depletion of energy resources, may result in dire consequences for the planet's future inhabitants.

The Ozone Layer

ozone layer—a thin layer in the earth's upper atmosphere. Unlike smog, this layer is beneficial, acting as a shield to prevent harmful ultraviolet light from reaching the earth's surface.

As mentioned earlier in this chapter, ozone is a primary component of the smog that often fouls the air in cities throughout the world. The earth's upper atmosphere also contains a thin layer of ozone. However, unlike the ozone in smog, this **ozone layer** is beneficial, even vital to all living things. It acts as a shield to prevent harmful ultraviolet light from reaching the earth's surface. Among the risks excess ultraviolet light poses for humans is an increase in the incidence of skin cancer and cataracts, a leading cause of blindness. Research also has indicated that excessive exposure to ultraviolet rays inhibits the immune response, reducing the ability of the body to fight viral disease.[29] Damage to the ozone layer affects the ability of the atmosphere to block these harmful ultraviolet rays, jeopardizing the health of humans as well as other plant and animal species.

Certain air pollutants, such as chlorofluorocarbons (CFCs), have been blamed for the damage being done to the ozone layer. Chlorofluorocarbons are used in refrigerators and air conditioners, in plastic foams and solvents, and as propellants in aerosol spray cans. The EPA ordered a 50 percent cutback in the production of CFCs beginning in 1989. This order—which relies on voluntary compliance by industries—will, if followed, bring the United States into compliance with a 1988 international agreement to protect the ozone layer.

Global Warming: The Greenhouse Effect

While there is still disagreement about this issue, many scientists have been predicting that rising levels of carbon dioxide (CO_2) and other gases in the atmosphere will create a *greenhouse effect*: like the glass roof of a greenhouse, they will trap heat, affecting the earth's atmosphere and causing a global warming trend.

The atmospheric level of CO_2, the primary greenhouse gas, has risen 25 percent since the 1850s.[30] Most of this increase is due to the combustion of wood and fossil fuels, including coal, natural gas, and gasoline. The rate of increase has accelerated since World War II, largely because of automobile exhaust. Chlorofluorocarbons contribute to the greenhouse effect as well as the destruction of the ozone layer.[31]

The EPA has estimated that the earth's overall temperature will rise as much as 8 degrees Fahrenheit over the next 50 or 60 years if the release of greenhouse gases continues unabated. According to experts, such a change would have a significant impact on the planet. The increased temperature would melt a substantial amount of ice at the north and south poles, raising sea levels and causing increased coastal flooding and the permanent inundation of some coastal areas. A temperature rise also has the potential to expand

People's efforts to develop the perfect tan are becoming dangerous as destruction of the ozone layer threatens to cause a severe increase in skin cancer rates. (Herb Snitzer/The Stock Shop)

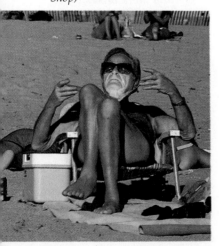

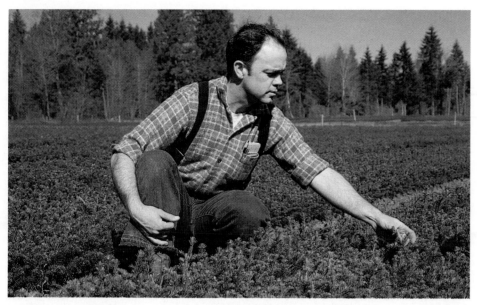

Careful forest management is a way to prevent the destruction of one of the most valuable natural resources—trees. (Porterfield-Chickering/Photo Researchers, Inc.)

the world's deserts by altering climate and rainfall patterns. Such changes could seriously impede the growth of crops and livestock in some areas and diminish world food supplies, putting the survival of large numbers of people at risk.

Dangers of Deforestation

Dealing with the greenhouse effect will require creative and sometimes difficult decisions. This is a major reason why environmentalists oppose the large-scale destruction of forests. While the burning or decay of trees releases carbon dioxide into the atmosphere, living trees and other plants are, along with oceans, the major consumers of atmospheric carbon dioxide. For this reason, some environmentalists suggest bans or limitations on lumbering, to be followed by massive tree-planting campaigns, as a way to deal with the greenhouse effect. At present, more forestland throughout the world is being destroyed than is being reforested. As a result, deforestation is turning forests into part of the global warming problem rather than part of the solution.[32]

In addition to their role in controlling carbon dioxide levels, forests serve other essential purposes. For example, forest growth helps prevent soil erosion; without tree roots to help anchor the soil, it is more easily eroded, leaving the land less able to support plant growth. Forests also play a role in preventing or lessening the effects of drought, as the evaporation of moisture from forest trees and plants helps generate rainfall. Tropical rain forests in particular are valuable because of the biological diversity they shelter. These forests provide a habitat for millions of plant and animal species, many of them unstudied. Many unique plants found there contain valuable medicinal and other compounds; if the forests are destroyed, these and other plants will be lost.

Unfortunately, deforestation is occurring rapidly in many places. The Amazonian rain forests of Brazil are being felled by people seeking land for farming or ranching. The monsoon forests in the Himalayan foothills have been stripped for firewood, cropland, and lumber. Other tropical forests are being denuded in Malaysia, East Africa, and northeast Australia.[33]

Deforestation is taking place in the northern hemisphere as well. In places such as the Pacific Northwest and the west coast of Canada, forests are being destroyed by land development and lumbering; other northern forests are

It takes a half million trees to produce Sunday newspapers for one weekend. Every ton of paper made from recycled materials saves 17 trees.

being damaged by acid rain. However, attempts to alleviate the situation *are* being made. The environmentalist movement is growing stronger both in Europe and in North America; in response, lumber companies are starting to research less destructive methods of harvesting trees for different wood-based products.

World Food Supplies

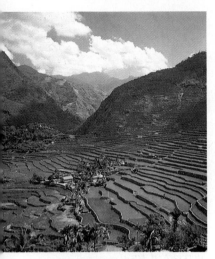

Conservationist approaches to farming have a long history. These terraced rice fields in the Philippines have been productive for centuries. (Blair Seitz/Photo Researchers, Inc.)

One of the most serious long-term threats to human life and health resulting from environmental degradation and destruction may be a shortage of food. In some parts of the world, especially in the poorer countries, food production has already been affected. In Africa, for example, per capita food production has fallen about 15 percent since 1970. Much of this decline can be attributed to environmental degradation coupled with increased population pressures on the land. In the future, *famine*—extreme shortages of food—may not be limited to the poorest countries, however. Even in the United States, the drought and summer heat of 1988 (which some scientists point to as a precursor to the greenhouse effect) kept farmers from producing as much grain as was consumed.[34]

A focus on obtaining immediate high crop yields rather than on long-term land use is ruining farmland in many countries. For example, the use of fertilizer often results in diminishing returns: the more fertilizer that is used, the less it helps.

Unfortunately, putting unused land to agricultural use is probably not a feasible solution to the problem of food supply. Much of the land that has not yet been cultivated or grazed is infertile or inaccessible. The oceans are also unlikely to offer a solution. Worldwide fish catches have been decreasing since the 1970s, and the effect of pollution on ocean ecosystems is to some extent still uncertain.

*Forty thousand babies under 1 year old die of starvation **each day** in third world countries.*

The situation is not hopeless, however. Human beings may be able to prevent widespread famine by reversing the trend toward depletion and destruction of agricultural and other food-producing resources. For example, some areas can still benefit from the use of improved farming techniques to increase crop yields; in other areas, farmland that has been overcultivated can be saved. Perhaps the most encouraging sign is a growing awareness that the earth cannot support an unlimited number of human beings.[35]

Unless world population growth is controlled, the point may be reached where the earth no longer has the capacity to feed its multitudes. Today, the world contains more than 5 billion people, and this number is expected to double in the next 100 years if population continues to grow at the present rate. In many of the poorer countries, populations are growing so fast that the land can no longer provide even the most basic levels of food, shelter, and fuel. People in these countries are overtaxing the soil, destroying forests, and turning grasslands into deserts. In India, for example, more than one-third of the country's 800 million people are unable to obtain the amount of food they need to sustain themselves.[36]

While the governments of many countries are committed to limiting population growth as a means of coping with food shortages, deeply held cultural values make population growth a continuing problem.[37]

Energy Use: The Global Outlook

Today most utility companies provide low-cost energy audits for residential homes. Such audits identify problems with heating systems and home insulation and can save both energy and dollars.

Most environmental experts urge more efficient energy use as a means of improving air quality and reducing the danger of a global greenhouse effect. More efficient use of energy can reduce the level of atmospheric carbon emissions, which are largely responsible for air pollution and global warming.

The United States's experience with energy conservation demonstrates that energy use can be reduced. Spurred by a gasoline shortage and soaring prices for petroleum products in the early 1970s, per capita energy consumption in this country fell 12 percent between 1973 and 1985. This effort reduced annual carbon emissions by millions of tons.[38]

According to the Worldwatch Institute, a similar effort to improve energy efficiency worldwide could reduce the amount of carbon emissions in the atmosphere by nearly one-third annually. The institute contends that the greatest potential for reducing carbon emissions lies in building cars that use fuel more efficiently. It also calls for improved public transportation, greater use of bicycles, taxes on all fossil fuels, and the use of energy-efficient electric lighting as additional means of reducing the level of carbon emissions in the atmosphere.[39]

Although new cars pollute less, the number of cars on the road continues to increase and more miles are driven per year. Traffic congestion problems are steadily growing worse. A study in 1985 showed that nearly 3 billion gallons of gas was wasted in the United States as a result of traffic congestion—about 4 percent of total consumption.

Alternatives to Fossil Fuels The Worldwatch Institute claims that reducing carbon emissions enough to stabilize the climate will require increased reliance on alternative energy sources such as solar power, wind power, and nuclear power in place of fossil fuels and wood.[40]

Solar power and wind power are gaining in popularity in some parts of the world. By 1986, California was using wind generators to produce more than twice as much energy as it had in previous years. Also in 1986, the Alabama Power Company opened a solar power plant that used the same technology that runs solar watches and calculators. Although the plant cost more to build than do conventional power plants, some analysts expect solar power to become economically competitive with other sources of energy for utilities in the 1990s.[41]

Methane gas is another alternative energy source that is being tested. The chief component of natural gas, methane is also produced from the decay of organic matter. When released into the atmosphere, methane adds substantially to the greenhouse effect. Using it as fuel, however, greatly reduces the damage to the atmosphere, and every home heated by methane is one that does not have to burn wood or petroleum. At present, several sites in the United States are collecting methane from landfills and using it as a heating fuel.[42]

Other potential energy sources are also available, including hydroelectric power, geothermal power, and tidal power. *Hydroelectric power*, in which water power is used to generate electricity, is already used widely in regions

Wind power and solar heating have been available for commercial use since the 1970s, but efforts to utilize these alternative energy sources have not been widespread. (Paul Conklin/ PhotoEdit; Tom McHugh/Photo Researchers, Inc.)

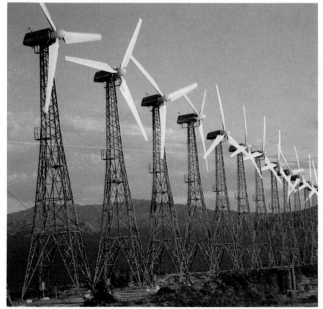
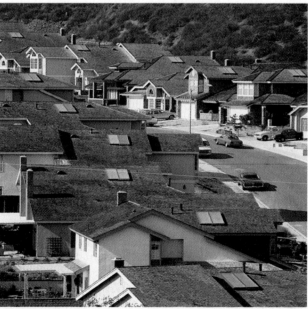

with an abundance of rivers and lakes that can be dammed. *Geothermal power* harnesses the heat generated deep within the earth; it is not widely used because of costs, limitations of technology, and limited access to sources of geothermal energy. *Tidal power*, which harnesses the energy of the ocean tides, also has very limited use at this time because of problems with cost and technology.

Nuclear Power Some people consider *nuclear power* to be the best solution to the fossil fuel crisis. Others see it as a growing menace that threatens the entire planet. Pronuclear groups point out that nuclear technology is already available and that power is being generated safely in many places—with no atmospheric pollution. France, for example, gets more than 70 percent of its electricity from nuclear power plants and has an impressive safety record.[43] Antinuclear groups point out the potential for dangerous nuclear accidents and the growing problem of the disposal of radioactive wastes.

The debate between the pronuclear and antinuclear forces has become more intense in recent years. The breakdown of the Three Mile Island nuclear reactor near Harrisburg, Pennsylvania, in 1979 raised serious questions about the future of the nuclear power industry in the United States. As a result of this incident and the ensuing controversy, no nuclear power plants were built in the United States during the 1980s.[44] In the Three Mile Island incident, a malfunction of the plant's cooling system caused by human and mechanical failure triggered a series of events that caused the powerful reactor to begin to self-destruct. For 16 hours large amounts of radioactive steam and gas were released into the atmosphere. Children and pregnant women were evacuated from the area. No one died at Three Mile Island, but the long-term effects on the health of those exposed to the radiation are still unknown.

In 1986 a worse incident occurred at a nuclear power plant at Chernobyl in the Soviet Union. The Chernobyl reactor probably failed because of a loss of coolant, as occurred in the Three Mile Island accident. Temperatures within the Chernobyl reactor climbed, setting off an explosion and fire that released radioactive gases into the air. Some plant workers died immediately as a result of the explosion and intense radiation, and many more people were placed at grave risk of developing radiation sickness or cancer. To make matters worse, shifting winds quickly spread dangerous levels of radiation across the Soviet Union and Eastern Europe. Progressively smaller concentrations were later detected in Western Europe and North America. Because of the slow, silent way in which radiation harms life, the full effects of the Chernobyl incident will not be known for years to come.

Besides the danger from accidents such as those at Three Mile Island and Chernobyl, nuclear power production generates radioactive wastes that pose a serious threat to human health and the environment. Overexposure to radiation can produce radiation sickness, with symptoms that include diarrhea, nausea, and vomiting, followed by hair loss, hemorrhaging, and ulcers, and finally by cataracts, susceptibility to infections, and leukemia (Table 20.3). Radiation is also a factor in genetic mutations, and significant doses are known to cause infertility, miscarriage, and birth defects. Higher than normal doses may also increase the risk of contracting cancer.

The disposal of radioactive wastes is a serious environmental problem. Much of the spent fuel and other debris from nuclear power plants will remain dangerously radioactive for hundreds and even thousands of years. In the United States alone thousands of tons of spent radioactive fuel and debris have been generated over the past few decades, and more is being produced all the time.[45]

No method for disposing of radioactive wastes has yet been proved safe, although scientists in several countries are searching for one. France is developing a process called *vitrification*, in which the radioactive materials are mixed with molten glass. The glass cools into a radioactive but stable solid

The exact effects of prolonged, intermittent exposure are not, however, well documented. Much of the knowledge about the effects of radiation comes from studies of the long-term effects of the bombs dropped on Hiroshima and Nagasaki, where the radiation was intense and relatively brief.

Injury caused by the nuclear accident at Chernobyl was immediate for some people, but many others who might have been affected will not know for many years. (Dr. Robert Gale/Sygma)

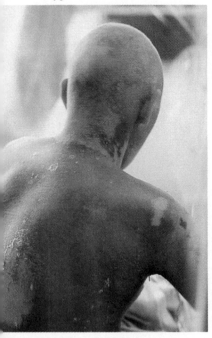

Table 20.3 Parts of the Body Where Components of Radioactive Fallout Lodge

Radioactive Substance	Part of Body
Gamma and x-rays, neutrons	Brain and nervous system
Iodine 131	Thyroid gland
Strontium 90, barium 140, lanthanum 140	Bones
Plutonium	Liver, bones, and sex organs
Insoluble radioactive airborne dust emitting alpha, beta, and gamma rays	Lungs
Ultrasmall insoluble radioactive particles	Bone marrow, liver, and spleen
Cesium 137	Lymph glands, blood
Krypton 85	Body fat
All soluble fission products (including some of the above)	Sex organs and kidneys

Source: Malcolm W. Browne, *"The Not-So-Clear but Present Danger,"* New York Times (May 18, 1986): sec. 4, p. 2. Copyright © 1986 by the New York Times Company. Reprinted by permission.

that can be buried deep below the earth's surface, according to the developers of the process. The United States is also pursuing a strategy of burying radioactive waste, though to date protests have ruled out several proposed burial sites.[46]

Taking Action to Protect the Environment

The United States has had a greater impact on the global environment than has any other nation. Although it has less than 5 percent of the total world population, the United States is the largest consumer of energy and natural resources. It consumes one-fourth of the world's energy and is responsible for one-fifth of all carbon emissions in the atmosphere. Because of its impact on the environment and its wealth and influence, this country must play a significant role in efforts to protect the environment. Success may ultimately depend on the willingness of Americans to lead the way both in dealing with their own problems and in helping other nations deal with theirs.[47]

The Need for Cooperative Action

The United States cannot act alone to solve the world's environmental problems. Environmental degradation is an international problem, and efforts by a single nation, no matter what that nation's impact, can have only a limited effect. Instead, there needs to be action on the part of all governments and a focus on international cooperation and standards. Even a single nation that refuses to cooperate can cause great damage.

Industry must respond to the challenge as well. Companies can no longer focus on short-term profits at the expense of long-term concerns such as the environment and public health. While economic profit is a vital concern for every business, all businesses must also concern themselves more with their impact on the environment and on human health.

Also very important is the responsibility of communities and individuals to help protect their local environments. People must begin to make choices that are based on how their actions will affect the quality of the air, water, and land on which all life depends. In democratic societies especially, individual choices can influence the actions of government and industry, prompting them to be more concerned about environmental issues. Community action can do even more: by communicating concerns to neighbors and friends and cooperating with them, people can ensure that major changes can be brought about even faster.

Being a Good Environmental Advocate

If you feel strongly about protecting the environment, what can you do in addition to acting responsibly? For instance, what can you do personally to fight industrial pollution, encourage recycling, and influence government policy? One approach is to devote time to environmental advocacy. You could join a group that works to protect the environment or take action on your own. The key is to communicate your feelings to those in business and government who make decisions that affect the environment.

People often feel powerless to protect the environment. You may wonder what difference one person can make. The fact is that companies *do* pay attention to what they hear. If the stockholders of a company receive letters about an action that affects the environment, if they are the target of negative publicity, or if they are criticized at public meetings, they are likely to reconsider their policies. By contrast, if no one protests a policy that is damaging the environment, the company may assume that no damage is being done or that no one cares. Elected government officials are also concerned about

public reaction to their actions. If a politician receives many letters urging a vote for environmental legislation, that politician has to consider what will happen in the next election if he or she ignores the letters.

Whether you speak out at a public meeting about building a new incinerator in your community, write a letter to your representative about a proposed law to stop ocean dumping of garbage, talk to your neighbors about recycling, or write to a company that produces chemicals that are harmful to the environment, you can take steps to make sure that your communication is effective. Before you speak or write, take some time to plan your approach. Be sure you understand who your audience is. If you are going to speak at a public meeting of your block association, you are talking to neighbors who have a common interest in maintaining a good quality of life in the neighborhood. If you are writing a letter to a local business about the use of nonbiodegradable containers, you are trying to reach a person or a group of people who are interested in making money selling products to your community. Tailor

Personal Action

Protecting the environment will require a great deal more thought than people ordinarily give to their daily routines and habits. For example, air pollution could be reduced significantly if drivers used their cars less. Sharing rides with friends and coworkers, using public transportation, and taking care of shopping in one trip rather than several can help accomplish this.

Since no one can live without utilizing the earth's resources, it is inevitable that people have an impact on the environment. A focus on conservation can result in a more efficient use of resources at a lower cost to the environment. Protecting the earth does not require that people stop using resources and technology but that they use them more carefully.

The decision that each person must make is whether the cost of an action is worth the benefit it provides. Take the purchase of a trash compactor, an appliance that compresses household trash into smaller, more convenient packages. Although this may be useful to the individual, when the compacted trash gets to a landfill, it presents a problem: the natural process of **biodegradation**—the breakdown and assimilation of organic material by microorganisms—is hampered because the trash is so compacted. What decision is to be made here? Is it better to accept the reduced effectiveness of the landfill in order to have compacted trash that is easy to handle? Or do people value the biodegradability of the trash over personal convenience?

Nearly all environmental issues involve such trade-offs. For example, with agricultural fertilizers, pesticides, and herbicides, the choice is often between

biodegradation—*the breakdown and assimilation of organic material by microorganisms.*

your message to a typical member of this audience. Try to find a way to appeal to that person's interests.

Whether you are speaking or writing, keep your communication brief and to the point. Start by deciding on your main point. Phrase it in a sentence or two: "We need to protect this park so our children can enjoy it." "We need to stop this pollution to protect the health of the community." "We must use recyclable materials so that we do not use up scarce resources and cause a solid waste disposal problem." If you are speaking to a group, state your main point right away and then repeat it as a summary at the end of the talk.

If you are writing, state the main point in the opening sentence and restate it at the conclusion of the letter. Find out the name and title of the person at the top of the company (perhaps the president or owner) and address the letter to that person. When possible, mention any group you represent. For example, it is more effective if you can say, "All my neighbors stand behind this position."

To make your basic point more telling, develop one or two hard-hitting arguments that support it. Select appropriate facts and statistics, being sure you understand them and present them clearly. Quantify when you can. It is more effective to say "The cancer rate is 10 percent higher in homes near the dump" than it is to say "People who live near the dump get sick more than other people in the community."

Try not to be too confrontational or negative in your communication. If you do that, you may alienate your audience. Make the assumption that they are reasonable people who would be ready to respond if they knew what you know. Instead of saying, "Your company is carelessly disregarding the health and safety of the community," you might say, "Your company has shown by its actions in supporting local charities that it cares about the community. I know that you will want to take action now to protect the health of the same people."

Adapted from Karen Berg and Andrew Gilman, *Get to the Point* (New York: Bantam, 1989); Rosemary T. Fruehlin and N. B. Oldham, *Write to the Point* (New York: McGraw-Hill, 1988).

higher crop yields and damage to the harmless insects and animals that inhabit the environment. Which choice is better? Obviously, there is no clear answer to this question. On the one hand, society values individual freedom—Americans believe that people should be free to manage their own affairs so long as they infringe only minimally on the rights of others. On the other hand, it is also important to consider the benefits of keeping the environment intact—benefits for people today, for the whole community, and for their descendants.

Almost all personal decisions can include environmental considerations. Is it better to buy an inexpensive plastic cutting board or a more expensive one made of wood? This is not merely a matter of taste or finances but also has environmental implications: the wood product is more environmentally sound. Is it better to buy frozen strawberries or fresh ones transported under refrigeration from another part of the country? Perhaps the fresh ones taste better, but refrigeration and transportation have negative environmental effects. The frozen berries, however, are no doubt packaged in plastic, which will end up in a landfill as nonbiodegradable garbage. The decision is not an easy one, and both choices require trade-offs.

Individual decisions can on occasion be personally beneficial. Choosing to walk or bicycle to the store rather than drive there is an environmentally sound decision. However, such a decision is also personally beneficial: walking or bicycling is a good form of exercise that can improve cardiovascular health and may even relieve stress and contribute to more positive emotional

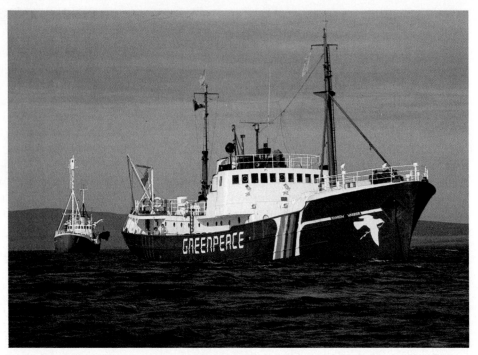

The ships of the Greenpeace organization are symbolic of the work this organization does to ensure a healthier environment in the future. (Julian Calder/Woodfin Camp & Associates, Inc.)

health. In such cases, making an environmentally sound decision provides long-term benefits for the individual as well as for society and all of humanity.

The Benefits of Commitment and Cooperation

Personal commitment to environmental issues becomes particularly meaningful when it can be translated into social awareness and action. While individual awareness and actions can accomplish a great deal, they gain strength when combined with the awareness and actions of others. Working together, people can do much to protect the environment and, in doing so, promote world health.

Taking action and working together on environmental issues are likely to affect not only physical health (by improving environmental quality) but also emotional, social, and spiritual health. Successful cooperation can contribute to emotional health by helping people develop feelings of self-efficacy and self-worth. It can also contribute to social health both for the individual and for the other people involved—shared concerns and support empower people to work for positive change and enable them to accomplish more than an individual could accomplish alone.

There are numerous opportunities for working with others on environmental concerns. Many organizations, such as the Sierra Club, the Wilderness Society, the World Wildlife Fund, and Greenpeace, actively deal with environmental issues and provide opportunities for more active involvement.

Because environmental issues touch on moral values, such as the sanctity both of human life and of other forms of life in nature, concern about environmental issues may also affect spiritual health. In the short run one may be brought into conflict with the views or rights of others and may challenge their moral, ethical, and spiritual values. In the long run a commitment to environmental causes is likely to contribute profoundly to spiritual health. Working selflessly for a belief and examining values help make a person spiritually stronger and more consistent.

In helping the environment, people are helping themselves. Although the task is daunting, the goal is worthwhile. People must not succumb to the feeling that they can do nothing. At stake is one's personal health as well as the health of billions of other people around the world.

Chapter Summary

- Environmental pollution can have a detrimental effect on physical health when it exposes people to toxic substances or affects the ability of the environment to provide for people's needs. Emotional, social, and spiritual health may also be deeply affected.

- The quality of the air is affected by contaminants and toxins, which can be detrimental to human health. Water quality also can be affected by the presence of contaminants and toxins and by thermal pollution and nutrient pollution. Uncontrolled dumping of hazardous wastes can severely damage health, and the proliferation of nonhazardous wastes can blight the environment and contribute to the pollution of land and water.

- Air quality can be improved by restricting the amount of pollutants discharged into the air, including pollutants from industry, small businesses, and individuals (most notably from automobiles). Water quality can be improved by limiting the discharge of pollutants into waterways. Treatment of polluted water before it is discharged into waterways can also reduce damage to the environment. Landfills and solid wastes cause difficult problems; one way to improve the situation is to enforce stringent controls over dumping and create safe and more reliable methods of treating and disposing of hazardous wastes. The solid waste problem can be alleviated by using alternative means of disposal such as incineration and, more important, by recycling and encouraging the manufacture and use of biodegradable products.

- The ozone layer in the upper atmosphere, which helps protect plant and animal life from harmful ultraviolet rays, is being damaged by chemical pollutants such as chlorofluorocarbons. The use of refrigerants, solvents, and aerosols contributes to this problem.

- Increasing levels of certain gases in the air may be contributing to the global warming known as the greenhouse effect. If such warming takes place, it may have disastrous effects on the environment, including increased flooding, inundation of coastal areas, and changes in climate and rainfall patterns that could affect agriculture and living conditions.

- Deforestation may contribute to global warming because trees consume carbon dioxide, the major greenhouse gas, and thus help control carbon dioxide levels. Deforestation can also increase soil erosion and eradicate potentially beneficial species of plant and animal life.

- World population growth is putting tremendous pressure on the environment. The more people there are in the world, the more those people can pollute the environment; overpopulation may also contribute to an increased incidence of famine as cultivated land becomes unable to support the population's need for food.

- Increased energy efficiency can help improve air quality by reducing the levels of pollutants discharged into the atmosphere. The use of alternative energy sources can also reduce the depletion of nonrenewable natural resources such as petroleum.

- Potential alternative energy sources include wind, hydroelectric, solar, geothermal, and tidal power. Each has certain advantages and disadvantages, and technologies for utilizing these forms of energy are at different stages of development.

- Nuclear power can be dangerous if accidents release radioactive material into the air, water, or soil. Radioactive waste materials produced as by-products of nuclear power generation are also dangerous to health and the environment; their disposal constitutes a serious environmental problem.

- The earth's environment is an interconnected and interdependent system. As a result, the solution of environmental problems requires a cooperative effort among governments, industry, and individuals. Such action is essential for arriving at successful solutions.

- People can personally help solve environmental problems by being aware of environmental issues, trying to lessen their impact on the environment, making environmentally sound choices in all aspects of their lives, and working with others to bring about positive change.

Key Terms

Pollution (page 509)

Ozone (page 511)

Carrying capacity
(page 514)

Chlorinated hydrocarbons
(page 514)

Polychlorinated biphenyls
(PCBs) (page 515)

Acid rain (page 515)

Eutrophication
(page 516)

Thermal pollution
(page 516)

Ozone layer (page 520)

Biodegradation
(page 526)

References

1. Arthur Strahler and Alan Strahler, *Elements of Physical Geography*, 3d ed. (New York: Wiley, 1984): 71.

2. U.S. Environmental Protection Agency, *Common Environmental Terms* (A-107) (November 1977): 2.

3. Daniel D. Chiras, *Environmental Science: A Framework for Decision Making* (Menlo Park, Calif.: Benjamin/Cummings, 1985): 428.

4. "Air Pollution: It's All Legal" *Newsweek* (July 24, 1989): p. 28.

5. *Ibid.*, p. 34.

6. "Are We Losing Ground in the Clean Air Battle?" *19th Environmental Quality Index* (Washington, D.C.: National Wildlife Federation, February–March 1987): 38.

7. *The State of the Environment 1985* (Paris: Organization for Economic Cooperation and Development, 1985): 39.

8. "Toxic Pollutants Pose a Far Greater Threat Than Anyone Imagined," *22nd Environmental Quality Index* (Washington, D.C.: National Wildlife Federation, February–March 1990): 47.

9. "Air Pollution: It's All Legal," op. cit., pp. 28–29, 33.

10. *The State of the Environment 1985*, op. cit., p. 38.

11. Bruce K. Ferguson, "Wither Water? The Fragile Future of the World's Most Important Resource," *The Futurist* (1983): 29–36.

12. "Ground Water Pollution Remains an Urgent Problem," op. cit., p. 39.

13. P. ReVelle and C. ReVelle, *The Environment: Issues and Choices for Society* (Boston: Willard Grant Press, 1984).

14. *Environment and Health* (Washington, D.C.: Congressional Quarterly, 1981): 21–22.

15. "Are We Losing Ground in the Clear Air Battle?" op. cit., p. 38.

16. *The State of the Environment 1985*, op. cit., p. 45.

17. "Are We Losing Ground in the Clean Air Battle?" op. cit., p. 39; Lester R. Brown et al., "No Time to Waste," *Worldwatch Agenda* (January–February 1989): 18.

18. Chiras, op. cit., pp. 475–476.

19. "Air Pollution: It's All Legal," op. cit., p. 35.

20. "Ground Water Pollution Remains an Urgent Problem," op. cit.

21. Chiras, op. cit., p. 527; Gordon F. Bloom, "The Hidden Liability of Hazardous Waste Cleanup," *Technology Review* (February–March 1986): 60.

22. *Environment and Health*, op. cit., pp. 35–36.

23. "Ground Water Pollution Remains an Urgent Problem," op. cit.

24. *Bloom*, op. cit., p. 61.

25. Material on hazardous waste treatment is from *Newsweek*, op. cit., pp. 37–40; *The State of the Environment 1985*, op. cit., pp. 167–168.

26. "Air Pollution: It's All Legal," op. cit., pp. 38, 40.

27. United Press International, "EPA Wants 25% of Trash Recycled by 1992 under 'Agenda for Action,'" September 23, 1988.

28. Kate Beardsley, *What We Can Do: Prescott's Practical Guide to Reducing Waste in Our Daily Lives* (Prescott, Ariz.: Beardsley, April 1988): 8.

29. Susan McKearney Bryan, "A Hole in the Sky," *Vim & Vigor* (Fall 1988): 24.

30. "Air Pollution: It's All Legal," op. cit., p. 41.

31. Michael D. Lemonick, "Feeling the Heat," *Time* (January 2, 1989): 38.

32. Eugene Linden, "The Death of Birth," *Time* (January 2, 1989): 37.

33. Ibid., p. 34.

34. Brown et al., op. cit., p. 10.

35. *National Geographic* (December 1988): 944.

36. Ibid., p. 917.

37. Anastasia Toufexis, "Too Many Mouths," *Time* (January 2, 1989): 49.

38. Ibid.

39. Brown et al., op. cit., pp. 10–19.

40. Ibid.

41. "Will America's Energy Conservation Gains Continue?" *19th Environmental Quality Index*, op. cit., p. 40.

42. Michael Lemonick, op. cit., p. 38.

43. Ibid., p. 39.

44. Brown et al., op. cit., pp. 11–13.

45. G. O. Barney, *The Global 2000 Report to the President of the United States*, vol. 1 (Elmsford, N.Y.: Pergamon Press, 1985): 37; McKearney Bryan, op. cit., p. 41.

46. Barney, op. cit., p. 37.

47. *Time* (January 2, 1989): 65.

Glossary

abortion—the termination of a pregnancy by removal of the uterine contents before the embryo or fetus is developed enough to survive on its own.

abscess—a pus-filled cavity formed as a result of destruction of local tissue in the inflammatory response.

acid rain—rain containing nitrogen and sulfur oxides discharged from motor vehicles and coal-burning power plants and factories, which react with moisture in the atmosphere.

active euthanasia—a situation in which something is done to a patient to cause death.

active immunity—long-lasting resistance to an infectious disease acquired through the production of antibodies as a result of having the disease or being vaccinated against it (compare with *passive immunity*).

active prevention—preventive measures that require individuals to do something to reduce the risk of injury, such as use a seat belt or wear a motorcycle helmet.

addiction—a compulsive pattern of drug use marked by both tolerance and psychic and physical dependence.

adenocarcinomas—cancers arising from glandular epithelial cells, such as the cells lining the milk ducts in the breast.

adjustment disorder—a nonpsychotic disorder in which the individual's response to a painful event is more extreme than would ordinarily be expected or considered normal.

aerobic exercise—sustained exercise of the whole body that increases the heart rate, done at a level that allows the body to meet its oxygen needs.

affective disorder—a serious disorder of mood or feeling.

agent factor—an organism that causes an infectious disease; includes bacteria, viruses, rickettsiae, fungi, and prions.

agility—the ability to change the position of the whole body quickly while controlling its movement.

alcoholic hepatitis—an alcohol-related disease in which the liver becomes swollen and inflamed.

allergy—an acquired overreaction to a specific substance by the immune system. Also called *hypersensitivity.*

Alzheimer's disease—a progressive, irreversible loss of mental and physical capacity associated with advancing age; the symptoms include severe memory loss, confusion, and depression.

amenorrhea—suppression of monthly menstrual periods for reasons other than pregnancy or menopause.

amniocentesis—a procedure in which a doctor withdraws amniotic fluid from a pregnant woman's uterus to test for certain genetic disorders in the fetus.

amnion (amniotic sac)—a fluid-filled sac within the uterus that encloses and protects the developing baby.

amphetamines—a group of synthetic stimulant drugs; the word *speed* is often used to refer to this group of drugs.

amyl nitrite—a prescription drug used to treat angina; it sometimes is used recreationally as a euphoriant and sexual stimulant.

anaerobic exercise—exercise in which the body's demand for oxygen exceeds its supply, producing oxygen debt.

anaphylactic shock—a life-threatening allergic reaction in which blood pressure can drop so low that a person dies.

anaplastic—refers to cancers whose cellular structure is so abnormal that they no longer resemble the cells of the tissue from which they originated.

angina pectoris—tightness, pressure, and intense pain in the chest caused by insufficient blood flow through partially blocked coronary arteries.

angioplasty—the process of increasing the diameter of the opening in a narrowed artery by expanding a balloon-like device.

anorexia nervosa—an eating disorder in which people severely limit the amount they eat, in effect starving themselves.

anorgasmia—the inability of a woman to experience an orgasm.

antibodies—chemical substances produced in response to an invading microorganism (the *antigen*) that can inactivate that microorganism.

antigen—part of an invading microorganism that stimulates the body to produce a chemical substance (*antibodies*) that can inactivate a microorganism.

antisocial personality disorder—a personality disorder marked by tantrums and behaviors which violate the rights of others; examples include vandalism, aggressive actions, and theft.

anxiety disorder—a nonpsychotic disorder involving a severe and persistent level of fear or worry that interferes with an individual's everyday functioning.

anxiolytics—sedative/hypnotic drugs used to reduce anxiety; some are also used as muscle relaxants and to control certain types of convulsive seizures.

aorta—the main artery of the circulatory system; carries blood from the heart to the arteries.

arrhythmia—an irregularity in the rhythm of the heartbeat.

arteries—blood vessels that carry blood from the heart to the various parts of the body.

arthritis—name for several diseases that affect the connective tissues of joints.

atherosclerosis—narrowing of the arteries caused by fatty deposits on the inner arterial walls.

atrophy—to waste away or grow smaller, usually as a result of inactivity.

autogenic training—a method of self-induced relaxation in which the person imagines certain relaxing sensations.

autonomic nervous system (ANS)—the part of the peripheral nervous system that coordinates involuntary muscles such as the heart.

bacteria (singular: **bacterium**)—a single-celled plantlike microorganism.

balance—the ability to maintain or regain upright posture, or equilibrium, while moving or standing still.

barbiturates—sedative/hypnotic drugs that are used primarily to treat insomnia and, less often, for daytime sedation; some also have anticonvulsant properties.

basal metabolism—the number of calories burned when the body is at rest but not sleeping.

basic health insurance—insurance that pays for hospitalization and for medical and surgical expenses.

behavior therapy—a therapy that attempts to alter a person's symptomatic behavior without attempting to discover its root causes.

benign tumor—a tumor that grows relatively slowly and remains localized.

benzopyrene—a chemical found in tobacco smoke, one of the deadliest carcinogens known.

bereavement—the loss of a loved or valued person.

biochemical individuality—the idea that some people need more of certain vitamins and minerals than others do.

biodegradation—the breakdown and assimilation of organic material by microorganisms.

bioelectrical impedance—a method of determining body composition in which a weak current is used to measure the body's water content.

biofeedback—a technique for developing conscious control over involuntary body processes such as blood pressure and heartbeat.

biotransform—to metabolize; to chemically alter a drug once it is inside the bloodstream so that it is a different compound when it leaves the bloodstream.

bipolar disorder—an affective disorder in which an individual exhibits mania with or without depressive episodes.

blood alcohol level (BAL)—the concentration of alcohol in the blood at a given time.

blood pressure—the force exerted by the blood on the walls of the arteries. It is measured by two separate figures taken when the heart is pumping and when it is at rest.

body composition—the proportion of fat in comparison with lean body tissue (muscle and bone) within the human body.

body leanness—the quality of having more than 75 to 80 percent of body composition as lean tissue (muscle and bone).

brain death—this occurs if an EEG (electroencephalogram) detects no brain activity for 24 hours, even though breathing and heart circulation are artificially maintained.

bulimia—an eating disorder characterized by eating binges followed by purges.

butyl nitrite—an analogue of amyl nitrite that is used recreationally as a euphoriant and presumed sexual stimulant.

bypass surgery—surgery during which a portion of a healthy blood vessel, usually from the patient's leg, is removed and used to replace (bypass) the section of the coronary artery that is blocked.

calcium—the most abundant mineral in the human body; essential for building bones and teeth and ensuring normal growth.

calorie—the amount of heat needed to raise 1 kilogram of water 1 degree Celsius; used to measure the energy potential of food.

cancer—a condition of abnormal cell growth; also known as *malignant neoplasm.*

capillaries—very small blood vessels that serve as a link between the smallest arteries and veins.

carbohydrate—a basic component of food that is found in bread, rice, potatoes, most fruits and vegetables, and certain other foods. Carbohydrates are the body's most immediate source of ready energy.

carbon monoxide—one of the most hazardous gases in tobacco smoke. It impairs the body's capacity to carry oxygen.

carcinogenic—cancer-producing.

carcinomas—cancers that arise from the epithelium.

cardiac arrest—any stoppage of the heartbeat.

cardiovascular fitness—the ability to exercise the whole body for long periods and have the circulatory system supply the fuel that the body needs to keep going.

carrier—a patient who has recovered from a disease but still gives off disease-causing organisms.

carrying capacity—the ability to support a human population of a certain size.

central nervous system (CNS)—the brain and spinal cord, which together regulate all bodily functions.

cerebral embolism—impaired blood flow to the brain caused by a mass of abnormal material clogging a cerebral blood vessel.

cerebral hemorrhage—impaired blood flow to the brain caused by rupture of a cerebral blood vessel.

cerebral thrombosis—impaired blood flow to the brain caused by a clot blocking a cerebral blood vessel.

cervix—the narrow lower end of the uterus; located at the upper end of the vagina.

cesarean section—delivery of a baby through surgical incisions made in the mother's abdomen and uterus.

chlorinated hydrocarbons—a group of chemicals that includes dangerous pesticides such as DDT, chlordane, and Kepone.

cholesterol—a fatlike substance (many researchers would not technically define it as a fat) that is found in all foods from animal sources and is also manufactured by the human body.

chorionic villi sampling—a new technique to test for genetic disorders in a fetus.

circumcision—surgical removal of the foreskin from the head of the penis.

cirrhosis of the liver—a chronic inflammatory disease in which healthy liver cells are replaced by scar tissue, impairing the liver's function.

classical conditioning theory—a theory that explores how sets of different objects or events (stimuli) become grouped, or associated, in an animal's mind and are evidenced by its behavior.

climacteric—see *menopause.*

clinical death—the brief period after heartbeat and

breathing have stopped, but before vital body cells decay irreversibly.

clinical disease—the phase in the pattern of a disease when characteristic symptoms appear and a specific diagnosis is possible.

clitoris—an extremely sensitive external female sexual organ located under a hood formed by the upper joining of the labia minora.

cocaine—a stimulant drug extracted from the leaves of the South American coca bush.

cognitive appraisal—a psychological and intellectual technique for analyzing stressors and learning different ways of responding to stress.

cohabitation—an arrangement in which two unrelated people live together in a sexual relationship without marrying.

collateral circulation—a system of smaller blood vessels which develop to provide alternative routes for blood when a main artery is blocked.

comfort level—the level of compromise a person feels comfortable making among different goals in order to maximize overall benefits.

complete protein—a protein of animal origin (meat, fish, poultry, eggs, dairy products) that contains all nine essential amino acids.

conditioned response theory—a basic, mechanistic account of how animals learn to perceive simple stimuli and react with consistent responses.

condom—a thin latex or natural skin sheath that is placed over the erect penis before intercourse to prevent conception.

congestive heart failure—a condition in which the heart cannot pump enough blood, resulting in congestion, or backing up, of blood in the lungs and other body tissues.

contraceptive implant—a device implanted under the skin that slowly releases chemicals to prevent menstruation.

convalescence—the final phase of a disease; the recovery period.

coordination—the ability to use the senses of vision and touch, together with kinesthetic (muscle) sense, to accomplish accurate, well-timed body movements.

coronal ridge—the rim of tissue between the glans and the shaft of the penis.

coronary embolism—blockage of a coronary artery that occurs when a piece of clotted material breaks away from the arterial wall and dams a narrowed coronary artery.

coronary thrombosis—a blood clot in a coronary artery.

Cowper's glands—two pea-sized organs just below the prostate gland that sometimes produce a few drops of fluid at the end of the penis during sexual arousal.

cross-sensitivity—a situation in which an allergy to one drug warns the user of possible similar reactions to other, chemically related ones.

decline stage—the phase of a disease when symptoms begin to subside and the patient may feel well enough to become more active.

defense mechanism—one of a number of mental strategies for preserving one's sense of self.

denial—a defense mechanism in which an individual covers up truths about the outer world, ignoring the things that threaten his or her self-esteem and create anxiety.

dependence—a condition in which users become so accustomed to a drug that they cannot, or feel they cannot, function without it; may be physical, psychic, or both.

depersonalization—a defense mechanism in which an individual refuses to recognize that other people are fully human, with human feelings and emotions, and thus protects himself or herself from feelings of guilt, disappointment, or obligation.

detoxification—the process of weaning a person from physical dependence on alcohol or some other drug and repairing the toxic effects of the drug in the body.

diabetes—a condition, caused by an insufficiency of insulin, in which the body is unable to metabolize sugars and other food materials efficiently.

diaphragm—a shallow rubber cup that is inserted into the vagina, where it completely covers the cervix, forming a mechanical barrier that prevents sperm from entering the uterus.

disability insurance—insurance that pays benefits to a person unable to work because of injury or illness.

distress—stress that has a negative effect.

drug—any nonnutritional substance that is *deliberately* introduced into the body to produce a physiological and/or psychological effect.

dyspareunia—a condition in which a woman experiences physical pain during sexual intercourse.

eclampsia—a severe form of toxemia; may cause convulsions and coma.

edema—swelling caused by fluid collecting in the tissues.

ejaculation—contractions of the urethra, penis, and prostate gland that usually accompany orgasm in the male, forcing semen out of the tip of the penis.

ejaculatory ducts—two structures formed by the ends of the seminal vesicles and the vas deferens that in turn join the urethra.

electroconvulsive therapy (ECT)—an organic therapy, also known as shock treatment, in which an electric current is applied to the brain to induce convulsions.

electroencephalogram (EEG)—the pattern of electrical waves that can be measured by placing electrodes on the skull.

electrolytes—substances that carry the electrical charges needed by cells to carry on their work. Potassium and sodium are the body's primary electrolytes.

embolism—a sudden blockage of a blood vessel by a blood clot (*embolus*).

embolus—a blood clot that breaks off an arterial wall, flows through the circulatory system, and becomes lodged in a smaller artery, where it blocks the flow of blood.

endocrine glands—structures that produce and secrete hormones directly into the bloodstream (ductless glands).

endogenous—pertaining to microorganisms that normally live on or within the human body, usually causing it no harm and often contributing to its welfare but sometimes causing disease.

endometrium—the inner lining of the uterus.

environmental factor—an extrinsic biological, social, or physical factor that influences the probability of contracting an infection.

enzyme—a type of protein that plays an important role in chemical reactions that break down cellular material in the body.

epididymis—a highly coiled network of tubing in the back of each testicle through which sperm cells travel as they mature.

episiotomy—a surgical incision made from a mother's vaginal opening into the perineum to prevent undue tearing of tissues during the delivery of a baby.

epithelium—the cells forming the skin, the glands, and the membranes that line the respiratory, urinary, and gastrointestinal tracts.

erogenous zone—any area of the body that is related to sexual desire or can be stimulated to produce sexual arousal.

essential amino acids—the nine amino acids that the body cannot manufacture in adequate amounts and that therefore must be present in the diet.

essential fat—fat that is necessary for the body's normal physiological functioning; it is involved in the storage and use of nutrients.

ethyl alcohol—the active ingredient in alcoholic beverages (distilled spirits, wine, beer) prepared from natural plant products such as fruits and grains.

eustress—stress that has a positive effect.

euthanasia—allowing or helping a person to die.

eutrophication—the depletion of oxygen in a body of water caused by an increase in its temperature, as by thermal pollution, which diminishes the ability of the water to support aquatic plant and animal life.

exogenous—referring to microorganisms that normally live outside the human body; many of these organisms can cause disease if they enter the body.

externality theory—the theory that overweight people eat primarily in response to external food-related cues rather than only to internal hunger caused by metabolic needs.

Fallopian tube (oviduct)—one of two tiny muscular tunnels that transport ova from the ovary to the uterus.

fat-soluble vitamins—vitamins that are stored in the fatty tissues and cannot be excreted.

fetal alcohol syndrome (FAS)—characteristic adverse effects (including mental retardation, slow growth before and after birth, and a wide range of physical defects) exhibited by children born to women who drink heavily during pregnancy.

flashbacks—brief, sudden, unexpected perceptual distortions and bizarre thoughts—similar to those experienced while on an LSD trip—that occur long after the immediate effects of a drug have worn off.

flexibility—the ability to use the joints fully and move them easily through the full range of possible motion.

foreplay—sexual activity leading to intercourse.

foreskin—the ring of tissue at the head of the penis.

frenulum—the triangular region on the underside of the penis.

fungi—many-celled plantlike organisms that lack chlorophyll and must therefore obtain food from organic material, in some cases from humans.

gamma globulin—certain blood proteins that contain antibodies.

general adaptation syndrome (GAS)—a three-stage process the body goes through in adapting to stress. The three stages are alarm, resistance, and exhaustion.

generalization—the association of the emotions involved in a particular experience with a whole category of objects and events.

generic name—the name of the chemical ingredient in a drug.

genes—inherited "code" chemicals found in every cell of the human body. They control many aspects of an individual's development and functioning.

gerontology—the study of aging.

glans—the head of the penis.

glucose—a type of sugar that is readily used by the body.

glycogen—a substance containing glucose that is stored in the liver and muscles and released into the bloodstream when blood sugar levels fall.

grief—the subjective, emotional response to bereavement.

group policy—a kind of insurance policy offered by employers to groups of employees.

hardiness—a personality trait which gives a person an optimistic and committed approach to life, so that he or she is able to weather life's ups and downs.

hashish—a concentrated and potent resin of *Cannabis sativa* (the hemp plant).

heart attack—the death of a portion of the heart muscle from lack of oxygen.

heroin—a narcotic analgesic derived from morphine and more than twice as powerful.

heterosexuality—a sexual or emotional preference for persons of the opposite sex.

homeostasis—the body's natural equilibrium, achieved through automatic mechanisms that control temperature, heart rate, blood pressure, and so on.

homosexuality—a sexual or emotional preference for persons of one's own sex.

hormones—chemical substances that act as messengers within the body to help regulate many bodily functions.

host factor—an attribute of an individual that may increase or decrease his or her susceptibility to certain diseases; includes genetics, immunity, and general state of health.

hydrostatic weighing method—underwater weighing; a technique for measuring the proportion of lean tissue to fat tissue in the body. It involves weighing a person out of the water and then in the water and then calculating body density.

hymen—a circular membrane that narrows the opening of the vagina in some women who have never had sexual intercourse.

hypertension—an elevation of blood pressure from the normal range; increases the risk of developing a cardiovascular disease.

hypochondriasis—a somatoform disorder in which a person imagines that every physical complaint is the first sign of a major illness.

iatrogenic—referring to an illness or injury caused by a doctor's carelessness, error, or poor judgment.

immunity—a group of mechanisms that help protect the body against specific diseases.

impotence—sexual dysfunction in which a man is unable to achieve or maintain an erection long enough to reach orgasm with a partner.

incomplete protein—a protein of plant origin (vegetables, seeds, grains, and nuts) that lacks one or more of the nine essential amino acids.

incubation period—the time between the first exposure to a virus or other disease-causing organism and the appearance of symptoms.

individual policy—an insurance policy bought primarily by single persons, couples, and families who are self-employed and do not have access to group plans.

inflammation—a general defense mechanism in the blood and tissues to ward off an irritant or foreign body. Also called the *inflammatory response.*

inhalants—a group of substances containing volatile chemical solvents that have psychoactive and other effects when breathed into the lungs.

injectable contraceptive—a contraceptive that releases synthetic hormones like those found in most oral contraceptives; it is effective for 2 or 3 months.

intellect—the thinking, problem-solving, rational side of human consciousness.

interferon—a substance produced by the body to help protect it against disease.

intramuscular—pertaining to the injection of a drug into a muscle.

intrauterine device (IUD)—a soft, flexible device that is inserted into the uterus to prevent pregnancy.

intravenous—pertaining to the injection of a drug into a vein.

iron—a trace mineral that is one of the most important nutrients; it is essential for the production of hemoglobin in red blood cells.

ischemia—narrowing of the arteries sufficient to cause inadequate blood supply to the body cells they serve.

isokinetic—referring to the strength training of muscles through the use of special apparatus that provides resistance that is equal to the force the user applies.

isometric—referring to the strength training of muscles by pushing or pulling against a fixed or an immovable object through a relatively narrow range of motion.

isotonic—referring to the strength training of muscles through exercises that involve muscle contractions throughout a complete range of motion.

labia—soft, sensitive folds of skin at either end of the opening of the vagina. The outer broad folds are called the *labia majora*; the inner, hairless lips are called the *labia minora.*

leukemias—cancers of blood-forming cells.

life expectancy—the average predicted length of life from birth to death.

life span—the maximum amount of time a person lives.

lifestyle—a person's overall way of living—the attitudes, habits, and behaviors of a person in daily life.

lipids—fats.

lipoproteins—substances containing both fat and protein that transport fat molecules through the body.

liposuction—a surgical procedure in which unwanted fat is sucked from the body through a tube.

long-term regulatory mechanism—a mechanism that monitors the body's nutrient levels over extended periods and controls food intake so that body weight is maintained within a relatively narrow range.

LSD (lysergic acid diethylamide)—a synthetic psychedelic/hallucinogen used recreationally; also called acid.

lymphocytes—protective white blood cells in the immune system that fight infection.

lymphomas—cancers arising from lymphatic cells.

macronutrients—nutrients the body needs in large amounts, such as proteins, carbohydrates, and fats.

major depression—an affective disorder in which an individual experiences a dysphoric mood, loses interest in all aspects of life, and may suffer from other incapacitating symptoms.

major medical insurance—medical insurance designed to protect against the high medical expenses that may accumulate if a person is seriously injured or ill for a long time.

malignant tumor—a tumor whose cells grow in abnormal ways and may break away and spread to other parts of the body.

mania—a mood of extreme excitement; an aspect of bipolar disorder.

marijuana—material from *Cannabis sativa* (the hemp plant); it is dried and prepared for smoking and has a variety of mind-altering and physiological effects.

masturbation—sexual self-stimulation.

maximum breathing capacity—the amount of air the lungs can take in over a period of time.

Medicaid—a federal-state health insurance program to assist people of any age who cannot pay for medical insurance.

Medicare—a federal health insurance program for people 65 and older and those who are disabled.

melanomas—cancers of the pigment-carrying cells of the skin.

menarche—the first menstrual period.

menopause—the gradual permanent cessation of a woman's menstruation and therefore of the reproductive phase of her life. Also known as the *climacteric.*

menstrual cycle—the monthly cycle in which the lining of the uterus first thickens and prepares to receive a fertilized ovum, then is discharged during menstruation if a pregnancy does not occur.

mescaline—a psychedelic/hallucinogen derived from the peyote cactus of the U.S. Southwest.

metabolism—the process by which the nutrients in food are converted into body tissue and energy.

metabolite—a substance produced when a drug biotransforms.

metastases—secondary tumors that form when cancerous cells break away from the original malignant tumor and are transferred to a new location in the body.

metastatic growth—the process by which cancerous cells break away from the original malignant tumor and are transferred to a new location in the body.

methadone—a synthetic drug that removes the desire for heroin and produces tolerance to its effects; used in the treatment of heroin addiction.

micronutrients—nutrients consisting of minerals and vitamins that the body needs in small amounts for its essential functions.

minerals—inorganic elements that humans need in trace amounts daily to help form tissues and various chemical substances.

mitosis—the orderly division of a cell into two new cells.

mons veneris—a sensitive cushion of fatty tissue covered with skin and hair; it is in the female vulva over the pubic bone.

morphine—a narcotic analgesic that is the active ingredient in opium.

mourning—all the culturally reinforced patterns of thought, feelings, and behaviors that individuals experience as a result of losing a loved one.

muscular endurance—the ability to use muscles continuously over a period of time.

muscular strength—the amount of external force the skeletal muscles can exert.

myocardial infarction—the death of a section of the heart muscle caused by a reduction in the supply of blood to that area.

myocardial ischemia—insufficient blood flow through partially blocked coronary arteries; starves a portion of the heart of oxygen.

myotonia—a generalized sexual response in which muscles throughout the body have an increase in tension.

narcissistic personality disorder—a personality disorder typified by an exaggerated sense of self-worth, a constant need for praise and attention, and a tendency to exploit others.

neoplasm—a group of cells growing in an uncontrolled fashion to form a tumor.

nicotine—a toxic element found in tobacco that acts as a stimulant and is responsible for many of the harmful effects of smoking.

nonpsychotic disorder—a mental disorder in which the individual's functioning is seriously inhibited but in which his or her thought processes are not so grossly distorted that the individual loses contact with reality.

normal aging—certain biological aging processes that seem time-related rather than being a function of disease, injury, or stress.

nosocomial—referring to an illness or injury caused by contact with a hospital or other health institution, ranging from a fall from a bed to an infection to a fatal surgical error.

operant conditioning theory—a theory that examines the conditions under which behaviors are learned.

opiate narcotics—group of narcotics made from the opium poppy; includes the opiates and opioids.

opiates—a group of narcotic analgesics that includes opium, morphine, and heroin.

opioids—a group of synthetic drugs, such as methadone and meperidine, that are chemically similar to the opiates.

opium—a narcotic analgesic substance made from the opium poppy; it is the parent substance of the opiate narcotics.

oral contraceptives (the pill)—synthetic equivalents of natural sex hormones that are prescribed to prevent ovulation and thus prevent conception.

organic therapy—a therapy that attempts to treat a person in a physical way rather than through learning or talking; the most common type of organic therapy involves the use of drugs.

orgasm—the climactic stage of sexual response.

osteoporosis—a chronic condition, most common among older women, that is marked by thin, brittle, easily fractured bones.

ovaries—two small internal female sexual organs that produce ova and female hormones.

overload—to work against a greater load than usual.

ovulation—the process by which ova periodically ripen and leave the ovaries.

ovum (plural: **ova**)—a female reproductive cell.

ozone—a form of oxygen created when sunlight reacts with gasoline fumes, other hydrocarbons, and nitrogen oxides; also present in the ozone layer of the upper atmosphere.

ozone layer—a thin layer in the earth's upper atmosphere. Unlike smog, this layer is beneficial, acting as a shield to prevent harmful ultraviolet light from reaching the earth's surface.

pacemaker—an electrical impulse center in the upper wall of the right atrium that regulates heartbeat by stimulating the heart muscles to pump in a coordinated fashion.

pancreatitis—inflammation of the pancreas associated with heavy alcohol intake.

panic disorder—a disorder characterized by episodes of extreme anxiety that may occur unpredictably or result from a specific situation.

parenteral—pertaining to the introduction of a drug in a manner other than through the digestive tract.

passive euthanasia—a situation in which no action is taken to prolong life even though action might enable a person to live longer.

passive immunity—short-term resistance to infectious disease acquired through the administration of antibodies formed by another person or an animal (compare with *active immunity*).

passive prevention—preventive measures that require little or no individual action on the part of those being protected; examples are automobile air bags and better street lighting.

passive smoking—the breathing in of air polluted by the tobacco smoke of others.

pathogen—an organism, such as a bacterium or virus, that can be the agent of an infectious disease.

pathological aging—a decrease in functioning caused by disease, illness, stress, injury, and other factors.

PCP (phencyclidine)—a psychedelic/hallucinogenic drug once used as an animal tranquilizer; also called angel dust.

pelvic inflammatory disease (PID)—inflammation of the pelvis; a painful condition that can damage the reproductive organs and cause infertility.

penis—the external male organ used in sexual intercourse and urination.

perineum—a hairless area of skin behind the genital area and in front of the anus.

peripheral nervous system (PNS)—all the nerves in the body other than those in the central nervous system; divided into the somatic nervous system and the autonomic nervous system.

personality disorder—a trait that impairs an individual's ability to function and cope with his or her environment; a counterproductive style of coping.

phagocytes—white blood cells that protect the body from infection by engulfing and digesting invading microorganisms, toxins, and other foreign substances.

pharmacokinetics—the movement of drugs through the body.

phobia—a type of anxiety disorder characterized by a persistent and irrational fear of a specific stimulus or activity, leading to a compelling desire to avoid it.

physical activity—any voluntary body movement that results in an expenditure of energy.

physical exercise—planned, structured, repetitive physical activities designed to improve or maintain one or more components of physical fitness.

placenta—a mass of tissue attached to the uterine lining that during pregnancy absorbs nutrients from the mother's bloodstream and transfers them to the bloodstream of the developing baby; it also carries away fetal wastes.

plaque—fatty deposits made up largely of cholesterol that can build up on the inner walls of blood vessels, narrowing them and eventually closing them completely.

pollution—any substance or energy that contributes to the development of undesirable environmental effects.

polychlorinated biphenyls (PCBs)—a group of hydrocarbons that, as water pollutants, have been linked to reproductive disorders, kidney damage, liver ailments, and eye irritation.

potassium—one of the two primary electrolytes in the body; found in beans, fruits, vegetables, whole grains, fish, lean meat, and potatoes.

power—the ability to do strength exercises quickly.

preeclampsia—a milder form of toxemia; the symptoms include hypertension and edema, or swelling, and protein in the urine.

premature ejaculation—unintentional ejaculation before, during, or immediately after insertion of the penis into the vagina.

premenstrual syndrome (PMS)—a pattern of physiological symptoms, irritability, lethargy, and depression that precedes menstruation in some women.

prenatal—before birth.

primary anorgasmia—a sexual dysfunction in which a woman has never experienced an orgasm by any method.

primary impotence—a sexual dysfunction in which a man has never been able to achieve an erection.

prion—a small protein capable of replicating itself within the cells of mammals.

priority—a need, want, or goal that is more important than another.

prodrome period—the second phase in the pattern of a disease; characterized by general symptoms such as headache, fever, runny nose, irritability, and generalized discomfort.

progression—the principle that once muscles adapt to an overload, the load should be increased slowly and gradually.

progressive relaxation—a technique for relieving muscle tension in which the individual tenses and relaxes various muscle groups in turn.

projection—a defense mechanism in which an individual attributes his or her undesirable motives and feelings to other people or even to inanimate objects.

prostaglandins—hormonelike substances secreted by various parts of the body into the bloodstream; excessive amounts of prostaglandins are suspected to be a cause of severe menstrual pain.

prostate gland—the male organ that surrounds the urethra and produces about 30 percent of the seminal fluid. Prostate problems are common as men grow older. Many men experience enlargement, or *hypertrophy*, a condition in which the prostate begins to enlarge and tighten around the urethra, often causing bladder and urination difficulties. This condition can usually be treated successfully.

protein—a basic component of food that is essential for growth and the repair of body tissues.

psilocybin—a psychedelic/hallucinogenic drug derived from a Mexican mushroom.

psychedelics/hallucinogens—a group of drugs that create illusions, distorting the user's mind by creating moods, thoughts, and perceptions that would otherwise take place only during the dream state.

psychic contactlessness—a defense mechanism in which an individual is unable to communicate with or become intimate with others.

psychoactive drug—a drug that acts primarily on the brain, producing altered states of mood, perception, consciousness, and central nervous system activity.

psychosomatic disease—a disease in which mental or psychological factors play an important role in the pathological process.

psychosurgery—an organic therapy in which small amounts of brain tissue are irreversibly destroyed using laser surgery techniques.

psychotic disorder—a mental disorder in which an individual has lost contact with reality.

pull school—a school of thought for explaining body composition problems; sees weight problems as primarily resulting from physiological factors.

push school—a school of thought for explaining body composition problems; sees weight problems as primarily resulting from psychological or social factors.

rationalization—a defense mechanism in which an individual does not admit that his or her motives are anything but the highest.

reaction time—the amount of time it takes to start moving once a person has decided to do so.

receptor sites—specific spots on cells where the molecules of a specific drug "fit."

refractory period—a temporary state following orgasm during which most males cannot respond to renewed sexual stimulation.

regenerate—to replace damaged cells on a regular basis.

regularity—the principle that exercise needs to be done frequently enough, with enough intensity, and for a sufficient period of time.

relaxation response—a method of stress management similar to meditation; involves muscular relaxation and conscious breathing.

repression—a defense mechanism in which an individual has no conscious awareness of threatening thoughts, feelings, memories, or wishes.

retarded ejaculation—a condition in which a man takes overly long to reach the point of ejaculation, possibly causing pain to his partner.

Rh factor—a substance in the red blood cells which, if lacking in the mother and inherited by the first baby from the father, can cause the mother's blood to produce antibodies that result in a blood disorder called *erythroblastosis fetalis* in second and later children.

rheumatic fever—an inflammatory disease that affects the connective tissues of the body, especially in the brain, the joints, and the heart.

rickettsiae—infectious organisms that grow in the intestinal tract of insects and insectlike creatures and can be transmitted to humans through insect bites.

route of administration—the way a drug is introduced into the body.

sarcomas—cancers that arise from supporting or connective tissues, such as bone, cartilage, and the membranes covering muscles and fat.

saturated fat—a fat that is usually solid at room temperature; found in meat, butter, whole milk, and some oils.

schizoid personality disorder—a personality disorder that involves a lack of desire to have social relationships.

schizophrenia—a psychotic disorder of the thinking processes in which the individual seems to be totally removed from reality.

scrotum—the loose pouch of skin that hangs behind the penis and contains the testicles.

secondary anorgasmia—a sexual dysfunction in which a woman frequently has difficulty achieving an orgasm.

secondary impotence—a sexual dysfunction in which a man who has previously been able to achieve an erection is now unable to do so in some or all sexual encounters.

sedatives/hypnotics—drugs that have both sedative (calming) and hypnotic (sleep-inducing) effects.

self-concept—all the perceptions that a person has about himself or herself; the result of thinking about oneself and evaluating what others think of one.

self-efficacy—confidence in one's ability to plan and control one's behavior and lifestyle components.

self-esteem—a person's feelings of worth and dignity.

semen—the sperm-carrying liquid expelled from the penis during ejaculation; also called *seminal fluid*.

seminal vesicles—two small structures located at the base of the bladder that produce about 70% of the seminal fluid.

setpoint theory—a theory in which the basic idea is that each person has a given weight range, or setpoint, that is natural to his or her body. Depending on their setpoints, some people stay thin and others stay fat regardless of what they eat.

sex—gender (maleness or femaleness); the physical expression of affectionate or erotic feeling which sometimes culminates in sexual intercourse.

sexual dysfunction—a problem that prevents a person from engaging in sexual relations or reaching orgasm.

sexuality—masculinity or femininity; the ways in which gender—male or female—is integrated into a person's personality and behavior.

sexually transmitted disease (STD)—an infectious disease that is almost always transmitted during sexual intercourse, homosexual relations, or other sexual activity.

shock—a condition in which the body loses control of blood flow.

short-term regulatory mechanism—a mechanism that signals the body when to eat and when to stop eating.

side effects—effects of a drug that are unwanted and unrelated to its essential purpose.

situational anorgasmia—a condition in which a woman is able to experience orgasm in certain situations but not in others.

skinfold measurement—a method of measuring body composition using calipers to measure the fat under the skin.

social learning theory—a learning model based on the notion that behavior is learned by observing the experiences and actions of others.

sodium—one of the two primary electrolytes in the body. It is found in table salt and in many processed foods and also occurs naturally in many foods.

somatic nervous system (SNS)—the part of the peripheral nervous system that controls the voluntary muscles; it consists of nerves that run between the sensory and motor organs.

somatoform disorder—a mental disorder that manifests itself in the form of physiological symptoms; hypochondriasis is a well-known example.

specificity—the principle that to develop a component of fitness, one must work on that particular component.

speed—the ability to perform a movement or cover a distance in a short time.

sperm—the male reproductive cells.

spermatic cords—muscular structures from which the testicles are suspended within the scrotum.

spermatogenesis—the continual process of sperm production.

spontaneous abortion—the expulsion of an improperly implanted or defective embryo or fetus from the uterus; commonly called *miscarriage*.

stimulants—drugs that activate the sympathetic division of the autonomic nervous system, causing a person to feel restless, talkative, more lively, and often unable to sleep.

storage fat—fat deposited under the skin and around the internal organs to protect them; some storage fat is used for heat production and energy.

stress—an individual's psychological and physiological response to any stimulus that is perceived as threatening.

stressor—a threatening event or stimulus that causes stress.

stroke—also called a cerebrovascular accident or cerebrovascular occlusion; a sudden loss of brain function resulting from interference with the blood supply to a part of the brain.

subcutaneous—pertaining to the administration of a drug under the skin.

sublimation—a defense mechanism in which an individual substitutes socially acceptable behavior for unacceptable impulses, for example, conformity for hostility.

synergism—a type of drug interaction in which two drugs taken at the same time or in rapid sequence have more powerful effects than the two drugs would have if taken alone.

synesthesia—a blending of senses in which a person "hears" colors or "sees" sounds.

tar—a sticky residue from burning tobacco consisting of more than 200 chemicals, many of which are hazardous.

teratogenic—pertaining to a drug which, if taken by a pregnant woman, can interfere with the crucial stages of a baby's prenatal development and is thus associated with birth defects.

testes (testicles)—the male organs that produce sperm and male hormones.

thanatology—the study of death.

therapeutic index—the safety margin between the effective dose of a drug and a lethal dose.

thermal pollution—an undesirable increase in the temperature of a body of water, as by the introduction of warm waste water from a factory.

thrombosis—the development of a blood clot within an artery that severely constricts or blocks the flow of blood.

thrombus—a blood clot.

tissue—a collection of cells in the body that are specialized to perform certain functions.

tolerance—a situation in which the body becomes adapted to a drug so that increasingly larger doses are needed to produce the desired effect.

toxemia—the presence of toxins in the bloodstream during pregnancy.

toxoids—modified toxins which are no longer poisonous; used to induce the production of antibodies that will inactivate specific microbial disease-producing toxins.

trade-off—a need, want, or goal that has to be delayed, postponed, or given up in order for a priority to be accomplished.

transient ischemic attack (TIA)—a mild stroke that causes only temporary dizziness or slight weakness or numbness; such a stroke is often ignored.

triglycerides—fatty acids into which excess glucose is converted and stored by the body's fat tissue.

tubal ligation—a surgical sterilization technique for women in which the Fallopian tubes are severed or tied.

tumor—a swelling or mass formed by a group of cells within a tissue that grow to an abnormal size and shape and multiply in an uncontrolled fashion.

umbilical cord—a ropelike tissue that links the developing fetus to the placenta nourishing its blood supply.

unsaturated fat—a fat that is usually liquid at room temperature. Most vegetable oils are unsaturated fats.

urethra—the tube from the urinary bladder through which urine is passed out of the body.

uterus—the womb; a hollow muscular internal female sexual organ that contributes to sexual response and shelters and nourishes the fetus during pregnancy.

vaccine—killed or weakened viruses that are taken orally or by injection to stimulate the body to produce antibodies that give immunity to the specific disease caused by a virus.

vagina—the canallike structure of the female body that extends from the bottom of the uterus to the vulva; it receives the penis during sexual intercourse and acts as a passageway for a baby during birth.

vaginal condoms—a prelubricated latex receptacle designed to be worn by women during sexual intercourse.

vaginal rings—rings which, when placed in the vagina, release a chemical that prevents ovulation or makes the cervical mucus impermeable to sperm.

vaginismus—a sexual dysfunction involving involuntary muscle spasms that cause the vagina to shut so tightly that penetration by a penis is impossible or painful.

vas deferens—long tubes that carry sperm from the epididymis to the seminal vesicles.

vasectomy—a surgical sterilization technique for men in which a section of each vas deferens is removed.

vasocongestion—the increase of blood flow to the genital region during the first stage of sexual excitement.

vector—a carrier of an infectious disease; insects, ticks, and rats are vectors for some human diseases.

veins—blood vessels that carry blood from the body back to the heart.

ventricular fibrillation—an arrhythmia in which the ventricles beat irregularly at an extremely fast rate.

virus—a microorganism that can reproduce only in living cells.

vital capacity—the amount of air the lungs can take in and breathe out at one time.

vitamins—substances found in food; they are needed in only very small amounts but are essential for triggering vital bodily functions.

vulva—the external genital region surrounding the opening of the vagina.

water-soluble vitamins—vitamins that dissolve in water and that the body can excrete.

withdrawal—a method of contraception in which the man withdraws his penis from the woman's vagina before he ejaculates; also known as *coitus interruptus*.

withdrawal syndrome—an unpleasant and possibly painful condition that an individual who is physically dependent on a drug experiences when deprived of that drug.

Index

*Note: Feature, diagram, and table references are indicated by **bold face** type.*

health and, 10–17
heart attack and changes in, **299**, 300, **308**
self-assessment of, **11**, 22–24
self-efficacy and, 17
stress baseline of, **35**
two-income, **422**
life-support systems, right to die and, 472–473
light drinker, 377
limbic system, **57**, **351**
lipids (fats), *see* fats (lipids)
lipoproteins, 115–116, 295
high-density, **88**, 96, 295, 302, 306
low-density, 295, 302, 306
liposuction, 149
liver
alcoholism and damage to, 379–381
cirrhosis of, 380–381
hepatitis and, 266–267, 381
"living will," 473
local environment, quality of, 510–519
lockjaw, 264
longevity, weight and, 139–140
longevity-determining genes, 449
long-range health, 25
long-term goals, 20
long-term regulatory mechanism, 151
Los Angeles, smog in, 510
lovastatin, 302
love, 172–173, 188
Love Canal disaster, 517
low blood pressure, 291
low-density lipoproteins (LDLs), 295, 302, 306
low-impact aerobic exercise, 97
LSD (lysergic acid diethylamide, "acid"), 364, 365
lumpectomy, 323
lung cancer, 320, 323, 361, 395, 491–492
lung diseases, death from, 395
lungs, 95, **393**
lupus, 274
luteinizing hormone (LH), 227
Lyme disease, 259, 264
lymphatic system, 315
lymphocytes, 43, 270–271, **271**, 279
lymphomas, 316
lysergic acid diethylamide (LSD), 364, 365

Maalin, Ali, **273**
macrominerals (electrolytes), 117, 119
macronutrients, 112–117
magnetic resonance imaging (MRI) systems, 302, **494–495**
major depression, 69

major medical insurance, 503, **504**
Make Today Count, 332
malaria, 259
male reproductive system, **203**, 203–204, **230**, 230–231, **231**
malignant neoplasm (malignant tumor), 314, 315
see also cancer
malnutrition, alcoholism and, 382
malpractice suits, **15**
mammogram (breast x-ray), 491, 492
mania, 69–70
marijuana (cannabis), 343, 348, 360–362
marriage, 169–178
alternatives to, 173–177
compatibility for, assessing, 173–174
developing successful relationship, 188–192
divorce and, 177–178, 184
love, romance, and attraction in, 171–172
meeting each other's needs in, **189**
reasons for, 171
see also parenthood
Maslow, Abraham, 18–19
Massachusetts Judicial Court, 473
massive bleeding, 425
mast cells, 274
mastectomy, 323
Masters, William, 206, 209, **218**
masturbation, 209, 210
maximum breathing capacity, 95
mechanical energy, 408
media, sex-role expectations and, **201**
Medicaid, 505
medical care, 483–507
complementary approaches to health care, 498–501
costs of, **494–495**, **501**, 501–506
health-activation and, 483–487, 492, 496, 506
institutions, 497–498
medical self-care, 487–492
providers of, 493–497
socialized, **502**
medical clearance for exercise program, 104
medical progress, disease patterns and, 259
medical technology, 472, **494–495**
Medicare, 503–505
medications, *see* drug(s); drug use and abuse
medicenters, 497
medicine chest, home, **489**, 489–490
meditation, 46–47
medulla oblongata, **351**
megadoses, vitamin, 122

megesterol acetate, 329
melanomas, 316, 323, 324
Memorial Sloan-Kettering Cancer Center, 42
memory, 71, 73, 301, 442
men, sexual dysfunction in, 216–217
see also father; marriage; parenthood; sexuality
menarche, 226
menopause, 229, 441, 445
menstrual cycle, 227–229, **228**
menstrual extraction (vacuum aspiration), 247–249
menstruation, 209, 227, **229**, 243–244
mental disorders, stress and, 44
see also specific disorders
mental health, working on, 75–81
mercury, 514, 515
mescaline, 364–365
mesothelioma, 320
metabolism, 112, **113**, 113, 115–116, **126**
basal, 152–153
metabolites, 348
metastases, metastatic growth, 315, **316**
methadone, 366
methamphetamine, 356
methane gas, 523
Metropolitan Life Insurance Company, **7**
micronutrients, 112, 117–122
middle age, 439
midwife, **251**
Minamata Bay, mercury poisoning in, 515
mind, dimensions of human, 55–56
see also emotion(s); intellect
mineralocorticoids, 36
minerals, 117–119, **125**
minor depression, 63–64, 69
minority groups, *see* race
minor tranquilizers, 78
miscarriage (spontaneous abortion), 246–247, 276
mitosis, 315
molecule, 343–345
money, problems over, 190
moniliasis, **275**
monogamy, 280
mononucleosis ("mono"), 267
monounsaturated fats, 116
mons veneris, 204
mood swings, suicide and extreme, 81
Mormons, health of, 8–9
"morning-after" pills, 247
morning sickness, 246
morphine, 363, 364
mothers
bereavement of, 478

retina, cancer of, 318
retirement communities, 452
Retrovir (zidovudine), 282–283
rheumatic fever, 263–264
rheumatic heart disease, 304
rheumatoid arthritis, 274
Rh hemolytic disease (erythroblastosis fetalis), 244
rhinoviruses, 265
rhythm method of birth control, 237
riboflavin, **120**
ribonucleic acid (RNA), 112
rickettsiae, 267
right(s)
  to die, 472–473
  of nonsmokers, 397, 398
  patient's bill of, 498, **499**
  reproductive, **248**
risk factors
  for cancer, 42, 318–322
  in cardiovascular disease (CVD), 305–309
  danger of multiple, 307–309
  see also diet and nutrition; drug use and abuse; environment; lifestyle
RISKO score for heart disease risks, **292–293**
rituals surrounding death, 474–475
Ritvo, Robert, **47**
Rocky Mountain spotted fever, 259, 267
Roe v. *Wade*, **248**, 249
roles
  gender, 199
  sex, **201**
romantic love, 172
roughage (fiber), 114, 122–123
route of administration, 346–347, **347**
Royal Society of London, **272**
RU 486 (morning-after pill), 247
rubella (German measles), 245, 274, 304

Safe Drinking Water Act (1986), 516
safety of health care institutions, 498
saline abortion, 249
San Diego Naval Health Research Center, 33
sanitation workers, injuries of, 412
sarcomas, 280, 316, 363
saturated fats, 116
scarlet fever, 263
schizoid personality disorder, 68
schizophrenia, 44, 70–71, 478
scrotum, 203, 206, 207, 230
secondary anorgasmia, 219
secondary impotence, 217
second-degree burns, 430

"secret survivors," 476
security, emotional development and, 180
sedatives/hypnotics ("downers"), 350, 352–353
seizures, first aid for, 430
self-acceptance, 141
self-assessment of one's health, 21–24, **22**
self-care, medical, 487–492
self-concept, 76
self-efficacy, 63
  health activation and, 483
  lifestyle and, 17
  parents and development of, 181
  will to live and, 466
self-esteem
  assessing your, **74–75**
  body image and, 141
  defined, 76
  depression and, 63
  exercise and, 89
  low, **79**
self-examination for cancer, 323–325
self-help groups, 78
Selye, Hans, 33
semen (seminal fluid), 207, 208, 216, 231
seminal vesicles, 231
sensory perception, aging and, 442
septum, 289
Service Council of Retired Executives, 453
setpoint theory of weight management, 151–153, 154, 155, 163
Seventh-Day Adventists, health of, 9
sewage treatment plants, 516
sex
  attitudes about, 199–202, **212–213**
  compatibility in marriage and, 173–174
  defined, 197
  after heart attack, 300
  oral, 212, 280
  premarital, 175
  relationship problems over, 191
sex education classes, **200**, 200
sex hormones, 197, 198, 214, 229, 230, 234
sex roles, 201
sex skin, 206
sex therapy, **218**, 220
sexual abuse of children, 215–216
sexual fantasies, 210
sexual intercourse, 211
sexuality, 197–223
  aging and, 441
  arousal, 202–205
  attitudes toward sex, 199–202, **212–213**

basis of, 197–199
defined, 197
physiology of sexual response, 206–209
responsible approach to sex, 220–221, 232–241
sexual anatomy, 202–205, 226–231
sexual expression, forms of, 210–216
sexual problems and dysfunction, 216–220, **217**
unacceptable sexual behavior, 214–216
see also reproduction
sexually transmitted diseases (STDs), 225, 232, **275**, 275–283
  AIDS, *see* acquired immune deficiency syndrome (AIDS)
  chlamydia, **275**, 279
  condyloma, **275**, 278
  contraceptive methods and, 232, 234, 235, 236, 239, 280–281
  defined, 275
  fetal health and, 245
  gonorrhea, **275**, 278, 279
  herpes genitalis, **275**, 276–277
  risks, symptoms, and treatment, **275**
  sexual responsibility and, 221
  syphilis, **275**, 277–278
sexual orientation, **201**, 213–214
shock
  anaphylactic, 345
  first aid for, 426
short-term goals, 20
short-term memory, 301
short-term regulatory mechanism, 151
sickle-cell anemia, 241
side effects, drug, 345–346, 349, 353, 357–358
Sierra Club, 528
silent ischemia, 296
silent suicide, 448
single living, 174–175
single parenthood, 184–185
situational anorgasmia, 219
situational drug use, 341
situational stressors, 30–31
skill-related components of fitness, 90–91
skin
  as first line of defense, 268
  self-examination of, 324
skin cancer, 318, 323
skin disorders, stress and, 44
skinfold measurement, 144, **145**
skin popping, 364
sleep, coping with stress and, **46**
smallpox, 258, 259, **272–273**
smog, 510
smokeless tobacco, 390, 392, 400

vertebrae, adjusting alignment of, 500
vertebral arteries, 290
vinyl chloride, 320, 514
violence
    alcohol and, 371, 376
    controlling, 422–423
    death rates due to, 414
    defined, 413
    domestic, 177, 185–187
    injury and, 413–414, 417–418
    in society, **422**
    television and, **422–423**
viruses, 41, 265–267, **271**, 271, 484
vital capacity, 95
vitamin deficiency, alcohol abuse and, 382
vitamin depletion, 130
vitamins, 119–122, **120–121**
    A, 119, 120
    B, 119, 130, 331
    C, 49, 120–121, **121**, 130
    D, 119
    E, 119
    K, 122
    RDAs for, **125**
vitamin supplements, 121–122
vitrification, 524–525
volatile solvents (inhalants), 362–363
volunteer organizations, 453
vulva, 204

waist-hip ratio, **143**
wants, 18–19, 21
warm-up activity, 92–93
wastes
    hazardous, **517**, 517–519
    nonhazardous, 519
    radioactive, 524–525
water in diet, 123
water pollution, 319, 514–516

water-soluble vitamins, 121
weather, exercise plan and, 105
weight disorders, 160–163
weight management
    achieving goals of, 164
    cardiovascular disease and, 307
    energy-balance equation and, 155, **157**
    longevity and, 139–140
    maintenance of weight loss, **161**
    methods of, 146–150, **161**, 356
    natural, 155–160
    setpoint theory of, 151–153, 154, 155, 163
    understanding problems of, 151–155
    see also body composition
weight-training programs, 95
weight-waist ratio, **143**
Weight Watchers, 149, **150**
well-being, health and, 4–10
white blood cells, 269, 270
whooping cough (pertussis), 274
widower or widow, 476
Wilderness Society, 528
will
    "living," 473
    making a, 470–472, **471**
will to live, 465–466
wind power, 523
withdrawal (coitus interruptus), **233**, 234
withdrawal syndrome (abstinence syndrome), 340, 353, 399–400
womb (uterus), 205, 207, 227
women
    anorexia nervosa and, 160–162
    benefits of exercise to, 87
    cocaine addiction among, 343
    divorce and changing status of, 177
    domestic violence and, 185, 186–187

ideas of intimacy, 190
money problems and, 190
osteoporosis in, 87, 119, 162, 229, 444–445
rape and, 214–215
risks of exercise to, 90
sexual dysfunction in, 217–219
single, 175
toxic shock syndrome in, 264
see also marriage; mothers; parenthood; sexuality
work
    air pollution at, 514
    cancer and disruption of, 318
    injuries at, 412–413
    stress at, costs of, 44
work force, mothers in, 182, 199
working style, 13
workplace chemicals, cancer and, 320
world food supplies, 522
world health care systems, **502**
World Health Organization, 5, **240**
World Health Organization Smallpox Reference Center, **273**
world hunger, **134–135**
Worldwatch Institute, 523
World Wildlife Fund, 528

Xanax, 78
x-rays, 302, 491, 492

yeast infections, **275**
young adulthood, 438–439
yo-yo effect, 151, 158

zero population growth, **240**
zidovudine (azathioprine [AZT] or Retrovir), 282–283